Pharmaceutical Dosage Forms and Drug Delivery Systems

D0117044

I am a Pharmacist

- *I am a specialist in medications*

  I supply medicines and pharmaceuticals to those who need them.

  I prepare and compound special dosage forms.

  I control the storage and preservation of all medications in my care.

- *I am a custodian of medical information*

  My library is a ready source of drug knowledge.

  My files contain thousands of specific drug names and tens of thousands of facts about them.

  My records include the medication and health history of entire families.

  My journals and meetings report advances in pharmacy from around the world.

- *I am a companion of the physician*

  I am a partner in the case of every patient who takes any kind of medication.

  I am a consultant on the merits of different therapeutic agents.

  I am the connecting link between physician and patient and the final check on the safety of medicines.

- *I am a counselor to the patient*

  I help the patient understand the proper use of prescription medication.

  I assist in the patient's choice of nonprescription drugs or in the decision to consult a physician.

  I advise the patient on matters of prescription storage and potency.

- *I am a guardian of the public health*

  My pharmacy is a center for health-care information.

  I encourage and promote sound personal health practices.

  My services are available to all at all times.

- *This is my calling* ♦ *This is my pride*

Pharmaceutical Dosage Forms and Drug Delivery Systems

Howard C. Ansel, Ph.D.
Panoz Professor of Pharmacy, Department of Pharmaceutics, College of Pharmacy
The University of Georgia

Nicholas G. Popovich, Ph.D.
Professor and Head, Department of Pharmacy Practice, School of Pharmacy and Pharmacal Sciences
Purdue University

Loyd V. Allen, Jr., Ph.D.
Professor and Chair, Department of Medicinal Chemistry and Pharmaceutics, College of Pharmacy
The University of Oklahoma

SIXTH EDITION

A Lea & Febiger Book

SANS TACHE

Williams & Wilkins

BALTIMORE • PHILADELPHIA • HONG KONG
LONDON • MUNICH • SYDNEY • TOKYO

A WAVERLY COMPANY

1995

Executive Editor: Donna M. Balado
Developmental Editor: Frances M. Klass
Production Coordinator: Peter J. Carley
Project Editor: Jessica Howie Martin

Copyright © 1995
Williams & Wilkins
200 Chester Field Parkway
Malvern, PA 19355 USA

All rights reserved. This book is protected by copyright. No part of this book may be reproduced in any form or by any means, including photocopying, or utilized by any information storage and retrieval system without written permission from the copyright owner.

Accurate indications, adverse reactions, and dosage schedules for drugs are provided in this book, but it is possible they may change. The reader is urged to review the package information data of the manufacturers of the medications mentioned.

Printed in the United States of America

Library of Congress Cataloging in Publication Data

94 95 96 97 98
1 2 3 4 5 6 7 8 9 10

Ansel, Howard C., 1933–
Pharmaceutical dosage forms and drug delivery systems / Howard C. Ansel, Nicholas G. Popovich, Lloyd V. Allen, Jr.—6th ed.
p. cm.
Includes bibliographical references and index.
ISBN 0-683-00193-0
1. Drugs—Dosage forms. 2. Drug delivery systems.
I. Popovich, Nicholas G. II. Allen, Loyd V. III. Title.
[DNLM: 1. Dosage Forms. 2. Drug Delivery Systems. QV 785 A618i 1995]
RS200.A57 1995
615′.1—dc20
DNLM/DLC
for Library of Congress 94-22471
CIP

The use of portions of the text of USP23/NF18, copyright 1994, is by permission of the USP Convention, Inc. The Convention is not responsible for any inaccuracy of quotation or for any false or misleading implication that may arise from separation of excerpts from the original context or by obsolescence resulting from publication of a supplement.

PRINTED IN THE UNITED STATES OF AMERICA

Print No. 4 3 2 1

Preface

There are many fine textbooks available within the realm of pharmaceutics that deal exclusively with specific subject areas, such as physical pharmacy, biopharmaceutics, pharmacokinetics, and industrial pharmacy. Also available are many definitive books and monographs that focus on specific dosage forms, such as tablets; on methods of drug delivery, such as targeted delivery; on pharmaceutical processes, such as microencapsulation; and on testing methods, such as drug stability testing. These areas, and many others, are important components of pharmaceutics and of the pharmacy curriculum. The extent to which each may be covered in a particular academic program depends upon the specific goals of the program, the instructional level, and the time allocated within the curriculum. For some of these areas, definitive coverage may be reserved for advanced or graduate study.

Purpose

The purpose of *Pharmaceutical Dosage Forms and Drug Delivery Systems* is to introduce beginning pharmacy students to the technologic and scientific principles underlying the preparation of dosage forms and drug delivery systems and to their use in patient care. Through an integrated presentation, students gain an understanding of the interrelationships between physical pharmacy principles, biopharmaceutics and pharmacokinetics, dosage form design, product formulation, small- and large-scale product manufacture, and the clinical application of pharmaceuticals in patient care.

The text is written at a level consistent with the requirements of the beginning pharmacy student. And, because of the entry level of its intended audience, it introduces such important topics as the heritage of pharmacy, the evolution of the scientific viewpoint in pharmacy, methods of drug discovery and product development, the history and use of the official compendia, and the role of the pharmacist in contemporary practice. Product examples and clinical applications are presented along with each type of dosage form.

Major Changes from Previous Edition

Two major changes have been made in the Sixth Edition. Physical Pharmacy Capsules highlight the physical pharmacy principles applicable to each chapter's content. Two new chapters have been added: "Biotechnology and Drugs" and "New Drug Development and Approval Process." These chapters contribute to the student's understanding of the preparation of various drug substances into dosage forms/drug delivery systems and the regulatory processes involved in their approval for marketing. All chapters and appendices carried over from the previous edition have been thoroughly revised and updated.

Organization

The first four chapters provide general professional and scientific underpinnings for each of the subsequent chapters, which are organized by dosage form/drug delivery system according to route of administration. Applicable methods of pharmaceutical technology, physical pharmacy principles, clinical applications, and product examples are included in each chapter.

Chapter 1, "Introduction to Drugs and Pharmacy," includes a synopsis of the heritage of pharmacy, a historical tracing of the development of the scientific viewpoint, and the pharmacist's contemporary role. Also included are the history and use of the *United States Pharmacopeia/National Formulary*, important federal laws and regulations governing drugs and pharmacy, and codes of ethics for pharmacy practitioners and for pharmaceutical scientists.

Chapter 2, "New Drug Development and Approval Process," introduces the process by which drugs are discovered, chemically and biologically characterized, investigated clinically, developed pharmaceutically, and examined through the federal regulatory process for approval for marketing. Included are considerations of preclinical studies, product development, clinical trials, and investigational (IND), new drug (NDA), abbreviated (ANDA), and supplemental (SNDA) new drug applications.

Chapter 3, "Dosage Form Design: Biopharmaceutic Considerations," introduces the general principles of drug absorption, the fate of drugs after absorption, principles of pharmacokinetics, pharmaceutic factor affecting bioavailability, standards of bioequivalence, and routes of drug administration and applicable dosage forms. Physical pharmacy principles such as dissociation constant, particle size and solubility, surface area, and dissolution rate are discussed.

Chapter 4, "Dosage Form Design: General Considerations, Pharmaceutic Ingredients, and Current Good Manufacturing Practice," presents the need for dosage forms/drug delivery systems and includes physical and chemical considerations of preformulation studies, characteristics and use of pharmaceutic ingredients, drug product stability and stability testing, types of pharmaceutical packaging, and general provisions of Current Good Manufacturing Practice standards for the manufacture of finished pharmaceuticals. Among the physical pharmacy principles included are stability kinetics and shelf-life determination.

Chapter 5 ("Peroral Solids, Capsules, Tablets, and Controlled-Release Dosage Forms"), Chapter 6 ("Oral Solutions, Syrups, and Elixirs"), and Chapter 7 ("Oral Suspensions, Emulsions, Magmas, and Gels") present the underlying physical pharmacy principles and the technologies used in the small- and large-scale production of orally administered dosage forms. Among the physical pharmacy principles included are micromeritics, particle size reduction, drug solubility and dissolution, surface area of globules, rheology, sedimentation rate, and the Stokes Equation.

Chapter 8, "Parenteral Medications and Sterile Fluids," covers the routes and methods of parenteral administration, the technology of product development, methods of sterilization, quality assurance programs for pharmacy-prepared sterile products, standards for and examples of small- and large-volume parenteral product types, immunizing biologic products, and physical pharmacy considerations of colligative properties, tonicity, and osmolality.

Chapter 9, "Biotechnology and Drugs," focuses on the recent advances in this area of pharmaceutical research and development. Products currently in use, as well as those in development, are discussed according to their general classification.

Chapter 10 ("Transdermal Drug Delivery Systems, Ointments, Creams, Lotions and Other Preparations"), Chapter 11 ("Ophthalmic, Nasal, Otic, and Oral Preparations Applied Topically"), Chapter 12 ("Suppositories and Other Rectal, Vaginal, and Urethral Preparations"), and Chapter 13 ("Aerosols, Inhalations, and Sprays") cover the dosage forms and drug delivery systems applicable to these types of pharmaceuticals. In each instance, methods of preparation, clinical application, and product examples are given. Physical Pharmacy Capsules include the pH of ophthalmic solutions and the density calculations for the preparation of suppositories.

Chapter 14, "Radiopharmaceuticals and Miscellaneous Preparations," includes discussion of radiopharmaceuticals as well as less commonly used pharmaceuticals including spirits, tinctures, and effervescent salts.

The appendices, "Definitions of Selected Drug Categories" and "Systems and Techniques of Pharmaceutical Measurement," provide useful definitions, metrology and techniques of pharmaceutical measurement, and basic methods of pharmaceutical calculations.

Acknowledgments

This sixth edition of *Pharmaceutical Dosage Forms and Drug Delivery Systems* brings together for the first time an integration of the methods of pharmaceutical technology, underlying principles of physical pharmacy, and applied aspects of pharmacy practice. Major credit for this approach is given to co-authors Nicholas G. Popovich and Loyd V. Allen, Jr. Through his expertise in the field of pharmaceutical care, Dr. Popovich has contributed important components throughout the text on the proper utilization of drugs and dosage forms in patient care. He also has completely revised the chapter "Parenteral Medications and Sterile Fluids" and written the new chapter "Products of Biotechnology." Dr. Allen, who joins the text as co-author with this edition, is well known for his expertise in pharmaceutical formulations and physical pharmacy. He has made a significant contribution to this work by creating the Physical Pharmacy Capsules that present physical pharmacy principles and are carefully positioned throughout the text. This textbook's integrated format provides a needed resource for the academic curriculum in pharmaceutics and establishes a new direction for future revisions of this text.

The authors are grateful to colleagues and students who have shared their thoughts regarding the content and format of this text. Their suggestions are reflected here. Special gratitude is extended to H. Douglas Johnson for the definitions of drug categories in the appendix; to Glen J. Sperandio for the inspiring statement "I am a Pharmacist" that appears in the front of the book; to William B. French, Southwestern Oklahoma State University; Seamus Mulligan, Elan Corporation; Danny A. Shive, Burroughs Wellcome Company; Lee C. Schramm, Smith Kline Beecham; Jeanne H. Van Tyle, Butler University; Steven L. Brown, Medical University of South Carolina; Glynn G. Raymond, The University of New Mexico; Beverly Sandmann, Butler University; and P. L. Madan, St. John's University, who participated in the review of the text and provided updated figures; and to Williams & Wilkins' Frances M. Klass and Lisa Stead, development editors, and Maria Laraio, editorial assistant, who contributed to the preparation and production of this new edition.

HOWARD C. ANSEL
Athens, Georgia

Contents

1

Introduction to Drugs and Pharmacy

A DRUG is defined as an agent intended for use in the diagnosis, mitigation, treatment, cure, or prevention of disease in man or in other animals. One of the most astounding qualities of drugs is the diversity of their actions and effects on the body. Drugs categorized as ecbolics or oxytocics stimulate the activity of the uterine muscle, whereas other drugs act as uterine muscle relaxants. Some drugs selectively stimulate the cardiac muscle, the smooth muscles, or the skeletal muscles; other drugs have the opposite effect. Mydriatic drugs dilate the pupil of the eye; miotics constrict or diminish pupillary size. Drugs can render blood more coagulable or less coagulable; they can increase the hemoglobin content of the erythrocytes, reduce serum cholesterol, or expand blood volume.

Drugs termed emetics induce vomiting, whereas antiemetic drugs have the opposite effect. Diuretic drugs increase the flow of urine, expectorant drugs increase respiratory tract fluid, and cathartics or laxatives promote the evacuation of the bowel. Other drugs decrease the flow of urine, diminish body secretions, or induce constipation.

Drugs are employed to reduce pain, fever, thyroid activity, rhinitis, insomnia, gastric acidity, motion sickness, blood pressure, and mental depression. Drugs can elevate the mood, the blood pressure, or the activity of the endocrine glands. Drugs can combat infectious disease, destroy intestinal worms, or act as antidotes against the poisoning effects of other drugs. Antineoplastic drugs provide one means of attacking the cancerous process; radioactive pharmaceuticals provide another.

Drugs may be used to diagnose diabetes, liver malfunction, tuberculosis, or pregnancy, or they may be employed to replenish a body deficient in antibodies, vitamins, hormones, electrolytes, protein, enzymes, or blood. Drugs may be used to prevent measles, poliomyelitis, or pregnancy or to assist the maintenance of pregnancy or to extend life itself.

Certainly the vast array of effective medicinal agents available today represents one of man's greatest scientific accomplishments. It would be frightening to conceive of our civilization devoid of these remarkable and beneficial agents. Through their use, many of the diseases which have plagued mankind throughout history, as smallpox and poliomyelitis, are now virtually extinct. Illnesses such as diabetes, hypertension, and mental depression are now effectively controlled with modern drugs. Today's surgical procedures would be virtually impossible without the benefit of general anesthetics, analgesics, antibiotics, blood transfusions, and intravenous fluids and nutrients.

The process of drug discovery and development is complex. It involves the collective contributions of many scientific specialists including organic, physical, and analytical chemists, biochemists, bacteriologists, physiologists, pharmacologists, toxicologists, hematologists, immunologists, endocrinologists, pathologists, biostatisticians, pharmaceutical scientists, clinical physicians and many others.

After a potential new drug substance is discovered and has undergone definitive chemical and physical characterization, a great deal of biological information must be gathered. The basic *pharmacology* or the nature and mechanism of action of the drug on the biological system must be determined including toxicologic features. A study must be made of the drug's site and rate of absorption, its pattern of distribution and concentration within the body, its duration of action, and the method and rate of its elimination or excretion. Information must be obtained on the drug's metabolic degradation and the activity of any of its metabolites. A comprehensive study must be made of the drug's short term and long term effects on various body cells, tissues, and organs. Highly specific information may be obtained, as the effect of the drug on the fetus of a pregnant animal or its ability to pass to a nursing baby through the breast milk of its mother. Many a promising new drug has been abandoned because of its potential to cause excessive or hazardous adverse effects.

A new drug's most effective routes of administration (e.g., oral, rectal, parenteral) must be determined and guidelines established concerning the dosage recommended for persons of varying ages, weights, and states of illness. To facilitate administration of the drug by the selected routes, appropriate *dosage forms* as tablets, capsules, injections, suppositories, ointments, aerosols, and others are formulated and prepared. Each of these dosage units is designed to contain a specified quantity of medication for ease and accuracy of dosage administration. These dosage forms are highly sophisticated pharmaceutical drug delivery systems. Their design, development, production, and use are a prime example of the application of the pharmaceutical sciences—the blending of the basic, applied, and clinical sciences with pharmaceutical technology.

Each particular pharmaceutical product is a formulation unique unto itself. In addition to the active therapeutic ingredients, a pharmaceutical formulation also contains a number of nontherapeutic or *pharmaceutic* ingredients. It is through their use that a formulation achieves its unique composition and characteristic physical appearance. Included are such materials as fillers, thickeners, vehicles, suspending agents, tablet coatings and disintegrants, stabilizing agents, antimicrobial preservatives, flavors, colorants, and sweeteners.

In order to assure the stability of a drug in a formulation and the continued effectiveness of the drug product throughout its usual shelf life, the principles of chemistry, physical pharmacy, microbiology, and pharmaceutical technology must be applied. The formulation must be such that all components are physically and chemically compatible, including the active therapeutic agents, the pharmaceutical ingredients and the packaging materials. The formulation must be preserved against decomposition due to chemical degradation and protected from microbial contamination and the destructive influences of excessive heat, light, and moisture. The therapeutic ingredients must be released from the dosage form in the proper amount and in such a manner that the onset and duration of the drug's action is that which is desired. The pharmaceutical product must lend itself to efficient administration and must possess attractive features of flavor, odor, color, and texture that enhance patient acceptance. Finally, the product must be effectively packaged and clearly and completely labeled according to existing legal regulations.

Once prepared, the pharmaceutical product must be properly administered if the patient is to receive maximum benefit. The medication must be taken in sufficient quantity, at specified intervals, and for an indicated duration of time. The effectiveness of the medication in achieving the prescriber's objectives should be reevaluated at regular intervals and necessary adjustments made in the dosage, *dosage regimen* or dosage schedule, dosage form, or indeed, in the choice of the drug administered. Patient expressions of disappointment in his rate of progress or complaints of side effects to the prescribed drug should be evaluated upon report and decisions made as to the continuance, minor adjustment, or major change in drug therapy. Prior to initially taking a medication, a patient should be warned of any expected side effects, and of foods, beverages, and/or other drugs which may interfere with the effectiveness of the medication or with the course of therapy.

Through professional interaction and communication with other health professionals the pharmacist is able to contribute greatly to patient care. The pharmacist's intimate knowledge of drug actions, drug therapy, dosage form design and utilization, available pharmaceutical products, and drug information sources makes him or her a vital member of the health care team. The pharmacist is entrusted with the legal responsibility for the procurement, storage, control and distribution of effective pharmaceutical products and for the compounding and filling of prescription orders. Utilizing extensive training and knowledge, the pharmacist serves the patient as an advisor on drugs and encourages their safe and proper utilization. The pharmacist delivers pharmaceutical services in a variety of community and institutional health care environments and effectively utilizes recordkeeping and monitoring techniques in safeguarding the public health.

To appreciate the progress that has been made in drug discovery and development and to provide background for the study of modern drugs and pharmaceutical dosage forms, it is important to examine pharmacy's heritage.

The Heritage of Pharmacy

Drugs, in the form of vegetation and minerals, have existed longer than man himself. Human disease and man's instinct to survive have, through the ages, led to their discovery. The use of drugs, crude though they may have been, undoubtedly dates back long prior to recorded history, for the instinct of primitive man to relieve the pain of a wound by bathing it in cool water or by soothing it with a fresh leaf or protecting it with mud is within the realm of belief. From experience primitive man would learn that certain therapy was more effective than others, and from the beginnings the practice of drug therapy began.

Among many early races, disease was believed to be caused by the entrance of demons or evil spirits into the body. The treatment quite naturally involved ridding the body of the supernatural intruders. From the earliest records of history it is evident that the primary methods of doing so were through the use of spiritual incantations, the application of noisome materials, and the administration of specific herbs or plants.

The First Apothecary

Before the days of the priestcraft, the wise man or woman of the tribe, whose knowledge of the healing qualities of plants had been gathered through experience or handed down by word of mouth, was called upon to attend to the sick or wounded and prepare the remedy. It was in the preparation of the medicinal materials that the art of the apothecary originated.

The art of the apothecary has always been associated with the mysterious, and its practitioners were believed to have connection with the world of spirits and thus performed as intermediaries between the seen and the unseen. The belief that a drug had magical associations meant that its action, for good or for evil, did not depend upon its natural qualities alone. The compassion of a god, the observance of ceremonies, the absence of evil spirits, and the healing intent of the dispenser were individually and collectively needed to make the drug therapeutically effective. Because of this, the tribal apothecary was one to be feared, respected, trusted, sometimes mistrusted, worshipped, and revered, for it was through his potions that spiritual contact was made and upon which the cures or failures depended. Throughout history the knowledge of drugs and their application to disease has always meant power. In the Homeric epics, the term *pharmakon* (Gr.) from which our word *pharmacy* was derived connotes a charm or a drug that can be used for good or for evil purposes. Many of the tribal apothecary's failures were doubtless due to impotent medicines, inappropriate medicines, underdosage, overdosage, and even poisoning. His successes may be attributed to an appropriate drug based on his experience, coincidence of proper therapy, inconsequential effect of the therapy for an individual with a nonfatal illness, or *placebo effects,* that is, successful treatment due to psychologic rather than therapeutic effects. Even today, placebo therapy with nonpotent or inconsequential chemicals is successfully employed in the treatment of individual patients and is a routine practice in the clinical evaluation of new drugs where subjects' responses to the effects of the actual drug and the placebo are compared and evaluated.

As time passed, the art of the apothecary became combined with priestly functions, and among the early civilizations the priest-magician or priest-physician became the healer of the body as well as of the soul. Pharmacy and medicine are indistinguishable in their early history, since their practice was generally the function of the tribal religious leaders.

Early Drugs

Due to the patience and intellect of the archeologist, the types and specific drugs employed in the early history of drug therapy are not as indefinable as one might suspect. Numerous ancient tablets, scrolls, and other relics dating as far back as 3000 B.C. have been uncovered and deciphered by archeologic scholars to the delight of historians of both medicine and pharmacy, for contained in these ancient documents are specific associations with our common heritage (Fig. 1–1).

Perhaps the most famous of these surviving memorials is the *Papyrus Ebers,* a continuous scroll some 60 feet long and a foot wide dating back to the 16th century before Christ. This document, which is now preserved at the University of Leipzig, is named for the noted German Egyptologist, Georg Ebers, who discovered it in the tomb of a mummy and partly translated it during the last half of the nineteenth century.

Fig. 1–1. *Sumerian clay tablet from the third millennium* B.C. *on which are believed to be the world's oldest written prescriptions. Among them are a preparation of the seed of "carpenter plant," gum resin of markhazi, and thyme, all pulverized and dissolved in beer, and a combination of powdered roots of "Moon plant," and white pear tree, also dissolved in beer. (Courtesy of the University Museum, University of Pennsylvania.)*

Since that time, many scholars have participated in the translation of the document's challenging hieroglyphics, and although they are not unanimous in their interpretations there is little doubt that by 1550 B.C. the Egyptians were using some drugs and dosage forms still employed today.

The text of the Ebers Papyrus is dominated by drug formulas, with more than 800 formulas or prescriptions being described and over 700 different drugs being mentioned. The drugs referred to are chiefly botanic, although mineral and animal drugs are also noted. Such botanic substances as acacia, castor bean (from which we express castor oil), and fennel are mentioned along with apparent references to such minerals as iron oxide, sodium carbonate, sodium chloride, and sulfur. Animal excrements were also employed in drug therapy.

The formulative vehicles of the day were beer, wine, milk, and honey. Many of the pharmaceutical formulas employed two dozen or more different medicinal agents, a type of preparation later referred to as a "polypharmacal." Mortars, hand mills, sieves, and balances were commonly used by the Egyptians in their compounding of suppositories, gargles, pills, inhalations, troches, lotions, ointments, plasters, and enemas.

Introduction of the Scientific Viewpoint

Throughout history many individuals have contributed to the advancement of the health sciences. Notable among those whose genius and creativeness had a revolutionary influence on the development of pharmacy and medicine were Hippocrates (ca. 460–377 B.C.), Dioscorides (1st century A.D.), Galen (ca. 130–200 A.D.), and Paracelsus (1493–1541 A.D.).

Hippocrates was a Greek physician who is credited with the introduction of scientific pharmacy and medicine. He rationalized medicine, systematized medical knowledge, and put the practice of medicine on a high ethical plane. His thinking on the ethics and science of medicine dominated the medical writings of his and successive generations, and his concepts and precepts are embodied into the now renowned Hippocratic oath of ethical behavior for the healing professions. His works included the descriptions of hundreds of drugs, and it was during this period that the term *pharmakon* came to mean a purifying remedy for good only, transcending the previous connotation of a charm or drug for good or for evil purposes. Because of his pioneering work in medical science and his inspirational teachings and advanced philosophies that have become a part of modern medicine, Hippocrates is honored by being called the "Father of Medicine."

Dioscorides, a Greek physician and botanist, was the first to deal with botany as an applied science of pharmacy. His work, *De Materia Medica,* is considered a milestone in the development of pharmaceutical botany and in the study of naturally occurring medicinal materials. This area of study is today known as pharmacognosy, a term formed from two Greek words, *pharmakon,* drug, and *gnōsis,* knowledge. Some of the drugs described by Dioscorides, as opium, ergot, and hyoscyamus, continue to have use in medicine. His descriptions of the art of identifying and col-

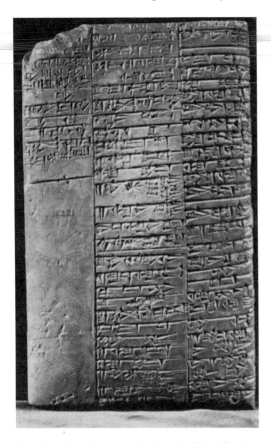

lecting natural drug products, the methods of their proper storage, and the means of detecting adulterants or contaminants were the standards of the period and established the need for additional work and the guidelines for future investigators.

Claudius Galen, a Greek pharmacist-physician who attained Roman citizenship, aimed to create a perfect system of physiology, pathology, and treatment and formulated doctrines that were followed for 1500 years. He was one of the most prolific authors of his or any other era, having been credited with 500 treatises on medicine and some 250 others on subjects of philosophy, law, and grammar. His medical writings include descriptions of numerous drugs of natural origin with a profusion of drug formulas and methods of compounding. He originated so many preparations of vegetable drugs by mixing or melting the individual ingredients that the area of pharmaceutical preparations was once commonly referred to as "Galenic pharmacy." Perhaps the most famous of his formulas is one for a cold cream, called Galen's Cerate, which has similarities in formulation to some in use today.

Pharmacy remained a function of medicine until the increasing variety of drugs and the growing complexity of compounding demanded specialists who could devote full attention to the art. Pharmacy was officially separated from medicine for the first time in 1240 A.D. when a decree of the German Emperor Frederick II regulated the practice of pharmacy within that part of his kingdom called the Two Sicilies. His edict separating the two professions acknowledged that pharmacy required special knowledge, skill, initiative, and responsibility if adequate care to the medical needs of the people was to be guaranteed. Pharmacists were obligated by oath to prepare reliable drugs of uniform quality according to their art. Any exploitation of the patient through business relations between the pharmacist and the physician was strictly forbidden. Between that time and the evolution of chemistry as an exact science, pharmacy and chemistry became united somewhat as pharmacy and medicine had been.

Perhaps no person in history exercised such a revolutionary influence on pharmacy and medicine as did Aureolus Philippus Theophrastus Bombastus von Hohenheim, a Swiss physician and chemist who called himself Paracelsus. He influenced the transformation of pharmacy from a profession based primarily on botanic science to one based on chemical science. Some of his chemical observations were astounding for his time and for their anticipation of later discoveries. He believed that it was possible to prepare a specific medicinal agent for use in combating each specific disease and introduced a host of chemical substances to internal therapy.

Early Research

As the knowledge of the basic sciences increased, so did their application to pharmacy. The opportunity was presented for the investigation of medicinal materials on a firm scientific basis, and the challenge was accepted by numerous pharmacists who conducted their research in the backrooms and basements of their pharmacies. Noteworthy among them was Karl Wilhelm Scheele (1742–1786), a Swedish pharmacist who is perhaps the most famous of all pharmacists because of his scientific genius and dramatic discoveries. Among his discoveries were the chemicals lactic acid, citric acid, oxalic acid, tartaric acid, and arsenic acid. He identified glycerin, invented new methods of preparing calomel and benzoic acid, and discovered oxygen a year prior to Priestley.

The isolation of morphine from opium by the German pharmacist Friedrich Sertürner (1783–1841) in 1805 prompted a series of isolations of other active materials from medicinal plants by a score of French pharmacists. Joseph Caventou (1795–1877) and Joseph Pelletier (1788–1842) combined their talents and isolated quinine and cinchonine from cinchona, and strychnine and brucine from nux vomica. Pelletier together with Pierre Robiquet (1780–1840) isolated caffeine, and Robiquet independently separated codeine from opium. Methodically one chemical after another was isolated from plant drugs and identified as an agent responsible for the plants' medicinal activity. Today we are still engaged in this fascinating activity as we probe nature for more useful and more specific therapeutic agents. An example is the drug taxol, derived from the Pacific yew tree and used in the treatment of ovarian cancer.

Throughout Europe during the late 18th century and the beginning of the 19th century, pharmacists like Pelletier and Sertürner were held in great esteem by their communities because of their intellect and technical abilities. They applied the art and the science of pharmacy to the preparation of drug products that were of the highest standards of purity, uniformity, and efficacy possible at that time. The extraction and isolation of various active constituents from crude or unprocessed drugs were major breakthroughs in the development of concentrated dosage forms of uniform strength containing singly effective therapeutic agents of natural origin. Many pharmacists of the period began to manufacture quality pharmaceutical products on a small but steadily increasing scale to meet the growing drug needs of their communities. Some of today's largest pharmaceutical research and manufacturing companies developed from these progressive prescription laboratories of almost two centuries ago.

Although many of the drugs indigenous to America and first used by the American Indian were adopted by the settlers, the vast majority of drugs needed in this country before the 19th century were imported from Europe, either as the raw materials or as finished pharmaceutical products. With the Revolutionary War, however, it became more difficult to import drugs, and the American pharmacist was stimulated to acquire the scientific and technologic expertise of his European contemporary. From this period until the Civil War, pharmaceutical manufacture was in its infancy in this country, but some of the pharmaceutical firms established during that period are still in existence. Three firms are known to have been established before 1826, with 22 additional ones having their origin in the subsequent half century. In 1821, Philadelphia College of Pharmacy was established as the nation's first school of pharmacy.

Drug Standards

As the scientific basis for drugs and drug products developed, so did the need for uniform standards to ensure quality.

The United States Pharmacopeia and the National Formulary[1,2]

The term *pharmacopeia* comes from the Greek, *pharmakon*, meaning "drug," and *poiein*, meaning "make," and the combination indicates any recipe or formula or other standards required to make or prepare a drug. The term was first used in 1580 in connection with a local book of drug standards in Bergamo, Italy. From that time on there were countless city, state, and national pharmacopeias published by various European pharmaceutical societies. As time passed, the value of a uniform set of national drug standards became apparent. In England, for example, three city pharmacopeias—the London, the Edinburgh, and the Dublin—were official throughout the kingdom until 1864, when they were replaced by the British Pharmacopoeia (BP).

In the United States drug standards were first provided on a national basis in 1820, when the first *United States Pharmacopeia* (USP) was published. The need for drug standards was recognized, however, in this country long before the first USP was published. For convenience and because of their familiarity with them, colonial physicians and apothecaries used the pharmacopeias and other references of their various homelands. The first American pharmacopeia was the so-called "Lititz Pharmacopeia," published in 1778 at Lititz, Pennsylvania, for use by the Military Hospital of the United States Army. It was a 32-page booklet containing information on 84 internal and 16 external drugs and preparations.

During the last decade of the 18th century, several attempts were made by various local medical societies to collate drug information, set appropriate standards, and prepare an extensive American pharmacopeia of the drugs in use at that time. In 1808 the Massachusetts Medical Society published a 272-page pharmacopeia containing information or monographs on 536 drugs and pharmaceutical preparations. Included were monographs on many drugs indigenous to America, which were not described in the European pharmacopeias of the day.

On January 6, 1817, Dr. Lyman Spalding, a physician from New York City, submitted a plan to the Medical Society of the County of New York for the creation of a national pharmacopeia. Dr. Spalding's efforts were later to result in his being recognized as the "Father of the United States Pharmacopeia." He proposed dividing the United States as then known into four geographical districts—Northern, Middle, Southern, and Western. The plan provided for calling a convention in each of these districts, to be composed of delegates from all medical societies and medical schools within them. Where there was as yet no incorporated medical society or medical school, voluntary associations of physicians and surgeons were invited to assist in the undertaking. Each district's convention was to draft a pharmacopeia and appoint delegates to a general convention to be held later in Washington, D.C. At the general convention, the four district pharmacopeias were to be compiled into a single national pharmacopeia.

Draft pharmacopeias were submitted to the convention by only the Northern and Middle districts. These were reviewed, consolidated, and adopted by the first United States Pharmacopeial Convention assembled in Washington, D.C., on January 1, 1820. The first *United States Pharmacopeia* was published on December 15, 1820, in English and also in Latin, then the international language of medicine, to render the book more intelligible to physicians and pharmacists of any nationality. Within its 272 pages were listed 217 drugs considered worthy of recognition, many of them taken from the Massachusetts Pharmacopeia, which is considered by some to be the precursor to the USP. The objective of the first USP was clearly stated in its preface and remains important. It reads in part:

> It is the objective of a Pharmacopeia to select from among substances which possess medicinal power, those, the utility of which is most fully established and best understood; and to form from them preparations and compositions, in which their powers may be exerted to the greatest advantage. It should likewise distinguish those articles by convenient and definite names, such as may prevent trouble or uncertainty in the intercourse of physicians and apothecaries.

Before adjourning, the Convention adopted a Constitution and Bylaws, with provisions for subsequent meetings of the Convention leading to a revised *United States Pharmacopeia* every 10 years. As many new drugs entered into drug therapy, the need for more frequent issuance of standards became increasingly apparent. In 1900, the Pharmacopeial Convention granted authority to issue supplements to the currently official USP whenever necessary to maintain satisfactory standards. At the 1940 meeting of the Convention, it was decided to revise the Pharmacopeia every 5 years while maintaining the use of periodic supplements.

The first United States Pharmacopeial Convention was composed exclusively of physicians. In 1830, and again in 1840, prominent pharmacists were invited to assist in the revision, and recognition of their contributions pharmacists were awarded full membership in the Convention of 1850 and have participated regularly ever since. Indeed, by 1870 the *Pharmacopeia* was so nearly in the hands of pharmacists that vigorous efforts were required to revive interest in it among physicians. The present Constitution and Bylaws of The United States Pharmacopeial Convention provide for accredited delegates representing educational institutions, professional and scientific organizations, designated divisions of the Federal Government, and public members.[3] Of the seven elected members of the Board of Trustees, at least two must be representatives of the medical science, two others must be representatives of the pharmaceutical sciences, and at least one must be a public member.

After the appearance of the first USP, the art and science of both pharmacy and medicine changed remarkably. Prior to 1820, the drugs employed in the treatment of disease had been much the same for centuries. The *Pharmacopeia* of 1820 reflected the fact that the apothecary of that day was competent at collecting and identifying botanic drugs and preparing from them the mixtures and preparations required by the physician. The individual pharmacist seemed quite fulfilled as he applied his total art to the creation of elegant pharmaceutical preparations from crude botanic materials. It was a time that would never be seen again because of the impending upsurge in technologic capabilities and the steady development of the basic sciences, particularly synthetic organic chemistry.

The second half of the 19th century brought great and far-reaching changes. The United States was now under the full impact of the industrial revolution. The steam engine, which used water power to turn mills that powdered crude botanic drugs, was replaced by the gas, diesel, or electric motor. New machinery was substituted for the old whenever possible, and often machinery from other industries was adapted to the special needs of pharmaceutical manufacturing. Mixers from the baking industry, centrifugal machines from the laundry industry, and sugarcoating pans from the candy industry were a few examples of the type of improvisations made. Production increased rapidly, but the new industry had to wait for the scientific revolution before it could claim newer and better drugs for mankind. A symbiosis was needed between science and the advancing technology.

By 1880, the industrial manufacture of chemicals and pharmaceutical products had become well established in this country, and the pharmacist was relying heavily upon commercial sources for his drug supply. Synthetic organic chemistry began to have its influence on drug therapy. The isolations of some active constituents of plant drugs had led to knowledge of their chemical structure. From this arose methods of synthetically duplicating the same structures, as well as manipulating molecular structure to produce organic chemicals yet undiscovered in nature. In 1872 the synthesis of salicylic acid from phenol inaugurated the synthesis of a group of analgesic compounds. Other new chemicals synthesized for the first time were phenolphthalein, a laxative, and sleep-producing derivatives of barbituric acid called "barbiturates." A new source of drugs, synthetic organic chemistry, welcomed the turn into the 20th century.

Until this time, drugs created through the genius of the synthetic organic chemist relieved a host of maladies, but none had been found to be curative—none, that is, until 1910, when arsphenamine, a specific agent against syphilis, was introduced to medical science. This was the start of an era of *chemotherapy,* an era in which the diseases of mankind became curable through the use of specific chemical agents. The concepts, discoveries, and inspirational work that led mankind to this glorious period are credited to Paul Ehrlich, the German bacteriologist who together with a Japanese colleague, Sahachiro Hata, discovered arsphenamine. Today most of our new drugs, whether they be curative or palliative, originate in the flask of the synthetic organic chemist.

The advancement of science, both basic and applied, led to drugs of a more complex nature and to more of them. The drug standards advanced by the USP were more than ever needed to protect the public by ensuring the purity and uniformity of the drugs administered.

When the American Pharmaceutical Association was organized in 1852, the only authoritative and generally recognized book of drug standards available was the third revision of the *United States Pharmacopeia.* In order to serve as a therapeutic guide to the medical profession, its scope, then as now, was restricted to drugs of established therapeutic merit. Because of this policy of strict selectivity, many drugs and formulas that were widely accepted and used by the medical profession were not granted admission to early revisions of the *Pharmacopeia.* As a type of a protest, and in keeping with the original objectives of the American Pharmaceutical Association to establish standardization of drugs and formulas, certain pharmacists, with the sanction of their national organization, prepared a formulary containing many of the popular drugs and formulas denied admission to the *Pharmacopeia.* The first edition was published in 1888 under the title *National Formulary of Unofficial Preparations.* The designation *Unofficial Preparations* reflected the protest mood of the authors, since the *Pharmacopeia* had earlier adopted the term "official" as applying to the drugs for which it provided standards. The title was changed to *National Formulary* on June 30, 1906 when President Theodore Roosevelt signed into law the first federal Pure Food and Drug Act, designating both the USP and NF as establishing legal standards for medicinal and pharmaceutic substances. Thus the two publications became *official compendia.* Among other things, the law required that whenever the designations "USP" or "NF" were used or implied on drug labeling that the products must conform to the physical and chemical standards set forth in the compendium monograph.

The early editions of the *National Formulary* served mainly as a convenience to practicing pharmacists by providing uniform names of drugs and preparations and working directions for the small-scale manufacture of popular pharmaceutical preparations prescribed by physicians. Prior to 1940, the NF, as the USP, was revised every 10 years. After that date, new editions appeared every 5 years, with supplements issued periodically as necessary.

In 1975, the United States Pharmacopeial Convention, Inc. purchased the National Formulary, unifying the official compendia and thereby provided the mechanism for a single, national compendium.

The first combined compendium, representing the USPXX and NFXV became official on July 1, 1980. All monographs on therapeutically active drug substances appeared in the USP section of the volume, whereas all monographs on pharmaceutic agents appeared in the NF section. This format has been continued with the most recent revision, the *United States Pharmacopeia 23/National Formulary 18,* which became official on January 1, 1995, and for the first time dropped the use of roman numerals to indicate the book's edition. This official compendium of legal standards, which contains over 3,500 drug monographs, is now published both in print and on computer disks.

The standards advanced by the *United States Pharmacopeia* and the *National Formulary* are put to active use by all members of the health care industry who share the responsibility and enjoy the public's trust for assuring the availability of quality drugs and pharmaceutical products. Included in this group are pharmacists, physicians, dentists, veterinarians, nurses, producers and suppliers of bulk chemicals for use in drug production, large and small manufacturers of pharmaceutical products, drug procurement officers of various private and public health agencies and institutions, drug regulatory and enforcement agencies, and many others.

USP and NF Monographs

The *United States Pharmacopeia* and the *National Formulary* adopt standards for drug substances, pharmaceutic ingredients, and dosage forms reflecting the best in the current practices of medicine and pharmacy and provide suitable tests and assay procedures for demonstrating compliance with these standards. In fulfilling this function, the compendia become legal documents, every statement of which must be of a high degree of clarity and specificity.

The USP includes detailed monographs on drug substances and dosage forms, whereas the NF contains monographs on pharmaceutic ingredients. These monographs represent the established standards and constitute the basis for maintaining quality.

It should be noted that many pharmaceutical products on the market, especially those which are combinations of therapeutic ingredients, are not represented by formulation or dosage form monographs in the official compendia. However, the individual components in these products are either represented by monographs in the compendia or are otherwise approved as a part of the manufacturer's drug applications and listings with the Food and Drug Administration and thus together with the approved product meet the designated standards.

An example of a typical monograph for a drug substance appearing in the USP is shown in Figure 1–2. This monograph demonstrates the type of information generally appearing for organic medicinal agents.

The initial part of the monograph consists of the official title (*generic* or *nonproprietary* name) of the drug substance. This is followed by its graphic or structural formula, its empirical formula, molecular weight, established chemical names, and the drug's Chemical Abstracts Service (CAS) Registry Number. The CAS Registry Number identifies each compound uniquely in the CAS computer-oriented information retrieval system. Appearing next in the monograph is a statement of chemical purity, a cautionary statement which reflects the toxic nature of the agent, packaging and storage recommendations, and chemical and physical tests and the prescribed method of assay to substantiate the identification and purity of the chemical.

In each monograph, the standards set forth are specific to the individual therapeutic agent, pharmaceutic material, or dosage form preparation to assure purity, potency, and quality.

The USP Drug Research and Testing Labora-

Chlorambucil

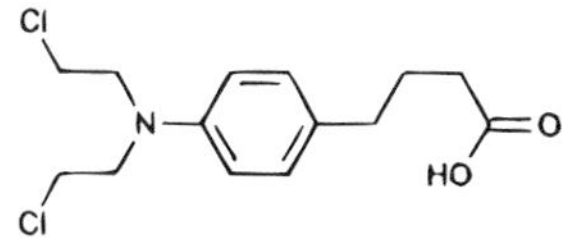

$C_{14}H_{19}Cl_2NO_2$ **304.22 Benzenebutanoic acid, 4-[bis(2-chloroethyl)amino]-4-[*p*[**Bis(2-chloroethyl)amino] phenyl]butyric acid [*305-03-3*].

▸ Chlorambucil contains not less than 98.0% and not more than 101.0% of $C_{14}H_{19}Cl_2NO_2$, calculated on the anhydrous basis.

Caution—Great care should be taken to prevent inhaling particles of Chlorambucil and exposing the skin to it.

Packaging and storage—Preserve in tight, light-resistant containers.

Reference standard—*USP Chlorambucil Reference Standard—[Caution—Avoid contact]*—Dry over silica gel for 24 hours before using.

Identification—

A: The infrared absorption spectrum of a 1 in 125 solution in carbon disulfide, in a 1-mm cell, exhibits maxima only at the same wavelengths as that of a similar solution of USP Chlorambucil RS.

B: Dissolve 50 mg in 5 mL of acetone, and dilute with water to 10 mL. Add 1 drop of 2 *N* sulfuric acid, then add 4 drops of silver nitrate TS: no opalescence is observed immediately *(absence of chloride ion)*. Warm the solution on a steam bath: opalescence develops *(presence of ionizable chlorine)*.

Melting range (741): between 65° and 69°.

Water, *Method I* (921): not more than 0.5%.

Assay—Dissolve about 200 mg of Chlorambucil, accurately weighed, in 10 mL of acetone, add 10 mL of water, and titrate with 0.1 *N* sodium hydroxide VS, using phenolphthalein TS as the indicator. Each mL of 0.1 *N* sodium hydroxide is equivalent to 30.42 mg of $C_{14}H_{19}Cl_2NO_2$.

Fig. 1–2. *Chlorambucil*

tory provides direct laboratory assistance to the *United States Pharmacopeia* and the *National Formulary*. The Laboratory's main functions are the evaluation of USP Reference Standards and the evaluation and development of analytical methods to be used in the compendia.

USP DI

As an aid to health care professionals and the public, the United States Pharmacopeial Convention publishes print and computer database versions of the three-volume set, *USP Drug Information* (USP DI).[3] Volume I, "Drug Information for the Health Care Professional," contains authoritative information on pharmaceutical products, including their indications, pharmacology, side effects, and dosage; Volume II, "Advice for the Patient," provides guidance in layman's language on the proper use of pharmaceutical products; and Volume III, "Approved Drug Products and Legal Requirements," presents legal requirements for dispensing pharmaceutical products, including information on product equivalence. The volumes serve as a resource to the health professional doing patient consultation. They also serve as the basis for printed or computer-generated USP DI Patient Education Leaflets, which may be provided to patients as a part of medication counseling.

Other Pharmacopeias and Drug Standards

In addition to the USP and the NF, other references to drug standards such as the *Homeopathic Pharmacopeia of the United States* (HPUS) and the *International Pharmacopeia* (IP) provide additional guidelines for drug quality required by certain practitioners and agencies. The *Homeopathic Pharmacopeia* is used in practice by pharmacists and homeopathists and is utilized by law enforcement agencies that must ensure the quality of homeopathic drugs. The term *homeopathy* was coined by Samuel Hahnemann (1755–1843) from the Greek *homoios,* meaning similar, and *pathos,* meaning disease. In essence, the philosophy of homeopathy is that like cures like: that is, a drug that produces in healthy persons the effects or set of symptoms of the illness present will cure the disease. Embodied in the homeopathic approach are (1) the testing of a drug on healthy persons to find the drug's effects so that it may be employed against the same symptoms manifesting a disease in an ill person, (2) the use of only minute doses of drugs in therapy, employed in dilutions expressed as "1x" (a 1:10 dilution), "2x" (a 1:100 dilution), etc., (3) the administration of not more than one drug at a time, and (4) the treatment of the entire symptom complex of the patient, not just one symptom.[4] The *Homeopathic Pharmacopeia* is essential for pharmacists who prepare drugs to be used in the practice of homeopathy.

The *Pharmacopeia Internationalis,* or *International Pharmacopoeia,* is published by the World Health Organization (WHO) of the United Nations with the cooperation of member countries. It is intended as a recommendation to national pharmacopeial revision committees to modify their respective pharmacopeias according to the international standards adopted. It has no legal authority, only the mutual respect and recognition accorded it by the participating countries in their joint effort to provide acceptable drug standards on an international basis. The first volume of the *Pharmacopoeia Internationalis* was published in 1951. It has been revised periodically since that time.

A number of countries publish their own pharmacopeias, including Great Britain, France, Italy, Japan, India, East Germany, Norway, and the former Union of Soviet Socialist Republics. Many of these pharmacopeias are utilized by multinational companies who develop and market products on an international basis. Countries not having a national pharmacopeia frequently adopt one of another country for their use in setting and regulating drug standards. The pharmacopeia selected is usually one based on geographic proximity, a common heritage or language, or a similarity of drugs and pharmaceutical products used.

In the United States, in addition to the official compendia, important drug standards are provided by means of the specifications set forth in individual New Drug and Antibiotic Applications (see Chapter 2) approved by the Food and Drug Administration. The approved standards for individually marketed drugs must be rigidly adhered to by the manufacturer, thereby maintaining the established quality of the product.

Drug Regulation and Control

The first Federal law in the United States designed to regulate drug products manufactured domestically was the Food and Drug Act of 1906. The law required drugs marketed through interstate commerce to comply with their claimed standards for strength, purity, and quality. Manufacturers' claims of therapeutic benefit were not regulated until 1912, when the passage of the Sherley Amendment specifically prohibited false claims of therapeutic effects, declaring such products "misbranded."

The Federal Food, Drug, and Cosmetic Act of 1938

The need for additional drug standards was tragically demonstrated in 1938. The then-new wonder drug, sulfanilamide, which was not soluble in most commonly used pharmaceutical solvents of the day, was prepared and distributed by a reputable manufacturer as an elixir, solubilized with diethylene glycol. Before the product could be removed from the market, over 100 persons had lost their lives due to the toxic effects of the formulation's solvent, diethylene glycol. The necessity for proper product formulation and for thorough pharmacologic and toxicologic testing of the therapeutic agent and of the completed pharmaceutical product was painfully recognized. Congress responded with passage of the Federal Food, Drug, and Cosmetic Act of 1938 and the creation of the Food and Drug Administration (FDA) to administer and enforce it. Included in the Act is a provision that prohibits the use of any new drug without the prior filing of a New Drug Application (NDA) with the Food and Drug Administration. The officials of the FDA grant or deny permission to distribute a new product after reviewing the applicant's filed data on the product's ingredients, manufacturing processes, toxicologic studies on animals, therapeutic claims, and clinical trials on human beings. Although the Act of 1938 required pharmaceutical products to be safe for human use, it should be noted that it did not require them to be efficacious.

Kefauver-Harris Amendments of 1962

Another major drug tragedy, which occurred in 1960, led to the passage of the Kefauver-Harris Amendments to the Federal Food Drug and Cosmetic Act of 1938. A new synthetic drug, called thalidomide, recommended as a sedative and tranquilizer, was being sold in Europe without the requirement of a physician's prescription. It was a drug of especial interest due to its apparent lack of toxicity even at extreme dosage levels. It was hoped that it would replace the barbiturates in popularity as a sedative and therefore prevent the frequent deaths caused from accidental and intentional overdosage with barbiturates. An American firm was awaiting FDA approval for marketing in this country when reports of a strange effect of the drug's use began to filter in from Europe. Thalidomide given to women during pregnancy produced phocomelia or an arrested development of the limbs of the newborn infant. Thousands of children were affected to various extents.[5] Some were born with neither arms nor legs; others, with partially formed limbs. The more fortunate were born with only disfigurations of the nose, eyes, and ears. Those more severely afflicted died, the result of internal malformation of the heart or gastrointestinal tract. This drug catastrophe, which for the most part did not affect American citizens, spurred Congress to strengthen the existing laws regarding new drugs. Without dissent, on October 10, 1962, the Kefauver-Harris Drug Amendments to the Food, Drug, and Cosmetic Act of 1938 were passed by both houses of Congress. The purpose of the enactment was to ensure a greater amount of safety in the drugs made available to our citizens, and for the first time the manufacturer was required to prove the drug efficacious before it would be granted FDA approval for marketing.

Under the Food, Drug, and Cosmetic Act as amended, the sponsor of a new drug (usually a drug manufacturer, but occasionally a research institution, an individual or a group of medical researchers) is required to file with the FDA an Investigational New Drug Application (IND) before a drug may be clinically tested on human beings. The Center for Drug Evaluation and Research of the FDA is charged with the responsibility of reviewing and evaluating the IND application. Following carefully designed and structured phases of human clinical trials, in which a proposed drug is evaluated for safety and effectiveness, the drug's sponsor may submit to the FDA a New Drug Application (NDA) seeking approval for marketing. The requirements for an IND, NDA, other submissions, and the FDA review process are presented in Chapter 2.

Additional Standards for Safety and Effectiveness

Following the full implementation of the procedures required for the evaluation of new drugs, the FDA turned its attention to the examination of products which had entered the marketplace between 1938 and 1962 and thus were never reviewed and "approved" under the same criteria for safety and efficacy as were the drugs marketed after 1962. The FDA initiated this Drug Efficacy Study in 1966 through an agreement reached with the National Academy of Sciences-National Research Council (NAS/NRC) for the review for safety and efficacy of some 4000 drug products then on the market. The NAS/NRC review was conducted by 30 panels of physicians, all experts in their fields. The drug products reviewed were primarily prescription drugs; however, over 400 nonprescription drugs were included in the study. In 1969, upon receipt of the NAS/NRC findings, a special task force of the FDA's Bureau of Drugs, called the Drug Efficacy Study Implementation (DESI) Project Office, reviewed the NAS/NRC recommendations. Products that were found to comply with the statutory requirements for safety and efficacy and bore correct labeling were allowed to remain on the market. Those that did not comply were either removed from the market by regulatory action or required to make the necessary changes in labeling, formulation, or submission of suitable additional data as was considered necessary to conform to the regulatory requirements. Through a 1970 FDA regulation, the opportunity for a drug sponsor to submit an Abbreviated New Drug Application (ANDA) was established. It provides an expeditious review and approval process for those drug products that were initially marketed in the period 1938–1962 and for which the FDA has information on the drug substance/product on file. The ANDA enables the manufacturer to expeditiously market a new dosage form of the approved drug or alter its formulation. Generally, the clinical investigations are not required to be repeated.

Drug Price Competition and Patent Term Restoration Act of 1984

Changes to speed up the process of approval of generic drugs were a major component of the Drug Price Competition and Patent Restoration Act of 1984. Under the provisions of the legislation, generic copies of a pioneer drug (originally approved drug) can be approved through an Abbreviated New Drug Application (ANDA) if the FDA determines that it is sufficiently equivalent to the pioneer drug not to require additional animal or human studies for safety and efficacy. The legislation also provides an extension of patent-life for patented drugs, equal to the time required for NDA approval, plus half the time spent in the testing phase, for a maximum of 5 years.

Another major effort of the Food and Drug Administration in achieving the goals of the 1962 Drug Amendments involved the massive review of nonprescription drug products. This effort involved the use of expert scientific panels to review the safety, effectiveness, and labeling of the various categories of nonprescription drugs. As was the case with prescription drugs, products not conforming to the established standards were to be removed from the market unless they were reformulated, relabeled or otherwise changed to meet the prevailing standards.

Drug Listing Act

The Drug Listing Act of 1972 was enacted to provide the Food and Drug Administration with the legislative authority to compile a list of currently marketed drugs to assist the Agency in the enforcement of Federal laws requiring that drugs be safe and effective and not adulterated or misbranded. Under the regulations of the Act, each firm which manufactures or repackages drugs for ultimate sale or distribution to patients or consumers must register with the FDA and submit appropriate information for listing. All foreign drug manufacturing and distributing firms whose products are imported into the United States are also included in this regulation. Exempt from the registration and listing requirement are hospitals, clinics, and the various health practitioners who prepare pharmaceutical products for use in their respective institutions and practices. Also exempt are research and teaching institutions in which drug products are prepared for purposes other than sale. Each registrant is assigned a permanent registration number, following the format of the National Drug Code (NDC) numbering system. Under this system, the first 4 numeric characteristics of 10-character code identify the manufacturer or distributor and are referred to as the "Labeler Code." The last 6 numeric characters of the 10-character code identify the drug formulation and the trade package size and type. The segment which identifies the drug formulation is known as the "Product Code," and the segment which identifies the trade package size and type is called the "Package Code." The manufacturer or distributor determines the ratio of use of the last 6 digits for the two codes, as a 3-to-3 digit Product-Code-Package Code configuration (e.g., 542-112) or a 4-to-2 digit configuration (e.g., 5421-12). Only one such type of configuration may be selected for use by a manufacturer or distributor who then assigns a code number to each of his products to be included in the drug listing. A final code number is presented as the example: "NDC 0081-5421-12."

The FDA requests that the National Drug Code number appear on all drug labeling, including the label of any prescription drug container furnished to a consumer. In some instances, manufacturers imprint the NDC number directly on the dosage units, as capsules and tablets, for rapid and positive identification when the number is matched in the *National Drug Code Directory* or against a decoding list provided by the manufacturer. Once a number is assigned to a drug product it is a permanent assignment. Even in instances in which a drug manufacturer discontinues the manufacture and distribution of a product, the number may not be used again. If a drug product is substantially changed, as through an alteration in the active ingredients, dosage form, or product name, a new NDC number is assigned to the product by the registrant and the FDA advised accordingly.

The product information received by the FDA is processed and stored by computer to provide easy access to the following types of information:

1. A list of all drug products.
2. A list of all drug products broken down by labeled indications or pharmacologic category.
3. A list of all drug products, broken down by manufacturer.
4. A list of a drug product's active ingredients.
5. A list of a drug product's inactive ingredients.
6. A list of drug products containing a particular ingredient.
7. A list of drug products newly marketed or remarketed.
8. A list of drug products discontinued.
9. All labeling of drug products.
10. All advertising of drug products.

The drug listing program enables the FDA to monitor the quality of all drugs on the market in this country.

In a continuing effort to assure the standards for drug quality control, the Food and Drug Administration's regulations provide not only for the inspection and certification of pharmaceutical manufacturing procedures and facilities, but also for the field surveillance and assay of products obtained from the shelves of retail distributors.

In instances in which it is found that a manufacturer is not meeting the established standards for drug product quality, that manufacturer will be denied permission to continue to produce products for distribution until compliance with the standards is attained.

Classification of Drugs

Drugs approved for marketing by the Food and Drug Administration are categorized according to the manner in which they may be legally obtained by the patient. Drugs deemed safe enough for use by the layman in the self-treatment of simple conditions for which competent medical care is not generally sought are classified as "over-the-counter" (O.T.C.) drugs and may be sold without the requirement of a physician's prescription. This status assigned to a drug product by the FDA may be changed should more stringent control over the drug's distribution and use later be warranted. Other drugs that are considered useful only after expert diagnosis or too dangerous for use in self-medication are made available only on the prescription of a licensed practitioner. These drugs are referred to as "Legend" drugs, because it is a requirement of their labeling to bear the legend: "Caution: Federal Law Prohibits Dispensing Without Prescription," under the provisions of the Durham-Humphrey Amendment of 1952 to the Federal Food, Drug, and Cosmetic Act. Drugs so designated may also change legal status from time to time according to the judgments of the Food and Drug Administration and the firm that distributes the product. New drugs that have not been shown to be safe in self-medication are generally limited to prescription dispensing until such time that they are considered useful and safe enough for the layman to use at his discretion.

According to the Durham-Humphrey Amendment, prescriptions for Legend drugs may not be refilled (dispensed again after the initial filling of the prescription) without the express consent of the prescriber. The refill status of prescriptions for certain Legend drugs known to be subject to public abuse was further regulated with the passage of the Drug Abuse Control Amendments of 1965 and then by the Comprehensive Drug Abuse Prevention and Control Act of 1970.

The Comprehensive Drug Abuse Prevention and Control Act of 1970 served to consolidate and codify drug control authority into a single statute. Under its provisions, the Drug Abuse Control Amendments of 1965, the Harrison Narcotic Act of 1914, and other related laws governing stimulants, depressants, narcotics and hallucinogenics were repealed and replaced by regulatory framework now administered by the Drug Enforcement Administration (DEA) in the Department of Justice.

The Comprehensive Drug Abuse Prevention and Control Act of 1970 established five "Schedules" for the classification and control of drug substances which are subject to public abuse. These schedules provide for decreasing levels of control from Schedule I drugs to those classified as Schedule V drugs. The drugs in the five Schedules may be described as follows:

Schedule I—Drugs with no accepted medical use, or other substances, with a high potential for abuse. In this category are heroin, LSD, and similar items, but virtually any non-medical substance that is being abused can be placed in this category.

Schedule II—Drugs with accepted medical uses and a high potential for abuse which, if abused, may lead to severe psychological or physical dependence.

Schedule III—Drugs with accepted medical uses and a potential for abuse less than those listed in Schedules I and II which, if abused, may lead to moderate psychological or physical dependence.

Schedule IV—Drugs with accepted medical uses and low potential for abuse relative to those in Schedule III which, if abused, may lead to limited physical dependence or psychological dependence relative to drugs in Schedule III.

Schedule V—Drugs with accepted medical uses and low potential for abuse relative to those in Schedule IV and which, if abused, may lead to limited physical dependence or psychological dependence relative to drugs in Schedule IV.

It should be noted that in all instances, local and state laws may strengthen the Federal drug laws but may not be used to weaken them.

Drug Product Recall

In instances in which it is found by the FDA or by a manufacturer that a marketed product presents a threat or a potential threat to consumer safety, that product may be "recalled" or sought for return to the manufacturer from its depth of distribution. The pharmaceutical manufacturer is legally bound to report serious unlabeled adverse reactions to the FDA within 15 working days of learning of an adverse drug reaction. The FDA/USP Drug Product Problem Reporting (DPPR) Program, which began in 1970, is designed as an aid in the protection of the public health, to the monitoring of manufacturer compliance with Current Good Manufacturing Practices (CGMP) and to detect problem products in the marketplace. The pharmacist can report a problem with any drug product or medical device by telephone or written report. Problems may include and are not limited to product adulteration, container leakage, improper labeling and/or unexpected reactions, among others.

A drug product recall may be initiated by the FDA or by the manufacturer, the latter case being termed a "voluntary recall." A numerical classification, as follows, indicates the degree of consumer hazards associated with the product being recalled.

Class I is a situation in which there is a reasonable probability that the use of, or exposure to, a violative product will cause serious, adverse health consequences or death.

Class II is a situation in which the use of, or exposure to, a violative product may cause temporary or medically reversible adverse health consequences or where the probability of serious adverse health consequences is remote.

Class III is a situation in which the use of, or exposure to, a violative product is not likely to cause adverse health consequences.

The "depth of recall," or the level of market removal or correction (as wholesaler, retailer, consumer), depends upon the nature of the product, the urgency of the situation, and depth to which the product has been distributed. The lot numbers of packaging control numbers on the containers or labels of the manufactured products help in identifying the specific lot or batch of product to be recalled.

Prescription Drug Marketing Act of 1987

The Prescription Drug Marketing Act of 1987, passed by Congress and signed into law by the President, became effective on July 21, 1988. The legislation, amending the Federal Food, Drug, and Cosmetic Act, established new safeguards on the integrity of the nation's supply of prescription drugs. Because of its author, Representative John Dingell, and its purpose to prevent drug diversion, the Act has often been referred to as the "Dingell Bill," and the "Drug Diversion Act." The Act is intended to reduce the risks of adulterated, misbranded, repackaged, or mislabeled drugs entering the legitimate marketplace through "secondary sources." The primary sections of the Act are summarized as follows:

1. *Reimportation.* Prohibits the reimportation of drug products manufactured in the United States except by the manufacturer of the product.
2. *Sales Restrictions.* Prohibits selling, trading, purchasing, or the offer to sell, trade or purchase a drug sample. It also prohibits resales by health care institutions of pharmaceuticals purchased explicitly for the use of the institution. Charitable institutions that receive drugs at reduced prices or no cost cannot resell the drugs.
3. *Distribution of Samples.* Samples may only be distributed to: (a) practitioners licensed to prescribe such drugs and, (b) at the written request of the practitioner, to pharmacies of hospitals or other health care institutions. Sample distribution must be made through mail or common carrier and not directly by employees or agents of the manufacturer.
4. *Wholesale Distributors.* Manufacturers are required to maintain a list of their authorized distributors. Wholesalers who desire to distribute a drug for which they are not authorized distributors must inform their wholesale customers, prior to the sale, the name of the person from whom they obtained the goods and all previous sales.
5. *Penalties.* Severe penalties are imposed for the violation of the Act.

Code of Federal Regulations and *The Federal Register*

Title 21 of the Code of Federal Regulations (CFR) consists of eight volumes containing all regulations issued under the Federal Food, Drug and Cosmetic Act and other statutes administered by the Food and Drug Administration. A ninth volume contains regulations issued under statutes administered by the Drug Enforcement Administration. The volumes are updated each year to incorporate all regulations issued during the preceding 12-month period. *The Federal Register* (FR), is issued each workday by the Superintendent of Documents, U.S. Government Printing Office, and contains proposed and final regulations and legal notices issued by Federal agencies, including the Food and Drug Administration and the Drug Enforcement Administration. These publications provide the most definitive information on Federal laws and regulations pertaining to drugs.

The Pharmacist's Contemporary Role

Pharmacists perform capably in numerous settings in which the basic pharmaceutical sciences, the clinical sciences, and professional training and experiences are applied.

A majority of pharmacists practice within an ambulatory care/community pharmacy setting. In this setting, the pharmacist plays an active role in the patient's use of prescription and nonprescription medication, diagnostic agents, durable medical equipment and devices, and other health-related products. The pharmacist develops patient medication profiles and counsels patients on their health status and use of drug and nondrug measures.

Because of accessibility, the pharmacist also exercises a vital health education role through community service and participation in public education forums and programs. By serving as a source of drug information to the patient, physician, and allied health professionals, the community pharmacist enjoys the opportunity to influence directly or indirectly the selection and use of drug therapies.

A significant number of pharmacists practice in institutional settings, including hospitals, extended care facilities, and Health Maintenance Organizations (HMO). Practice in these settings may include the provision of professional and clinical services, e.g., nuclear pharmacy, intravenous admixture services, patient monitoring, the provision of educational and technical services, e.g., drug information and poison control, and/or the provision of research and support services, e.g., pharmacokinetic consult service, investigational drug studies division. In addition to maintaining a safe drug distribution and control system, the pharmacist is asked to apply his knowledge in a variety of ways, including drug regimen review and participation on patient-care review committees.

Some graduate pharmacists participate in postgraduate *residency* and/or *fellowship* programs to enhance their practice and/or research skills. A pharmacy residency is defined as: *an organized, directed postgraduate training program in a defined area of practice.* The chief purpose of pharmacy residencies is to train pharmacists in professional practice and management skills.

Residency programs are conducted primarily in institutional practice settings. A fellowship is focused toward developing competency in scientific research. It is defined as: *a directed, highly individualized postgraduate program designed to prepare the participant to become an independent researcher.* Both pharmacy residencies and fellowships generally last 12 months or longer and require the close direction of a qualified preceptor.

Pharmacists working for pharmaceutical research, manufacturing, and distributing firms become involved in virtually every phase of drug product development, clinical testing, production, marketing, and management functions. Their knowledge of the basic and pharmaceutical sciences, dosage form design, and the technical aspects of production fits well with this major function of industrial pharmacy firms. Pharmacists with advanced degrees in the basic or pharmaceutical sciences, or in other areas of health care administration, marketing, law, or medicine contribute to their industrial employers in their respective areas of expertise.

In addition to the areas of drug research, product development, and production, many pharmacists in industry work in such varied areas as drug materials procurement; in public, trade, or professional relations; as scientific, technical, or professional information specialists; in liaison work with governmental agencies, educational or research institutions, or professional organizations; or in marketing, advertising, promotion, or pharmaceutical sales.

In government service, pharmacists perform professional and administrative functions, as in the development and implementation of health care programs in the design and enforcement of regulations involving drug quality standards, good manufacturing practices, and drug distribution and utilization practices. Pharmacists also practice their profession in government supported hospitals, clinics, and specialized health care institutions.

Career opportunities for pharmacists in government service at the Federal level include positions in the military service, in the Public Health Service, and in such Civil Service agencies as the Food and Drug Administration, Veterans Administration, Department of Health and Human Services, Drug Enforcement Administration of the Department of Justice, National Institutes of Health, and others. At the state and local level, many pharmacists find rewarding careers in developing programs for drug procurement, distribution and utilization in the various health departments, welfare departments or agencies, drug investigation and regulatory agencies, clinics and health-care institutions, and also with state boards of pharmacy.

A number of pharmacists serve their profession in positions with various professional organizations, as state and national pharmaceutical associations.

Schools of pharmacy utilize pharmacists, some with and some without advanced degrees, to teach in the professional curriculum, to conduct pharmaceutical research, and to participate in the service and continuing education functions of the school. Although most of the educators working full time for the school do so within the classrooms and laboratories of the academic institution, many others provide professional instruction in the practice or clinical setting. Part-time pharmacist-educators also are employed by schools of pharmacy to provide professional instruction within the academic institution or in affiliated teaching hospitals, medical specialty clinics, hospital pharmacies, drug information centers, nursing homes and extended care facilities, drug abuse clinics, health departments, mental health hospitals or clinics, community pharmacies, and other places in which pharmaceutical services are delivered. Many community and institutional pharmacy practitioners serve educational institutions as "preceptors," and provide pharmacy students with educational experiences within the scope and their own daily practice of pharmacy.

The Mission of Pharmacy

In 1990, the Board of Trustees of the American Pharmaceutical Association adopted the following mission statement for pharmacy[7]:

The mission of pharmacy is to serve society as the profession responsible for the appropriate use of medications, devices, and services to achieve optimal therapeutic outcomes.

The elements of the statement were defined as follows:

Pharmacy is the health profession that concerns itself with the knowledge system that results in the discovery, development, and use of medications and medication information in the care of patients. It encompasses the clinical, scientific, economic, and educational aspects of the profession's knowledge base and its communication to others in the health-care system.

Society encompasses patients, other health-care providers, health-policy decision makers, corporate health benefits managers, the healthy public, and other individuals and groups to whom health care and medication use are important.

Appropriate refers to the pharmacist's responsibility to ensure that a medication regimen is specifically tailored for the individual patient, based on accepted clinical and pharmacological parameters. Further, the pharmacist should evaluate the regimen to assure maximum safety, cost-effectiveness, and compliance by the patient.

Medications refers to legend and nonlegend agents used in the diagnosis, treatment, prevention, and/or cure of disease. The term is specifically and purposefully used and is distinguished from the term *drug,* which has a negative and nontherapeutic public image.

Devices refers to the equipment, process, biotechnological entities, diagnostic agents, or other products that are used to assist in effective management of the medication regimen.

Services refers to patient, health professional and public education services, screening and monitoring programs, medication-regimen management, and related activities that contribute to effective medication use by patients.

Optimal therapeutic outcomes declares the profession's ultimate contribution to public health. Pharmacy asserts it unique rights, privileges, and responsibilities—and accepts the attendant liabilities—associated with medication use. Pharmacy recognizes the need effectively to integrate its health-care role with the complementary roles of the patient and other health care professionals.

Definition of Pharmaceutical Care

The role of the pharmacist in practice is the delivery of *pharmaceutical care.* The contemporary definition of *pharmaceutical care,* presented by Hepler and Strand[8] in 1989, is as follows:

Pharmaceutical care is the responsible provision of drug therapy for the purpose of achieving definite outcomes that improve a patient's quality of life. These outcomes are: *(i)* cure of a disease; *(ii)* elimination or reduction of a patient's symptomatology; *(iii)* arresting or slowing of a disease process; or *(iv)* preventing a disease or symptomatology.

Pharmaceutical care involves the process through which a pharmacist cooperates with a patient and other professionals in designing, implementing and monitoring a therapeutic plan that will produce specific therapeutic outcomes for the patient. This in turn involves three major functions: *(i)* identifying potential and actual drug-related problems; *(ii)* resolving actual drug-related problems; and *(iii)* preventing potential drug-related problems.

Pharmaceutical care is a necessary element of health care, and should be integrated with other elements. Pharmaceutical care is, however, provided for the direct benefit of the patient, and the pharmacist is responsible directly to the patient for the quality of that care. The fundamental relationship in pharmaceutical care is a mutually beneficial exchange in which the patient grants authority to the provider, and the provider gives competence and commitment (accepts responsibility) to the patient.

The fundamental goals, processes, and relationships of pharmaceutical care exist regardless of practice setting.

Pharmacy Practice Standards

The scope of pharmacy practice is established in each state through laws and regulations promulgated generally by the Board of Pharmacy. Together with Federal laws pertaining to pharmacy activities, they constitute the basis for the legal practice of pharmacy.

Over the years, various professional associations in pharmacy have jointly or separately developed documents termed *standards of practice.* One such document, "Practice Standards of the American Society of Hospital Pharmacists," is updated and published annually.[9] In 1991, the American Pharmaceutical Association (APhA), the American Association of Colleges of Pharmacy (AACP), and the National Association of Boards of Pharmacy (NABP) engaged a study of the *scope of pharmacy practice* to revalidate the *Standards of Practice for the Profession of Pharmacy* (which were published in 1979 and updated in 1986 as *Competency Statements for Pharmacy Practice*[10]). They can be summarized as follows.

General Management and Administration of the Pharmacy: Selects and supervises pharmacists and non-professionals for pharmacy staff; establishes a pricing structure for pharmaceutical services and products; administers budgets and negotiates with vendors; develops and maintains a purchasing and inventory system for all drugs and pharmaceutical supplies; initiates a formulary system. In general, establishes and administers pharmacy management, personnel and fiscal policy.

Activities Related to Processing the Prescription: Verifies prescription for legality, and physical and chemical compatibility; checks patient record before dispensing prescription; measures quantities needed to dispense prescription; performs final check of finished prescription; dispenses prescription.

Patient Care Functions: Clarifies patient's understanding of dosage; integrates drug-related with patient-related information; advises patient of potential drug-related conditions; refers patient to other health care resources; monitors and evaluates therapeutic response of patient; reviews and/or seeks additional drug-related information.

Education of Health Care Professionals and Patients: Organizes, maintains and provides drug information to other health care professionals; organizes and/or participates in "in pharmacy" education programs for other pharmacists; makes recommendations regarding drug therapy to physician or patient; develops and maintains system for drug distributions and quality control.

Each of the areas of responsibility were further broken down in the document with specific tasks reflecting the desired standards of practice.

The works referred to capture the contemporary aspects of the professional practice of pharmacy. By definition, a profession is founded upon an art, built upon specialized intellectual training, and has as its primary objective the performing of a service. The principles upon which the professional practice of pharmacy is based are embodied in the Code of Ethics of the American Pharmaceutical Association.

Omnibus Budget Reconciliation Act of 1990

Included in the Omnibus Budget Reconciliation Act of 1990 (OBRA 90) was the requirement for the establishment of state drug use review (DUR) programs to improve the quality of pharmaceutical care provided to patients covered by the Federal medical assistance (Medicaid) program.[11,12] The OBRA regulations, first implemented in 1993, provide for retrospective and prospective drug review, the development and application of quality drug use standards, and appropriate educational programs. The program is designed to ensure that prescriptions are appropriate, medically necessary, and not likely to result in adverse medical effects. The statute requires that each state's plan provide for a review of drug therapy before each prescription is filled and delivered to an eligible patient. Certain patient care environments, such as nursing home facilities, are exempt from this requirement.

The regulations require *patient medication monitoring* for therapeutic appropriateness, therapeutic duplication, overutilization, underutilization, drug-disease contraindications, drug-drug interactions with other prescribed and over-the-counter medications, drug-allergy interactions, correct drug dosage and duration of treatment, and clinical abuse or misuse. They also require that pharmacists offer *therapeutic counseling* to each recipient of a prescription, or the recipient's caregiver, regarding the drug, dosage and duration of use, route of administration, side effects, contraindications, techniques for self-monitoring drug therapy, proper storage, refill information, and action to be taken in the event of a missed dose. Pharmacists are to maintain patient medication profiles and therapeutic counseling records.

In designing the DUR programs, state boards of pharmacy have commonly included the Federal requirements in the state's pharmacy practice regulations, thereby applying them to each recipient of a prescription—not only to patients receiving benefits under the Medicaid program.

*Code of Ethics for Pharmacists—American Pharmaceutical Association**

The Code of Ethics for Pharmacists of the American Pharmaceutical Association has been revised over the years to reflect dynamic changes in the profession. The current version, revised in 1994, is as follows.[7]

Preamble

Pharmacists are health professionals who assist individuals in making the best use of medications. This Code, prepared and supported by pharmacists, is intended to state publicly the principles that form the fundamental basis of the roles and responsibilities of pharmacists. These principles, based on moral obligations and virtues, are established to guide pharmacists in relationships with patients, health professionals, and society.

I. A pharmacist respects the covenantal relationship between the patient and pharmacist.

Considering the patient-pharmacist relationship as a covenant means that a pharmacist has moral obligations in response to the gift of trust

* Copyright by the American Pharmaceutical Association. Reprinted with permission of the American Pharmaceutical Association.

received from society. In return for this gift, a pharmacist promises to help individuals achieve optimum benefit from their medications, to be committed to their welfare, and to maintain their trust.

II. A pharmacist promotes the good of every patient in a caring, compassionate, and confidential manner.

A pharmacist places concern for the well-being of the patient at the center of professional practice. In doing so, a pharmacist considers needs stated by the patient as well as those defined by health science. A pharmacist is dedicated to protecting the dignity of the patient. With a caring attitude and a compassionate spirit, a pharmacist focuses on serving the patient in a private and confidential manner.

III. A pharmacist respects the autonomy and dignity of each patient.

A pharmacist promotes the right of self-determination and recognizes individual self-worth by encouraging patients to participate in decisions about their health. A pharmacist communicates with patients in terms that are understandable. In all cases, a pharmacist respects personal and cultural differences among patients.

IV. A pharmacist acts with honesty and integrity in professional relationships.

A pharmacist has a duty to tell the truth and to act with conviction of conscience. A pharmacist avoids discriminatory practices, behavior or work conditions that impair professional judgment, and actions that compromise dedication to the best interests of patients.

V. A pharmacist maintains professional competence.

A pharmacist has a duty to maintain knowledge and abilities as new medications, devices, and technologies become available and as health information advances.

VI. A pharmacist respects the values and abilities of colleagues and other health professionals.

When appropriate, a pharmacist asks for the consultation of colleagues or other health professionals or refers the patient. A pharmacist acknowledges that colleagues and other health professionals may differ in the beliefs and values they apply to the care of the patient.

VII. A pharmacist serves individual, community, and societal needs.

The primary obligation of a pharmacist is to individual patients. However, the obligations of a pharmacist may at times extend beyond the individual to the community and society. In these situations, the pharmacist recognizes the responsibilities that accompany these obligations and acts accordingly.

VIII. A pharmacist seeks justice in the distribution of health resources.

When health resources are allocated, a pharmacist is fair and equitable, balancing the needs of patients and society.

Code of Ethics—American Association of Pharmaceutical Scientists

Like pharmacy practitioners, pharmaceutical scientists recognize their special obligation to society and to the public welfare. Members of the American Association of Pharmaceutical Scientists (AAPS) adopted the following Code of Ethics in 1991.[13]

In their scientific pursuits, they:

- Conduct their work in a manner that adheres to the highest principles of scientific research so as to merit the confidence and trust of peers and the public in particular regarding the rights of human subjects and concern for the proper use of animals involved and provision for suitable safeguards against environmental damage.
- Avoid scientific misconduct and expose and condemn it when recognized. This includes: knowingly misrepresenting data, experimental procedures or data analysis; plagiarism, improper inclusion or exclusion of authors and willful exclusion of acknowledgments for previous contributions.
- Recognize latitude for differences of scientific opinion in the interpretation of scientific data and that such differences of opinion do not constitute unethical conduct.
- Disclose sources of external financial support for, or significant financial interests in the content of, research reports/publications and avoid the manipulation of the release of such information for illegal financial gain.
- Report results accurately, stating explicitly any known or suspected bias, opposing efforts to improperly modify data or conclusions and offering professional advice only on those subjects concerning which they themselves regard themselves competent through scientific education, training, or experience.
- Respect the known ownership rights of others in scientific research and seek prior authorization from the owner before disclosure or use

of such information including the contents of manuscripts submitted for pre-publication review.

- Support in their research and among their employers the participation and employment of all qualified persons regardless of race, gender, creed, or national origin.

References

1. History of the Pharmacopeia of the United States, in *United States Pharmacopeia,* 23rd revision, Rockville, MD, United States Pharmacopeial Convention, Inc., 1995.
2. History of National Formulary, in *National Formulary,* 18th edition, Rockville, MD, United States Pharmacopeial Convention, Inc., 1995.
3. United States Pharmacopeial Convention, Inc., Rockville, MD.
4. Conditions Under Which Homeopathic Drugs May be Marketed, in *National Pharmacy Compliance News, 10:*2, 1989, National Association of Boards of Pharmacy Foundation, Inc., Park Ridge, IL.
5. The Thalidomide Tragedy—25 Years Ago. *FDA Consumer, 21 (1):*14–17, 1987.
6. *Am. J. Hosp. Pharm. 44:*1142–1144, 1987.
7. American Pharmaceutical Association, Washington, DC.
8. Hepler, C.D. and Strand, L.M.: Opportunities and Responsibilities in Pharmaceutical Care. *Am. J. Pharm. Ed. 53:*7S–15S, 1989.
9. American Society of Hospital Pharmacists, Bethesda, MD.
10. Pancorbo, S.A., Campagna, K.D., Davenport, J.K., Garnett, W.R., and Littlefield, L.C.: Task Force Report of Competency Statements for Pharmacy Practice. *Am. J. Pharm. Ed., 51:*196–206, 1987.
11. Medicaid Program: Drug Use Review Program and Electronic Claims Management System for Outpatient Drug Claims. Health Care Financing Administration, Department of Health and Human Services, *Federal Register 57 (212):*49397–49412, November 2, 1992.
12. Brushwood, D.B., Catizone, C.A., and Coster, J. M.: OBRA 90: What it Means to Your Practice. *U.S. Pharmacist 17:*64–73, 1992.
13. American Association of Pharmaceutical Scientists, Alexandria, VA.

2

New Drug Development and Approval Process

THE FEDERAL Food, Drug, and Cosmetic Act, as regulated through Title 21 of the U.S. Code of Federal Regulations,[1] requires a new drug to be approved by the Food and Drug Administration (FDA) before it may be legally introduced in interstate commerce. The regulations apply to drug products manufactured domestically as well as those imported into the United States.

In order to gain approval for marketing, a drug's sponsor (as a pharmaceutical company) must demonstrate, through supporting scientific evidence, that the new drug/drug product is safe and effective for its proposed use. The sponsor must also demonstrate that the various processes and controls utilized in producing the drug substance and in manufacturing, packaging, and labeling the drug product are properly controlled and validated, to ensure the production of a product that meets established standards of quality.

The process and time-course from drug discovery to approval for marketing can be lengthy and tedious, but are well defined and understood within the pharmaceutical industry. A schematic representation of the process for new drug development is shown in Figure 2–1 and the usual time-course is depicted in Figure 2–2. Following the discovery (e.g., synthesis) of a proposed new drug, the agent is biologically characterized for pharmacologic and toxicologic effects and for potential therapeutic application. Preformulation studies are initiated to define the physical and chemical properties of the agent. Formulation studies follow, to develop the initial features of the proposed pharmaceutical product or dosage form. To obtain the required evidence that will demonstrate the drug's safety and effectiveness for its proposed use, a carefully designed and progressive sequence of preclinical (e.g., animal) and clinical (human) studies are undertaken.

Only when the requisite series of preclinical studies demonstrate adequate safety and the new agent shows promise as a useful drug will the drug's sponsor file an Investigational New Drug Application (IND), seeking the FDA's allowance of initial testing in humans. If, in these initial human studies, termed *Phase 1*, the drug demonstrates acceptable levels of toxicity, progressive human trials through Phases 2 and 3 are undertaken to assess both safety and efficacy. As the clinical trials progress, laboratory work continues toward defining the agent's basic and clinical pharmacology and toxicology, product design and development, manufacturing scale-up and process controls, analytical methods development, proposed labeling and package design, and initial plans for marketing. At the completion of the carefully designed preclinical and clinical studies, the drug's sponsor may complete and file a New Drug Application (NDA).

Permission to market a drug product occurs at the time of the FDA's approval of the NDA, indicating that the body of scientific evidence submitted demonstrates that the drug/drug product is safe and effective for the proposed clinical indications; that there is adequate assurance of its proper manufacture and control; and that the final labeling accurately presents the necessary information, guidelines, and conditions for its proper use.

A product's approved labeling, represented by the package insert, is a demonstration of the entire drug development process, since by regulation it contains a summary of the essential chemistry, pharmacology, toxicology, indications and contraindications for use, adverse effects, formulation composition, dosage, and storage requirements, as ascertained during the research and development process.

In addition to the new drug approval process described above, alternative regulations apply in certain instances. For example, certain new drugs designed to treat serious or life-threaten-

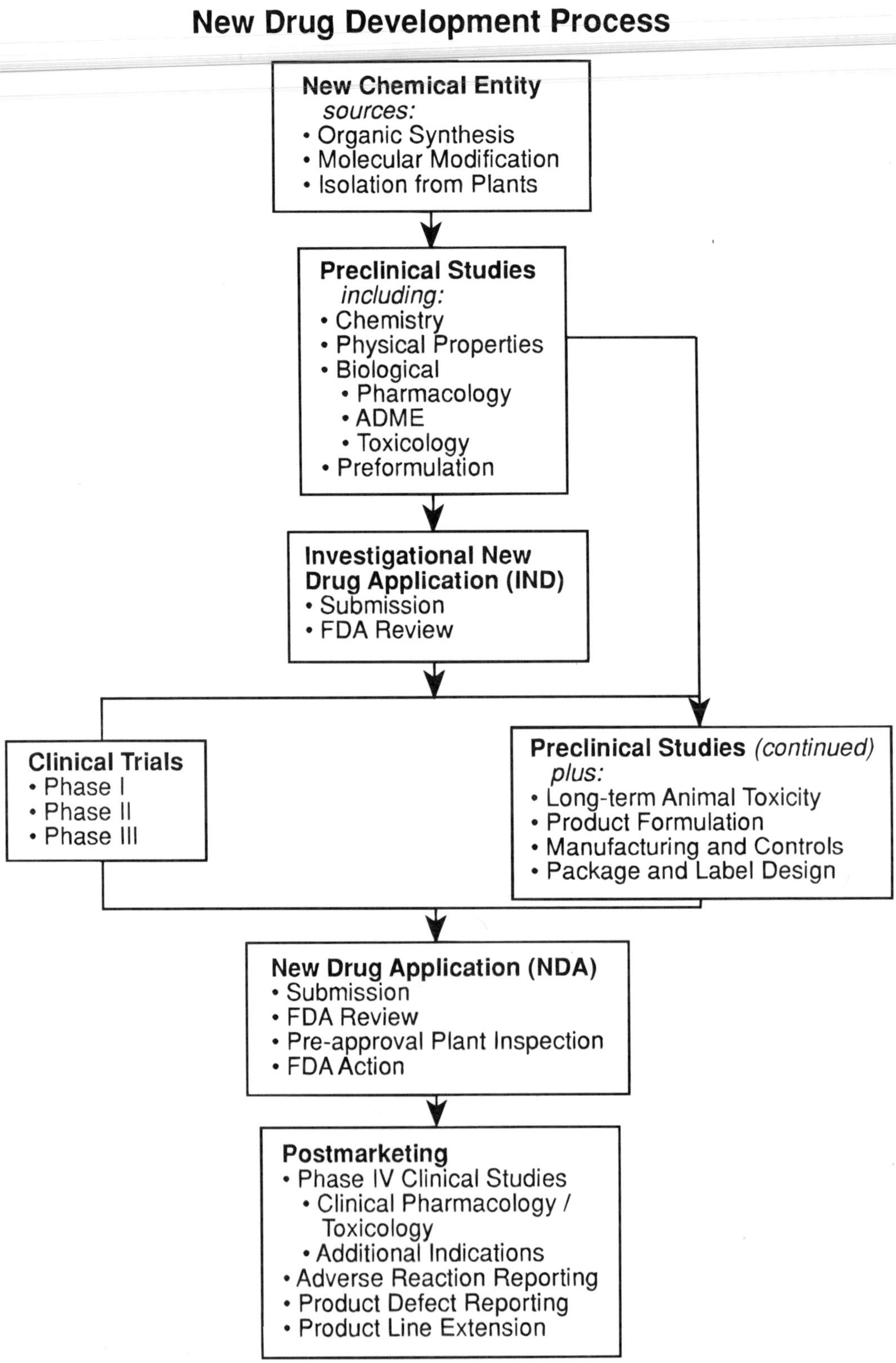

Fig. 2–1. *Schematic representation of the new drug development process, from drug discovery, through preclinical and clinical studies, FDA review of the new drug application, and postmarketing activities.*

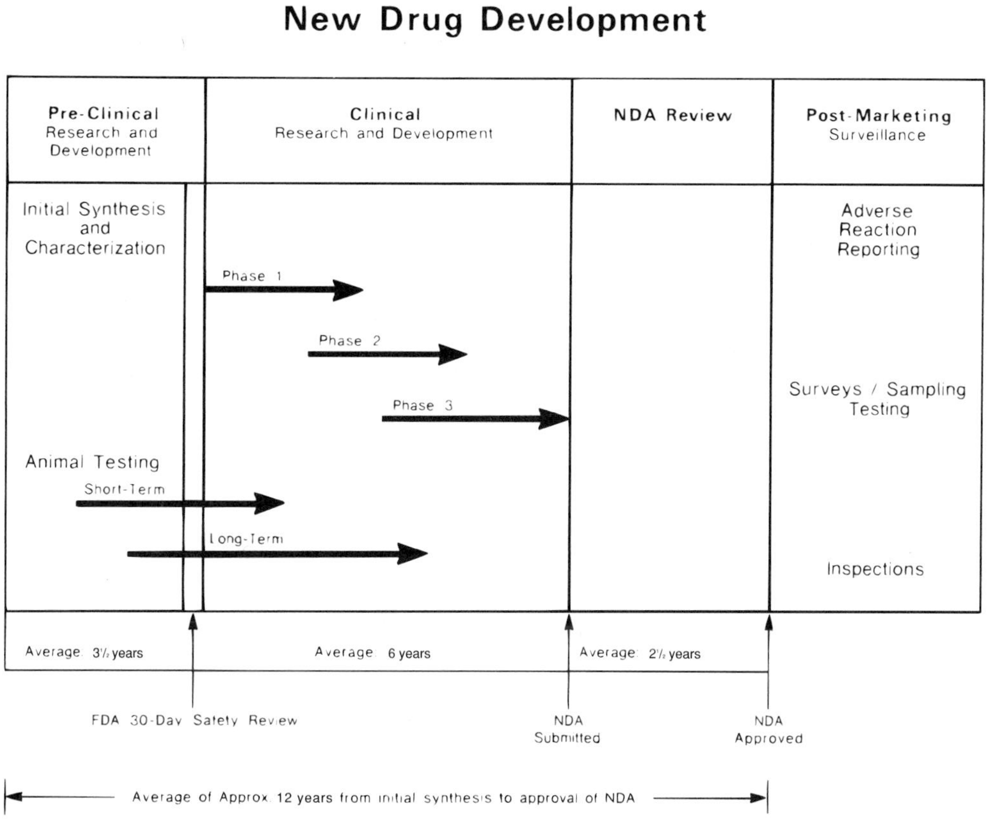

Fig. 2–2. *Time course for the development of a new drug. (Adapted from FDA Consumer, 21:5, 1987.)*

ing illnesses for which there are no satisfactory approved-drug alternatives may be placed on an accelerated program for approval, with special protocols issued for use of the drug in some patients prior to general marketing. Similarly, the early use of drugs may be approved for "orphan drugs," which are targeted for small numbers of patients who have rare conditions or diseases for which there are no satisfactory alternative treatments.

For certain changes in a previously approved NDA, such as a labeling or formulation change, a manufacturer is required to submit for approval a Supplemental New Drug Application (SNDA). An Abbreviated New Drug Application (ANDA) may be utilized by manufacturers to gain approval to market a duplicate product (usually a competing product) to one that had been approved previously and marketed by the pioneer, or original sponsor, of the drug. In these instances, nonclinical laboratory studies and reports of clinical investigations (undertaken by the pioneer sponsor) generally need not be repeated, except for bioavailability studies of the proposed product to demonstrate biologic equivalency to the original product[2] (discussed in Chapter 3).

Federal regulations are also varied for antibiotic drugs[3]; for biologics, such as human blood products and vaccines, which require approval of a Product Licensing Application (PLA) for product distribution[4]; for over-the-counter (OTC) drugs[5]; and for animal drugs, which may require a New Animal Drug Application (NADA) or a Supplemental New Animal Drug Application (SNADA).[6] Medical devices, such as catheters and cardiac pacemakers, follow a separate premarket approval process as defined in the *Code of Federal Regulations.*[7]

The following sections are intended to serve as an overview of the new drug development and approval process. More specific and detailed information may be obtained directly from the referenced *Code of Federal Regulations* Titles,[1–7] from relevant entries in the *Federal Register*,[8] and from other treatises on the topic.[9–13]

Drug Discovery and Drug Design

The discovery of new drugs and their development into commercial products takes place across the broad scope of the pharmaceutical industry. The basic underpinning for this effort is the cumulative body of scientific and biomedical information generated worldwide in research institutes, academic centers, and industry. The combined efforts of chemists, biologists, pharmacologists, toxicologists, statisticians, clinicians, pharmacists and pharmaceutical scientists, engineers, and many others are involved in the drug discovery and development process.

Some pharmaceutical firms focus their research-and-development activities on new prescription drugs for human use, whereas other firms concentrate on the development of over-the-counter medications, generic drugs, biotechnology products, animal health-care drugs, diagnostic products, and/or medical devices. Many of the large pharmaceutical companies develop and manufacture products of various types, with some firms having subsidiary companies for specialized functions and products.

The pharmaceutical industry in the United States grew phenomenally during World War II and in the years immediately following. The upsurge in the domestic production of drugs and pharmaceutical products stemmed in part from the wartime hazards and consequent undependability of overseas shipping, the unavailability of drugs from former sources in the enemy camp or control, and the increased need for drugs of all kinds, especially those of life-saving capabilities. One such drug is penicillin, which became commercially available in 1944, some 15 years after serendipitous discovery in England by Sir Alexander Fleming. The delay in the development of penicillin was in part due to a poor appreciation for its potential, and thus for many years it was not investigated with the required vigor.

After the war, other antibiotics were developed and today there is a host of them, some effective against limited types of microorganisms with others having a broad range of activity against pathogens. The postwar boom in drug discovery continued and has provided many drugs important to the conquest of disease. Vaccines, such as those effective in preventing poliomyelitis, measles, and influenza, have been as beneficial to mankind in preventing disease as have the antibiotic drugs in curing disease. New pharmacologic categories of drugs were developed in this period, including oral hypoglycemic drugs effective against certain types of diabetes mellitus, antineoplastic drugs active against the cancerous process, immunosuppressive agents which assist the body's acceptance of organ transplants, oral contraceptives, which prevent pregnancy, and a host of tranquilizers and antidepressant drugs that provide assistance to the emotionally distraught or distressed.

In recent years, many new and important innovative pharmacologic agents have been developed and approved by the FDA, including drugs to treat: acquired immunodeficiency syndrome, AIDS (zidovudine, Retrovir); refractory benign prostatic hyperplasia (finasteride, Proscar); migraine headaches (sumatriptan, Imitrex); ovarian carcinoma (paclitaxel, Taxol); gastric ulcers (H_2 receptor antagonist cimetidine, Tagamet); hyperlipidemia (gemfibrozil, Lopid); hypertension (calcium channel-blocking agent diltiazem, Cardizem; angiotensin-converting enzyme (ACE) inhibitor captopril, Capoten); arthritis (nonsteroidal antiinflammatory agent (NSAIA) nedocromil, Tilade); and many other therapeutic categories and agents. Each year, approximately thirty new molecular entities (NME) receive FDA approval for marketing. In addition, many new formulations of older drugs, generic drugs, and new biologics are also approved.

Not all drugs are discovered, developed, and first approved for marketing in the United States. In fact, many drugs originate in other countries. It is important to recognize that there are many domestic and foreign pharmaceutical companies involved in drug research and development. Many of the world's largest pharmaceutical companies are multinational and have facilities for research and development, regulatory affairs, manufacturing, and distribution in countries around the world. Without regard to country of origin, a drug may be proposed by its sponsor for regulatory approval for marketing in the United States and in other countries. These approvals do not occur simultaneously, as they are subject to the laws, regulations, and requirements peculiar to each country's governing authority. However, there is an effort under way toward international harmonization of regulatory requirements.[14]

Sources of New Drugs

New drugs may be discovered from a variety of natural sources or created synthetically in the laboratory. They may be found quite by accident or as the result of many years of tireless pursuit.

Throughout history, plant materials have served as a reservoir of potential new drugs. Only a small portion of the plant species thus far identified have been investigated for medicinal agents. Certain major contributions to modern drug therapy may be attributed to the successful conversion of botanic folklore remedies into modern wonder drugs. The chemical reserpine, a tranquilizer and hypotensive agent, is an example of a medicinal chemical isolated by design from the folklore remedy *Rauwolfia serpentina*. Another plant drug, periwinkle or *Vinca rosea*, was scientifically investigated as a result of its reputation in folklore as an agent useful in the treatment of diabetes mellitus. Plant extractives yielded two potent drugs, which when screened for pharmacologic activity surprisingly exhibited antitumor capabilities. These two materials, vinblastine and vincristine, since have been used successfully in the treatment of certain types of cancer including acute leukemia, Hodgkin's disease, lymphocytic lymphoma, and other malignancies. The drug Taxol (paclitaxel), extracted from the Pacific yew tree *(Taxus brevifolia)*, was recently developed and approved for the treatment of ovarian cancer.

After the isolation and structural identification of active plant constituents, organic chemists may recreate them by total synthesis in the laboratory or more importantly use the natural chemical as the starting material in the creation of slightly different chemical structures through molecule manipulation procedures. The new structures, termed semisynthetic drugs, may have a slightly or vastly different pharmacologic activity than the starting substance, depending upon the nature and extent of chemical alteration. Other plant constituents which in themselves may be inactive or rather unimportant therapeutically may be employed in the semisynthetic process to yield important drugs with profound pharmacologic activity. For example, the various species of *Dioscorea*, popularly known as Mexican yams, are rich in the chemical *steroid* structure from which hormonal chemicals like cortisone and estrogens, the female sex hormones, are semisynthetically produced.

Animals have served man in his search for drugs in a number of ways. They not only have yielded to drug testing and biologic assay procedures but also have provided drugs fashioned from their own tissues or through their biologic processes. Hormonal substances such as thyroid extract, insulin, and pituitary hormone obtained from the endocrine glands of cattle, sheep, and swine are lifesaving drugs employed daily as replacement therapy in the human body. The urine of pregnant mares is a rich source of estrogens. Knowledge of the structural architecture of the individual hormonal substances has led to the production of a variety of synthetic and semisynthetic compounds with hormone-like activity. The synthetic chemicals in oral contraceptive agents are a notable example. The use of animals in the production of various biologic products, including serums, antitoxins, and vaccines, has been of lifesaving significance ever since the pioneering work of Dr. Edward Jenner on the smallpox vaccine in England in 1796. Today, the poliomyelitis vaccine is prepared in cultures of renal monkey tissue, the mumps and influenza vaccines in fluids of chick embryo, the rubella (German measles) vaccine in duck embryo and the smallpox vaccine from the skin of bovine calves inoculated with vaccinia virus. Tomorrow, vaccines for diseases as AIDS and cancer may be developed through the utilization of cell and tissue cultures.

Today we are witnessing a new era in the development of pharmaceutical products due to the advent of genetic engineering, the sub-microscopic manipulation of the "double helix," the spiral DNA chain of life. Through this process, will come more abundant and vastly purer antibiotics, vaccines, and yet unknown chemical and biological products to combat human disease.

There are two basic technologies that drive the genetic field of drug development; they are recombinant DNA (rDNA) and monoclonal antibody (MoAB) production.[15–17] Common to each technique is the ability to manipulate and produce proteins, the building blocks of living matter. Proteins represent an almost infinite source of drugs. Made up of long chains of amino acids, their sequence and spatial configuration offer a staggering number of possibilities. Both recombinant DNA and monoclonal antibody production techniques influence cells in their ability to produce proteins.

The more fundamental of the two techniques is recombinant DNA. It can potentially produce almost any protein. It is possible to transplant genetic material from higher species such as man into a lowly bacterium. This so-called "gene splicing" can induce the lower organism to make proteins it would not otherwise have made. Such drug products as human insulin, human growth hormone, hepatitis B vaccine, epoetin alpha, and interferon are being produced in this manner.

Whereas recombinant DNA techniques involve the manipulation of proteins within the cells of lower animals, monoclonal antibody production is conducted entirely within the cells of higher animals, including the patient. The technique exploits the ability of cells that have the potential to produce a desired antibody and stimulates an unending stream of pure antibody production. These antibodies then have the capacity to combat the specific target.

Monoclonal antibodies have an enormous potential to change the face of medicine and pharmacy in the next decade and applications for their use are already in progress. Diagnostically, for example, monoclonal antibodies are used in home pregnancy testing products. Their use ensures that a woman can perform the test easily, in a short period of time, with high reproducibility, and in an inexpensive manner. In these tests, the monoclonal antibody is highly sensitive to binding upon one site on the human chorionic gonadotropin (HCG) molecule, a specific marker to pregnancy because in healthy women, HCG is synthesized exclusively by the placenta. In medicine, monoclonal antibodies are being used to stage and to localize malignant cells of cancer, and it is anticipated that they will be used in the future to combat disease such as lupus erythematosus, juvenile-onset diabetes, and myasthenia gravis.

Human gene therapy, used to prevent, treat, cure, diagnose, or mitigate human disease caused by genetic disorders, represents another promising new technology. Gene therapy is a medical intervention based on the modification of the genetic material of living cells. Cells may be modified outside the body (ex vivo) for subsequent administration, or they may be modified within the body (in vivo) by gene therapy products given directly to the patient. In either case, gene therapy involves the transfer of new genetic material to the cells of a patient afflicted with a genetic disease. The genetic material, usually cloned DNA, may be transferred into the patient's cells physically, as through microinjection, through chemically mediated transfer procedures, or through disabled retroviral gene transfer systems that integrate genetic material directly into the host cell chromosomes.[18] Gene therapy is being examined for a number of genetic-based blood and immunologic diseases including sickle cell anemia, Cooley's anemia, malignant melanoma, renal cell cancer, and familial hypercholesteremia.

However, today's most usual source of potential drugs is the flask of the synthetic organic chemist. Through his art he creates not only chemical modifications of known structures but also totally new synthetic organic compounds.

A "Goal Drug"

In theory, a "goal drug" would produce the specifically desired effect, be administered by the most desired route (generally orally) at minimal dosage and dosing frequency, have optimal onset and duration of activity, exhibit no side effects, and following its desired effect would be eliminated from the body efficiently, completely, and without residual effect. It would also be easily produced at low cost, be pharmaceutically elegant, and physically and chemically stable under various conditions of use and storage. Although not completely attainable in practice, these qualities and features are sought in drug and dosage form design.

Methods of Drug Discovery

Although some drugs may be the result of fortuitous discovery, most drugs nowadays are the result of carefully designed research programs of screening, molecular modification, and mechanism-based drug design.[19]

Random or nontargeted screening involves the testing of large numbers of synthetic organic compounds or substances of natural origin for the purpose of detecting biologic activity. Random screens may be employed initially as a means to (a) detect an unknown activity of the test compound or substance, and (b) identify the most promising compounds to be studied by more sophisticated *nonrandom or targeted* screens, to determine more specific activity.

To detect and evaluate biological activity, *bioassays* are used to differentiate the effect and potency (strength of the effect) of the test agent compared to controls of known action and effect. The initial screens may be performed in vitro using cell cultures to test the new agent's effect against enzyme systems or tumor cells, whereas subsequent screens may be performed in vivo and involve more expensive and disease-specific animal model systems.

Although random and nonrandom screening programs are generally effective in examining a host of new compounds for activity, sometimes promising compounds may be overlooked if the screening models are not sensitive enough to reflect accurately the specific disease against which the agent, or its metabolites, may be useful.[20]

Molecular modification involves the chemical alteration of a known and previously characterized organic compound (frequently a *lead compound*; see the following) for the purpose of enhancing its usefulness as a drug. This could mean: enhancing its specificity for a particular body target site; increasing its potency; improving its rate and extent of absorption; modifying to advantage its time-course in the body; reducing its toxicity; or changing its physical or chemical properties (e.g., solubility) to provide pharmaceutically desired features.[19] The molecular modifications may be slight or substantial, involving changes in functional groups, ring structures, or configuration. Knowledge of chemical structure–pharmacologic activity relationships (SAR) plays an important role in designing new drug molecules. Through molecular modification, new chemical entities (NCEs) and improved therapeutic agents result. Figures 2–3A and 2–3B present the molecular modifications that led to the discoveries of the first commercial beta blocker, propranolol, and the first commercial histamine H_2-receptor blocking agent, cimetidine.

Mechanism-based drug design involves molecular modification in designing a drug that interferes specifically with the known or suspected biochemical pathway or mechanism of a disease process. The intention is the interaction of the drug with specific cell receptors, enzyme systems, or the metabolic processes of pathogens or tumor cells, resulting in a blocking, disruption, or reversal of the disease process. In designing drugs on this basis, therefore, it is essential to understand the biochemical basis of the disease process and the manner in which it is regulated. *Molecular graphics,* that is, the use of computer graphics to represent and manipulate the structure of the drug molecule to "fit" the simulated molecular structure of the receptor site, is a useful and emerging complementary tool in drug molecule design.

A "Lead Compound"

A "lead compound" is a prototype chemical compound which has a fundamental desired biologic or pharmacologic activity. Although active, the lead compound may not possess *all* of the features desired—potency, absorbability, solubility, toxicity, and so forth. Thus the medicinal chemist may seek to modify the lead compound's basic chemical structure in an effort to improve the desired features while reducing the undesired ones. The chemical modifications produce analogs having additional or different functional chemical groups, altered ring structures, or different chemical configurations. The results are modified chemical compounds capable of having different interactions with the body's receptors, thereby eliciting different actions and intensities of action.

The synthesis of derivatives of the prototype chemical may ultimately lead to successive "generations" of new compounds of the same pharmacologic type. This may be exemplified by the many modifications of the original penicillin structure to yield many new semisynthetic penicillins; the similar development of new generations of cephalosporin antibiotics; additional H_2 antagonists from the pioneer drug cimetidine, Tagamet; and the large series of antianxiety drugs derived from the benzodiazepine structure and the innovator drug chlordiazepoxide, Librium.

Most drugs exhibit secondary activities (side effects) in addition to their primary, or most desired, pharmacologic action. It is not uncommon to take advantage of a secondary activity (such as drowsiness) by developing new lead compounds for the secondary use of the drug through the molecular modification.

Overall, drug discovery includes the identification of active substances from natural sources, the creation of new drug prototype compounds, and the extension of that knowledge in developing additional and improved drug modifications. The *core team* involved in this process largely consists of chemists and biologists.

Prodrugs

Prodrug is a term used to describe a compound that requires metabolic biotransformation following administration to yield the desired pharmacologically active compound. The conversion of an inactive prodrug to an active compound may occur through nonenzymatic action as chemical hydrolysis, but occurs primarily

A **BETA-BLOCKERS**

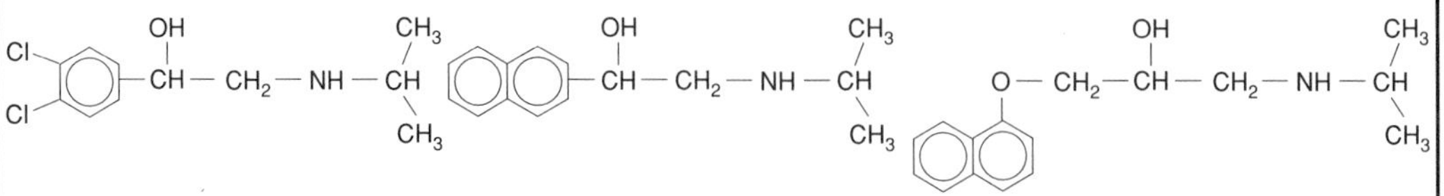

Dichloroisoproterenol 1957 → **Pronethalol 1962** → **Propranolol* 1964**

Progress leading to the first commercial beta-blocker. Dichloroisoproterenol—first compound with beta-adrenoceptor blocking action; had partial agonist (sympathomimetic) activity. Pronethalol—beta-adrenoceptor blocking agent, relatively free from sympathomimetic activity. Clinical use limited by side effects, including light-headedness, incoordination, nausea and vomiting. Propranolol—beta-adrenoceptor blocking agent, free of sympathomimetic activity, and lacking side effects of pronethalol in humans.

B **H_2 ANTAGONISTS**

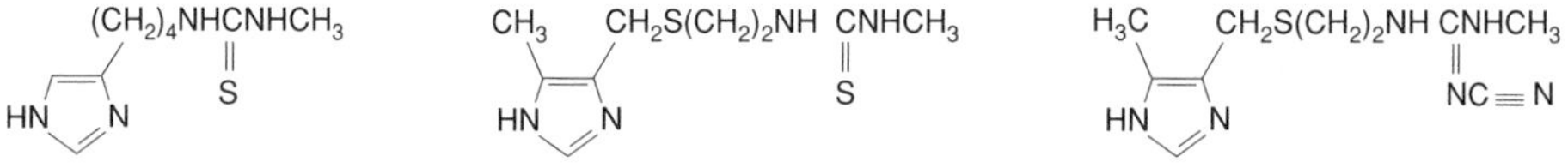

Burimamide 1972 → **Metiamide 1973** → **Cimetidine* 1975**

Progress leading to the first commercial ulcer drug. Burimamide—first histamine H_2-receptor blocking agent, poor oral availability. Metiamide—histamine H_2-receptor blocking agent, good oral bioavailability. Produced reversible agranulocytosis in some people. Cimetidine—histamine H_2-receptor blocking agent, good oral bioavailability. No agranulocytosis in man.

*Final Compound

Fig. 2–3A and B. *Molecular modifications leading to the development of the first commercial beta blocker, propranolol, and the first commercial histamine H_2-receptor blocking agent, cimetidine. (From Maxwell, R.A.: The State of the Art of the Science of Drug Discovery.* Drug. Dev. Res. *4:375–389, 1984; through "Pharmaceutical Research: Therapeutic and Economic Value of Incremental Improvements," 1990, p. 12. Courtesy of National Pharmaceutical Council, Reston, VA).*

through enzymatic biochemical cleavage. Depending upon the specific prodrug-enzyme interaction, the biotransformation may occur anywhere along the course of drug transit or at the body site where the requisite enzymes are sufficiently present.

Prodrugs may be designed preferentially for the following, and other, reasons.[19]

SOLUBILITY. A prodrug may be designed with solubility advantages over the active drug, enabling the formulation and use of specifically desired dosage forms and routes of administration. For example, if an active drug is insufficiently soluble in water to prepare a desired intravenous injection, a water-soluble prodrug could be prepared through the addition of a functional group that later would be detached by the metabolic process to yield, once again, the active drug molecule.

ABSORPTION. A drug may be made more water- or lipid-soluble, as desired, to facilitate absorption from the intended route of administration.

The prodrug would be designed most ideally if the added chemical group(s) were enzymatically removed following optimal absorption and transport to the site of action.

BIOSTABILITY. It is important that a drug reach its site of action of the desired effects. If a drug is prematurely destroyed by biochemical or enzymatic processes, the design of a prodrug may be useful in protecting the drug during transport. If, in addition, the prodrug is metabolized (to yield the active drug) by enzymes inherent at the desired site of action, the use of the prodrug could result in site-specific action of greater potency.

PROLONGED RELEASE. Depending on a prodrug's rate of metabolic conversion to active drug, it may be useful in providing prolonged drug release and extended therapeutic activity.

FDA's Definition of a New Drug[1]

The term *new drug* means any drug that has not been generally recognized, among experts qualified by scientific training and experience, as safe and effective under the conditions recommended.

A drug need not be a new chemical entity to be considered new by the Food and Drug Administration and therefore subject to the requirements for proof of safety and efficacy. A well-known chemical formulated in a new manner with different excipients, coatings, solvents, vehicles, or other formulative materials results in a pharmaceutical product that has not been examined for safety and efficacy and therefore constitutes "newness" under the law. It is well recognized that different methods of manufacture or different formulative additives can alter the therapeutic efficacy of a product through chemical or physical interference with the therapeutic agents. Thus the *reformulation* of an approved product by the originator company, or a new formulation of the same drug by another manufacturer not having previously received FDA approval to market that product, would constitute newness.

A new combination of two or more old drugs or a change in the usual proportions of drugs in an established combination product can be considered "new" if a question of safety or efficacy is introduced by the alteration. A proposed new use for an old drug, a new dosage schedule or regimen, a proposed new route of administration, or a new dosage form all cause an old drug to be reconsidered for safety and efficacy.

Drug Nomenclature

When first synthesized, or identified from a natural source, an organic compound is represented by an *empirical formula*, as $C_{14}H_{19}Cl_2NO_2$ for chlorambucil, which indicates the number and the relationship of the atoms comprising the molecule. As knowledge of the relative locations of these atoms is gained, the compound receives a *systematic chemical name*, as 4-[bis(2-chloroethyl)amino] - 4 - [*p*-[Bis(2-chloroethyl)amino]phenyl]-butyric acid. To be adequate and fully specific, the name must reveal every part of the compound's molecular structure, so that it describes only the compound concerned and no other. The systematic name is generally so formidable that it soon is replaced in scientific communication by a condensed name, which, although less descriptive chemically, is understood to refer only to that chemical compound. This new name may be the first attempt at assigning a *nonproprietary* name, or it may be a *code number*.

Today many companies give their new compounds code numbers prior to the assignment of a nonproprietary name. These code numbers generally take the form of an identifying prefix letter or letters that identify the drug's sponsor, followed by a number that further identifies the test compound (for example, SQ 14,225, the investigational code number for the drug *captopril*, initially developed by Squibb). The code number generally stays with a compound from its initial preclinical laboratory investigation through human clinical trials.

When the results of testing indicate that a compound shows sufficient promise of becoming a drug, the sponsor may propose a *nonproprietary* (or *generic*) name and may also apply to the U.S. Patent Office (and foreign agencies as well) for a *proprietary* or trademark name. Should the drug receive recognition in an official compendium, the nonproprietary name established during the period of the drug's early usage is generally adopted. It should be pointed out that nonproprietary names are issued only for single agents whereas proprietary or trademark names may be associated with a single chemical entity or with a mixture of chemicals comprising a specific proprietary product.

The task of designating appropriate nonproprietary names for chemical agents rests primarily with the United States Adopted Names Council (USAN Council). This organized effort at coining nonproprietary names for drugs was inaugurated in 1961 as a joint project of the American Medical Association and the United States Pharmacopeial Convention. They were joined in 1964 by the American Pharmaceutical Association to form the USAN Council; in 1967, the Food and Drug Administration was invited to take part in the work of the Council.

The United States Pharmacopeial Convention publishes the *USAN* and the *USP Dictionary of Drug Names*. In addition to listing the US Adopted Names, the reference also includes brand names of research-oriented firms, investigational drug code designations, official names of USP and NF articles with their chemical names and graphic formulas, and international nonproprietary names (INN) published by the World Health Organization (WHO). This reference of drug names now includes over 18,000 entries.

A proposal for a USAN usually originates from a firm or an individual who has developed a substance of potential therapeutic usefulness to the point where there is a distinct possibility of its being marketed in the United States. Occasionally, the initiative is taken by the USAN Council in the form of a request to parties interested in a substance for which a nonproprietary name appears to be lacking. Proposals are expected to conform to the Council's guidelines for coining nonproprietary names. In general, the name should (1) be short and distinctive in sound and spelling and not be such that it is easily confused with existing names, (2) indicate the general pharmacologic or therapeutic class into which the substance falls or the general chemical nature of the substance if the latter is associated with the specific pharmacologic activity, (3) embody the syllable or syllables characteristic of a related group of compounds.

When general agreement on a name has been reached between the Council and the drug's sponsor, it is announced as a "Proposed USAN." This indicates the Council's intention to adopt the name and serves notice on those who wish to protest the selection. The tentatively adopted USAN is then submitted for consideration by various American and foreign drug regulatory agencies, including the World Health Organization, the British Pharmacopoeia Commission, the French Codex, the Nordic Pharmacopeia, the United States Pharmacopeia and National Formulary, and the U.S. Food and Drug Administration. Under the 1962 Drug Amendments, the Secretary of the Department of Health and Human Services has authority to designate the nonproprietary name for any drug in the interest of usefulness or simplicity. The authority is generally delegated to the Commissioner of the Food and Drug Administration within the Department. If no objections are raised, adoption is considered final, and the USAN is published in the various literature of the medical and pharmaceutical professions. With the creation of the USAN Council and the cooperation of the interested parties on a worldwide basis, nonproprietary drug nomenclature has been standardized.

Biological Characterization

Prospective drug substances must undergo preclinical testing for biologic activity in order to assess their potential as useful therapeutic agents. These studies fall into the general areas of pharmacology, drug metabolism, and toxicology, and involve many types of biologic scientists including general biologists, microbiologists, molecular biologists, biochemists, geneticists, pharmacologists, physiologists, pharmacokineticists, pathologists, toxicologists, statisticians, and others. Their work leads to the determination of whether a chemical agent possesses adequate features of safety and sufficient promise of usefulness to pursue as a prospective new drug.

To judge whether a drug is safe and effective, information must be gained on how it is absorbed, distributed throughout the body, stored, metabolized, and excreted, and how it affects the action of the body's cells, tissues, and organs. Scientists have developed studies that may be conducted outside the living body (in vitro), by using cell and tissue culture and computer programs that stimulate human and animal systems. Cell cultures are being used increasingly to screen for toxicity before progressing to whole-animal testing. Computer models help to predict the properties of substances and their probable actions in living systems. Although these nonanimal systems have reduced dependence on the use of animals in drug studies, they have not completely replaced the need to study drugs in whole animals as a safeguard prior to their administration to humans.

Pharmacology

In its broad definition, *pharmacology* embraces the physical and chemical properties, biochemical and physiological effects, mechanisms of action, absorption, distribution, biotransformation and excretion, and therapeutic and other uses of drugs.[21] From this basic field of study come such subareas as *pharmacodynamics,* which is the study of the biochemical and physiological effects of drugs and their mechanisms of action; *pharmacokinetics,* which deals with the absorption, distribution, metabolism or biotransformation, and excretion (ADME) of drugs; and *clinical pharmacology,* which applies pharmacologic principles to the study of the effects and actions of drugs in humans.

Different drug substances, because of their unique chemical structures, exert their own individual effects on the biological system. In general, drugs exert their effects by one of the following means: (1) through physical action, as the protective effects of ointments upon topical application; (2) by reacting chemically, as antacids that reduce excess gastric acidity; (3) by modifying the metabolic activity of invading pathogens, as antibiotics, or (4) by modifying the biochemical or metabolic process of the body's cells or enzyme systems to change the course of a disease process.

Today's emphasis in the development of new drugs is on the fourth method—that is, on the design of drug molecules capable of interfering with a particular disease process. Although we do not understand the action precisely for every disease, it is generally known that most diseases arise from an endogenous biochemical imbalance, an abnormal and aberrant proliferation of cells, or an exogenous chemical toxin or invasive pathogen. An understanding of the cause of a particular disease or illness can provide the basis for the development of agents effective against it.

The processes of life and metabolism within the body's cells involve intricate enzymatic reactions. Each component of these complex enzyme systems is vital to the normal functioning of the cell. Drug agents that interact with enzyme systems may affect the course of a disease arising from *abnormal* enzymatic function. Enzymes are protein substances that catalyze specific reactions in biologic systems, transforming substrates into metabolic products. A drug that is an enzyme inhibitor reduces or blocks the enzyme's action. Understanding of the role of enzymes in the process of certain diseases can therefore lead to the design of new drug agents that have the capacity to interfere with the course of the disease process. For example, the drug *captopril,* an antihypertensive agent, was designed to interact with a specific enzyme system. The drug binds to the angiotensin-converting enzyme (ACE) as a specific competitive inhibitor, preventing conversion of angiotensin I to angiotensin II, and thereby reducing the formation of a substance that has the capacity to constrict blood vessels and elevate blood pressure. Captopril is the lead drug in a growing class of ACE inhibitors. In the case of excessive cell growth (a tumor), inhibition of an essential enzyme or enzyme system can interfere with the metabolic process required for cell replication and tumor growth.

The action of most drugs takes place at the molecular level with the drug molecules interacting with the molecules of the cell structure or its contents.

The selectivity and specificity of drugs for a certain body tissue—for example, drugs that act primarily on the nerves, heart, or kidney—are related to specific sites on or within the cells, receptive only to chemicals of a particular chemical structure and configuration. This is the basis for *structure-activity relationships (SAR)* defined for drugs and for families of drugs within therapeutic categories. As noted earlier, the synthesis of analogs of a lead compound is undertaken primarily to create compounds that, through their structural modification, are more specific, more potent, and present fewer side effects than the lead compound, while retaining the basic structure-activity relationship. Studies of the pharmacologic activities of a series of analogs having varied functional groups and side chains can be useful in revealing the most specific structure for a given drug-cell or drug-enzyme interaction.

The cellular component directly involved in the action of a drug is termed its *receptor.* The chemical groups that participate in the drug-receptor combination and the adjacent portions of the receptor that favor or hinder access of the drug to these active groups are known as *receptor groups* or *receptor sites* (Fig. 2–4).

Although receptors for most drugs have yet to be identified, they, like the active centers of enzymes, are thought to be carboxyl, amino, sulfhydryl, phosphate, and similar reactive groups oriented on or in the cell in a pattern complementary to that of the drugs with which they react. The binding of a drug to the receptor is thought to be accomplished mainly by ionic, covalent, and other relatively weak reversible bonds. Occasionally, firm covalent bonding is involved, and the drug effect is then very slowly reversible.

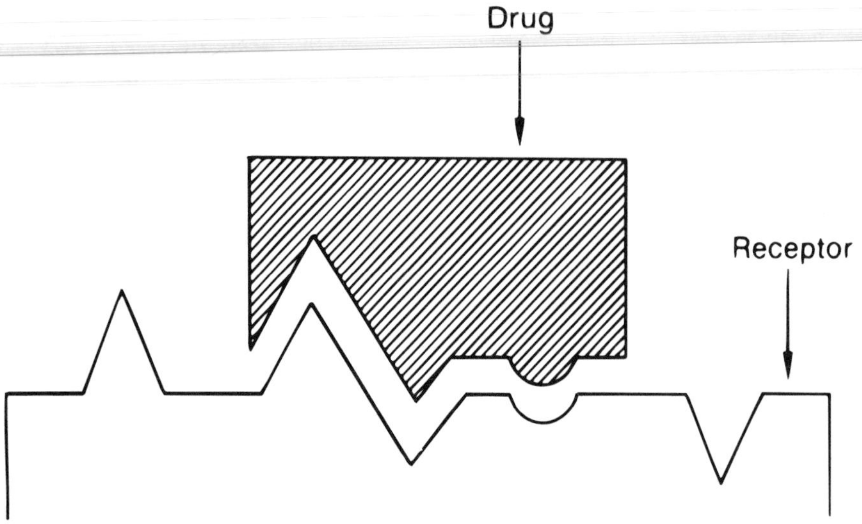

Fig. 2–4. *Schematic drawing of receptor site and substrate (drug). (From "How Modern Medicines are Discovered," Frank H. Clark, Ed., Courtesy of Futura Publishing Company, Inc.)*

There is a relationship between the quantity of drug molecules *available* for interaction and the *capacity* of the specific receptor site. For instance, following a dose of drug and its transit to the site of action, the cell's receptors may or may not become fully saturated with interacting drug. When the receptors are saturated, the effects of the specific interaction are maximized. Any additional drug present and not participating in the interaction may serve as a reservoir to replace drug molecules that become released from the complex. Two drugs, when present in a biologic system, may *compete* for the same binding sites, with the drug having the stronger bonding attraction for the site generally prevailing. Already-bound molecules of the more weakly bound drug may be replaced from the binding site and left free in the circulation as unbound drug.

Certain cells within the body are capable of binding drugs without eliciting a drug effect. These cells act as *carriers* and are important in drug transport to active sites or to sites of their biotransformation and elimination.

Because receptor sites bind chemicals with specific chemical groupings and orientation, many chemicals that are but slight modifications of a parent compound possess the same pharmacologic effect. Thus, based on the knowledge of the receptor size, shape, stereospecificity and arrangements of reactive groups, a drug can be redesigned to improve specificity and selectivity. The process of designing chemical structures to interact most effectively with receptors and enzymes has been enhanced in recent years through the use of *molecular graphics* techniques, using computer graphics to represent and manipulate molecular structures to "fit" receptor sites and enzymes.[19,20] The method is not a replacement for the other methods of drug discovery and design, but is complementary to them.

A prime example of a drug discovered through rational drug design is the antiulcer drug cimetidine, Tagamet. Through bioassay it was discovered that histamine stimulates acid secretion. This knowledge led to the discovery that histamine binds to two receptors: H_1, which evokes allergic and hypersensitivity reactions; and H_2, which stimulates acid secretion. Antihistamine drugs were well known to block or antagonize the H_1 receptor activity, but not the H_2 activity. After much research and the synthesis and testing of over 200 compounds, the first effective H_2 antagonist, cimetidine, was developed.[19]

The process of evaluating chemical compounds for biologic activity and the determination of their mechanisms of action is the responsibility of the pharmacologist. In vitro cultures of cells and enzymes systems, and in vivo animal models are utilized in defining a chemical's *pharmacologic profile.*

To define a pharmacologic profile, pharmacologists progress stepwise through increasingly sophisticated levels of evaluation, based on the test compound's success in prior studies. Whole-animal studies are generally reserved for test compounds that have demonstrated reasonable potential as a drug candidate.

Among the early studies undertaken are the determination of a compound's selectivity for various receptor sites and its activity against select enzyme systems, based on the molecular design and reasoned structure-activity relationship of the compound. Studies of cell function are then performed to detect evidence of efficacy and determine whether the compound is an agonist or antagonist. These are followed by studies with isolated tissues to define further the compound's activity and selectivity. Whole-animal studies are employed to evaluate the pharmacologic effects of the agent on specific organ systems, and against animal models of human disease for which the compound is considered a drug candidate.

The majority of animal testing is done initially utilizing small animals, usually rodents (mouse, rat) for a number of reasons including cost, availability, the small amount of drug required for study, the ease of administration by various routes (oral, inhalation, intravenous), and experience with drug testing in these species. However, in final pharmacologic and toxicologic development studies, two or more animal species generally are required, including a rodent and a nonrodent.

The primary objective of the animal studies is to obtain basic information on the drug's effects that may be used to predict safe and effective use in humans. This is a difficult task because of species variation and the fact that animals are not absolute predictors of human response. However, a number of animal models have been developed to mimic certain human diseases, and these are used effectively. For instance, there are animal models for type I diabetes and hypertension, using genetically diabetic and hypertensive animals, respectively, and for tumor growth, using tumor transplants into various species. Certain animal species have been determined to be best for certain studies of organ systems, or as disease models, including: the dog and rat for hypertension; the dog and guinea pig for respiratory effects; the dog for diuretic activity; the rabbit for blood coagulation; and the mouse and rat for central nervous system studies.[22,23] Unfortunately, useful animal models are not available for every human disease. Drugs are studied in the test animals at various dose levels to determine effect, potency, and safety.

As a drug candidate progresses in its preclinical pharmacologic evaluation, drug metabolism and toxicity tests are initiated.

Drug Metabolism

A series of animal studies of a proposed drug's absorption, distribution, metabolism, and elimination (ADME) are undertaken to determine: (1) the *extent* and *rate* of drug absorption following various routes of administration, including the one intended for human use; (2) the rate of distribution of the drug through the body, and the site(s) and duration of the drug's residence while in the body; (3) the rate, primary and secondary sites, and mechanism of the drug's metabolism in the body, and the chemistry and pharmacology of any metabolites; and (4) the proportion of administered dose eliminated from the body, and its rate and route of elimination. In these studies, a minimum of two animal species are employed (generally the same as used in the pharmacologic and toxicologic studies), a rodent and a nonrodent, usually a dog.

The biochemical transformation or metabolism of drug substances is the body's means of transforming nonpolar drug molecules into polar compounds that are more readily eliminated. Specific and nonspecific enzymes participate in drug metabolism, primarily in the liver, but also in the kidneys, lung, and gastrointestinal tract. Drugs that enter the hepatic circulation following absorption from the gut, as after oral administration, are particularly exposed to rapid drug metabolism. This transit through the liver and exposure to the hepatic enzyme system is termed the *first pass effect.* If especially undesirable, the first-pass effect may be avoided by other routes of administration (buccal, rectal) that allow the drug to be absorbed into the systemic circulation through blood vessels other than hepatic.

Drug metabolism or biotransformation results in the production of one or more metabolites of the administered drug, some of which may be pharmacologically active compounds, others not. As noted previously, drug metabolism may be essential to convert prodrugs to active compounds. For reasons of drug safety, it is important to determine whether a drug's metabolic products are toxic or nontoxic to the animal—and later, the human. When metabolites are found, they are chemically and biologically characterized for activity and toxicity. Some new drugs have been discovered as metabolic byproducts or metabolites of parent compounds.

ADME studies are performed in a highly quantitative fashion through the timely collection and analysis of urine, blood, and feces samples, and through a careful examination of tissues and organs upon autopsy. In addition, special studies are undertaken to determine: the presence, if any, of a test drug or its metabolites in the milk of lactating animals; the ability of the drug to cross the placental barrier and enter the fetal blood supply; and the long-term retention of drug or metabolites in the body. In studying the formation and disposition of metabolites, a radioactive label is commonly incorporated into the parent compound prior to administration and traced in the animal's waste products and tissues.

Refer to the next chapter for additional material on drug absorption, distribution, metabolism, and elimination as they relate to drug product development.

Toxicology

Toxicology is the area of pharmacology that deals with the adverse, or undesired, effects of drugs.[21] In the development of a new drug, the ability to predict with reasonable assurance its safe use in humans is essential. However, the extrapolation of preclinical animal safety data to humans is not certain, because of species variation, different dose-response relationships, immunologic differences, subjective reactions nondeducible in animals (such as headache), and other reasons.[23] Although many adverse reactions that occur in humans cannot be predicted through animal studies, the more animal species that demonstrate a toxic effect, the greater the likelihood the effect will also be seen in humans.

No chemical or drug can be deemed entirely safe. All drugs carry some risk and should be taken with a clear understanding of the benefits weighed against the possible risks. Safety is only relative, and is based on a drug's proper and appropriate use, with the understanding that a definable portion of the population may experience adverse effects ranging from relatively minor to serious, even fatal, as a result of a drug's inherent action, patient idiosyncrasy, or drug allergy.

In drug development programs, *initial* toxicology studies are conducted on rodents for the reasons stated previously for pharmacology studies. Following successful initial testing, a nonrodent species, usually a dog, is added to the testing program to develop the requisite toxicology profile. The toxicology profile includes acute or short-term toxicity; subacute or subchronic toxicity; chronic toxicity; carcinogenicity testing; reproduction studies; and mutagenicity screening.[9,24] Figure 2–1 showed that short-term and long-term toxicity studies span the entire program of drug development, from preclinical studies through clinical trials, and continue during the market life of a drug product as a part of postmarketing surveillance.

Acute or *short-term* toxicity studies are designed to determine the toxic effects of a test compound when administered in a single dose and/or in multiple doses over a short period of time, generally a single day. Although various routes of administration may be used (such as lavage dosing via gastric tube), the studies must represent the intended route for human use. The test compound is administered at various dose levels, with toxic signs observed for onset, progression or reversal, severity, mortality, and rates of incidence. Doses are ranged, in order to find the largest single dose of the test compound that will *not* produce a toxic effect; the dose level at which severe toxicity occurs; and intermediate toxicity levels. The animals are observed and compared to controls for eating and drinking habits, weight change, toxic effects, psychomotor changes, and any other signs of untoward effects, generally over a 30-day postdose period. Feces and urine specimens are collected and clinical laboratory tests performed to detect clinical chemistry and other changes that could indicate toxicity. Any animal deaths are recorded, studied by histology and pathology, and statistically evaluated on the basis of dose-response, gender, age, intraspecies, interspecies, and against laboratory controls.

In designing a toxicology program, the requirements for human clinical testing must be borne in mind. Animal toxicity studies of a minimum of two weeks duration of daily drug administration at three or more dosage levels to two animal species are required to support the initial administration of a single dose in human clinical testing.[9] These studies are termed *subacute* or *subchronic*. The initial human dose is generally one-tenth of the highest nontoxic dose (usually on a milligram-per-kilogram weight basis) shown during the animal studies. For drugs intended to be given to humans for a week or more, animal studies of 90 to 180 days in length must be provided to demonstrate safety. These are termed *chronic toxicity* studies. And, if the drug is to be used for a chronic human illness, long-term animal studies of one year or longer must support human use. Some animal toxicity studies last two years or longer and may be used to corroborate findings obtained during the course of human clinical trials.

Included in the subchronic and chronic studies are comparative data of test and control animal species, strain, sex, age, dose levels and ranges, routes of administration, duration of treatment and study, observed effects, mortality, body weight changes, food/water consumption, physical examinations (e.g., ECG, ophthalmic), hematology, clinical chemistry, organ weights, gross pathology, neoplastic pathology, histopathology, urinalysis, ADME data, and other.[24]

Carcinogenicity testing is usually a component of chronic testing and is undertaken when the compound has shown sufficient promise as a drug to enter human clinical trials. The studies are long term (18–24 months), with animals sacrificed and studied at defined weeks during the test period. The study results include data on animal death or sacrifice, tumor incidence, type, and site, necropsy reports, and statistical evaluation. *Reproduction* studies include fertility and reproductive performance, teratology, perinatal and postnatal, and multigenerational effects. The maternal parent, fetus, neonates, and weaning offspring are evaluated for anatomical abnormalities, growth, and development. *Mutagenicity* studies are undertaken in vitro to determine if the test compound can affect gene mutation, or cause chromosome or DNA damage. These data are related to any teratologic or carcinogenic effects of the drug.[9]

Early Formulation Studies

As a promising compound is characterized for biologic activity, it is also evaluated with regard to those chemical and physical properties that have a bearing on its ultimate and successful formulation into a stable and effective pharmaceutical product or dosage form. This is the area of responsibility of pharmaceutical scientists and formulation pharmacists trained in the field of *pharmaceutics.* When sufficient information is gleaned on the compound's physical and chemical properties, initial formulations are developed of the dosage form proposed for use in human clinical trials. During the course of the clinical studies, the proposed product is developed further, from initial formulation to final formulation, and from pilot plant (or small-scale production) to scale-up studies, in preparation for large-scale manufacturing.

In order to provide sufficient quantities of the bulk chemical (drug) compound for the sequence of preclinical studies, clinical trials, and both small-scale and large-scale dosage form production, the careful planning, scheduling, and implementation of chemical production plant scale-up must be undertaken by chemical engineers. Quality control and quality assurance must be built into each step of the process.

Full documentation of the chemistry, manufacturing, and controls is an essential part of all drug applications filed with the FDA.[25]

Preformulation Studies

Each drug substance has fundamental chemical and physical characteristics that must be considered prior to the development of a drug formulation or dosage form. Among these characteristics are the drug's solubility, partition coefficient, dissolution rate, physical form, and stability. Each of these and other factors are considered more fully in Chapter 4, but their importance is briefly noted here.

DRUG SOLUBILITY. A drug substance administered by any route must possess some aqueous solubility for systemic absorption and therapeutic response. Poorly soluble compounds (e.g., less than 10 mg/mL aqueous solubility) may exhibit either incomplete or erratic absorption and thus produce a minimal response at desired dosage. Enhanced aqueous solubility may be achieved through the preparation of more soluble derivatives of the parent compound, such as salts or esters, through chemical complexation, or through drug particle-size reduction.

PARTITION COEFFICIENT. To produce a pharmacologic response, a drug molecule must first cross a biologic membrane of protein and lipid, which acts as a lipophilic barrier to many drugs. The ability of a drug molecule to penetrate this barrier is based, in part, on its preference for lipids (lipophilic) versus its preference for an aqueous phase (hydrophilic). A drug's partition coefficient is a measure of its distribution in a lipophilic/hydrophilic phase system, and is indicative of its ability to penetrate biologic multiphase systems.

DISSOLUTION RATE. The speed, or rate, at which a drug substance dissolves in a medium is called its *dissolution rate.* Dissolution rate data, when considered along with data on a drug's solubility, dissolution constant, and partition coefficient, can provide an indication of the drug's absorption potential following administration. For a chemical entity, its acid, base, or salt forms, as well as its physical form (as particle size), may result in substantial differences in the dissolution rate.

PHYSICAL FORM. The crystal or amorphous forms and/or the particle size of a powdered drug have been shown to affect the dissolution rate, and thus the rate and extent of absorption, for a number of drugs. For example, by increasing powder fineness and therefore the surface area of a poorly soluble drug, its dissolution rate in the gut is enhanced (through greater drug/gastrointestinal fluid exposure) and its biologic absorption increased. Small and controlled particle size is also critical for drugs administered to the lung by inhalation. The smaller the particle, the deeper is the penetration into the alveoli. Thus, by selective control of the physical parameters of a drug, biologic response may be optimized.

STABILITY. The chemical and physical stability of a drug substance alone, and when combined with formulation components, is critical in preparing a successful pharmaceutical product. For a given drug, one type of crystal structure may provide greater stability than other structures and may therefore be preferred. For certain drugs susceptible to oxidative decomposition, the addition of antioxidant stabilizing agents to the formulation may be required to protect potency. For other drugs destroyed by hydrolysis, the avoidance of moisture in formulation, processing, and packaging may be required to prevent decomposition. In every case, drug stability testing at various temperatures, conditions of relative humidity (RH)—as 40°C 75% RH/30°C 60% RH—durations, and environments of light, air, and packaging is essential in assessing drug and drug product stability. Such information is vital in developing label instructions for use and storage, in assigning product expiration dating, and for proper packaging and shipping.

Initial Product Formulation and Clinical Trial Materials (CTM)

An initial product is formulated utilizing the knowledge gained during the preformulation studies and with consideration of the dose(s), dosage form, and route of administration desired for the clinical studies and for the proposed marketed product. Thus, depending upon the design of the clinical protocol and desired final product, formulation pharmacists are called upon to develop a specific dosage form (capsule, suppository, solution) of one or more dosage strengths for administration by the intended route of administration (oral, rectal, intravenous). Additional dosage forms for other than the initial route of administration may later be developed, depending on patient requirements, therapeutic utility, and marketing assessments.

The initial formulation prepared for clinical trials, although not as sophisticated and elegant as the final formulation, should be of high pharmaceutical quality, meet analytical specifications for composition, manufacturing, and control, and be sufficiently stable for the period of use. During the course of the human trials, studies of the drug's absorption, distribution, metabolism, and excretion are undertaken to obtain a profile of the drug's biologic availability from the formulation administered. Subsequently, differing formulations may be prepared and examined to develop the one deemed most proficient in meeting the desired bioavailability characteristics (see Chapter 3).

Clinical supplies, or *clinical trial materials,* refer to those dosage formulations used in the clinical evaluation, including the proposed new drug, *placebos* (nonmedicated forms for controlled studies), and drug products against which the new drug is to be clinically compared. They all must be prepared in indistinguishable dosage forms (look alike, taste alike, etc.) in order to reduce possible bias and meet the criteria for double-blind studies in which neither patient nor physician knows which product is being administered. At the conclusion of a clinical study, the product codes are broken and the results critically evaluated. Some pharmaceutical companies have special units for the preparation, analytical control, coding, packaging, labeling, shipping, and record maintenance of clinical supplies. Other companies integrate this activity within their existing operations. Still other companies employ contract firms specializing in this function to prepare and administer their clinical supply program. In all clinical study programs, the package label of the investigational drug must bear the statement "Caution: New Drug—Limited by Federal (or United States)

Law to Investigational Use." Once received by the investigator, the clinical supplies may be administered only to subjects included in the study. Records of the disposition of the drug must be maintained by patient number, dates, and quantities administered. The department of pharmacy at the site of the clinical study (e.g., university teaching hospital) frequently assists in the control and management of clinical supplies. If an investigation is terminated, suspended, discontinued, or completed, all unused clinical supplies must be returned to the sponsor and an accounting made.

The final formulation is developed during the early stages of clinical testing, with the final to-be-marketed version available no later than the end of Phase 2 and the start of Phase 3 clinical studies. All formulations, from those developed initially through the final marketed version, must be prepared under the conditions and procedures set out by the FDA in its Current Good Manufacturing Practice (CGMP) guidelines, as outlined in Chapter 4.

The Investigational New Drug (IND) Application

Under the Food, Drug, and Cosmetic Act as amended, the sponsor of a new drug is required to file with the FDA an Investigational New Drug Application (IND) before the drug may be given to human subjects. This is to protect the rights and safety of the human subjects and to ensure that the investigational plan is sound and is designed to achieve the stated objectives. The *sponsor* of an IND takes responsibility for and initiates a clinical investigation. The sponsor may be an individual (medical researcher), a pharmaceutical company, governmental agency, academic institution, or other private or public organization. The sponsor may be a *clinical investigator* who actually conducts the study or employs or designates other qualified persons to do so.

Following submission of the IND, the sponsor must delay use of the drug in human subjects for not less than 30 days from the date the FDA acknowledges receipt of the application. An IND automatically goes into effect following this period unless the FDA notifies the sponsor that, based on its review of the submission, the period is waived (and the sponsor may initiate the study early), or the investigation is being placed on a clinical hold.

A *clinical hold* is an order issued by the FDA to delay the start of a clinical investigation or, in the case of an ongoing investigation, to suspend the study. During a clinical hold, the investigational drug may not be issued to human subjects (unless specifically permitted by the FDA for individual patients in an ongoing study). A clinical hold is issued when there is concern that human subjects will be exposed to unreasonable and significant risk of illness or injury; where there is question over the qualifying credentials of the clinical investigators; or in instances in which the IND is considered incomplete, inaccurate, or misleading. If the concerns raised are addressed to the FDA's satisfaction, a clinical hold may be lifted and clinical investigations resumed; if not, an IND may be maintained in a clinical hold position, declared inactive, withdrawn by the sponsor, or terminated by the FDA.

Content of the IND

Among the items included in the IND are the following: the name and address of the sponsor of the drug; the name and chemical description of the drug substance to be investigated; a quantitative list of the active and inactive components of the dosage form to be administered; the source or supplier and method of preparation of the drug to be administered; a statement relating to the methods, facilities, and controls employed in the manufacture, processing, packaging and labeling of the new drug to ensure appropriate standards of identity, strength, quality, and purity; a thorough presentation of all preclinical (animal) studies of the drug including the names and qualifications of the investigators and the names and locations of the laboratories in which the work was performed; the relation between the preclinical studies and the proposed clinical studies; information on any clinical studies performed in other countries and any related bibliography of publications on the new drug; if the new drug is a combination of previously investigated components, a complete preclinical and clinical summary of these components when administered singly and any data or expectations relating to the effect when combined; copies of labeling and other pertinent information to be distributed to the proposed clinical investigators of the drug; the names and summaries of the training and experience of the proposed clinical investigators; the name of the persons following the progress of the study and collating and evaluating the data received from the investigators;

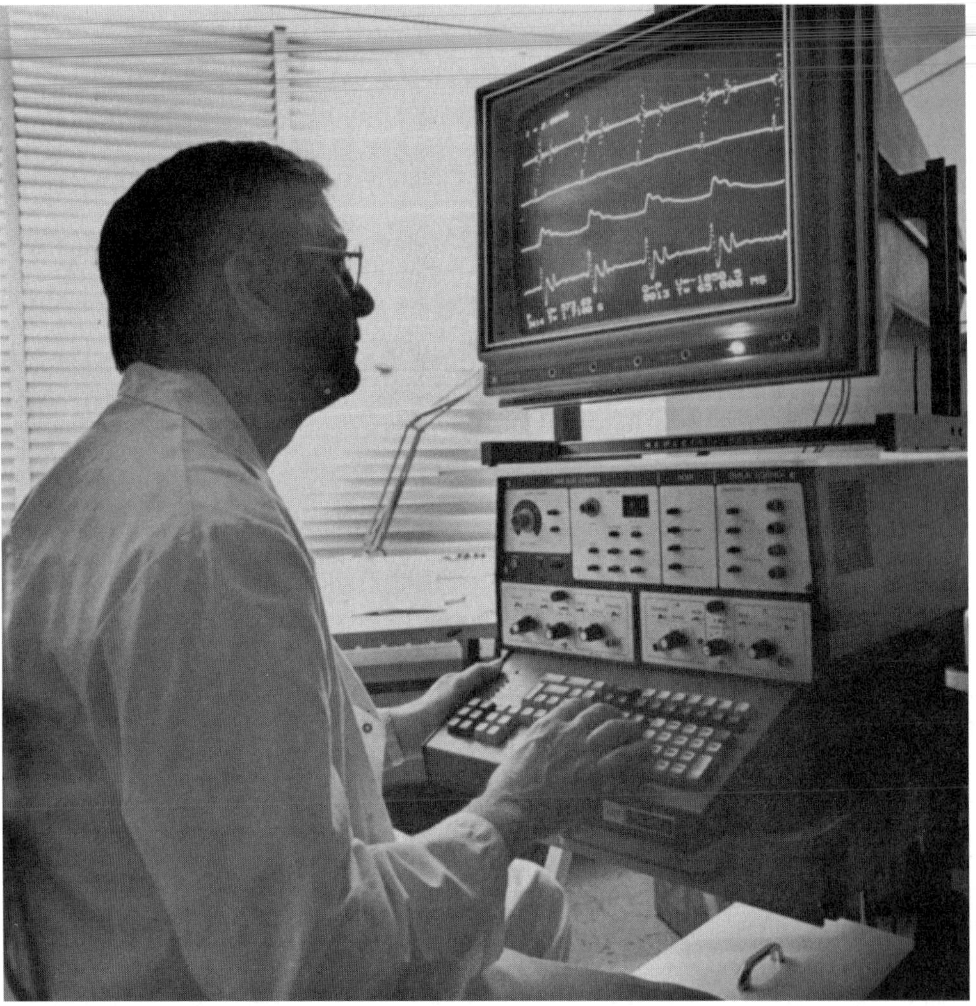

Fig. 2–5. *Monitoring the effects for cardiac function of an uninvestigational drug as a part of its clinical evaluation. (Courtesy of Eli Lilly and Company.)*

a description of the facilities in which the drug will be investigated; and a complete protocol on the methodology to be employed in the clinical investigation, including the method of selection of subjects for the investigation, the method and route of drug administration, the studies to be performed in the evaluation of the safety and effectiveness of the new drug, and the assurance of the safety and protection of the human subjects participating in the investigation (Fig. 2–5).

Pre-IND Meetings

On request, the FDA will advise the sponsor on scientific, technical, or formatting concerns relating to an IND. Examples include advice on the adequacy of technical data to support an investigational plan, on the design of a clinical trial, and on whether proposed investigations are likely to produce the data needed to meet requirements for a marketing application.

FDA Review of the IND Application

The Food and Drug Administration's primary objectives in reviewing an IND are to protect the safety and rights of the human subjects and to help ensure that the quality of the study permits the evaluation of the safety and effectiveness of the drug. This is fostered by the accuracy and completeness of the IND submission, the design and conduct of the investigational plan, and the expertise and diligence of the investigators.

When received by the FDA, the IND submission is stamped with the date of receipt, assigned an application number, and forwarded to the appropriate drug review division within the FDA's Center for Drug Evaluation and Research (CDER)—or the Center for Biologics Evaluation and Research (CBER) for biologic drugs. The current divisions of the CDER are:

- Division of Cardio-Renal Drugs
- Division of Gastrointestinal and Coagulation Drugs
- Division of Topical Drugs
- Division of Oncology and Pulmonary Drugs
- Division of Neuropharmacologic Drugs
- Division of Analgesic and Anti-Inflammatory Drugs
- Division of Metabolism and Endocrine Drugs
- Division of Anti-Infective Drugs
- Division of Anti-Viral Drugs
- Division of Medical Imaging, Surgical and Dental Drugs

Following assignment to one of these divisions, the content of application is thoroughly reviewed by experts in each discipline to determine whether the preclinical data (e.g., chemistry, pharmacology, toxicology) indicate that the drug has been shown to be sufficiently safe for administration to human subjects and that the proposed clinical studies are designed to provide the desired data on drug safety and efficacy while not exposing the human subjects to unnecessary risks. In addition to the divisions, there is a Pilot Drug Evaluation Staff charged to experiment with innovative drug review processes to improve and speed the review process.

Table 2–1. FDA Drug Classification System*

By chemical type:	
Type 1	New molecular entity; not marketed in the U.S.
Type 2	New ester, new salt, or other derivative of an approved active moiety
Type 3	New formulation of a drug marketed in the U.S.
Type 4	New combination of two or more compounds
Type 5	New manufacturer of a drug marketed in U.S.
Type 6	New therapeutic indication for an approved drug
Note: a drug may receive a single or multiple classification, as "3,4"	
By therapeutic classification:	
Type P	Priority review; a therapeutic gain
Type S	A standard review; similar to other approved drugs
Additional classifications:	
Type AA	For treatment of AIDS or HIV-related disease
Type E	For life-threatening or severely debilitating disease
Type F	Review deferred pending data validation
Type G	Data validated, removal of "F" rating
Type N	Nonprescription drug
Type V	Drug having orphan drug status
Note: a drug may receive a single or multiple classification, as "Type P, AA, V"	

* Adapted from information from references 9 and 26.

FDA Drug Classification System

Upon receipt and examination of an IND or NDA application, the FDA classifies the drug by chemical type and therapeutic potential, as shown in Table 2–1. The classification system allows the FDA to set review priorities according to greatest therapeutic advance or need.[26]

Clinical Protocols

Clinical protocols are submitted for each planned study to ensure the appropriate design and conduct of the investigation. Written clinical protocols include: a statement of the purpose and objectives of the study; an outline of the investigational plan and study design, including the kind of control group and methods to minimize bias on the part of the subjects, investigators, and analysts; an estimate of the number of patients to be involved; a description of human subject inclusion criteria and safety exclusions; a description of the dosing plan, including maximum dose and duration of patient exposure; a description of the patient observations, measurements, tests, and objective criteria to be used in the study; the clinical procedures, laboratory tests and monitoring to be used in minimizing patient risk; the names, addresses and credentials of the principal investigators and subinvestigators; the locations and descriptions of the research facilities to be used; and the approval of the authorized Institutional Review Board. Once an IND is in effect, a sponsor may submit an amendment for approval of any proposed changes. This may involve changes of dosing levels, testing procedures, the addition of new investigators, additional sites for the study, and so on.

For many years, women and the elderly were included only rarely in clinical drug investigations. Women of childbearing age were excluded from early drug tests out of fear that a female volunteer would become pregnant during the investigation with possible harm to the fetus. Exceptions were made only in cases of potentially lifesaving drugs. However, in recognition that the general exclusion of women from drug investigations results in inadequate data on any gender-based differences in a drug's effects, the FDA now requires gender-analysis studies on new drugs and greater inclusion of women. The FDA guidelines now encourage women to be enrolled in studies of new drugs in numbers adequate to allow detection of clinically significant differences in drug response and stress the importance of assessing possible pharmacokinetic differences between women and men. Pharmacokinetic differences could be particularly important in the case of a drug with a low therapeutic index, where the smaller average size of women might necessitate modified dosing. Other issues that must be considered are: the effects of the menstrual cycle and menopausal status on a drug's pharmacokinetics; the effects of concomitant estrogen supplementation or use of systemic contraceptive agents, including estrogen-progestin combinations and long-acting progesterones, on a drug's pharmacokinetics; and the influence of a drug on the effectiveness of oral contraceptives. To evaluate fully the potential for gender differences, the FDA urges that women of all ages be included in drug trials. There is no longer a restriction on the enrollment of women of childbearing potential in even the earliest phase of clinical trials. Instead, the FDA guideline calls for appropriate measures for minimizing the risk of fetal exposure, such as pregnancy testing, contraception, and provision of all information about potential fetal risks to prospective study subjects. In addition, when a proposed drug is likely to have significant use in the elderly, elderly patients are to be included in clinical studies. These studies yield data, analyzed according to age, of the drug's effectiveness and the occurrence of adverse effects. Older people handle a drug differently, not because of age itself, but because of altered body functions (such as diminished liver and kidney function, reduced circulation, and changes in drug absorption, distribution, metabolism, and excretion). Differentiation of a drug's activity in minority groups and their subpopulations is an added consideration in the full assessment of a drug's potential.

Each IND submission must have the prior approval of the *Institutional Review Board (IRB)* having jurisdiction over the site of the proposed clinical investigation. An IRB is a body of professional and public members that has the responsibility for reviewing and approving any study involving human subjects within the institution they serve. The purpose of the IRB is to protect the safety of human subjects by assessing a proposed clinical protocol, evaluating the benefits against potential risks, and ensuring that the plan includes all needed measures for subject protection.

Each clinical investigator receives from the sponsor an *Investigator's Brochure,* which contains all of the pertinent information developed during the preclinical studies, including summary information on the drug's chemistry, pharmacology, toxicology, pharmacokinetics, any known information related to the drug's safety and effectiveness, the clinical protocol and study design, criteria for patient inclusion and exclusion, laboratory and clinical tests to be performed, and drug control and record keeping information. Each study has defined criteria for *patient inclusion/exclusion.* These criteria may relate to age, sex, health status, and other factors deemed desirable for human subjects in a given phase of investigation. Each subject participating in a clinical investigation does so willingly. The sponsor of the study must certify that each person who will receive the investigational drug has given *informed consent*—that is, has been informed of the purpose and nature of the study, the procedures involved, the potential benefits (for patients), and the potential risks involved, and has agreed in writing to participate.

Any pertinent safety information observed during the clinical trials is required to be conveyed to each investigator. Investigators are responsible for ensuring that an investigation is conducted according to the investigational plan; for protecting the rights, safety, and welfare of human subjects under the investigator's care; for control of the investigational drug; for written records of case histories and clinical observations; and for timely submission of progress reports, safety reports, and a final report. Any serious, unexpected, life-threatening, or fatal adverse experience that can be associated with the use of the drug during a clinical investigation must be reported promptly to the sponsor and, subsequently, to the FDA for investigation. Depending upon the severity and assessment of the adverse experience, an alert notice may be sent to other investigators, a clinical hold may be placed on the study for further evaluation and assessment, or the IND may be withdrawn by the sponsor, placed on inactive status, or terminated by the FDA.

Phases of a Clinical Investigation

An IND may be submitted for one or more *phases* of a clinical investigation. The clinical investigation is generally divided into Phase 1, Phase 2, and Phase 3 (Figure 2–2; Table 2–2). Although in general the phases are conducted sequentially, they may overlap.

Phase 1 includes the initial introduction of an investigational drug into humans and is primarily for the purpose of assessing safety. The studies are closely monitored by clinicians expert in such investigations. The human subjects are usually healthy volunteers, although in certain protocols they may be patients. The total number of subjects included in Phase 1 studies varies with the drug, but is generally in the range of 20 to 100. The initial dose of the drug is usually quite low, usually one-tenth of the highest "no-effect dose" observed during the animal studies. If the first dose is well tolerated, the investigation is continued with the administration of progressively greater doses (to new subjects) until evidence of the drug's effects are observed. Phase 1 studies are designed to determine the metabolism and pharmacologic actions of the drug in humans, the side effects associated with increasing doses, and, if possible, to gain early evidence on effectiveness. Among the basic data collected during this time phase include the rate of the drug's absorption; the rate and level of its concentration in the blood; its rate and method of elimination from the body, and toxicological effect, if any, in body tissues and major organs; and changes in the blood forming organs or in the normal physiologic processes of the body. The subjects' ability to tolerate the drug are observed and any unpleasant effects of the drug are recorded. If Phase 1 is successful in demonstrating sufficient merit to the drug and if the order of toxicity remains low, Phase 2 of clinical testing is begun utilizing up to several hundred patients.

Patients suffering from a malady against which the new drug indicated promise through its pharmacological activity are treated in limited numbers and under close observation during *Phae* 2 of clinical testing. The main purpose of Phase 2 is to determine the efficacy of the new drug in treating the disease against which it is being tested and to detect side effects or toxicity symptoms not manifest in the animal studies or in studies with healthy volunteers.

Clinicians familiar with the disease being treated with the investigational drug are utilized during Phase 2 studies. During this phase, additional data are collected relating to the drug's patterns of absorption, distribution, and excretin, and drug metabolites which may be formed are identified. Each patient is monitored for the appearance of side effects while the dose of the drug is carefully increased to determine the minimal effective dose. Following this determination, the dose is extended beyond the minimally effective dose to ascertain the dosage level at

Table 2–2. Phases of Clinical Testing

	Number of Patients	*Length*	*Purpose*	*Percent of Drugs Successfully Completing**
Phase 1:	20–100	Several months	Mainly safety	67%
Phase 2:	Up to several hundred	Several months to 2 years	Some short-term safety, but mainly effectiveness	45%
Phase 3:	Several hundred to several thousand	1–4 years	Safety, effectiveness, dosage	5–10%

* For example, of 20 drugs entering clinical testing, 13 or 14 will successfully complete phase 1 trials and go on to phase 2; about nine will complete phase 2 and go to phase 3; only one or two will clear phase 3 and, on average, about one of the original 20 will ultimately be approved for marketing. (Reference: *FDA Consumer, 21*: 12, 1987.)

which a patient reveals extremely undesirable or intolerable toxic or adverse effects from the drug. The greater the range between the amount of drug determined to be minimally effective and that determined to cause severe side effects, the greater is the safety margin of the drug and the greater the promise for effective use in drug therapy.

If the clinical results of Phase 2 indicate continued promise for the new drug and if the margin of safety appears to be good, *end-of-Phase 2* meetings between the drug's sponsor and the FDA are generally held to resolve any questions and issues raised during the course of an investigation and to plan for Phase 3 studies. In these sessions, data from Phases 1 and 2 are carefully reviewed, investigational plans for Phase 3 discussed, and agreements reached. *Phase 3* studies involve the participation of additional clinicians and medical practitioners with the objective of determining the usefulness of the drug in an expanded patient base. Depending upon the drug and the disease against which it is being studied, this phase may involve a thousand or more patients.

"Treatment IND"

Special provisions have been established to expedite the development, evaluation, and marketing of new therapies intended to treat persons with life-threatening and severely debilitating illnesses where no satisfactory alternative therapy exists. The FDA has determined that physicians and patients are generally willing to accept greater risks or side effects from products used for such illness than for less serious illness. *Life-threatening* is defined as diseases or conditions where the likelihood of death is high unless the course of the disease is interrupted, and *severely debilitating* means diseases or conditions that cause major irreversible morbidity.[1] Such diseases are included as advanced cases of AIDS, herpes simplex encephalitis, advanced metastatic refractory cancers, bacterial endocarditis, Alzheimer's disease, advanced multiple sclerosis, advanced Parkinson's disease, and others.

For products considered under "Treatment INDs," sponsors meet with FDA–reviewing officials early in the drug development process to review and reach agreement on the design of necessary preclinical and Phase 1 clinical studies. When data from Phase 1 studies are available, additional meetings are held to review the findings and reach agreement on the design of Phase 2 controlled clinical trials, with the goal that such testing will be adequate to provide sufficient data on the drug's safety and effectiveness to support a decision on its approvability for marketing. During Phase 2, a sponsor may file a "treatment protocol" seeking *early availability* of the drug to physicians and patients, while the controlled clinical studies continue to gather data sufficient for the marketing application. In rendering its decision, the FDA applies a risk-benefit judgment, and considers whether the benefits of the drug outweigh the known and potential risks, taking into consideration the severity of the disease and the absence of alternative therapy. In an effort to make promising drugs available as early as possible to people with AIDS and HIV-related diseases, in 1992 the FDA instituted a "parallel track" program that allows one or more studies of these investigational drugs to be conducted without a concurrent control under a special study protocol.[27]

IND for an Orphan Drug

Under the Orphan Drug Act of 1983 as amended, an *orphan disease* is defined as a rare disease or condition that affects fewer than 200,000 people in the United States and for which there is no reasonable expectation that costs of research and development for the indication can be recovered by sales of the product in the United States. Examples of such illnesses are chronic lymphocytic leukemia, Gaucher's disease, cystic fibrosis, and conditions related to acquired immune deficiency syndrome (AIDS).

The FDA Office of Orphan Products Development was established to identify and facilitate the development of orphan products, including drugs, biologics (vaccines and diagnostic drugs), medical devices, and foods. To foster the necessary research and development, the FDA provides support grants to conduct clinical trials on safety and effectiveness. Applicants first request orphan status designation for the disease and file an investigational new drug (IND) or an investigational device exemption (IDE) with their grant application. In most cases, grants are awarded for Phase 2 and Phase 3 clinical studies based upon preliminary clinical research suggesting effectiveness and relative safety. Regular and Treatment IND protocols may be included in orphan drug clinical trials. An incentive to orphan product development is a provision for a seven-year period of exclusive marketing rights following regulatory approval of a product.

The New Drug Application (NDA)

If following the three phases of clinical testing the drug demonstrates sufficient safety and significant therapeutic effect, the sponsor of the drug may file a New Drug Application (NDA) with the Food and Drug Administration. This filing may be preceded by a pre–NDA meeting between the drug's sponsor and the FDA to discuss the content and format of the new drug application.

General Content of the NDA Submission

A complete NDA application may be several hundred volumes in length, and contains a highly organized and complete presentation of all of the preclinical and clinical data that the sponsor has obtained during his investigation of the drug, including a summary of human pharmacokinetics and bioavailability, microbiology data (for anti-infective agents only), a discussion of benefit and risk considerations in the use of the drug, and complete proposed product labeling. In recent years, a computer-assisted new drug application (CANDA) process has been implemented whereby the sponsor may interact by computer with the FDA reviewer to facilitate the application and review process.

Drug Dosage

A critical part of any clinical drug study is the determination of a drug's usual safe and effective dose. Accurate and dependable information on drug dosage is essential to sound medical practice and thus is a vital component of an NDA and of approved product labeling.

The most effective dose for an individual patient may vary, depending upon a number of factors including the person's age, body weight, general health status, pathologic condition(s), concomitant drug therapy, dosage form, and route of drug administration. These factors and others are considered in clinical studies and become important components of product labeling.

The determination of a drug's dosage also is integral to product formulation. For convenience of dosage administration, most products are formulated to contain a drug's usual dose within a single dosage unit (tablet, capsule), or within a specified volume of a liquid preparation. To serve varying dosage requirements, a manufacturer may prepare a drug in more than one dosage form and in more than one drug strength.

There are various terms in use regarding the dose of drug substances. The *usual dose* of a drug may be defined as that amount which may be expected to produce, in adults, the medicinal effect for which it is indicated. It serves as a guide to physicians who then may vary the dose depending upon the particular requirements of the patient. The *usual dosage range* for a drug indicates the quantitative range or amounts of the drug that may be prescribed within the framework of usual medical practice. Doses falling outside of the usual dosage range may be underdosage or overdosage, or may reflect a patient's special requirements. For drugs which may be administered to children, a *usual pediatric dose* is generally included in the product literature.

The schedule of dosage, or the *dosage regimen,* is also given in the drug literature. For instance, some drugs are best taken at specific intervals (e.g., every 8 hours) or at specific times (e.g., at bedtime, before meals, or on arising in the morning). Single doses are given for some drugs and daily doses for others, depending upon the drug substance, the dosage form, and the condition being treated. When a drug is taken for an extended period of time, as aspirin for arthritis, a daily dose is appropriate. When aspirin is taken occasionally as for a headache, a single dose is more appropriate.

For certain drugs, an *initial, priming,* or *loading* dose may be required to attain the desired concentration of the drug in the blood or tissues, which may then be maintained through the subsequent administration of regularly scheduled *maintenance doses.* Digoxin, a cardiotonic agent, is a good example of a drug which is administered in this way. The initial goal of digoxin therapy is to achieve the desired *digoxin level* in the patient through the initial administration of the drug four or more times a day. Then a single daily dose may be given to maintain the desired blood level of the drug.

Certain drugs may produce more than one effect, depending upon the dose administered. For example, a low dose of a barbiturate may produce a sedative effect, whereas a larger dose may produce hypnotic effects.

Certain biological products, as Tetanus Immune Globulin, may have two different usual doses, one the *prophylactic dose,* or that amount administered to protect the patient from contracting the illness, and the second, the *therapeutic dose* which is administered to a patient after exposure or contraction of the illness. The recommended doses of vaccines and other biological products including antibiotics and endocrine products are sometimes expressed in *units of activity* rather than in specific quantitative amounts of the drug substance. Units of activity derived from biological assay methods reflect a drug's potency and become necessary when suitable chemical assay methods are unavailable for a particular drug. The potency of a given drug is based on the comparison with an international reference standard of that drug. Insulin injection, for example, is prepared to contain 40, 100, or 500 Insulin units of activity in each milliliter of injection to meet all dosage requirements in a convenient amount of injection. Since the biological activities of different products, such as penicillin, poliomyelitis vaccine, and insulin, are so varied, the units of activity for each is specific for each drug and has no relation between the units of activity for another drug.

Today drug dosage is expressed almost exclusively in the metric system. Systems of weights and measures applicable to pharmacy are presented in the Appendix.

The dose of a drug has been appropriately described as an amount which is "enough but not too much," the idea being to produce the drug's optimum therapeutic effect in a particular patient with the lowest possible dose. The dose of a given drug is specific to the patient, with many factors contributing to its size and effectiveness. The correct dose of aspirin to relieve the pain of a headache would vary from individual to individual and, indeed, within the same individual from one occasion to another. The familiar bell-shaped curve, presented in Figure 2–6 shows that in a normal distribution of patients, a drug's usual dose will provide what might be called an average effect in the majority of individuals. In a portion of the patients, however, the drug will produce little effect, whereas in another group of similar size, the drug will produce an effect greater than the average effect. The amount of drug that will generally produce the desired effect in the majority of patients is considered the drug's usual dose and would likely be the initial dose for an individual taking the drug for the first time. From this initial dose the physician may, if necessary, increase or decrease subsequent doses to meet the particular requirements of the patient.

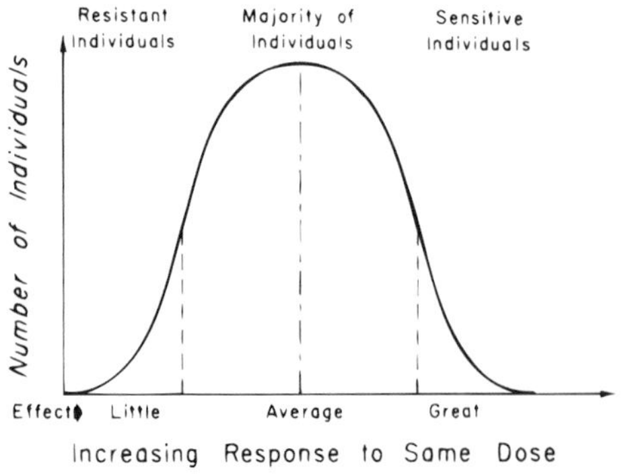

Fig. 2–6. *Drug effect in a population sample.*

In order for a drug to provide systemic effects, it must be absorbed from its route of administration at a suitable rate, be distributed in adequate concentration to the receptor sites, and remain there for a sufficient duration of time. One measure of a drug's absorption characteristics is the determination of its blood serum concentration at various time intervals following administration. For systemic drugs, a correlation can be made between their blood serum concentration and the presentation of drug effects. An average blood serum concentration of a drug can be determined that represents the minimum concentration that can be expected to produce the drug's desired effects in a patient. This concentration is referred to as the *Minimum Effective Concentration* (MEC). As shown in Figure 2–7, for a hypothetical drug, the serum concentration of the drug reaches the MEC 2 hours following its administration, achieves a peak concentration in 4 hours and decreases below the MEC in 10 hours. If it would be desired to maintain the drug serum concentration above the MEC for a longer period of time, a second dose of the drug would be required at approximately the 8-hour time frame. The time-blood level curve presented in Figure 2–7 is an example. In practice, the curve would vary, depending on the nature of the drug substance, its chemical and physical characteristics, the dosage form administered as well as pathological state of the patient, dietary and smoking habits, concomitant drug therapy, and other considerations. The second level of blood serum concentration of drug labeled MTC in Figure 2–7 refers to the *Minimum Toxic Concentration*. Drug serum concentrations above this level would produce dose-related toxic effects in the average individual and perhaps would negate the desirable effects of the drug, compromising the safety of the patient. Ideally, the serum drug concentration in a well-dosed patient would be maintained between the MEC and the MTC (the

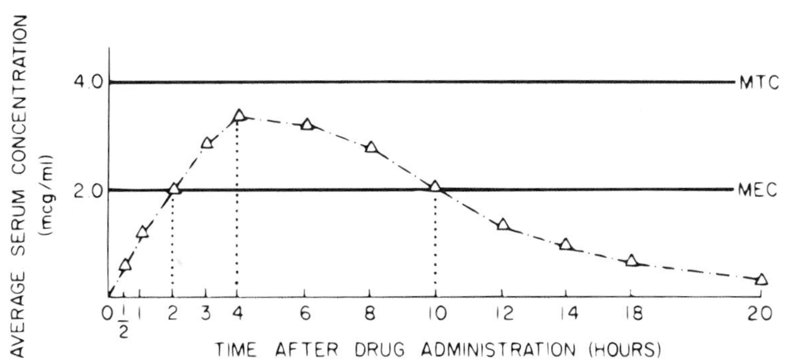

Fig. 2–7. *Example of a blood level curve for a hypothetical drug as a function of time following oral administration. MEC stands for* minimum effective concentration *and* MTC *for* minimum toxic concentration.

"therapeutic window" for the drug) for the period that drug effects are desired. Table 2–3 presents examples of therapeutic, toxic, and lethal concentrations for some drug substances.

The *median effective dose* of a drug is that amount which will produce the desired intensity of effect in 50% of the individuals tested. The *median toxic dose* is that amount which will produce a defined toxic effect in 50% of the individuals tested. The relationship between the desired and undesired effects of a drug is commonly expressed as the *therapeutic index* and is defined as the ratio between a drug's median toxic dose and its median effective dose, TD50/ED50. Thus, a drug with a therapeutic index of 15 would be expected to have a greater margin of safety in its use than a drug with a therapeutic index of 5. For certain drugs, the therapeutic index may be as low as 2 and extreme caution must be exercised in the administration of agents such as these. Table 2–4 presents the therapeutic indices of various drugs.

The therapeutic index must be viewed as a general guide to the margin of safety of a drug, with each patient considered separately. The therapeutic index does not take into account individual patient idiosyncrasy. Further, because the criteria for determining the therapeutic index

Table 2–3. Examples of Therapeutic and Toxic Blood Level Concentrations of Some Drug Substances*

	Drug Substance Concentration, mg/liter		
Drug Substance	*Therapeutic*	*Toxic*	*Lethal*
Acetaminophen	10–20	400	1500
Amitriptyline	0.5–0.20	0.4	10–20
Barbiturates:			
short acting	1	7	10
intermediate acting	1–5	10–30	30
long acting	~10	40–60	80–150
Dextropropoxyphene	0.05–0.2	5–10	57
Diazepam	0.5–2.5	5–20	>50
Digoxin	0.0006–0.0013	0.002–0.009	—
Imipramine	0.05–0.16	0.7	2
Lidocaine	1.2–5.0	6	—
Lithium	4.2–8.3	13.9	13.9–34.7
Meperidine	0.6–0.65	5	30
Morphine	0.1	—	0.05–4
Phenytoin	5–22	50	100
Quinidine	3–6	10	30–50
Theophylline	20–100	—	—

* Adapted from Winek, C.L.: *Clin. Chem.* 22:832, 1976, and Goth, A.: *Medical Pharmacology*, 11th ed, St. Louis, C. V. Mosby Co., 1984, pp. 757–759.

Table 2–4. Examples of Therapeutic Indices for Various Drug Substances*

Drug Substances with Therapeutic Indices		
Less than 5	*Between 5 and 10*	*Greater than 10*
Amitriptyline	Barbiturates	Acetaminophen
Chlordiazepoxide	Diazepam	Bromide
Diphenhydramine	Digoxin	Chloral hydrate
Ethchlorvynol	Imipramine	Glutethimide
Lidocaine	Meperidine	Meprobamate
Methadone	Paraldehyde	Nortriptyline
Procainamide	Primodone	Pentazocine
Quinidine	Thioridazine	Propoxyphene

* From Niazi, S.: *Textbook of Biopharmaceutics and Clinical Pharmacokinetics,* New York, Appleton-Century-Crofts, 1979, p. 254.

involve the use of median figures and intentionally narrow definitions of "effectiveness" and "toxicity," the index does not reflect extremes of the population sample and, depending upon the definitions of effectiveness and toxicity used, a number of therapeutic indices may be determined for a single drug. For instance, the median effective dose for aspirin can be determined for simple headache, arthritic pain, fever, or other conditions and a different ED50 and therapeutic index calculated. Some of the factors that can influence the proper dose of a drug for a given patient are considered briefly here.

1. AGE. The age of the patient is a consideration in the determination of drug dosage. It is particularly true in treating neonatal, prediatric and geriatric patients. Newborn infants, particularly those born prematurely, are abnormally sensitive to certain drugs because of the immature state of their hepatic and renal function by which drugs are normally inactivated and eliminated from the body. Failure to detoxify and eliminate drugs results in their accumulation in the tissues to a toxic level.

Before there was an understanding of the physiologic differences between adult and pediatric patients, the latter were treated with drugs as if they were merely miniature adults. Various rules of dosage in which the pediatric dose was a fraction of the adult dose, based on relative age, were created for youngsters. Today these rules are not in general use because age alone is no longer considered to be a singularly valid criterion for use in the determination of children's dosage, especially when calculated from a *usual* adult dose which itself provides wide clinical variations in response. Instead, the *usual pediatric dose,* determined for specific drugs and dosage forms by clinical evaluation, is most commonly utilized. These pediatric doses are included in drug literature and in pharmaceutical product labeling and are used as guidelines to be considered with other factors in the dosage determination for a specific pediatric patient. In instances in which dosage for a pediatric patient is calculated, methods using body weight and body surface area are most used (see below).

Elderly persons also present unique therapeutic and dosing problems which require special attention. Most physiologic functions begin to diminish in adults following their third decade of life. For example, cardiac output declines approximately 1% per year from age 20 to age 80. Glomerular filtration rate also falls progressively until at age 80, it may be only half of what it was at age 20. There is also a decrease in vital capacity, immune capacity and liver microsomal enzyme function.[28]

The decline in renal and hepatic function in the elderly may show drug clearance and increases the possibility of drug accumulation in the body and subsequent toxicity. Dosing of medication in the elderly must include this consideration. Elderly persons may also respond differently to drugs than younger patients because of changes in drug-receptor sensitivity or because of age-related alterations in target tissues or organs.[29] To assist the pharmacist in pediatric and geriatric patient dosing, the American Pharmaceutical Association annually publishes the *Pediatric Dosage Handbook* and the *Geriatric Dosage Handbook.*

Chronic conditions have largely replaced acute illnesses as the leading causes of death in the elderly population. Frequently, acute illnesses represent the terminal episode of a progressively debilitating chronic disorder. The chronic disorders present in the majority of geriatric patients include cardiovascular disease, cerebrovascular disease, malignant neoplasms, diabetes, and rheumatic disease. Frequently in the elderly patient, there are multiple medical problems which require concomitant treatment. An acute illness may present itself along with one or more chronic conditions, complicating drug therapy and raising the possibility of drug-drug interactions, adverse drug effects, and even therapeutic failure. The elderly patient, taking multiple mediations frequently faces difficulty in taking each one according to the prescribed schedule. The elderly have special problems in complying with therapeutic regimens. The hearing and sight of the elderly are frequently diminished. Because of these physical impairments, their ability to communicate is often affected. The pharmacist can be of special assistance in achieving patient compliance with medications through careful communications, skillful drug packaging and labeling techniques and patient monitoring.

2. **BODY WEIGHT.** The *usual doses* for drugs are considered generally suitable for 70 kg (150 pound) individuals. The ratio between the amount of drug administered and the size of the body influences the drug concentration in body fluids. Therefore, drug dosage may require adjustment from the usual adult dose for abnormally lean or obese patients. The determination of drug dosage for youngsters on the basis of body weight is considered more dependable than that based strictly on age.

For some drug substances, a pediatric dose may be based on a combination of age and weight. For example, the recommended dose for iron replacement in deficiency states is:

6 months to 2 years of age—up to 6 mg/kg/day
2 years to 12 years of age—3 mg/kg/day

As indicated, when dosage is based on body weight, it is frequently expressed on a *milligram* (drug) *per kilogram* (body weight) basis. Occasionally, a literature reference may express the dose of a drug based on a *milligram per pound* of body weight.

3. **BODY SURFACE AREA.** Other methods of determining drug dosage are used in preference to those based solely on age or weight. One such method has as its basis the recognition that a close correlation exists between a large number of physiological processes and body surface area (BSA). A formula for the determination of a child's dose based on relative body surface area and the adult dose is:

$$\frac{\text{Surface of child's body}}{\text{Surface area adult's body}} \times \text{Adult Usual Dose} = \text{Approximate Child's Dose}$$

The surface area of individuals may be determined from a nomogram composed of scales of height, weight, and surface area. Two such nomograms are presented in Fig. 2–8. Surface area is indicated where a straight line drawn to connect the height and weight of an individual intersects the surface area column. The administration of a total adult dose is considered appropriate when the body surface area reaches 1.7 square meters, thus this figure may be employed in the denominator of the equation.

For some drug substances, the dose may be indicated in terms of *milligrams per square meter.* For instance, the usual pediatric dose of chlorambucil based in BSA is 4.5 mg per square meter per day as a single dose or in divided doses. Using the nomogram for calculating the BSA of children and using the example of a child weighing 15 kg and measuring 100 cm in height, the surface area would be 0.64 square meter. Thus, the dose of chlorambucil for this child would be: 4.5 mg $\times$ 0.64 = 2.88 mg once a day or in divided daily doses.

4. **SEX.** Women are thought to be more susceptible to the effects of certain drugs than are men, and in some instances this difference is considered sufficient to necessitate reduction in dosage. During pregnancy, caution is necessary in the administration of drugs that might affect the uterus or fetus. A number of drugs have been shown to be readily transported from the maternal to the fetal circulation including such agents as: alcohol, anesthetic gases, barbiturates, narcotic and non-narcotic analgesics, anticoagulants, anti-infective agents, and many others.[30,31] Fetal exposure to agents such as these has resulting in death *in utero* or in congenital damage to the neonate. The fetus is apparently more sensitive to the effects of certain drugs than is the mother. For instance, respiration in the fetus may be halted at a level of general anesthesia that does not impair maternal respiration. Also, because of the undeveloped and thus ineffective drug detoxication and excretion mechanisms present in the fetus, concentrations of drugs may actually reach a higher level in the fetus than in the maternal circulation. The addiction of newborn infants to narcotic drugs such as heroin, cocaine, and morphine due to the maternal use of these agents during pregnancy is a common occurrence. The same result occurs when an infant is breast-fed by a narcotic-dependent mother. The transfer of drugs from the mother to the nursing infant through human milk may occur with a wide variety of drugs with the drug effects becoming manifest in the infant.[32,33] Thus, pregnant women and nursing mothers should

Nomogram for Calculating the Body Surface Area of Children[1]

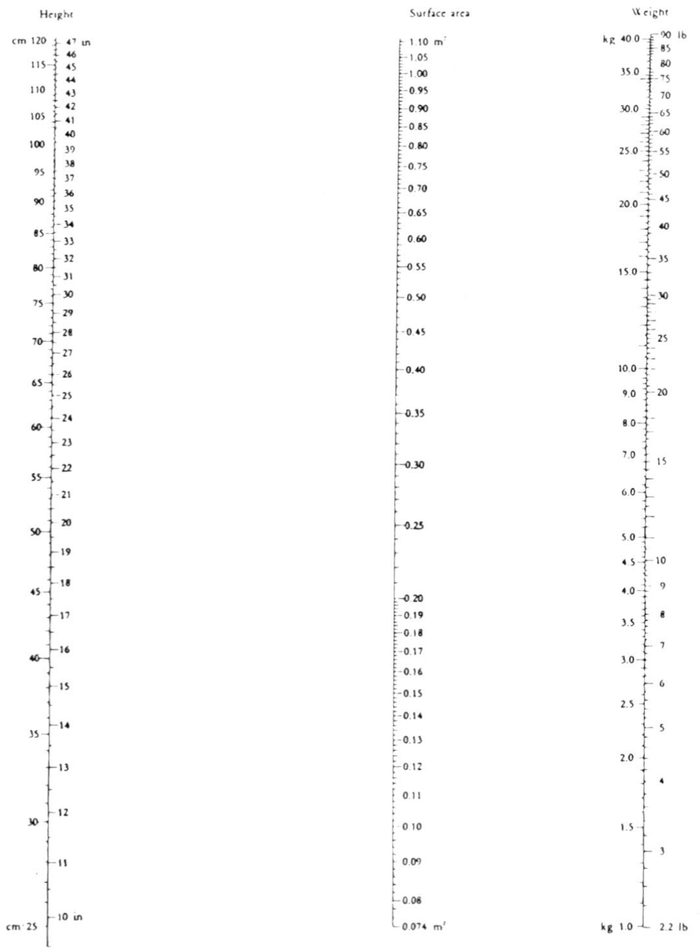

Nomogram for Calculating the Body Surface Area of Adults[1]

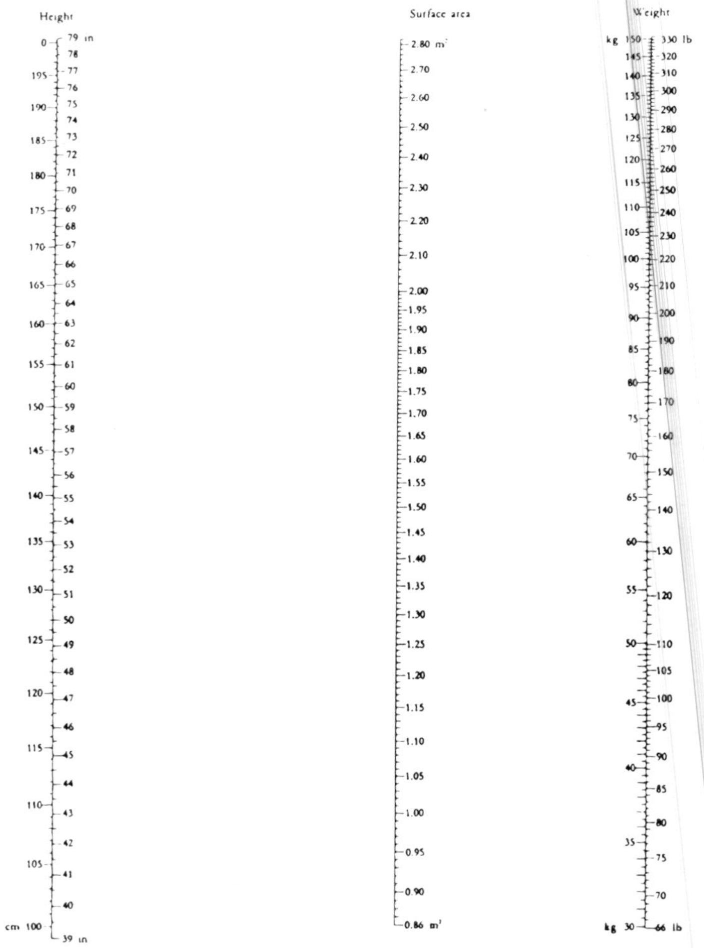

[1] From the formula of Du Bois and Du Bois, *Arch. intern. Med.* 17, 863 (1916): $S = W^{0.425} \times H^{0.725} \times 71.84$, or $\log S = 0.425 \log W + 0.725 \log H + 1.8564$ where S = body surface area in square centimeters, W = weight in kilograms, H = height in centimeters

Fig. 2–8. *Nomograms for calculating body surface area. (From* Documenta Geigy Scientific Tables, 6th ed., pp. 632–633. By permission of R.J. Geigy S.A.)

use medications only with the advice and under the guidance of their physician.

5. PATHOLOGIC STATE. The effects of certain drugs may be modified by the pathologic condition of the patient and must be considered in determining the drug to use as well as its proper dose. For example, if tetracycline HCl is used in the presence of renal impairment, it may lead to the excessive systemic accumulation of the drug and possible liver toxicity. Under such conditions, lower than usual doses are indicated, and if therapy is prolonged, blood serum levels of the drug should be taken and the patient monitored at regular intervals to assure the maintenance of non-toxic levels of the drug. Also, liver function tests may be performed to detect possible liver damage. Drugs having a high danger potential in a given therapeutic situation should be used only when the possible benefit to the patient exceeds the possible risk and when no other suitable drug with a lesser toxicity is available. Pharmacokinetic dosing, discussed in the next chapter, takes into consideration factors such as renal clearance in determining drug dosage.

6. TOLERANCE. The ability to endure the influence of a drug, particularly when acquired by a continued use of the substance, is referred to as drug *tolerance.* It is usually developed to a specific drug or to its chemical congeners; in the latter instance it is referred to as *cross-tolerance.* The effect of drug tolerance is that the drug dosage must be increased to maintain a given therapeutic response. Tolerance occurs commonly to the use of such drugs as antihistaminics, narcotic analgesics, and barbiturates. After the development of tolerance to a certain drug or type of drug, normal sensitivity may be regained only by suspending the drug's administration for a period of time. For most drugs, the development of tolerance can be minimized by initiating therapy with the lowest effective dose and by avoiding prolonged administration.

7. CONCOMITANT DRUG THERAPY. The effects of a drug may be modified by the prior or concurrent administration of another drug. Such interferences between drugs are referred to as *drug-drug interactions* and are due to the chemical or physical interaction between the drugs or to an alteration of the absorption, distribution, metabolism, or excretion patterns of one of the drugs. The effects of drug-drug interactions may be desirable and beneficial to the patient or they may be detrimental. An example of a beneficial interaction involves the drugs probenecid and penicillin or its derivatives. Given concomitantly, probenecid causes the prolongation of penicillin serum levels, enabling a reduction in the total dose of penicillin required as well as in the frequency of its administration. This has the effect of reducing the incidence of missed dosage administration by patients.

A detrimental interaction between drugs may be exemplified by that between certain metal ions and the antibiotic tetracycline or its derivations. Tetracyclines can combine with the metal ions calcium, magnesium, aluminum, and iron in the gastrointestinal tract to form complexes that are poorly absorbed. Many antacid drugs are particularly rich in calcium, magnesium, and aluminum and should be avoided during tetracycline administration. If offending antacids and tetracycline are both required in a patient, they should be given alternately according to a strict schedule which avoids their simultaneous presence during the period allowed for tetracycline absorption. Certain calcium-containing foods, as milk, cheese, and other dairy products must similarly be restricted during tetracycline administration.

Another example of drug-drug interaction which can alter the effectiveness of a given dose of drug involves the drug cimetidine and the anticoagulant drug warfarin. Cimetidine reduces liver microsomal enzymes which can result in the decreased rate of metabolism of a number of drugs including warfarin. Thus, a person stabilized on a specific dose of warfarin may require a decreased dosage level of that drug if cimetidine is subsequently added to the therapeutic regimen. Conversely, if a patient is stabilized on a level of warfarin while also being administered cimetidine, the dosage of the warfarin would likely need to be increased if the cimetidine therapy is discontinued.

A person's use of "social" agents may also interact with prescribed medications. Numerous studies have demonstrated that smoking can influence the rate of elimination of theophylline from the body. Cigarette and marijuana smoking stimulates the hepatic metabolism of theophylline and shortens its half-life, increases total body theophylline clearance, and reduces theophylline serum concentration levels. Smokers may require a 50 to 100% increase in theophylline dosage to accommodate this interaction and a period of time between 3 months to 2 years may be necessary to normalize the effects of smoking on theophylline kinetics. Interestingly, because of the smoking-induced reduction in serum theophylline levels smokers tend to encounter less adverse reactions to theophylline. When patients stop smoking, the smoking-induced metabolism of theophylline dissipates slowly over a period of time and downward adjustments in theophylline dosage are made accordingly. It has also been demonstrated that diabetic patients who smoke heavily may require insulin dosage one-third higher than normal. It is thought that this is due partly to the increased catecholamine and corticosteroid release caused by smoking. In addition, it has been demonstrated that smoking-induced peripheral vasoconstriction will reduce the rate of insulin absorption following subcutaneous injection.

8. TIME OF ADMINISTRATION. The time at which a drug is administered sometimes influences dosage. This is especially true for oral therapy in relation to meals. Absorption proceeds more rapidly if the stomach and upper portions of the intestinal tract are free of food, and an amount of a drug that is effective when taken before a meal may be ineffective if administered during or after eating. On the other hand, irritating drugs are better tolerated by the patient if food is present in the stomach to dilute the drug's concentration.

The proper schedule of a drug's dosage (as "four times a day," or "every 8 hours") is a factor of the illness and the body drug level desired, the physicochemical nature of the drug itself, the dosage form design, and the degree and rate of the drug's absorption, distribution, metabolism and elimination from the body.

9. DOSAGE FORM AND ROUTE OF ADMINISTRATION. The dosage of a given drug may vary, depending upon the dosage form employed and the route of administration utilized. This is due to the different rates and extents of absorption resulting from the various means of administering drugs. Drugs administered intravenously enter the blood stream directly and thus the full amount administered is present in the blood. In contrast, drugs administered orally are rarely, if ever, fully absorbed due to the various physical, chemical, and biologic barriers to their absorption, including interactions with the gastric and intestinal contents. Thus in many instances, a lesser parenteral (injectable) dose of a drug is required than the oral dose to achieve the same blood levels of drugs or clinical effects. This is not to say that adequate absorption cannot take place from the various body sites. Sufficient absorption of certain drugs can be achieved from the rectum, gastrointestinal tract, under the tongue, through the skin and from other sites. However, each drug has to be studied individually to determine the best routes of its administration and then suitable dosage forms and drug delivery systems designed to carry the necessary amount of drug to meet the desired clinical requirements.

Commercially prepared dosage forms contain fixed amounts of drugs designed to meet the *usual dosage* requirements of patients. The liquid dosage forms, as injections, syrups and elixirs, are flexible in that they permit the dosage administered to be easily adjusted simply by altering the volume of product used. Some tablets are *scored* or grooved to permit even breaking to facilitate the accurate administration of partial dosage units. However, some dosage forms as capsules and unscored tablets do not permit easy and accurate partial dosage unit administration. Thus, to provide greater flexibility in the selection and use of commercially prepared dosage forms, manufacturers generally prepare more than a single strength of a given drug product. For instance, phenobarbital tablets are commercially available containing 15, 30, 60, and 100 mg of phenobarbital. Information as to the available strengths of drug products is provided to the pharmacist by means of drug package inserts, drug literature, and reference books.

Drug Product Data in the NDA Submission

An NDA must contain the following information related to the drug product proposed for marketing: a list of all components used in manufacture of the product; a statement of the composition of the drug product; the specifications and analytical methods for each component, and those to ensure the identity, strength, quality, purity, and bioavailability of the drug product; specifications related to sterility, dissolution rate, containers, and closure systems; a description of the manufacturing and packaging procedures and in-process controls; stability data with proposed expiration dating; and the name and address of each manufacturer of the drug product. In addition, the sponsor must submit product samples for testing in FDA laboratories and copies of the proposed labeling and packaging. Prior to the final approval of an NDA application, the facilities where the product is to be manufactured undergo a *pre-approval inspection* by FDA field representatives to assure its capability to comply with all the quality standards contained in the application, as well as those broadly represented by the FDA's Current Good Manufacturing Practice Standards.

Drug Product Labeling

The labeling of all drug products distributed in the United States must meet the specific labeling requirements set forth in federal regulations[34] and approved for each product by the Food and Drug Administration. Labeling requirements differ for prescription drugs, nonprescription drugs, and animal drugs. In each instance, however, the objective is the same, to ensure the appropriate and safe use of the medication.

According to federal regulations, *drug labeling* includes not only the labels placed on an immediate container but also the information on the packaging, in package inserts, and in company literature, advertising, and promotional material. For prescription drugs, labeling represents a summary of all of the preclinical and clinical studies conducted over the period of years from drug discovery through product development to FDA approval. The essential prescribing information for a human prescription drug is provided in the package insert, which by law contains a balanced presentation of the usefulness and the risks associated with the product to enable safe and effective use. The package insert is required to contain the following summary information in the order listed.

1. *Description* of the product, including the proprietary and nonproprietary names, dosage form and route of administration, quantitative product composition, pharmacologic or therapeutic class of the drug, chemical name and structural formula of the drug compound, and important chemical and physical information (pH, sterility, etc.).
2. *Clinical Pharmacology,* including a summary of actions of the drug in humans, relevant in-vitro and animal studies essential to the biochemical and/or physiological basis for action, pharmacokinetic information on rate and degree of absorption, biotransformation and metabolite formation, degree of drug binding to plasma proteins, rate or half-time of elimination, uptake by a particular organ or fetus, and any toxic effects.
3. *Indications and Usage,* including the FDA–approved indications in the treatment, prevention, or diagnosis of a disease or condition, evidence of effectiveness demonstrated by results of controlled clinical trials, special conditions to the drug's use for short-term or long-term use.
4. *Contraindications,* stating those situations in which the drug should not be used because the risk of use clearly outweighs any possible beneficial effect. Included are contraindications associated with drug hypersensitivity, concomitant therapy, disease state, and/or factors of age or gender.
5. *Warnings,* including descriptions of serious adverse reactions and potential safety hazards, limitations to use imposed by them, and steps to be taken if they occur.
6. *Precautions,* including special care to be exercised by prescriber and patient in the use of the drug (drug/drug, drug/food, drug/laboratory test interactions, effects on fertility, use in pregnancy, use in nursing mothers, and use in pediatric patients.
7. *Adverse Reactions,* including predictable and potential unpredictable undesired (side) effects, categorized by organ system or severity of reaction and frequency of occurrence.
8. *Drug Abuse and Dependence,* including legal schedule if a controlled substance, types of abuse and resultant adverse reactions, psychological and physical dependence potential, and treatment of withdrawal.
9. *Overdosage,* including signs, symptoms, usual doses, and laboratory findings of acute overdosage, along with specifics or general principles of treatment.
10. *Dosage and Administration,* stating the recommended usual dose, the usual dosage range, the safe upper limit of dosage, duration of treatment, modification of dosage in special patient populations (children, elders, patients with kidney and/or liver dysfunction), and special rates of administration (as with parenteral medications).
11. *How Supplied,* including information on available dosage forms, strengths, and means of dosage form identification, as color, coating, scoring, and National Drug Code.

Note: Additional information on drug labeling and packaging is presented in Chapter 4.

FDA Review Decision, "Action Letters"

The completed New Drug Application is carefully reviewed by the Food and Drug Administration, which decides whether to allow the sponsor to market the drug, to disallow marketing, or to require additional data before rendering a judgment. By regulation, the Food and Drug Administration must respond within 180 days of receipt of an application. This 180-day period is called the *review clock.* This period is often extended by mutual agreement between the applicant and the FDA as additional information, studies, or clarifications are sought. After review of a completed application, the FDA sends one of the following *action letters.*

Approvable Letter. The agency will approve the application if specific additional data or other material is submitted, or specified conditions are met. This frequently pertains to development of approved final product labeling.

Approval Letter. Approval of the application permitting marketing.

Not Approvable Letter. The application is not considered approvable because of one or more deficiencies.

Should the sponsor of the drug be accorded a favorable decision, the FDA continues to require good manufacturing procedures, adequate scientific control over these procedures, continued receipt of information pertinent to the drug's side effects and toxicity, fairness in promotion and advertising, and above all the right to remove the drug from the market, temporarily or permanently, should further study later be justified. The time course from the initial synthesis of a new drug compound to approval for marketing by the FDA is shown in Figure 2–2. On average, approximately twelve years are required for this research and evaluation process, and only a small proportion of the drugs that enter human testing reach the market. The others are dropped from consideration because they have unacceptable toxicity, they fail to produce the desired therapeutic effects, or the potential market for sales has been determined to be insufficient to justify continued developmental expense.

Phase 4 Studies and Postmarketing Surveillance

The receipt of marketing status for a new drug product does not terminate a company's investigation of the activity of the drug. Continued clinical investigations, often referred to as *Phase 4* studies, add to the understanding of the mechanism of the drug's actions and frequently reveal new therapeutic applications or indications for the drug. Should the drug demonstrate usefulness in treating patients with diseases or illnesses other than that for which the drug was originally approved, the drug's sponsor can apply to the FDA for permission to promote and market the drug for the "new indication." The FDA would once again evaluate the new clinical data and make a determination. Postmarketing studies may continue as long as useful information is gathered on the safety and effectiveness of the product. As additional experience is gained with the drug, newly revealed adverse effects may also be generated and new cautions or restrictions to the use of the drug imposed.

A drug's sponsor is required to review and report to the FDA all adverse drug experience information received from any internal or external source (physicians, pharmacists, postmarketing studies). Health care professionals participate by providing information voluntarily on "Medication and Device Problem Report" forms provided by the FDA.[35] Manufacturers are required to report serious adverse drug experiences, defined as fatal or life-threatening, to the FDA as soon as possible, but no later than 15 working days after receipt of the information. This is termed a "15-Day Alert Report." All other adverse experiences must be reported to the FDA on a quarterly basis for three years following the date of approval of the marketing application and then annually thereafter. Depending upon the nature, causal relationship, and seriousness of the adverse reaction reports, the FDA may require revised product labeling to reflect the new findings; require the sponsor to issue special warning notices to prescribers and other health care professionals; undertake a review of available clinical data; issue a product recall notice; restrict the marketing of the product during a review period; or withdraw product approval for marketing.

Annual Reports

Each year the sponsor of an approved drug must file, with the FDA division responsible for the NDA review, a report containing the following information: an annual summary of significant new information that might affect the safety, effectiveness, or labeling of the drug product; data on the quantity of dosage units of the drug product distributed domestically and abroad; a sample of currently used professional labeling, patient brochures, or package inserts, and a summary of any changes since the previous report; reports of experiences, investigations, studies, or tests involving chemical or physical properties of the drug that may affect its safety or effectiveness; a full description of any manufacturing and controls changes (not requiring a Supplemental New Drug Application); copies of unpublished reports and summaries of published reports of new toxicologic findings in vitro and animal studies conducted or obtained by the sponsor; full or abstract reports on published clinical trials of the drug, including studies on safety and effectiveness; new uses; biopharmaceutic, pharmacokinetic, clinical pharmacologic, and epidemiologic reports; pharmacotherapeutic and lay press articles on the drug; summaries of unpublished clinical trials or prepublication manuscripts, as available, conducted or obtained by the sponsor; a statement on the current status of any postmarketing studies performed by, or on behalf of, the sponsor; and specimens of mailing pieces or other forms of promotion of the drug product. Failure to make required reports may lead to FDA withdrawal of approval for marketing.

Supplemental, Abbreviated, and Other Applications

As briefly described in the following, other Food and Drug Administration applications apply to certain approval requests.

Supplemental New Drug Application (SNDA)

A sponsor of an approved NDA may make changes in that application through the filing of a supplement. Depending on the changes proposed, some require FDA approval before implementing, others do not. Among the supplements requiring prior approval are: a change in the method of synthesis of the drug substance; use of a different facility to manufacture the drug substance where the facility has not been approved through inspection for Current Good Manufacturing Practice standards within the previous two years; change in the formulation, analytical standards, method of manufacture, or in-process controls of the drug product; use of a different facility or contractor to manufacture, process, or pack the drug product; change in the container and closure system for a drug product; extension of the expiration date for a drug product based on new stability data; any labeling change that does not add to or strengthen a previously approved label statement. Examples of changes that may be made without prior FDA approval are: minor editorial or other changes in the labeling that add to or strengthen an approved label section; any analytical changes made to comply with the USP/NF; an extension of the product's expiration date based upon full shelf-life data obtained from a protocol in the approved application; and a change in the size (not the type of system) of the container for a solid dosage form.

Abbreviated New Drug Application (ANDA)

An abbreviated application is one in which reports of nonclinical laboratory studies and reports of clinical investigations, except those pertaining to bioavailability, may be omitted. These applications are usually filed for duplicates (generic products) of drug products previously approved under a full NDA, and for which the FDA has determined that the exempted information is already available at the agency. ANDAs are frequently filed by competing companies following the expiration of patent term protection of the innovator drug/drug product.

Bioavailability and product bioequivalency are discussed in the following chapter.

Product License Application (PLA)

Product License Applications are submitted to the FDA's Center for Biologics Evaluation and Research (CBER) for manufacture of biological products (blood products, vaccines, toxins). Special regulations apply for the licensure of facilities as well as products.[4]

Animal Drug Applications

The Federal Food, Drug, and Cosmetic Act, as amended, contains specific regulations pertaining to the approval for marketing and labeling of drugs intended for animal use.[6] Regulations are in place for new animal drugs for investigational use, New Animal Drug Applications (NADA), and Supplemental New Animal Drug Applications (SNADA).

Medical Devices

The Food and Drug Administration has regulatory authority over the manufacture and licensing of medical devices, such as contact lenses, cardiac pacemakers, and breast implants.[7] Included in the regulations are standards and procedures for manufacturer registration, investigational studies, good manufacturing practices, and premarket approval.

References

1. *Code of Federal Regulations,* Title 21, Parts 300–314.
2. *Code of Federal Regulations,* Title 21, Part 320.
3. *Code of Federal Regulations,* Title 21, Part 430.
4. *Code of Federal Regulations,* Title 21, Parts 600–680.
5. *Code of Federal Regulations,* Title 21, Part 330.
6. *Code of Federal Regulations,* Title 21, Parts 510–555.
7. *Code of Federal Regulations,* Title 21, Parts 800–895.
8. *Federal Register,* U.S. Government Printing Office, Superintendent of Documents, Washington, DC.
9. Mathieu, M.: *New Drug Development: A Regulatory Overview.* PAREXEL International Corporation, Cambridge, MA, 1990.
10. Guarino, R.A.: *New Drug Approval Process.* Marcel Dekker, Inc., New York, 1987.
11. Smith, C.G.: *The Process of New Drug Discovery and Development.* CRC Press, Boca Raton, FL, 1992.
12. Sneader, W.: *Drug Development: From Laboratory to Clinic.* John Wiley & Sons, New York, 1986.
13. Spilker, B.: *Multinational Drug Companies. Issues in Drug Discovery and Development.* Raven Press, New York, 1989.
14. "Report of the FDA Task Force on International Harmonization," National Technical Information Service, U.S. Department of Commerce, Springfield, VA, 1993.
15. Wordell, C.J.: Biotechnology Update. *Hosp. Pharm. 26:*897–900, 1991.
16. Tami, J.A., Parr, M.D., Brown, S.A., and Thompson, J.S.: Monoclonal Antibody Technology. *Am. J. Hosp. Pharm. 43:*2816–2826, 1986.
17. Brodsky, F.M.: Monoclonal Antibodies as Magic Bullets. *Pharm. Res. 5:*1–9, 1988.
18. Morgan, R.A.: Human Gene Therapy. *BioPharm 6:* 32–35, 1993.
19. Silverman, R.B.: Drug Discovery, Design, and Development. *The Organic Chemistry of Drug Design and Drug Action,* Academic Press, New York, 1992, pp. 4–51.
20. Perun, T.J. and Propst, C.L., Eds.: *Computer-Aided Drug Design. Methods and Applications,* Marcel Dekker, Inc., New York, 1989.
21. Benet, L.Z., Mitchell, J.R., and Sheiner, L.B.: General Principles, in *Goodman and Gilman's The Pharmacologic Basis of Therapeutics,* Eighth Edition, Pergamon Press, New York, 1990, pp. 1–2.
22. Katzung, B.G.: *Basic and Clinical Pharmacology,* Appleton & Lange, Norwalk, CT, 1987, pp. 44–51.
23. Spilker, B.: Extrapolation of Preclinical Safety Data to Humans. *Drug News & Perspectives* 4:214–216, 1991.
24. *Guideline for the Format and Content of the Nonclinical/Pharmacology/Toxicology Section of an Application,* Food and Drug Administration, 1987.
25. *Guideline for the Format and Content of the Chemistry, Manufacturing, and Controls Section of an Application,* Food and Drug Administration, 1987.
26. Hunter, J.R., Rosen, D.L., and DeChristoforo, R.: How FDA Expedites Evaluation of Drugs for AIDS and Other Life-Threatening Illnesses. *Wellcome Programs in Hospital Pharmacy,* No. 67930093009, January 1993.
27. *Federal Register, 57:*1356, April 15, 1992.
28. Cohen, H.J.: The Elderly Patient, A Challenge to the Art and Science of Medicine. *Drug Therapy 13:* 41, 1983.
29. Futerman S.S.: The Geriatric Patient—Pharmacy Care Can Make a Difference. *The Apothecary, 94:*34, 1982.
30. Martin, E.W.: *Hazards of Medication.* J.B. Lippincott, Philadelphia, 1972, pp. 274–280.
31. Richardson, E.R.: Drugs and Pregnancy. *Wellcome Trends in Pharmacy, 7:*4, 1983.
32. Goldberg, R.J. and Cutie, A.J.: Drug Excretion into Human Milk, *Pharmacy Times,* May 1982, p 60.
33. The Transfer of Drugs and Other Chemicals into Human Breast Milk. *Am. Pharm. NS23:*29–36, 1983.
34. *Code of Federal Regulations,* Title 21, Part 201.
35. Draft Form for Reporting Suspect Adverse Events and Product Problems with Medications and Devices. *Federal Register, 58:*11768, February 26, 1993.

3

Dosage Form Design: Biopharmaceutic Considerations

AS DISCUSSED in the previous chapter, the biologic response to a drug is the result of an interaction between the drug substance and functionally important cell receptors or enzyme systems. The response is due to an alteration in the biologic processes that were present prior to the drug's administration. The magnitude of the response is related to the concentration of the drug achieved at the site of its action. This drug concentration depends upon the dosage of the drug administered, the extent of its absorption and distribution to the site, and the rate and extent of its elimination from the body. The physical and chemical constitution of the drug substance—particularly its lipid solubility, degree of ionization, and molecular size—determines to a great extent its ability to effect its biological activity. The area of study embracing this relationship between the physical, chemical, and biological sciences as they apply to drugs, dosage forms, and to drug action has been given the descriptive term *biopharmaceutics*.

In general, for a drug to exert its biologic effect, it must be transported by the body fluids, traverse the required biologic membrane barriers, escape widespread distribution to unwanted areas, endure metabolic attack, penetrate in adequate concentration to the sites of action, and interact in a specific fashion, causing an alteration of cellular function. A simplified diagram of this complex series of events between a drug's administration and its elimination is presented in Figure 3–1.

The absorption, distribution, biotransformation (metabolism), and elimination of a drug from the body are dynamic processes that continue from the time a drug is taken until all of the drug has been removed from the body. The *rates* at which these processes occur affect the onset, intensity, and the duration of the drug's activity within the body. The area of study which elucidates the time course of drug concentration in the blood and tissues is termed *pharmacokinetics*. It is the study of the kinetics of absorption, distribution, metabolism and excretion (ADME) of drugs and their corresponding pharmacologic, therapeutic, or toxic response in animals and man. Further, since one drug may alter the absorption, distribution, metabolism or excretion of another drug, pharmacokinetics also may be applied in the study of interactions between drugs.

Once a drug is administered and drug absorption begins, the drug does not remain in a single body location, but rather is distributed throughout the body until its ultimate elimination. For instance, following the oral administration of a drug and its entry into the gastrointestinal tract, a portion of the drug is absorbed into the circulatory system from which it is distributed to the various other body fluids, tissues, and organs. From these sites the drug may return to the circulatory system and be excreted through the kidney as such or the drug may be metabolized by the liver or other cellular sites and be excreted as metabolites. As shown in Figure 3–1, drugs administered by intravenous injection are placed directly into the circulatory system, thereby avoiding the absorption process which is required from all other routes of administration for systemic effects.

The various body locations to which a drug travels may be viewed as separate compartments, each containing some fraction of the administered dose of drug. The transfer of drug from the blood to other body locations is generally a rapid process and is reversible; that is, the drug may diffuse back into the circulation. The drug in the blood therefore exists in equilibrium with the drug in the other compartments. However, in this equilibrium state, the concentration of the drug in the blood may be quite different (greater or lesser) than the concentration of the drug in the other compartments. This is due

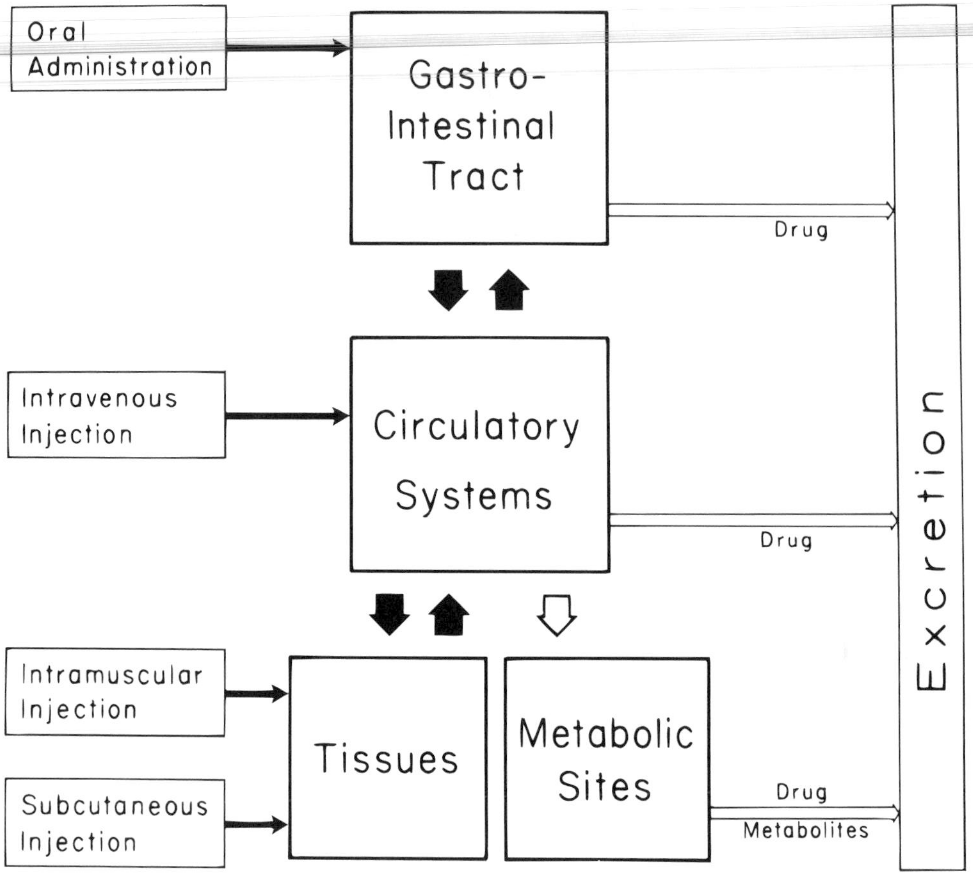

Fig. 3–1. *Schematic representation of events of absorption, metabolism, and excretion of drugs after their administration by various routes.*

largely to the physiochemical properties of the drug and its resultant ability to leave the blood and traverse the biological membranes. Certain drugs may leave the circulatory system rapidly and completely, whereas other drugs may do so slowly and with difficulty. A number of drugs become bound to blood proteins, particularly the albumins, and only a small fraction of the drug administered may actually be found at locations outside of the circulatory system at a given time. The transfer of drug from one compartment to another is mathematically associated with a specific rate constant describing that particular transfer. Generally, the rate of transfer of a drug from one compartment to another is proportional to the concentration of the drug in the compartment from which it exits; the greater the concentration, the greater is the amount of drug transfer.

Metabolism is the major process by which foreign substances, including drugs are eliminated from the body. In the process of metabolism a drug substance may be biotransformed into pharmacologically active or inactive metabolites. Often, both the drug substance and its metabolite(s) are active and exert pharmacologic effects. For example, the antianxiety drug prazepam (Centrax) metabolizes, in part, to oxazepam (Serax), which also has antianxiety effects. In some instances a pharmacologically inactive drug (termed a *prodrug*) may be administered for the known effects of its active metabolites. Dipivefrin, for example, is a prodrug of epinephrine formed by the esterification of epinephrine and pivalic acid. This enhances the lipophilic character of the drug, and as a consequence its penetration into the anterior chamber of the eye is 17 times that of epinephrine. Within the eye, dipivefrin HCl is converted by enzymatic hydrolysis to epinephrine.

The metabolism of a drug to inactive products is usually an irreversible process which culminates in the excretion of the drug from the body, usually via the urine. The pharmacokineticist may calculate an elimination rate constant (termed k_{el}) for a drug to describe its rate of elimination from the body. The term *elimination* refers to both metabolism and excretion. For drugs which are administered intravenously, and therefore involve no absorption process, the task is much less complex than for drugs administered orally or by other routes. In the latter instances, drug absorption and drug elimination are occurring simultaneously but at different rates.

General Principles of Drug Absorption

Before an administered drug can arrive at its site of action in effective concentrations, it must surmount a number of barriers. These barriers are chiefly a succession of biologic membranes such as those of the gastrointestinal epithelium, lungs, blood, and brain. Body membranes are generally classified as three main types: (a) those composed of several layers of cells, as the skin; (b) those composed of a single layer of cells, as the intestinal epithelium; and (c) those of less than one cell in thickness, as the membrane of a single cell. In most instances a drug substance must pass more than one of these membrane types before it reaches its site of action. For instance, a drug taken orally must first traverse the gastrointestinal membranes (stomach, small and large intestine), gain entrance into the general circulation, pass to the organ or tissue with which it has affinity, gain entrance into that tissue, and then enter into its individual cells.

Although the chemistry of body membranes differs one from another, the membranes may be viewed in general as a bimolecular lipoid (fat-containing) layer attached on both sides to a protein layer. Drugs are thought to penetrate these biologic membranes in two general ways: (1) by passive diffusion and (2) through specialized transport mechanisms. Within each of these main categories, more clearly defined processes have been ascribed to drug transfer.

Passive Diffusion

The term *passive diffusion* is used to describe the passage of (drug) molecules through a membrane which behaves inertly in that it does not actively participate in the process. Drugs absorbed according to this method are said to be *passively absorbed*. The absorption process is driven by the concentration gradient (i.e., the differences in concentration) existing across the membrane, with the passage of drug molecules occurring primarily from the side of high drug concentration. Most drugs pass through biologic membranes by diffusion.

Passive diffusion is described by *Fick's first law*, which states that the rate of diffusion or transport across a membrane (dc/dt) is proportional to the difference in drug concentration on both sides of the membrane:

$$-\frac{dc}{dt} = P(C_1 - C_2)$$

in which C_1 and C_2 refer to the drug concentrations on each side of the membrane and P is a permeability coefficient or constant. The term C_1 is customarily used to represent the compartment with the greater concentration of drug and thus the transport of drug proceeds from compartment one (e.g., absorption site) to compartment two (e.g., blood).

Because the concentration of drug at the site of absorption (C_1) is usually much greater than on the other side of the membrane, due to the rapid dilution of the drug in the blood and its subsequent distribution to the tissues, for practical purposes the value of $C_1 - C_2$ may be taken simply as that of C_1 and the equation written in the standard form for a first order rate equation:

$$-\frac{dc}{dt} = PC_1$$

The gastrointestinal absorption of most drugs from solution occurs in this manner in accordance with *first order kinetics* in which the rate is dependent upon drug concentration, i.e., doubling the dose doubles the transfer rate. The magnitude of the permeability constant, depends on the diffusion coefficient of the drug, the thickness and area of the absorbing membrane, and the permeability of the membrane to the particular drug.

Because of the lipoid nature of the cell membrane, it is highly permeable to lipid soluble substances. The rate of diffusion of a drug across the membrane depends not only upon its concentration but also upon the relative extent of its affinity for lipid and rejection of water (a high lipid partition coefficient). The greater its affinity for lipid and the more hydrophobic it is, the faster will be its rate of penetration into the lipid-rich membrane. Erythromycin base, for example, possesses a higher partition coefficient than other erythromycin compounds, e.g., estolate, gluceptate. Consequently, the base is the preferred agent for the topical treatment of acne where penetration into the skin is desired.

Because biologic cells are also permeated by water and lipid-insoluble substances, it is thought that the membrane also contains water-filled pores or channels that permit the passage of these types of substances. As water passes in bulk across a porous membrane, any dissolved solute molecularly small enough to traverse the pores passes in by *filtration*. Aqueous pores vary in size from membrane to membrane and thus in their individual permeability characteristics for certain drugs and other substances.

The majority of drugs today are weak organic acids or bases. Knowledge of their individual ionization or dissociation characteristics is important, because their absorption is governed to a large extent by their degrees of ionization as they are presented to the membrane barriers. Cell membranes are more permeable to the unionized forms of drugs than to their ionized forms, mainly because of the greater lipid solubility of the unionized forms and to the highly charged nature of the cell membrane which results in the binding or repelling of the ionized drug and thereby decreases cell penetration. Also, ions become hydrated through association with water molecules, resulting in larger particles than the undissociated molecule and again decreased penetrating capability.

The degree of a drug's ionization depends both on the pH of the solution in which it is presented to the biologic membrane and on the pK_a, or dissociation constant, of the drug (whether an acid or base). The concept of pK_a is derived from the Henderson-Hasselbalch equation and is:

For an acid:

$$pH = pK_a + \log \frac{\text{ionized conc. (salt)}}{\text{unionized conc. (acid)}}$$

For a base:

$$pH = pK_a + \log \frac{\text{unionized conc. (base)}}{\text{ionized conc. (salt)}}$$

Since the pH of body fluids varies (stomach, ≃ pH 1; lumen of the intestine, ≃ pH 6.6; blood plasma, ≃ pH 7.4), the absorption of a drug from various body fluids will differ and may dictate to some extent the type of dosage form and the route of administration preferred for a given drug.

By rearranging the equation for an acid:

$$pK_a - pH = \log \frac{\text{unionized concentration (acid)}}{\text{ionized concentration (salt)}}$$

one can theoretically determine the relative extent to which a drug remains unionized under various conditions of pH. This is particularly useful when applied to conditions of body fluids. For instance, if a weak acid having a pK_a of 4 is assumed to be in an environment of gastric juice with a pH of 1, the left side of the equation would yield the number 3, which would mean that the ratio of unionized to ionized drug particles would be about 1000 to 1, and gastric absorption would be excellent. At the pH of plasma the reverse would be true, and in the blood the drug would be largely in the ionized form. Table 3–1 presents the effect of pH on the ionization of weak electrolytes, and Table 3–2 offers some representative pK_a values of common drug substances.

From the equation and from Table 3–1, it may be seen that a drug substance is half ionized at

Table 3–1. The Effect of pH on the Ionization of Weak Electrolytes*

	% Unionized	
pK_a-pH	*If Weak Acid*	*If Weak Base*
−3.0	0.100	99.9
−2.0	0.990	99.0
−1.0	9.09	90.9
−0.7	16.6	83.4
−0.5	24.0	76.0
−0.2	38.7	61.3
0	50.0	50.0
+0.2	61.3	38.7
+0.5	76.0	24.0
+0.7	83.4	16.6
+1.0	90.9	9.09
+2.0	99.0	0.99
+3.0	99.9	0.100

* From Doluisio, J.T., and Swintosky, J.V.; *Amer. J. Pharm., 137*:149, 1965.

Table 3–2. pK_a Values for Some Acidic and Basic Drugs

		pK_a
Acids:	Acetylsalicylic acid	3.5
	Barbital	7.9
	Benzylpenicillin	2.8
	Boric acid	9.2
	Dicoumarol	5.7
	Phenobarbital	7.4
	Phenytoin	8.3
	Sulfanilamide	10.4
	Theophylline	9.0
	Thiopental	7.6
	Tolbutamide	5.5
	Warfarin	4.8
Bases:	Amphetamine	9.8
	Apomorphine	7.0
	Atropine	9.7
	Caffeine	0.8
	Chlordiazepoxide	4.6
	Cocaine	8.5
	Codeine	7.9
	Guanethidine	11.8
	Morphine	7.9
	Procaine	9.0
	Quinine	8.4
	Reserpine	6.6

a pH value which is equal to its pK_a. Thus pK_a may be defined as the pH at which a drug is 50% ionized. For example, phenobarbital has a pK_a value of about 7.4, and in plasma (pH 7.4) it is present as ionized and unionized forms in equal amounts. However, a drug substance cannot reach the blood plasma for distribution throughout the body unless it is placed there directly through intravenous injection or is favorably absorbed from a site along its route of entry, as the gastrointestional tract, and allowed to pass into the general circulation. Utilizing Table 3–2 it may be easily seen that phenobarbital, a weak acid, with a pK_a of 7.4 would be largely undissociated in the gastric environment of pH 1, and would likely be well absorbed. A drug may enter the circulation rapidly and at high concentrations if membrane penetration is easily accomplished or at a low rate and low level if the drug is not readily absorbed from its route of entry. The pH of the drug's current environment influences the rate and the degree of its further distribution, since it becomes more or less unionized and therefore more or less lipid-penetrating under some condition of pH than under another. If an unionized molecule is able to diffuse through the lipid barrier and remain unionized in the new environment, it may return to its former location or go on to a new one. However, if in the new environment it is greatly ionized due to the influence of the pH of the second fluid, it likely will be unable to cross the membrane with its former ability. Thus a concentration gradient of a drug usually is reached at equilibrium on each side of a membrane due to different degrees of ionization occurring on each side. *A summary of the concepts of dissociation/ionization is found in the accompanying Physical Pharmacy Capsule.*

It is often desirable for pharmaceutical scientists to make structural modifications in organic drugs and thereby favorably alter their lipid solubility, partition coefficients, and dissociation constants while maintaining the same basic pharmacologic activity. These efforts frequently result in increased absorption, better therapeutic response, and lower dosage.

Specialized Transport Mechanisms

In contrast to the passive transfer of drugs and other substances across a biologic membrane, certain substances, including some drugs and biologic metabolites, are conducted across a membrane through one of several postulated *specialized transport* mechanisms. This type of transfer seems to account for those substances, many naturally occurring as amino acids and glucose, that are too lipid-insoluble to dissolve in the boundary and too large to flow or filter through the pores. This type of transport is thought to involve membrane components that may be enzymes or some other type of agent capable of forming a complex with the drug (or other agent) at the surface membrane, after which the complex moves across the membrane where the drug is released, with the carrier returning to the original surface. Figure 3–2 presents the simplified scheme of this process. Specialized transport may be differentiated from passive transfer in that the former process may become "saturated" as the amount of carrier present for a given substance becomes completely bound with that substance resulting in a delay in the "ferrying" or transport process. Other features of specialized transport include the specificity by a carrier for a particular type of chemical structure so that if two substances are transported by the same mechanism one will competitively inhibit the transport of the other. Further, the transport mechanism is inhibited in general by substances that interfere with cell metabolism. The term *ac-*

Dissociation Constants

Among the physicochemical characteristics of interest is the extent of dissociation/ionization of drug substances. This is important because the extent of ionization has an important effect on the formulation and pharmacokinetic parameters of the drug. The extent of dissociation/ ionization is, in many cases, highly dependent on the pH of the medium containing the drug. In formulation, often the vehicle is adjusted to a certain pH in order to obtain a certain level of ionization of the drug for solubility and stability purposes. In the pharmacokinetic area, the extent of ionization of a drug is an important affector of its extent of absorption, distribution, and elimination. For the practicing pharmacist, it is important in predicting precipitation in admixtures and in the calculating of the solubility of drugs at certain pH values. The following discussion will present only a brief summary of dissociation/ionization concepts.

The dissociation of a weak acid in water is given by the expression:

$$HA \leftrightarrow H^+ + A^-$$
$$K_1[HA] \leftrightarrow K_2[H^+][A^-]$$

At equilibrium, the reaction rate constants K_1 and K_2 are equal. This can be rearranged, and the dissociation constant defined as

$$K_a = \frac{K_1}{K_2} = \frac{[H^+][A^-]}{[HA]}$$

where K_a is the acid dissociation constant.

For the dissociation of a weak base that does not contain a hydroxyl group, the following relationship can be used:

$$BH^+ \leftrightarrow H^+ + B$$

The dissociation constant is described by:

$$K_a = \frac{[H^+][B]}{[BH^+]}$$

The dissociation of a hydroxyl-containing weak base,

$$B + H_2O \leftrightarrow OH^- + BH^+$$

The dissociation constant is described by:

$$K_b = \frac{[OH^-][BH^+]}{[B]}$$

The hydrogen ion concentrations can be calculated for the solution of a weak acid using:

$$[H^+] = \sqrt{K_a c}$$

Similarly, the hydroxyl ion concentration for a solution of a weak base is approximated by:

$$[OH^-] = \sqrt{K_b c}$$

Some practical applications of these equations are as follows.

EXAMPLE 1

The K_a of lactic acid is 1.387×10^{-4} at 25°C. What is the hydrogen ion concentration of a 0.02 M solution?

$$[H^+] = \sqrt{1.387 \times 10^{-4} \times 0.02} = 1.665 \times 10^{-3} \text{ G-ion/L.}$$

EXAMPLE 2

The K_b of morphine is 7.4×10^{-7}. What is the hydroxyl ion concentration of a 0.02 M solution?

$$[OH] = \sqrt{7.4 \times 10^{-7} \times 0.02} = 1.216 \times 10^{-4} \text{ G-ion/L.}$$

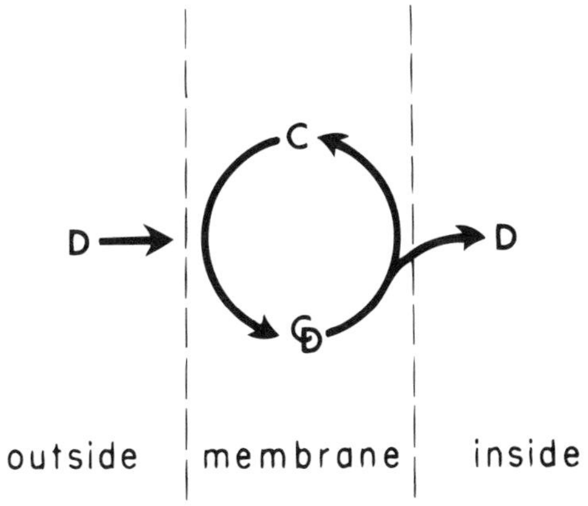

Fig. 3–2. *Active transport mechanism. D represents a drug molecule; C represents the carrier in the membrane. (After O'Reilly, W.J.: Aust. J. Pharm., 47:568, 1966.)*

tive transport, as a subclassification of specialized transport, denotes a process with the additional feature of the solute or drug being moved across the membrane against a concentration gradient, that is, from a solution of lower concentration to one of a higher concentration or, if the solute is an ion, against an electrochemical potential gradient. In contrast to active transport, *facilitated diffusion* is a specialized transport mechanism having all of the above characteristics except that the solute is not transferred against a concentration gradient and may attain the same concentration inside the cell as that on the outside.

Many body nutrients, as sugars and amino acids, are transported across the membranes of the gastrointestinal tract by carrier processes. Certain vitamins, as thiamine, niacin, riboflavin and vitamin B_6, and drug substances as methyldopa and 5-fluorouracil, require active transport mechanisms for their absorption.

Investigations of intestinal transport have often utilized *in situ* (at the site) or *in vivo* (in the body) animal models or *ex vivo* (outside the body) transport models; however, recently cell culture models of human small-intestine absorptive cells have become available to investigate transport across intestinal epithelium.[1] Both passive and transport-mediated studies have been conducted to investigate mechanisms as well as rates of transport.

Dissolution and Drug Absorption

In order for a drug to be absorbed, it must first be dissolved in the fluid at the absorption site. For instance, a drug administered orally in tablet or capsule form cannot be absorbed until the drug particles are dissolved by the fluids at some point within the gastrointestinal tract. In instances in which the solubility of a drug is dependent upon either an acidic or basic medium, the drug would be dissolved in the stomach or intestines respectively (Fig. 3–3). The process by which a drug particle dissolves is termed *dissolution.*

As a drug particle undergoes dissolution, the drug molecules on the surface are the first to enter into solution creating a saturated layer of drug-solution which envelops the surface of the solid drug particle. This layer of solution is referred to as the *diffusion layer.* From this diffusion layer, the drug molecules pass throughout the dissolving fluid and make contact with the biologic membranes and absorption ensues. As the molecules of drug continue to leave the diffusion layer, the layer is replenished with dissolved drug from the surface of the drug particle and the process of absorption continues.

If the process of dissolution for a given drug particle is rapid, or if the drug is administered as a solution and remains present in the body as such, the rate at which the drug becomes absorbed would be primarily dependent upon its ability to traverse the membrane barrier. However, if the rate of dissolution for a drug particle

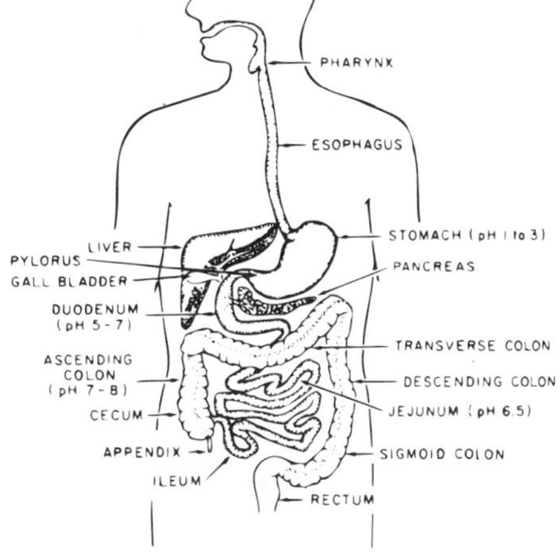

Fig. 3–3. *Anatomical diagram showing the digestive system including the locations involved in drug absorption and their respective pHs.*

is slow, as may be due to the physiochemical characteristics of the drug substance or the dosage form, the dissolution process itself would be a rate-limiting step in the absorption process. Slowly soluble drugs such as digoxin, may not only be absorbed at a slow rate, they may be incompletely absorbed, or, in some cases largely unabsorbed following oral administration, due to the natural limitation of time that they may remain within the stomach or the intestinal tract. Thus, poorly soluble drugs or poorly formulated drug products may result in a drug's incomplete absorption and its passage, unchanged, out of the system via the feces.

Under normal circumstances a drug may be expected to remain in the stomach for 2 to 4 hours (*gastric emptying time*) and in the small intestines for 4 to 10 hours, although there is substantial variation between people, and even in the same person on different occasions. Various techniques have been used to determine gastric emptying time and the gastrointestinal passage of drug from various oral dosage forms, including the tracking of dosage forms labeled with gamma-emitting radionuclides through gamma scintigraphy.[2,3] The gastric emptying time for a drug is most rapid with a fasting stomach, becoming slower as the food content is increased. Changes in gastric emptying time and/or in intestinal motility can affect drug transit time and thus the opportunity for drug dissolution and absorption.

These changes can be effected by drugs the patient may be taking. Certain drugs with anticholinergic properties, e.g., dicyclomine HCl, amitriptyline HCl, have the ability to slow down gastric emptying. This can enhance the rate of absorption of drugs normally absorbed from the stomach, and reduce the rate of absorption of drugs that are primarily absorbed from the small intestine. Alternatively, drugs which enhance gastric motility, e.g., laxatives, may cause some drugs to move so quickly through the gastrointestinal system and past their absorptive site at such a rate to reduce the amount of drug actually absorbed. This effect has been demonstrated with digoxin, whose absorption is significantly decreased by accelerating gastrointestinal motility.

The aging process itself may also influence gastrointestinal absorption. In the elderly, gastric acidity, the number of absorptive cells, intestinal blood flow, the rate of gastric emptying and intestinal motility are all decreased. It appears, however, that drugs for which absorption is dependent upon passive processes are not affected by these factors as much as those that are dependent upon active transport mechanisms, e.g., calcium, iron, thiamine, sugars. A decrease in gastric emptying time would be advantageous for those drugs that are absorbed from the stomach but disadvantageous for those drugs which are prone to acid degradation, e.g., penicillins, erythromycin, or inactivated by stomach enzymes, e.g., L-dopa.

The dissolution of a substance may be described by the modified Noyes-Whitney equation:

$$\frac{dc}{dt} = kS(c_s - c_t)$$

in which dc/dt is the rate of dissolution, k is the dissolution rate constant, S is the surface area of the dissolving solid, c_s is the saturation concentration of drug in the diffusion layer (which may be approximated by the maximum solubility of the drug in the solvent since the diffusion layer is considered saturated), and c_t is the concentration of the drug in the dissolution medium at time t ($c_s - c_t$ is the concentration gradient). The rate of dissolution is governed by the rate of diffusion of solute molecules through the diffusion layer into the body of the solution. The equation reveals that the dissolution rate of a drug may be increased by increasing the surface area (reducing the particle size) of the drug, by increasing the solubility of the drug in the diffusion layer, and by factors embodied in the dissolution rate constant, k, including the intensity of agitation of the solvent and the diffusion coefficient of the dissolving drug. For a given drug, the diffusion coefficient and usually the concentration of the drug in the diffusion layer will increase with increasing temperature. Also, increasing the rate of agitation of the dissolving medium will increase the rate of dissolution. A reduction in the viscosity of the solvent employed is another means which may be used to enhance the dissolution rate of a drug. Changes in the pH or the nature of the solvent which influence the solubility of the drug may be used to advantage in increasing dissolution rate. Effervescent, buffered aspirin tablet formulations use some of these principles to their advantage. Due to the alkaline adjuvants in the tablet, the solubility of the aspirin is enhanced within the diffusional layer and the evolution of carbon dioxide agitates the solvent system, i.e., gastric juices. Consequently, the rate of aspirin absorbed into the bloodstream is faster than that achieved from a conventional aspirin tablet formulation. If this dosage form is acceptable to the patient, it provides a quicker means for the patient to gain relief from a troublesome headache. Many manufacturers will utilize a particular amorphous, crystalline, salt or ester form of a drug that will exhibit the solubility characteristics needed to achieve the desired dissolution characteristics when administered. Some of these factors which affect drug dissolution briefly are discussed in the following paragraphs, whereas others will be discussed in succeeding chapters in which they are relevant.

It is important to remember that the chemical and physical characteristics of a drug substance that can affect drug/drug product safety, efficacy, and stability must be carefully defined by appropriate standards in an application for FDA approval and then substained and controlled throughout product manufacture.

Surface Area

When a drug particle is reduced to a larger number of smaller particles, the total surface area created is increased. For drug substances that are poorly or slowly soluble, this generally results in an increase in the *rate* of dissolution. The actual solubility of a pure drug remains the same.

Increased therapeutic response to orally administered drugs due to smaller particle size has been reported for a number of drugs, among them theophylline, a xanthine derivative used to treat bronchial asthma; griseofulvin, an antibiotic with antifungal activity; sulfisoxazole, an anti-infective sulfonamide, and nitrofurantoin, a urinary anti-infective drug. To achieve increased surface area, pharmaceutical manufacturers frequently use *micronized* powders in their solid dosage form products. Micronized powders consist of drug particles reduced in size to about 5 microns and smaller. The use of micronized drugs is not confined to oral preparations. For example, ophthalmic ointments and topical ointments utilize micronized drugs for their preferred release characteristics and nonirritating quality after application.

Due to the different rates and degrees of absorption obtainable from drugs of various particle size, it is conceivable that products of the same drug substance prepared by two or more reliable pharmaceutical manufacturers may result in different degrees of therapeutic response in the same individual. A classic example of this occurs with phenytoin sodium capsules where there are two distinct forms. The first is the rapid-release type, i.e., Prompt Phenytoin Sodium Capsules, USP, and the second is the slow-dissolution type, i.e., Extended Phenytoin Sodium Capsules, USP. The former has a dissolution rate of not less than 85% in 30 minutes and is recommended for patient use 3 to 4 times per day. The latter has a slower dissolution rate, e.g., 15 to 35% in 30 minutes, which lends itself for use in patients who could be dosed less frequently. Because of such differences in formulation for a number of drugs and drug products, it is generally advisable for a person to continue taking the same brand of medication, provided it produces the desired therapeutic effect. Patients who are stabilized on one brand of drug should not be switched to another unless necessary. However, when a change is necessary, appropriate blood or plasma concentrations of the drug should be monitored until the patient is stabilized on the new product.

Occasionally, a rapid rate of drug absorption is not desired in a pharmaceutical preparation. Research pharmacists, in providing sustained rather than rapid action in certain preparations, may employ agents of varying particle size to provide a controlled dissolution and absorption process. *Summaries of the physical chemical principles of particle size reduction and the relation of particle size to surface area, dissolution, and solubility may be found in the accompanying Physical Pharmacy Capsules.*

Crystal or Amorphous Drug Form

Solid drug materials may occur as pure crystalline substances of definite identifiable shape or as amorphous particles without definite structure. The amorphous or crystalline character of a drug substance may be of considerable importance to its ease of formulation and handling, its chemical stability, and, as has been recently shown, even its biological activity. Certain medicinal agents may be produced to exist in either a crystalline or an amorphous state. Since the amorphous form of a chemical is usually more soluble than the crystalline form, different extents of drug absorption may result with consequent differences in the degree of pharmacologic activity obtained from each. Experiences with two antibiotic substances, novobiocin and chlor-

Particle Size, Surface Area and Dissolution Rate

Particle size has an effect on dissolution rate and solubility. As shown in the Noyes-Whitney equation:

$$\frac{dC}{dT} = kS(C_s - C_t)$$

where dC/dT is the rate of dissolution (concentration with respect to time),
k is the dissolution rate constant
S is the surface area of the particles,
C_s is the concentration of the drug in the immediate proximity of the dissolving particle, i.e., the solubility of the drug,
C_t is the concentration of the drug in the bulk fluid.

It is evident that the "C_s" cannot be significantly changed, the "C_t" is often under sink conditions (an amount of the drug is used that is less than 20% of its solubility) and "k" comprises many factors such as agitation, temperature. This leaves the "S," surface area, as a factor that can affect the rate of dissolution.

An increase in the surface area of a drug will, within reason, increase the dissolution rate. Circumstances when it may decrease the rate would include a decrease in the "effective surface area," i.e., a condition in which the dissolving fluid would not be able to "wet" the particles. Wetting is the first step in the dissolution process. This can be demonstrated by visualizing a 0.75 inch diameter by ¼ inch thick tablet. The surface area of the tablet can be increased by drilling a series of 1/16 inch holes in the tablet. However, even though the surface area has been increased, the dissolution fluid, i.e., water, would not necessarily be able to penetrate into the new holes due to surface tension, etc., and displace the air. Adsorbed air and other factors can decrease the effective surface area of a dosage form, including powders. This is the reason that particle size reduction does not always result in an increase in dissolution rate. One can also visualize a powder that has been comminuted to a very fine state of subdivision and when it is placed in a beaker of water, the powder floats due to the entrapped and adsorbed air. The "effective surface area" is not the same as the actual "surface area" of the resulting powder.

amphenicol palmitate, have revealed that these materials are essentially inactive when administered in crystalline form, but when they are administered in the amorphous form, absorption from the gastrointestinal tract proceeds rapidly with good therapeutic response. In other instances, crystalline forms of drugs may be used because of greater stability than the corresponding amorphous forms. For example, the crystalline forms of Penicillin G as either the potassium or sodium salt are considerably more stable than the analogous amorphous forms. Thus, in formulation work involving Penicillin G, the crystalline forms are preferred and result in excellent therapeutic response.

The hormonal substance insulin presents another striking example of the different degree of activity that may result from the use of different physical forms of the same medicinal agent. Insulin is the active principle of the pancreas gland and is vital to the body's metabolism of glucose. The hormone is produced by two means. The first is by extraction procedures from either beef or pork pancreas. The second process involves a biosynthetic process with strains of *Escherichia coli,* i.e., recombinant DNA. Insulin is used by man as replacement therapy, by injection, when his body's production of the hormone is insufficient. Insulin is a protein, which, when combined with zinc in the presence of acetate buffer, forms an extremely insoluble zinc-insulin complex. Depending upon the pH of the acetate buffer solution, the complex may be an amorphous precipitate or a crystalline material. Each type is produced commercially to take advantage of their unique absorption characteristics.

The amorphous form, referred to as *semilente insulin* or Prompt Insulin Zinc Suspension, USP, is rapidly absorbed upon intramuscular or subcutaneous (under the skin) injection. The larger

Particle Size and Solubility

In addition to dissolution rate, surface area can affect actual solubility, within reason. For example, in the following relationship:

$$\log \frac{S}{S_0} = \frac{2\gamma V}{2.303\ RTr}$$

where "S" is the solubility of the small particles,
"S_0" is the solubility of the large particles,
γ is the surface tension
V is the molar volume
R is the gas constant
T is the absolute temperature
r is the radius of the small particles.

The equation can be used to estimate the decrease in particle size required to result in an increase in solubility. For example, for a desired increase in solubility of 5%, this would require an increase in the S/So ratio to 1.05, that is, the left term in the equation would become "log 1.05." If an example is used for a powder with a surface tension of 125 dynes/cm, the molar volume is 45 cm^3 and the temperature is 27°C, what is the particle size required to obtain the 5% increase in solubility?

$$\log 1.05 = \frac{(2)(125)(45)}{(2.303)(8.314 \times 10^7)(300)r}$$

$$r = 9.238 \times 10^{-6} \text{ cm or } 0.09238\mu$$

A number of factors are involved in actual solubility enhancement and this is only a basic introduction of the general effects of particle size reduction.

crystalline material, called *ultralente insulin* or Extended Insulin Zinc Suspension, USP, is more slowly absorbed with a resultant longer duration of action. By combining the two types in various proportions, a physician is able to provide his patients with intermediate acting insulin of varying degrees of onset and duration of action. A physical mixture of 70% of the crystalline form and 30% of the amorphous form, called *lente insulin* or Insulin Zinc Suspension, USP, is commercially available and provides an intermediate acting insulin preparation that meets the requirements of many diabetics.

Some medicinal chemicals that exist in crystalline form are capable of forming different types of crystals, depending upon the conditions (temperature, solvent, time) under which crystallization is induced. This property, whereby a single chemical substance may exist in more than one crystalline form, is known as "polymorphism." It is known that only one form of a pure drug substance is stable at a given temperature and pressure with the other forms, called metastable forms, converting in time to the stable crystalline form. It is therefore not unusual for a metastable form of a medicinal agent to change form even when present in a completed pharmaceutical preparation, although the time required for a complete change may exceed the normal shelf-life of the product itself. However, from a pharmaceutical point of view, any change in the crystal structure of a medicinal agent may critically affect the stability and even the therapeutic efficacy of the product in which the conversion takes place.

The various polymorphic forms of the same chemical generally differ in many physical properties, including their solubility and dissolution characteristics, which are of prime importance to the rate and extent of drug absorption into the body's system. These differences are manifest so long as the drug is in the solid state. Once solution is effected, the different forms are indistinguishable one from another. Therefore, differences in drug action, pharmaceutically and therapeutically, can be expected from polymorphs contained in solid dosage forms as well as in liquid suspension. The use of metastable forms generally results in higher solubility and dissolution rates than the respective stable crystal forms of the same drug. If all other factors remain constant, more rapid and complete drug absorption will likely result from the metastable forms than from the stable form of the same drug. On the other hand, the stable polymorph is generally more resistant to chemical degradation and because of its lower solubility is frequently preferred in pharmaceutical suspensions of insoluble drugs. If metastable forms are employed in the preparation of suspensions, their gradual conversion to the stable form may be accompanied by an alteration in the consistency of the suspension itself, thereby affecting its permanency. In all instances, the advantages of the metastable crystalline forms in terms of increased physiologic availability of the drug must be balanced against the increased product stability when stable polymorphs are employed. Sulfur and cortisone acetate are two examples of drugs that exist in more than one crystalline form and are frequently prepared in pharmaceutical suspensions. In fact, cortisone acetate is reported to exist in at least five different crystalline forms. It is possible for the commercial products of two manufacturers to differ in stability and in the therapeutic effect, depending upon the crystalline form of the drug used in the formulation.

Salt Forms

The dissolution rate of a salt form of a drug is generally quite different from that of the parent compound. Sodium and potassium salts of weak organic acids and hydrochloride salts of weak organic bases dissolve much more readily than do the respective free acids or bases. The result is a more rapid saturation of the diffusion layer surrounding the dissolving particle and the consequent more rapid diffusion of the drug to the absorption sites.

Numerous examples could be cited to demonstrate the increased rate of drug dissolution due to the use of the salt form of the drug rather than the free acid or base, but the following will suffice: the addition of the ethylenediamine moiety to theophylline increases the water solubility of theophylline 5-fold. The use of the ethylenediamine salt of theophylline has allowed the development of oral aqueous solutions of theophylline and diminished the need to use hydroalcoholic mixtures, e.g., elixirs.

Other Factors

The *state of hydration* of a drug molecule can affect its solubility and pattern of absorption. Usually the anhydrous form of an organic molecule is more readily soluble than the hydrated form. This characteristic was demonstrated with the drug ampicillin, when the anhydrous form was shown to have a greater rate of solubility than the trihydrate form.[4] It was also shown that the rate of absorption for the anyhdrous form was greater than that for the trihydrate form of the drug.

Once swallowed, a drug is placed in the gastrointestinal tract where its solubility can be affected not only by the pH of the environment, but by the normal components of the tract and the foodstuffs which may be present. A drug may interact with one of the other agents present to form a chemical complex which may result in reduced drug solubility and decreased drug absorption. The classic example of this complexation phenomenon is that which occurs between tetracycline analogues and certain cations, e.g., calcium, magnesium, aluminum, resulting in a decreased absorption of the tetracycline derivative. Also, if the drug becomes *ad*sorbed onto insoluble material in the tract, its availability for absorption may be correspondingly reduced.

Bioavailability and Bioequivalence

The term *bioavailability* describes the *rate* and *extent* to which an active drug ingredient or therapeutic moiety is absorbed from a drug product and becomes available at the site of drug action. The term *bioequivalence* refers to the *comparison* of bioavailabilities of different formulations, drug products, or batches of the same drug product.

The availability to the biologic system of a drug substance formulated into a pharmaceutical product is integral to the goals of dosage form design and paramount to the effectiveness of the medication. The study of a drug's bioavailability depends upon the drug's absorption or entry into the systemic circulation, and studying the pharmacokinetic profile of the drug or its metabolite(s) over time in the appropriate biologic system, e.g., blood, plasma, urine. Graphically, bioavailability of a drug is portrayed by a concentration-time curve of the administered drug in an appropriate tissue system, e.g., plasma (Fig. 3–4). Bioavailability data are used to determine: (1) the amount or proportion of drug absorbed from a formulation or dosage form; (2) the rate at which the drug was absorbed; (3) the duration of the drug's presence in the biologic fluid or tissue; and, when correlated

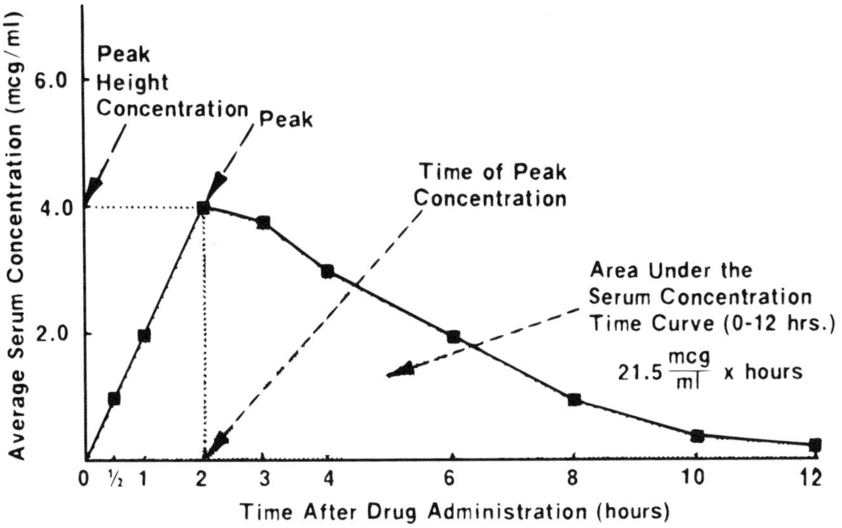

Fig. 3–4. *Serum concentration-time curve showing peak height concentration, time of peak concentration, and area under the curve. (Courtesy of D.J. Chodos and A.R. DiSanto, The Upjohn Company.)*

with patient response, (4) the relationship between drug blood levels and clinical efficacy and toxicity.

During the product development stages of a proposed drug product, pharmaceutical manufacturers employ bioavailability studies to compare different formulations of the drug substance to ascertain the one which allows the most desirable absorption pattern. Later, bioavailability studies may be used to compare the availability of the drug substance from different production batches of the product. They may also be used to compare the availability of the drug substance from different dosage forms (as tablets, capsules, elixirs, etc.), or from the same dosage form produced by different (competing) manufacturers.

FDA Bioavailability Submission Requirements[5]

The FDA requires bioavailability data submissions in the following instances.

1. *New Drug Applications (NDAs).* A section of each NDA is required to describe the human pharmacokinetic data and human bioavailability data, or information supporting a waiver of the bioavailability data requirement (see waiver provisions following).
2. *Abbreviated New Drug Applications (ANDAs).* In vivo bioavailability data are required unless information is provided and accepted supporting a waiver of this requirement (see waiver provisions following).
3. *Supplemental Applications.* In vivo bioavailability data are required if there is a change in the:
   a. manufacturing process, product formulation or dosage strength, beyond the variations provided for in the approved NDA.
   b. labeling, to provide for a new indication for use of the drug product and, if clinical studies are required, to support the new indication.
   c. labeling, to provide for a new or additional dosage regimen for a special patient population (e.g., infants) if clinical studies are required to support the new or additional dosage regimen.

Conditions under which the FDA *may* waive the in-vivo bioavailability requirement include:

1. The product is a solution intended solely for intravenous administration, and contains the same active agent, in the same concentration and solvent, as a product previously approved through a full NDA.
2. The drug product is administered by inhalation as a gas or vapor, and contains the same active agent, in the same dosage form, as a product previously approved through a full NDA.

3. The drug product is an oral solution, elixir, syrup, tincture or similar other solubilized form and contains the same active agent in the same concentration as a previously approved drug product through a full NDA, and contains no inactive ingredient known to significantly affect absorption of the active drug ingredient.
4. The drug product is a topically applied preparation (e.g., ointment) intended for local therapeutic effect.
5. The drug product is an oral dosage form that is not intended to be absorbed (e.g., antacid or radiopaque medium).
6. The drug product is a solid oral dosage form that has been demonstrated to be identical, or sufficiently similar, to a drug product that has met the in-vivo bioavailability requirement.

Most of the bioavailability studies have been applied to drugs contained in solid dosage forms intended to be administered orally for systemic effects. The emphasis in this direction has been primarily due to the proliferation of competing products on the market in recent years, particularly the nonproprietary (generic) capsules and tablets, and the knowledge that certain drug entities when formulated and manufactured differently into solid dosage forms are particularly prone to variations in biologic availability. Thus, the present discussions will be centered around solid dosage forms. However, this is not to imply that systemic drug absorption is not intended from other routes of administration or other dosage forms, or that bioavailability problems may not exist from these products as well. Indeed, drug absorption from other routes is affected by the physicochemical properties of the drug and the formulative and manufacturing aspects of the dosage form design.

Blood (or Serum or Plasma) Concentration-Time Curve

Following the oral administration of a medication, if blood samples are drawn from the patient at specific time intervals and analyzed for drug content, the resulting data may be plotted on ordinary graph paper to yield the type of drug blood level curve presented in Figure 3–4. The verical axis of this type of plot characteristically presents the concentration of drug present in the blood (or serum or plasma) and the horizontal axis presents the time the samples were obtained following the administration of the drug. When the drug is first administered (time zero), the blood concentration of the drug should also be zero. As the drug passes into the stomach and/or intestine, it is released from the dosage form, eventually dissolves, and is absorbed. As the sampling and analysis continue, the blood samples reveal increasing concentrations of drug until the maximum (peak) concentration (C_{max}) is reached. Then, the blood level of the drug progressively decreases and, if no additional dose is given, eventually falls to zero. The diminished blood level of drug after the peak height is reached indicates that the rate of drug elimination from the blood stream is greater than the rate of drug absorption into the circulatory system. It should be understood that drug absorption does not terminate after the peak blood level is reached, but may continue for some time. Similarly the process of drug elimination is a continuous one. It begins as soon as the drug first appears in the blood stream and continues until all of the drug has been eliminated. When the drug leaves the blood it may be found in various body tissues and cells for which it has an affinity until ultimately it is excreted as such or as drug metabolites in the urine or via some other route (see Fig. 3–5). A urinalysis for the drug or its metabolities may be used to indicate the extent of drug absorption and/or the rate of drug elimination from the body.

Parameters for Assessment and Comparison of Bioavailability

In discussing the important parameters to be considered in the comparative evaluation of the blood level curves following the oral administration of single doses of two formulations of the same drug entity, Chodos and DiSanto[6] list the following:

1. The Peak Height Concentration (C_{max})
2. The Time of the Peak Concentration (T_{max})
3. The Area Under the Blood (or serum or plasma) Concentration-Time Curve (AUC)

Using Figure 3–4 as an example, the height of the peak concentration is equivalent to 4.0 μg/mL of drug in the serum; the time of the peak concentration is 2 hours following administration; and the area under the curve from 0 to 12 hours is calculated as 21.5 μg/mL × hours. The meaning and use of these parameters are further explained as follows.

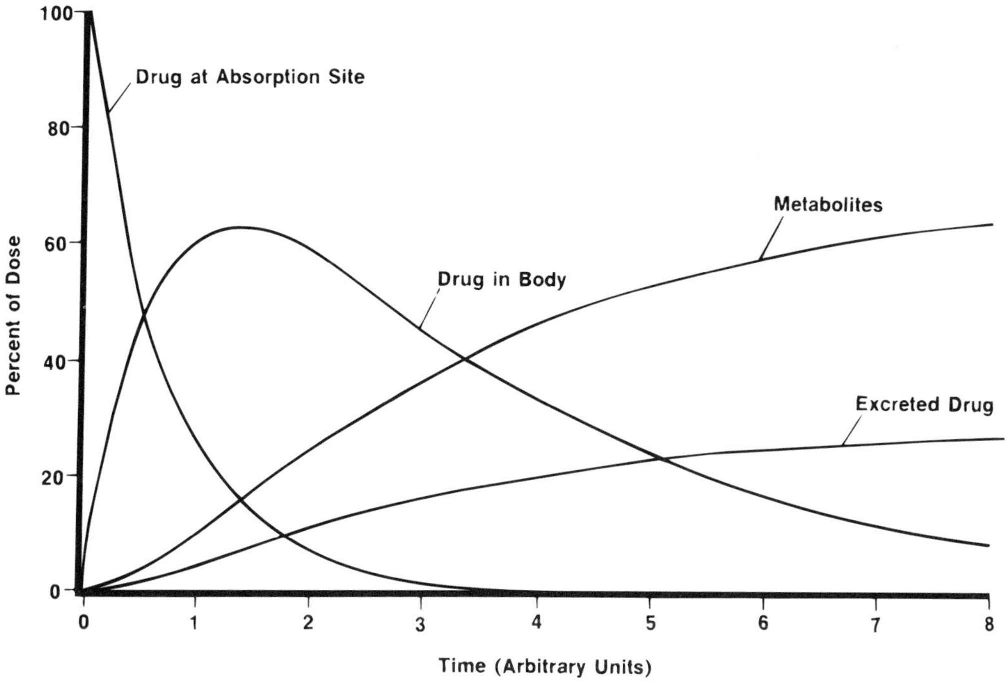

Fig. 3–5. *Time course of drug in the body. (From Rowland, M., and Tozer, T.N.:* Clinical Pharmacokinetics. *2nd Ed., Philadelphia, Lea & Febiger, 1989.)*

PEAK HEIGHT. Peak height concentration is the maximum drug concentration (C_{max}) observed in the blood plasma or serum following a dose of the drug. For conventional dosage forms, as tablets and capsules, the C_{max} will usually occur at only a single time point, referred to as T_{max}. The amount of drug is usually expressed in terms of its concentration in relation to a specific volume of blood, serum, or plasma. For example, the concentration may be expressed as g/100 mL, mcg/mL or mg% (mg/100 mL). Figure 3–6 depicts concentration-time curves showing different peak height concentrations for *equal* amounts of drug from two different formulations following oral administration. The horizontal line drawn across the figure indicates that the minimum effective concentration (MEC) for the drug substance is 4.0 mcg/mL. This means that in order for the patient to exhibit an adequate response to the drug, this concentration in the blood must be achieved. Comparing the blood levels of drug achieved after the oral administration of equal doses of formulations "A" and "B" in Figure 3–6, it is apparent that formulation "A" will achieve the required blood levels of drug to produce the desired pharmacologic effect whereas the administration of formulation "B" will not. On the other hand, if the minimum effective concentration for the drug was 2.0 mcg/mL and the mimimum toxic concentration (MTC) was 4.0 mcg/mL as depicted in Figure 3–7, equal doses of the two formulations would result in toxic effects produced by formulation "A" but only desired effects by formulation "B." The objective in the individual dosing of a patient is to achieve the MEC but not the MTC.

The *size* of the dose administered influences the blood level concentration and C_{max} for that drug substance. Figure 3–8 depicts the influence of dose on the blood level time curve for a hypothetical drug administered by the same route and in the same dosage form. In this example, it is assumed that all doses are completely absorbed and eliminated at the same rates. It is evident that as the dose increases, the C_{max} is proportionately higher and the area-under-the-curve (AUC) proportionately greater. The peak time, T_{max}, if the same for each dose.

TIME OF PEAK. The second parameter of importance in assessing the comparative bioavailability of two formulations is the time required to achieve the maximum level of drug in the blood

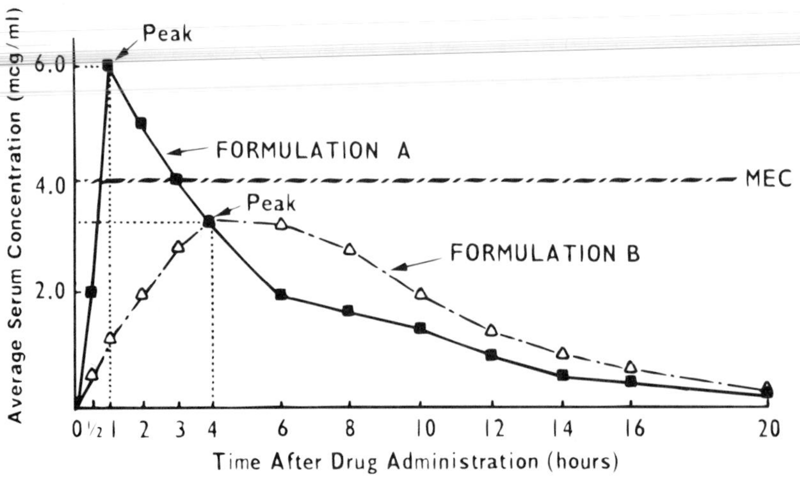

Fig. 3–6. *Serum concentration-time curve showing different peak height concentrations for equal amounts of drug from two different formulations following oral administration. (Courtesy of D.J. Chodos and A.R. DiSanto, The Upjohn Company.)*

(T_{max}). In Figure 3–6, the time required to achieve the peak serum concentration of drug is 1 hour for formulation "A" and 4 hours for formulation "B." This parameter reflects the *rate* of drug absorption from a formulation. It is the rate of drug absorption that determines the time needed for the minimum effective concentration to be reached and thus for the initiation of the desired pharmacologic effect. The rate of drug absorption also influences the period of time over which the drug enters the blood stream and therefore affects the duration of time that the drug is maintained in the blood. Looking at Figure 3–7, formulation "A" allows the drug to reach the MEC within 30 minutes following administration and a peak concentration in 1 hour. Formulation "B" has a slower rate of drug release. Drug from this formulation reached the MEC 2 hours after administration and its peak concentration 4 hours after administration. Thus

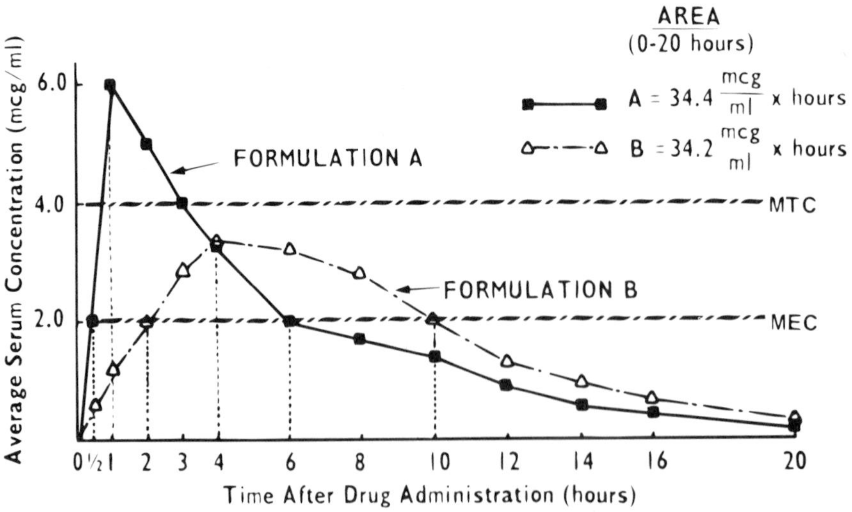

Fig. 3–7. *Serum concentration-time curve showing peak height concentrations, peak height times, times to reach minimum effective concentration (MEC) and areas under the curves for equal amounts of drug from two different formulations following oral administration. (Courtesy of D.I. Chodos and A.R. DiSanto, The Upjohn Company.)*

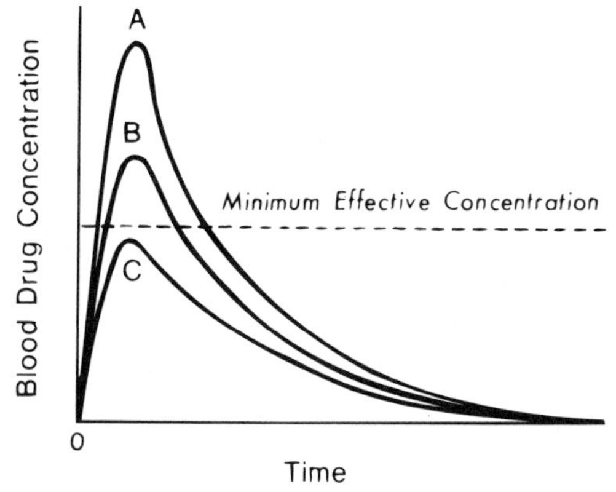

Fig. 3–8. *The influence of dose size on the resultant blood drug concentration-time curves when three different doses of the same drug are administered and the rates of drug absorption and elimination are equal after the three doses. A = 100 mg, B = 80 mg, C = 50 mg. (From C.T. Ueda, "Concepts in Clinical Pharmacology. Essentials of Bioavailability and Bioequivalence," 1979, The Upjohn Company, Reproduced with permission.)*

formulation "A" permits the greater rate of drug absorption; it allows drug to reach both the MEC and its peak height sooner than drug formulation "B." On the other hand, formulation "B" provides the greater duration of time for drug concentrations maintained above the MEC, 8 hours (from 2 to 10 hours following administration) to 5½ hours (from 30 minutes to 6 hours following administration) for formulation "A." Thus, if a rapid onset of action is desired, a formulation similar to "A" would be preferred, but, if a longer duration of action is desired rather than a rapid onset of action, a formulation similar to "B" would be preferred.

In sum, changes in the *rate* of drug absorption will result in changes in the values of both C_{max} and T_{max}. Each product has its own characteristic rate of absorption. When the *rate* of absorption is decreased, the C_{max} is lowered and T_{max} occurs at a later time. If the doses of the drugs are the same and presumed completely absorbed, as in Figure 3–7, the AUC for each is essentially the same.

AREA UNDER THE SERUM CONCENTRATION-TIME CURVE. The area under the curve (AUC) of a concentration-time plot (Fig. 3–4) is considered representative of the total amount of drug absorbed into the circulation following the administration of a single dose of that drug. Equivalent doses of a drug, when fully absorbed, would produce the same AUC. Thus, two curves much unalike in terms of peak height and time of peak, as those in Figure 3–7, may be much alike in terms of area under the curve, and thus in the amount of drug absorbed. As indicated in Figure 3–7, the area under the curve for formulation "A" is 34.4 mcg/mL × hours and for formulation "B" is 34.2 mcg/mL × hours, essentially the same. If equivalent doses of drug in different formulation produce *different* AUC values, differences exist

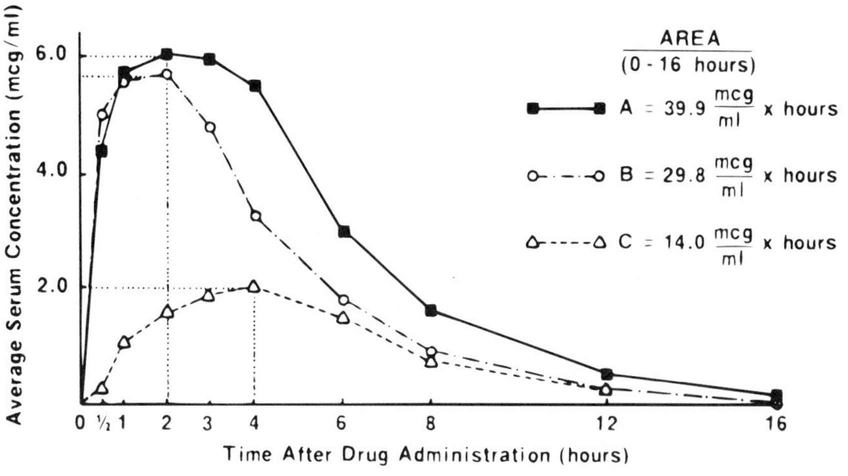

Fig. 3–9. *Serum concentration-time curve showing peak height concentrations, peak height times, and areas under the curves for equal amounts of drugs from three different formulations following oral administration. (Courtesy of D.J. Chodos and A.R. DiSanto, The Upjohn Company.)*

in the *extent* of absorption between the formulations. Figure 3–9 depicts concentration-time curves for three different formulations of equal amounts of drug with greatly different areas under the curve. In this example, formulation "A" delivers a much greater amount of drug to the circulatory system than do the other two formulations. In general, the smaller the AUC, the less drug absorbed.

The area under the curve may be measured mathematically, using a technique known as the trapezoidal rule, and is reported in amount of drug/volume of fluid × time (e.g., mcg/mL × hours; g/100 × hours; etc.).

According to the trapezoidal rule, the area beneath a drug concentration-time curve can be estimated through the assumption that the AUC can be represented by a series of trapezoids (quadrilateral planes having two parallel and two nonparallel sides). The total AUC would be the sum of the areas of the individual trapezoids. The area of each trapezoid is calculated taking $\frac{1}{2}(C_{n+1} + C_n)(t_n - t_{n-1})$, where C_n and t_n are drug concentrations in the blood plasma, or serum, and time, respectively. Ueda demonstrates the use of the trapezoid by the data reproduced in Table 3–3 and plotted into a plasma drug concentration-time curve as shown in Figure 3–10.

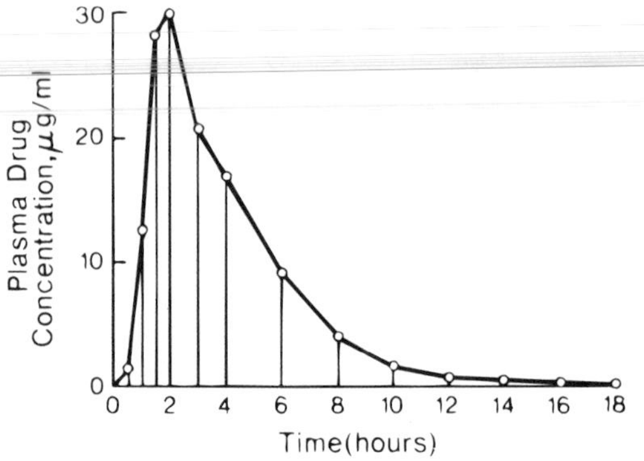

Fig. 3–10. *Estimation of area under the drug concentration-time curve using the trapezoidal rule (see Table 4–3 for raw data). (From C.T. Udea, "Concepts in Clinical Pharmacology. Essentials of Bioavailability and Bioequivalence," 1979, The Upjohn Company, Reproduced with permission.)*

The fraction (F) (or bioavailability) of an orally administered drug may be calculated by comparison of the AUC after oral administration with that obtained after intravenous administration:

$$F = (AUC)_{oral}/(AUC)_{intravenous}$$

In practice, it would be rare for a drug to be

Table 3–3. Determination of AUC Using the Trapezoidal Rule for the Following Plasma Drug Concentration-Time Data*

Sample (n)	*Time (hr)*	*Plasma Concentration (µg/mL)*	*$AUC/t_n t_{n-1}$ (µg/mL × hr)*
1	0	0	½(0 + 1)(0.5 − 0) = 0.25
2	0.5	1	½(1 + 11)(1 − 0.5) = 3.00
3	1.0	11	½(11 + 28)(1.5 − 1) = 9.75
4	1.5	28	½(28 + 30)(2 − 1.5) = 14.50
5	2	30	½(30 + 21)(3 − 2) = 25.50
6	3	21	½(21 + 17)(4 − 3) = 19.00
7	4	17	½(17 + 9)(6 − 4) = 26.00
8	6	9	½(9 + 4)(8 − 6) = 13.00
9	8	4	½(4 + 2)(10 − 8) = 6.00
10	10	2	½(2 + 1)(12 − 10) = 3.00
11	12	1	½(1 + 0)(18 − 12) = 3.00
12	18	0	
			AUC = 123.00

* From C. T. Ueda, "Concepts in Clinical Pharmacology. Essentials of Bioavailability and Bioequivalence," 1979, The Upjohn Company, Reproduced with permission.

completely absorbed into the circulation following oral administration. As noted earlier, many drugs undergo the first-pass effect resulting in some degree of metabolic degradation before entering the general circulation. In addition, factors of drug product formulation, drug dissolution, chemical and physical interactions with the gastrointestinal contents, gastric emptying time, intestinal motility, and others contribute to the incomplete absorption of an administered dose of a drug. The oral dosage strengths of many commerical products are based on considerations of the proportion of the dose administered that is expected to be absorbed and available to its site of action in order to produce the desired drug blood level and/or therapeutic response. The absolute bioavailability following oral dosing is generally compared to intravenous dosing. As examples, the mean oral absorption of a dose of verapamil (Calan) is reported to be 90%; enalapril (Vasotec) 60%; diltiazem (Cardizem) about 40%, and lisinopril (Zestril) about 25%. However, there is large intersubject variability, and the absorbed doses may vary patient-to-patient.

Bioequivalence of Drug Products

A great deal of discussion and scientific investigation has been devoted recently to the problem of determining the equivalence between drug products of competing manufacturers.

It has become well established that the rate and extent to which a drug in a dosage form becomes available for biologic absorption or utilization depends in great measure upon the materials utilized in the formulation and also on the method of manufacture. Thus, the same drug when formulated in *different* dosage forms may be found to possess different bioavailability characteristics and hence exhibit different clinical effectiveness. Further, two seemingly "identical" or "equivalent" products, of the same drug, in the same dosage strength and in the *same* dosage form type, but differing in formulative materials or method of manufacture, may vary widely in bioavailability and thus in clinical effectiveness.

Dissolution requirements for capsules and tablets are included in the USP and are integral to bioavailability. Experience has shown that where bioinequivalence has been found between two supposedly equivalent products, dissolution testing can help to define the product differences. According to the USP, significant bioavailability and bioinequivalence problems may be revealed through dissolution testing and are generally the result of one or more of the following causal factors: the drug's particle size; excessive amounts of the lubricant magnesium stearate in the formulation; coating materials, especially shellac; and inadequate amounts of tablet or capsule disintegrants.

The following terms are used by the Food and Drug Administration to define the type or level of "equivalency" between drug products.[5]

Pharmaceutical equivalents are drug products that contain identical amounts of the identical active drug ingredient, i.e., the same salt or ester of the same therapeutic moiety, in identical dosage forms, but not necessarily containing the same inactive ingredients, and that meet the identical compendial or other applicable standard of identity, strength, quality, and purity, including potency and, where applicable, content uniformity, disintegration times, and/or dissolution rates.

Pharmaceutical alternatives are drug products that contain the identical therapeutic moiety, or its precursor, but not necessarily in the same amount or dosage form or as the same salt or ester. Each such drug product individually meets either the identical or its own respective compendial or other applicable standard of identity, strength, quality, and purity, including potency and, where applicable, content uniformity, disintegration times, and/or dissolution rates.

Bioequivalent drug products are pharmaceutical equivalents or pharmaceutical alternatives whose rate and extent of absorption do not show a significant difference when administered at the same molar dose of the therapeutic moiety under similar experimental conditions, either single dose or multiple dose. Some pharmaceutical equivalents or pharmaceutical alternatives may be equivalent in the extent of their absorption but not in their rate of absorption, and yet may be considered bioequivalent because such differences in the rate of absorption are intentional and are reflected in the labeling, are not essential to the attainment of effective body drug concentrations on chronic use, or are considered medically insignificant for the particular drug product studied.

In addition, the term *therapeutic equivalents* has been used to indicate pharmaceutical equivalents which, when administered to the same individuals in the same dosage regimens, will provide essentially the same therapeutic effect.

Differences in bioavailability have been demonstrated for a number of products involving the following and other drugs: tetracycline, chloramphenicol, digoxin, phenylbutazone, warfarin, diazepam, levodopa, and oxytetracycline. Not only has bio*in*equivalence been shown to exist in products of different manufacturers but there have also been variations in the bioavailability of different batches of drug products from the same manufacturer. Variations in the bioavailability of certain drug products have resulted in some therapeutic failures in patients who have taken two inequivalent drug products in the course of their therapy.

The most common experimental plan to compare the bioavailability of two drug products is the simple *crossover design study*. In this method, each of the 12 to 24 individuals in the group of carefully matched subjects (usually healthy adult males between 18 and 40 years of age of similar height and weight) is administered both products under fasting conditions and essentially serves as his own control. To avoid bias of the test results, each test subject is randomly assigned one of the two products for the first phase of the study. Once the first assigned product is administered, samples of blood or plasma are drawn from the subjects at predetermined times and analyzed for the active drug moiety and its metabolites as a function of time. The same procedure is then repeated (*crossover*) with the second product after an appropriate interval of time, i.e., a washout period to ensure that there is no residual amount of drug from the first administered product that would artificially inflate the test results of the second administered product. Afterward, the patient population data are tabulated and the parameters used to assess and compare bioavailability, i.e., C_{max}, T_{max}, AUC, are then analyzed with statistical procedures. Statistical differences in bioavailability parameters may not always be clinically significant in therapeutic outcome.

It should be recognized that there are inherent differences in individuals which result in different patterns of drug absorption, metabolism and excretion. These differences must be statistically analyzed to separate them from the factors of bioavailability related to the products themselves. The value in the crossover-designed experiment is that each individual serves as his own control by taking each of the products. Thus, inherent differences as mentioned between individuals is minimized.

Absolute bioequivalency between drug products rarely, if ever, occurs. Such absolute equivalency would yield serum concentration-time curves for the products involved that would be exactly superimposable. This simply is not expected of products which are made at different times, in different batches, or indeed by different manufacturers. However, some expectations of bioequivalency are expected of products which are considered to be of equivalent merit for therapy.

In most studies of bioavailability, the originally marketed product (frequently referred to as the "prototype," "pioneer," or "innovator" drug product) is recognized as the established product of the drug and is utilized as the standard for the bioavailability comparative studies.

As a result of the implementation of the Drug Price Competition and Patent Term Restoration Act of 1984, many additional drugs became available in generic form. Prior to the 1984 act, only those drugs marketed before 1962 could be processed by an Abbreviated New Drug Application (ANDA). The ANDA process does not require the sponsor to repeat costly clinical research on active ingredients already found to be safe and effective. The 1984 Act extended the eligibility for ANDA processing to drugs first marketed after 1962, making generic versions immediately possible for many additional off-patent drugs previously available only as brand name (pioneer) products.

According to the FDA, a generic drug is considered bioequivalent if the rate and extent of absorption do not show a significant difference from that of the pioneer drug when administered at the same molar dose of the therapeutic ingredient under the same experimental conditions.[7] Because, in the case of a systemically absorbed drug, blood levels even if from an identical product may vary in different subjects, in bioequivalence studies each subject receives both the pioneer and the test drug and thus serves as his own control.

Under the 1984 act, to gain FDA approval a generic drug product must:

- -Contain the same active ingredients as the pioneer drug (inert ingredients may vary)
- -Be identical in strength, dosage form, and route of administration
- -Have the same indications and precautions for use and other labeling instructions
- -Be bioequivalent

-Meet the same batch-to-batch requirements for identity, strength, purity, and quality
-Be manufactured under the same strict standards of FDA's Current Good Manufacturing Practice regulations as required for pioneer products.

In the design and evaluation of bioequivalence, the FDA employs the "80/20 rule." This rule requires that a study be large enough to provide an 80% probability to detect a 20% difference in average bioavailability. The allowance of a statistical variability of ±20% in bioequivalence applies to both reformulated pioneer drugs and generics. If a pioneer manufacturer reformulates an FDA-approved product, the subsequent formulation must meet the same bioequivalency standards that are required of generic manufacturers of that product (i.e., the approved bioavailability standard for that product).

The FDA recommends generic substitution only among products that it has evaluated to be therapeutically equivalent. Since 1980, the Agency has published an annual *Approved Drug Products with Therapeutic Equivalence Evaluations* (also known as the "Orange Book"). This publication is updated monthly and contains information on about 10,000 approved prescription drug products. About 7,500 of these are available from more than a single manufacturer, with only about 10% considered therapeutically *in*equivalent to the pioneer products. For example, the FDA rates all conjugated estrogens and esterified estrogen products as "not therapeutically equivalent," because no manufacturer to date has submitted an acceptable in vivo bioequivalence study. Therefore, the FDA does not recommend that these products be substituted for each other.

The variables that can contribute to the differences between products are many (Table 3–4). For instance in the manufacture of a tablet, different materials or amounts of such formulative components as fillers, disintegrating agents, binders, lubricants, colorants, flavorants and coatings may be used. The particle size or crystalline form of a therapeutic or pharmaceutic component may vary between formulations. The tablet may vary in shape, size, and hardness depending upon the punches and dies selected for use by the manufacturer and the compression forces utilized in the process. During packaging, shipping and storage the integrity of the tablets may be altered by physical impact, or changes in conditions of humidity, temperature, or through interactions with the components of the container. Each of the factors noted may have an effect on the rates of tablet disintegration, drug dissolution, and consequently on the rate and extent of drug absorption. Although the bioequivalency problems are perhaps greater among tablets than for other doage forms because of the multiplicity of variables, the same types of problems exist for the other dosage forms and must be considered in bioequivalency evaluations.

Table 3–4. Some Factors Which Can Influence the Bioavailability of Orally Administered Drugs

I. *Drug Substance Physiochemical Properties*
  A. Particle Size
  B. Crystalline or Amorphous Form
  C. Salt Form
  D. Hydration
  E. Lipid/Water Solubility
  F. pH and pK_a
II. *Pharmaceutic Ingredients and Dosage Form Characteristics*
  A. Pharmaceutic Ingredients
    1. Fillers
    2. Binders
    3. Coatings
    4. Disintegrating Agents
    5. Lubricants
    6. Suspending Agents
    7. Surface Active Agents
    8. Flavoring Agents
    9. Coloring Agents
    10. Preservative Agents
    11. Stabilizing Agents
  B. Disintegration Rate (Tablets)
  C. Dissolution Time of Drug in Dosage Form
  D. Product Age and Storage Conditions
III. *Physiologic Factors and Patient Characteristics*
  A. Gastric Emptying Time
  B. Intestinal Transit Time
  C. Gastrointestinal Abnormality or Pathologic Condition
  D. Gastric Contents
    1. Other drugs
    2. Food
    3. Fluids
  E. Gastrointestinal pH
  F. Drug Metabolism (Gut and during first passage through liver).

There are situations in which even therapeutically equivalent drugs may not be equally suitable for a particular patient. For example, a patient may be hypersensitive to an inert ingredient in one product (brand name or generic) that another product does not contain. Or a patient may become confused or upset if dispensed an alternate product that differs in color, flavor, shape, or packaging from that to which he or she has become accustomed. Switching between products can generate concern, and thus pharmacists need to be prudent in both initial product selection and in product interchange.

Routes of Drug Administration

Drugs may be administered by a variety of dosage forms and routes of administration, as presented in Tables 3–5 and 3–6. One of the fundamental considerations in dosage form design is whether the drug is intended for local or systemic effects. *Local* effects are achieved from direct application of the drug to the desired site of action, such as the eye, nose, or skin. *Systemic* effects result from the entrance of the drug into the circulatory system and its subsequent transport to the cellular site of its action. For systemic effects, a drug may be placed directly into the blood stream via intravenous injection or absorbed into the venous circulation following oral, or other routes of administration.

Table 3–5. Routes of Drug Administration

Term	*Site*
oral	mouth
peroral (per os[1])	gastrointestinal tract via mouth
sublingual	under the tongue
parenteral	other than the gastrointestinal tract (by injection)
intravenous	vein
intraarterial	artery
intracardiac	heart
intraspinal or intrathecal	spine
intraosseous	bone
intraarticular	joint
intrasynovial	joint-fluid area
intracutaneous or intradermal	skin
subcutaneous	beneath the skin
intramuscular	muscle
epicutaneous (topical)	skin surface
transdermal	skin surface
conjunctival	conjunctiva
intraocular	eye
intranasal	nose
aural	ear
intrarespiratory	lung
rectal	rectum
vaginal	vagina
urethral	urethra

[1] The abbreviation "p.o." is commonly employed on prescriptions to indicate to be swallowed.

Table 3–6. Dosage Form/Drug Delivery System Application

Route of Administration	*Primary Dosage Forms*
oral	tablets capsules solutions syrups elixirs suspensions magmas gels powders
sublingual	tablets troches or lozenges
parenteral	solutions suspensions
epicutaneous/ transdermal	ointments creams infusion pumps pastes plasters powders aerosols lotions transdermal patches, discs, solutions
conjunctival	contact lens inserts ointments
intraocular/ intraaural	solutions suspensions
intranasal	solutions sprays inhalants ointments
intrarespiratory	aerosols
rectal	solutions ointments suppositories
vaginal	solutions ointments emulsion foams tablets inserts, suppositories, sponge
urethral	solutions suppositories

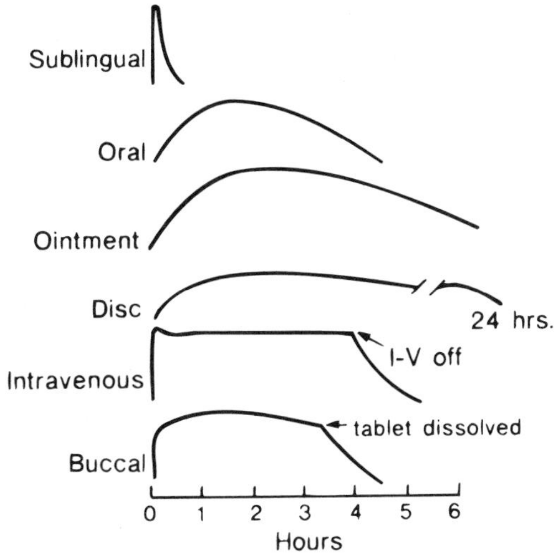

Fig. 3–11. *Blood-level curves of nitroglycerin following administration of dosage forms by various routes. (From Abrams, J.: Nitroglycerin and Long-Acting Nitrates in Clinical Practice.* The American Journal of Medicine, *Proceedings of a Symposium: First North American Conference on Nitroglycerin Therapy, June 27, 1983. Reprinted with Permission.)*

An individual drug substance may be formulated into multiple dosage forms which result in different drug absorption rates and times of onset, peak, and duration of action. This is demonstrated by Figure 3–11 and Table 3–7, for the drug nitroglycerin in various dosage forms. The sublingual, intravenous, and buccal forms present extremely rapid onsets of action whereas the oral (swallowed), topical ointment and topical disc present slower onsets of action but greater durations of action. The disc provides the longest duration of action, up to 24 hours following application of a single patch to the skin. The transdermal nitroglycerin disc allows a single daily dose, whereas the other forms require multiple dosing to maintain drug levels within the therapeutic window.

The difference in drug absorption between dosage forms is a function of the formulation and the route of administration. For example, a problem associated with the oral administration of a drug is that once absorbed through the lumen of the gastrointestinal tract into the portal vein, the drug may pass directly to the liver and undergo the *first-pass effect.* In essence a portion or all of the drug may be metabolized by the liver. Consequently, as the drug is extracted by the liver, its bioavailability to the body is decreased. Thus, the bioavailable fraction is determined by the fraction of drug that is absorbed from the gastrointestinal tract and the fraction that escapes metabolism during its first pass through the liver. The bioavailable fraction (f) is the product of these two fractions as follows:

$$f = \text{Fraction of drug absorbed} \times \text{Fraction escaping first-pass metabolism}$$

The bioavailability is lowest, then, for those drugs that undergo a significant first-pass effect. For these drugs, a hepatic extraction ratio, or the fraction of drug metabolized, E, is calculated. The fraction of drug that enters the system circulation and is ultimately available to exert its effect then is equal to the quantity (1 − E). Table 3–8 lists some drugs according to their pharmacologic class that undergo a significant first-pass effect when administered by the oral route.

To compensate for this marked effect, the drug manufacturer may consider other routes of drug administration, e.g., intravenous, intramuscular, sublingual, that avoid the first-pass effect. With these routes there will be a corresponding decrease in the dosage required when compared to oral administration.

Table 3–7. Dosage and Kinetics of Nitroglycerin in Various Dosage Forms[1]

Nitroglycerin, Dosage Form	*Usual Recommended Dosage (mg)*	*Onset of Action (Minutes)*	*Peak Action (Minutes)*	*Duration (Minutes/hours)*
Sublingual	0.3–0.8	2–5	4–8	10–30 minutes
Buccal	1–3	2–5	4–10	30–300 minutes[Δ]
Oral	6.5–19.5	20–45	45–120	2–6 hours[Ω]
Ointment (2%)	½–2 inches	15–60	30–120	3–8 hours
Discs	5–10	30–60	60–180	Up to 24 hours

[Δ] Effect persists so long as tablet is intact.

[Ω] Some short-term dosing studies have demonstrated effects to 8 hours.

[1] From Abrams, J.: Nitroglycerin and Long-Acting Nitrates in Clinical Practice. *The American Journal of Medicine,* Proceedings of a Symposium: First North American Conference of Nitroglycerin Therapy, June 27, 1983, p. 88.

Table 3–8. Examples of Drugs that Undergo Significant Liver Metabolism and Exhibit Low Bioavailability when Administered by First-pass Routes

Drug Class	*Examples*
Analgesics	Aspirin, meperidine, pentazocine, propoxyphene
Antianginal	Nitroglycerin
Antiarrhythmics	Lidocaine
Beta-adrenergic blockers	Labetolol, metoprolol, propranolol
Calcium channel blockers	Verapamil
Sympathomimetic amines	Isoproterenol
Tricyclic antidepressants	Desipramine, imipramine, nortriptyline

Another consideration centers around the metabolites themselves, and whether they are pharmacologically active or inactive. If they are inactive, a larger oral dose will be required to attain the desired therapeutic effect when compared to a lower dosage in a nonfirst-pass effect route. The classic example of drug that exhibits this effect is propranolol. If, on the other hand, the metabolites are the active species, the oral dosage must be carefully tailored to the desired therapeutic effect. First-pass metabolism in this case will result in a quicker therapeutic response than that achieved by a nonfirst-pass effect route.

One must remember also that the flow of blood through the liver can be decreased under certain conditions. Consequently, the bioavailability of those drugs that undergo a first-pass effect then would be expected to increase. For example, during cirrhosis the blood flow to the kidney is dramatically decreased and efficient hepatic extraction by enzymes responsible for a drug's metabolism also falls off. Consequently, in cirrhotic patients the dosage of drug that undergoes a first-pass effect from oral administration will have to be reduced to avoid toxicity.

Oral Route

Drugs are most frequently taken by oral administration. Although a few drugs taken orally are intended to be dissolved within the mouth, the vast majority of drugs taken orally are swallowed. Of these, most are taken for the *systemic* drug effects that result after absorption from the various surfaces along the gastrointestinal tract. A few drugs, such as antacids, are swallowed for their local action within the confines of the gastrointestinal tract.

Compared with alternate routes, the oral route is considered the most natural, uncomplicated, convenient, and safe means of administering drugs. Disadvantages of the oral route include slow drug response (when compared with parenterally administered drugs); chance of irregular absorption of drugs, depending upon such factors as constitutional make-up, the amount or type of food present within the gastrointestinal tract; and the destruction of certain drugs by the acid reaction of the stomach or by gastrointestinal enzymes.

DOSAGE FORMS APPLICABLE. Drugs are administered by the oral route in a variety of pharmaceutical forms. The most popular are tablets, capsules, suspensions, and various pharmaceutical solutions. Briefly, *tablets* are solid dosage forms prepared by compression or molding and contain medicinal substances with or without suitable diluents, disintegrants, coatings, colorants, and other pharmaceutical adjuncts. Diluents are fillers used in preparing tablets of the proper size and consistency. Disintegrants are used for the break-up or separation of the tablet's compressed ingredients. This ensures prompt exposure of drug particles to the dissolution process thereby enhancing drug absorption, as shown in Figure 3–12. Tablet coatings are of several types and for several different purposes. Some called *enteric coatings* are employed to permit safe pas-

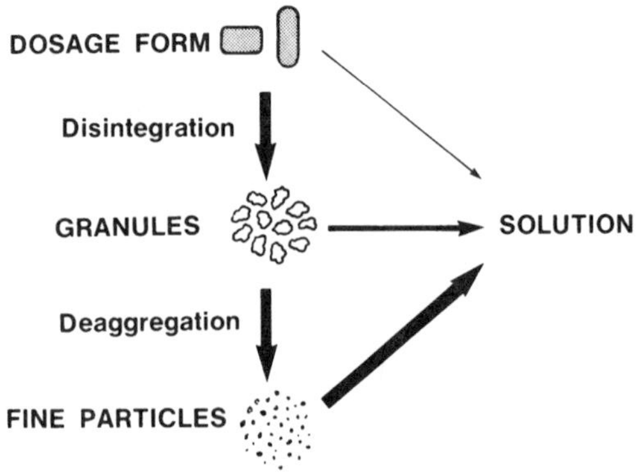

Fig. 3–12. *Schematic drawing showing disintegration of a tablet dosage form and direct availability of the contents in a capsule dosage form for dissolution and drug absorption after oral administration. (From Rowland, M., and Rozer, T.N.:* Clinical Pharmacokinetics. *2nd Ed., Philadelphia, Lea & Febiger, 1989.)*

sage of a tablet through the acid environment of the stomach where certain drugs may be destroyed, to the more suitable juices of the intestines where tablet dissolution safely takes place. Other coatings are employed to protect the drug substance from the destructive influences of moisture, light, and air throughout their period of storage or to conceal a bad or bitter taste from the taste buds of a patient. Commercial tablets, because of their distinctive shapes, colors, and frequently employed monograms of company symbols and code numbers facilitate identification by persons trained in their use and serve as an added protection to public health.

Capsules are solid dosage forms in which the drug substance and appropriate pharmaceutical adjuncts as fillers are enclosed in either a hard or a soft "shell," generally composed of a form of gelatin. Capsules vary in size, depending upon the amount of drug to be administered, and are of distinctive shapes and colors when produced commercially. Generally, drug materials are released from capsules faster than from tablets. Capsules of gelatin, a protein, are rapidly disfigured within the gastrointestinal tract, permitting the gastric juices to permeate and reach the contents. Because unsealed capsules have been subject to tampering by unscrupulous individuals, many capsules nowadays are sealed by fusion of the two capsule shells. Also, capsule-shaped and coated tablets, called "caplets," are increasingly utilized. These are easily swallowed but their contents are sealed and protected from tampering like tablets.

Suspensions are preparations of finely divided drugs held in suspension throughout a suitable vehicle. Suspensions taken orally generally employ an aqueous vehicle, whereas those employed for other purposes may utilize a different vehicle. Suspensions of certain drugs to be used for intramuscular injection, for instance, may be maintained in a suitable oil. To be suspended, the drug particles must be insoluble in the vehicle in which they are placed. Nearly all suspensions must be shaken before use because they tend to settle. This ensures not only uniformity of the preparation but more importantly the administration of the proper dosage. Suspensions are a useful means to administer large amounts of solid drugs that would be inconveniently taken in tablet or capsule form. In addition, suspensions have the advantage over solid dosage forms in that they are presented to the body in fine particle size, ready for the dissolution process immediately upon administration. However, not all oral suspensions are intended to be dissolved and absorbed by the body. For instance, Kaolin Mixture with Pectin, an antidiarrheal preparation, contains suspended kaolin, which acts in the intestinal tract by adsorbing excessive intestinal fluid on the large surface area of its particles.

Drugs administered in aqueous solution are generally absorbed much more rapidly than those administered in solid form, because the processes of disintegration and dissolution are not required. Pharmaceutical solutions may differ in the type of solvent employed and therefore in their fluidity characteristics. Among the solutions frequently administered orally are *elixirs,* which are solutions in a sweetened hydroalcoholic vehicle and are generally more mobile than water; *syrups,* which generally utilize sucrose solutions as the sweet vehicle resulting in a viscous preparation; and *solutions* themselves, which officially are preparations in which the drug substance is dissolved predominantly in an aqueous vehicle and do not for reasons of their method of preparation (e.g., injections, which must be sterilized) fall into another category of pharmaceutical preparations.

ABSORPTION. Absorption of drugs after oral administration may occur at the various body sites between the mouth and rectum. In general, the higher up a drug is absorbed along the length of the alimentary tract, the more rapid will be its action, a desirable feature in most instances. Because of the differences in the chemical and physical nature among drug substances, a given drug may be better absorbed from the environment of one site than from another within the alimentary tract.

The oral cavity is used on certain occasions as the absorption site of certain drugs. Physically, the oral absorption of drugs is managed by allowing the drug substance to be dissolved within the oral cavity with infrequent or no swallowing until the taste of the drug has dissipated. This process is accommodated by providing the drug as extremely soluble and rapidly dissolving uncoated tablets. Drugs capable of being absorbed in the mouth present themselves to the absorbing surface in a much more concentrated form than when swallowed, since drugs become progressively more diluted with gastrointestinal secretions and contents as they pass along the alimentary tract.

Currently the oral or *sublingual* (beneath the

tongue) administration of drugs is regularly employed for only a few drugs, with nitroglycerin and certain steroid sex hormones being the best examples. Nitroglycerin, a coronary vasodilator used in the prophylaxis and treatment of angina pectoris, is available in the form of tiny tablets which are allowed to dissolve under the tongue, producing therapeutic effects in a few minutes after administration. The dose of nitroglycerin is so small (usually 400 mcg) that if it were swallowed the resulting dilute gastrointestinal concentration may not result in reliable and sufficient drug absorption. Even more important, however, is the fact that nitroglycerin is rapidly destroyed by the liver throught the *first-pass effect*. Many sex hormones have been shown to be absorbed materially better from sublingual administration than when swallowed. Although the sublingual route is probably an effective absorption route for many other drugs, it has not been extensively used, primarily because other routes have proven satisfactory and more convenient for the patient. Retaining drug substances in the mouth is unattractive because of the bitter taste of most drugs.

Drugs may be altered within the gastrointestinal tract to render them less available for absorption. This may result from the drug's interaction with or binding to some normal constituent of the gastrointestinal tract or a foodstuff or even another drug. For instance, the absorption of the tetracycline group of antibiotics is greatly interfered with by the simultaneous presence of calcium. Because of this, tetracycline drugs must not be taken with milk or other calcium-containing foods or drugs.

In some instances it is the intent of the pharmacist to prepare a formulation that releases the drug slowly over an extended period of time. There are many methods by which slow release is accomplished, including the complexation of the drug with another material, the combination of which is only slowly released from the dosage form. An example of this is the slow-release waxy matrix potassium chloride tablets. These are designed to release their contents gradually as they are shunted through the gastrointestinal tract. Because their contents are leached out gradually there is less incidence of gastric irritation. The intermingling of food and drug generally results in delayed drug absorption. Since most drugs are absorbed more effectively from the intestines than from the stomach, when rapid absorption is intended, it is generally desirable to have the drug pass from the stomach into the intestines as rapidly as possible. Therefore, gastric emptying time is an important factor in effecting drug action dependent upon intestinal absorption. Gastric emptying time may be increased by a number of factors, including the presence of fatty foods (more effect than proteins, which in turn have more effect than carbohydrates), lying on the back when bedridden (lying on the right side facilitates passage in many instances), and the presence of drugs (for example, morphine) that have a quieting effect on the movements of the gastrointestinal tract. If a drug is administered in the form of a solution, it may be expected to pass into the intestines more rapidly than drugs administered in solid form. As a rule, large volumes of water taken with medication facilitate gastric emptying and passage into the intestines.

The pH of the gastrointestinal tract increases progressively along its length from a pH of about 1 in the stomach to approximately pH 8 at the far end of the intestines. pH has a definite bearing on the degree of ionization of most drugs, and this in turn affects lipid solubility, membrane permeability and absorption. Because most drugs are absorbed by passive diffusion through the lipoid barrier, the lipid/water partition coefficient and the pK_a of the drugs are of prime importance to both their degree and site of absorption within the gastrointestinal tract. As a general rule, weak acids are largely *un*ionized in the stomach and are absorbed fairly well from this site, whereas weak bases are highly ionized in the stomach and are not significantly absorbed from the gastric surface. Alkalinization of the gastric environment by artificial means (simultaneous administration of alkaline or antacid drugs) would be expected to decrease the gastric absorption of weak acids and to increase that of weak bases. Strong acids and bases are generally poorly absorbed due to their high degrees of ionization.

The small intestine serves as the major absorption pathway for drugs because of its suitable pH and the great surface area available for drug absorption within its approximate 20-foot length extending from the pylorus at the base of the stomach to the junction with the large intestine at the cecum. The pH of the lumen of the intestine is about 6.5 (see Fig. 3–3) and both weakly acidic and weakly basic drugs are well absorbed from the intestinal surface, which behaves in the ionization and distribution of drugs between it and the plasma on the other side of the membrane as though its pH were about 5.3.

Rectal Route

Some drugs are administered rectally for their local effects and others for their systemic effects. Drugs given rectally may be administered as solutions, suppositories, or ointments. *Suppositories* are defined as solid bodies of various weights and shapes intended for introduction into a body orifice (usually rectal, vaginal, or urethral) where they soften, melt, or dissolve, release their medication, and exert their drug effects. These effects simply may be the promotion of laxation (as with glycerin suppositories), the soothing of inflamed tissues (as with various commercial suppositories used to relieve the discomfort of hemorrhoids), or the promotion of systemic effects (as antinausea or antimotion sickness). The composition of the suppository base, or carrier of the medication, can greatly influence the degree and rate of drug release and should be selected on an individual basis for each drug. The use of rectal ointments is generally limited to the treatment of local conditions. Rectal solutions are usually employed as enemas or cleansing solutions.

The rectum and the colon are capable of absorbing many soluble drugs. Rectal administration for systemic action may be preferred for those drugs destroyed or inactivated by the environments of the stomach and intestines. The administration of drugs by the rectal route may also be indicated when the oral route is precluded because of vomiting or when the patient is unconscious or incapable of swallowing drugs safely without choking. It is estimated that about 50% of a dose of drug absorbed from rectal administration is likely to bypass the liver, an important factor when considering those orally administered drugs that are rapidly destroyed in the liver by the first-pass effect. On the negative side, compared with oral administration, rectal administration of drugs is inconvenient, and the absorption of drugs from the rectum is frequently irregular and difficult to predict.

Parenteral Route

The term *parenteral* is derived from the Greek words *para,* meaning beside, and *enteron,* meaning intestine, which together indicate something done outside of the intestine and not by way of the alimentary tract. A drug administered parenterally is one injected through the hollow of a fine needle into the body at various sites and to various depths. Th
parenteral administra
tramuscular (I.M.), a
though there are othe
intraspinal.

Drugs destroyed or
testinal tract or too poorly absorbed to provide satisfactory response may be parenterally administered. The parenteral route is also preferred when rapid absorption is essential, as in emergency situations. Absorption by the parenteral route is not only faster than after oral administration, but the blood levels of drug that result are far more predictable, because little is lost after subcutaneous or intramuscular injection, and virtually none by intravenous injection; this also generally permits the administration of smaller doses. The parenteral route of administration is especially useful in treating patients who are uncooperative, unconscious, or otherwise unable to accept oral medication.

One disadvantage of parenteral administration is that once the drug is injected, there is no retreat. That is, once the substance is within the tissues or is placed directly into the blood stream, removal of the drug warranted by an untoward or toxic effect or an inadvertent overdose is most difficult. By other means of administration, there is more time between drug administration and drug absorption, which becomes a safety factor by allowing for the extraction of unabsorbed drug (as by the induction of vomiting after an orally administered drug). Also, because of the strict sterility requirements for all injections, they are generally more expensive than other dosage forms and require competent trained personnel for their proper administration.

DOSAGE FORMS APPLICABLE. Pharmaceutically, injectable preparations are usually either sterile suspensions or solutions of a drug substance in water or in a suitable vegetable oil. In general, drugs in solution act more rapidly than drugs in suspension, with an aqueous vehicle providing faster action in each instance than an oleaginous vehicle. As in other instances of drug absorption, a drug must be in solution to be absorbed, and a suspended drug must first submit to the dissolution process. Also, because body fluids are aqueous, they are more receptive to drugs in an aqueous vehicle than those in an oily one. For these reasons, the rate of drug absorption can be varied in parenteral products by selective combinations of drug state and supporting vehicle. For instance, a suspension of a drug in a vegetable ely would be much more slowly absorbed n an aqueous solution of the same drug. Slow absorption generally means prolonged drug action, and when this is achieved through pharmaceutical means, the resulting preparation is referred to as a *depot* or *repository* injection, because it represents a storage reservoir of the drug substance within the body from which it is slowly removed into the systemic circulation. In this regard, even more sustained drug action may be achieved through the use of subcutaneous implantation of compressed tablets, termed pellets which are only slowly dissolved from their site of implantation, releasing their medication at a rather constant rate over a period of several weeks to many months. The repository type of injection is mainly limited to the subcutaneous or intramscular route. It is obvious that drugs injected intraveously do not encounter absorption barriers and thus produce only rapid drug effects. Preparations for intravenous injection must not interfere with the blood components or with circulation and therefore, with few exceptions, are aqueous solutions.

SUBCUTANEOUS INJECTIONS. The subcutaneous (hypodermic) administration of drugs involves their injection through the layers of skin into the loose subcutaneous tissue. Generally, subcutaneous injections are prepared as aqueous solutions or as suspensions and are administered in relatively small volumes of 2 mL or less. Insulin is an example of a drug administered by the subcutaneous route. Subcutaneous injections are generally given in the forearm, upper arm, thigh, or nates. If the patient is to receive frequent injections, it is best to alterate injection sites to reduce tissue irritation. After injection, the drug comes into the immediate vicinity of blood capillaries and permates them by diffusion or filtration. The capillary wall is an example of a membrane that behaves as a lipid pore barrier, with lipid-soluble substances penetrating the membrane at rates varying with their oil/water partition coefficients. Lipid-insoluble (generally more water-soluble) drugs penetrate the capillary membrane at rates which appear to be inversely related to their molecular size, with smaller molecules penetrating much more rapidly than larger ones. All substances, whether lipid-soluble or not, cross the capillary membrane at rates that are much more rapid than the rates of their transfer across other body membranes. The blood supply to the site of injection is an important factor in considering the rate of drug absorption, consequently the more proximal capillaries are to the site of injection, the more prompt will be the drug's entrance into the circulation. Also, the more capillaries, the more surface area for absorption, and the faster the rate of absorption. Some substances have the capability of modifying the rate of drug absorption from a subcutaneous site of injection. The addition of a vasconstrictor to the injection formulation (or its prior injection) will generally diminish the rate of drug absorption by causing constriction of the blood vessels in the area of injection and thereby reducing blood flow and the capacity for absorption. This principle is utilized in the administration of local anesthetics by employing the vasoconstrictor epinephrine. Conversely, vasodilators may be employed to enhance subcutaneous absorption by increasing blood flow to the area. Physical exercise can also influence the absorption of drug from an injection site. Diabetic patients who rotate subcutaneous injection sites and then do physical exercise, e.g., jogging, must realize the onset of insulin activity might be influenced by the selected site of administration. Because of the movement of the leg and blood circulation to it during running, the absorption of insulin from a thigh injection site would be expected to be faster than that from an abdominal injection site.

INTRAMUSCULAR INJECTIONS. Intramuscular injections are performed deep into the skeletal muscles, generally the gluteal or lumbar muscles. The site is selected where the danger of hitting a nerve or blood vessel is minimal. Aqueous or oleaginous solutions or suspensions may be used intramuscularly. Certain drugs, because of their inherent low solubilities, provide sustained drug action after an intramuscular injection. For instance, one deep intramuscular injection of a suspension of penicillin G benzathine results in effective blood levels of the drug for seven to ten days.

Drugs which are irritating to subcutaneous tissue are often administered intramuscularly. Also, greater volumes (2 to 5 mL) may be administered intramuscularly than subcutaneously. When a volume greater than 5 mL is to be injected, it is frequently administered in divided doses using two injection sites. Injection sites best are rotated when a patient is receiving repeated injections over a period of time.

INTRAVENOUS INJECTIONS. In the intravenous administration of drugs, an aqueous solution is injected directly into the vein at a rate commensurate with efficiency, safety, comfort to the patient, and the desired duration of drug response. Drugs may be administered intravenously as a single, small-volume injection or as a large-volume, slow intravenous drip infusion (as is common following surgery). Intravenous injection allows the desired blood level of drug to be achieved in an optimal and quantitative manner. Intravenous injections are usually made into the veins of the forearm and are especially useful in emergency situations where immediate drug response is desired. It is essential that the drug be maintained in solution after injection and not be precipitated within the circulatory system, an event that might produce emboli. Because of a fear of the development of pulmonary embolism, oleaginous bases are not usually intravenously administered. However, an intravenous fat emulsion is used therapeutically as a caloric source for patients receiving parenteral nutrition whose caloric requirements cannot be met by glucose. It may be administered either through a peripheral vein or a central venous catheter at a distinct rate to help prevent the occurrence of untoward reactions.

INTRADERMAL INJECTIONS. These injections are administered into the corium of the skin, usually in volumes of about a tenth of a milliliter. Common sites for the injection are the arm and the back. The injections are frequently performed as diagnostic measures, as in tuberculin and allergy testing.

Epicutaneous Route

Drugs are administered topically, or applied to the skin, for their action at the site of application or for systemic drug effects.

In general, drug absorption via the skin is enhanced if the drug substance is in solution, if it has a favorable lipid/water partition coefficient, and if it is a nonelectrolyte. Drugs that are absorbed enter the skin by way of the pores, sweat glands, hair follicles, sebaceous glands, and other anatomic structures of the skin's surface. Because blood capillaries are present just below the epidermal cells, a drug that penetrates the skin and is able to traverse the capillary wall finds ready access to the general circulation.

Among the few drugs currently employed topically to the skin surface for percutaneous absorption and systemic action are nitroglycerin (antianginal), nicotine (smoking cessation), estradiol (estrogenic hormone), clonidine (antihypertensive), and scopolamine (antinausea/anti-motion sickness). Each of these drugs is available for use in the form of transdermal delivery systems fabricated as an adhesive disc or patch which slowly releases the medication for percutaneous absorption. Additionally, nitroglycerin is available in an ointment form of application to the skin's surface for systemic absorption. Nitroglycerin is employed therapeutically for ischemic heart diease, with the transermal dosage forms becoming increasingly popular because of the benefit in patient compliance through their long-acting (24 hours) characteristics. The nitroglycerin patch is generally applied to the arm or chest, preferably in a hair-free or shaven area. The transdermal scopolamine sytem is also in the form of a patch to be applied to the skin; in this case, behind the ear. The drug system is indicated for the prevention of nausea and vomiting associated with motion sickness. The commercially available product is applied to the postauricular area several hours before need (as prior to an air or sea trip) where it releases its medication over a period of 3 days. The concepts of transdermal therapeutic systems are discussed further in Chapter 10.

For the most part, pharmaceutical preparations applied to the skin are intended to serve some local action and as such are formulated to provide prolonged local contact with minimal absorption. Drugs applied to the skin for their local action include antiseptics, antifungal agents, anti-inflammatory agents, local anesthetic agents, skin emollients, and protectants, against environmental conditions, as the effects of the sun, wind, pests, and chemical irritants. For these purposes drugs are most commonly administered in the form of ointments and related semisolid preparations such as creams and pastes, as solid dry powders, aerosol sprays or as liquid preparations such as solutions and lotions.

Pharmaceutically, ointments, creams, and pastes are semisolid preparations in which the drug is contained in a suitable base (ointment base) which is itself semisolid and either hydrophilic or hydrophobic in character. These bases play an important role in the proper formulation of semisolid preparations, and there is no single base universally suitable as a carrier of all drug substances or for all therapeutic indications. The proper base for a drug must be determined individually to provide the desired drug release rate, staying qualities after application, and texture. Briefly, *ointments* are simple mixtures of drug substances in an ointment base, whereas *creams* are semisolid emulsions and are generally less viscid and lighter than ointments. Creams are considered to have greater esthetic appeal due to their nongreasy character and their ability to "vanish" into the skin upon rubbing. *Pastes* contain more solid materials than do ointments and are therefore stiffer and less penetrating. Pastes are usually employed for their protective action and for their ability to absorb serous discharges from skin lesions. Thus when protective rather than therapeutic action is desired, the formulation pharmacist will favor a paste, but when therapeutic action is required, he will prefer ointments and creams. Commerically, many therapeutic agents are prepared in both ointment and cream form and are dispensed and used according to the particular preference of the patient and the prescribing practitioner.

Medicinal powders are intimate mixtures of medicinal substances usually in an inert base as talcum powder. Depending upon the particle size of the resulting blend, the powder will have varying dusting and covering capabilities. In any case, the particle size should be small enough to ensure against grittiness and consequent skin irritation. Powders are most frequently applied topically to relieve such conditions as diaper rash, chafing, and athlete's foot.

When topical application is desired in liquid form other than solution, lotions are most frequently employed. *Lotions* are generally suspensions of solid materials in an aqueous vehicle, although certain emulsions and even some true solutions have been designated as lotions because of either their appearance or application. Lotions may be preferred over semisolid preparations because of their nongreasy character and their increased spreadability over large areas of skin.

Ocular, Oral, and Nasal Routes

Drugs are frequently applied topically to the eye, ear, and the mucous membranes of the nose. In these instances, ointments, suspensions, and solutions are generally employed. Ophthalmic solutions and suspensions are sterile aqueous preparations with other quantities essential to the safety and comfort of the patient. Ophthalmic ointments must be sterile, and also free of grittiness. Innovative new delivery systems for ophthalmic drugs continue to be investigated. One dosage form, the Ocusert, is an elliptically shaped unit designed for continuous release of pilocarpine following its placement into the cul-de-sac of the eye. Further, case reports of the ability of soft contact lenses to absorb drug from the eye have spawned research in the development of soft contact lenses impregnated with drug for therapeutic application in the eye. Nasal preparations are usually solutions or suspensions administered by drops or as a fine mist from a nasal spray container. Current research is directed toward the feasibility of the nasal administration of insulin for diabetes mellitus. Otic, or ear preparations are usually viscid so that they have prolonged contact with the affected area. They may be employed simply to soften ear wax, to relieve an earache, or to combat an ear infection. Eye, ear, and nose preparations are not generally employed for systemic effects, and although ophthalmic and otic preparations are not usually absorbed to any great extent, nasal preparations *may* be absorbed, and systemic effects after the intranasal application of solution are not unusual.

Other Routes

The lungs provide an excellent absorbing surface for the administration of gases and for aerosol mists of very minute particles of liquids or solids. The gases employed are mainly oxygen and the common general anesthetic drugs administered to patients entering surgery. The rich capillary area of the alveoli of the lungs, which in man covers nearly a thousand square feet, provides rapid absorption and drug effects comparable in speed to those following an intravenous injection. In the case of drug particles, their size largely determines the depth to which they penetrate the alveolar regions; their solubility, the extent to which they are absorbed. After contact with the inner surface of the lungs, an insoluble drug particle is caught in the mucus and is moved up the pulmonary tree by ciliary action. Soluble drug particles that are approximately 0.5 to 1.0 micron in size reach the minute alveolar sacs and are most prompt and efficient in providing systemic effects. Particles that are smaller than 0.5 micron are expired to some extent, and thus their absorption is not total but variable. Particles from 1 to 10 microns in size effectively reach the terminal bronchioles and to some extent the alveolar ducts and are favored for local therapy. Therefore, in the pharmaceutical manufacture of aerosol sprays for inhalation therapy, the manufacturers not only must attain the proper drug particle size but also must ensure their uniformity for consistent penetration of the pulmonary tree and uniform effects.

In certain instances and generally for local effects, drugs are inserted into the vagina and the urethra. Drugs are generally presented to the vagina in tablet form, as suppositories, ointments, emulsion foams, or solutions, and to the urethra as suppositories or solutions. Systemic drug effects, which may result after the vaginal or urethral application of drugs due to absorption of the drug from the mucous membranes of these sites, are generally undesired.

Fate of Drug after Absorption

After absorption into the general circulation from any route of administration, a drug may become bound to blood proteins and delayed in its passage into the surrounding tissues. Many drug substances may be highly bound to blood protein and others little-bound. For instance, when in the blood stream, naproxen is 99% bound to plasma proteins, penicillin G is 60% bound, amoxicillin only 20% bound, and minoxidil is unbound.

The degree of drug binding to plasma proteins is usually expressed as a percentage or as a fraction (termed *alpha,* or α) of the bound concentration (C_b) to the total concentration (C_t), bound plus unbound (C_u) drug:

$$\alpha = \frac{C_b}{C_u + C_b} = \frac{C_b}{C_t}$$

Thus, if one knows two of the three terms in the equation, the third may be calculated. Drugs having an alpha value of greater than 0.9 are considered highly bound (90%); those drugs with an alpha value of less than 0.2 are considered to be little (20% or less) protein bound. Table 3–9 presents approximate serum protein binding characteristics for representative drugs present in the blood under conditions associated with usual therapy. The drug-protein complex is reversible and generally involves albumin, although globulins are also involved in the binding of drugs, particularly some of the hormones. The binding of drugs to biologic materials generally involves the formation of relatively weak bonds (e.g., van der Waals, hydrogen, and ionic bonds). The binding capacity of blood proteins is limited, and once they are saturated, additional drug absorbed into the blood stream remains unbound unless bound drug is released, creating a vacant site for another drug molecule to attach.

Table 3–9. Examples of Drug Binding to Plasma Proteins

Drug	*Percent Bound*[1]
Naproxen (Naprosyn, Syntex)	>99
Chlorambucil (Leukeran, B/W)	99
Etodolac (Lodine, Wyeth-Ayerst)	99
Warfarin (Coumadin, DuPont)	97
Fluoxetine (Prozac, Lilly)	95
Cloxacillin (Tegopen, Apothecon)	95
Ceftriaxone (Rocephin, Roche)	85–95
Cefoperazone (Cefobid, Roerig)	82–93
Cefonicid (Monocid, SKB)	>90
Indomethacine (Indocin, MSD)	90
Spironolactone (Aldactone, Searle)	90
Digitoxin (Crystodigin, Lilly)	90
Cyclosporine (Sandimmune, Sandoz)	90
Sulfisoxazole (Gantrisin, Roche)	85
Diltiazem (Cardizem, MMD)	70–80
Penicillin V (Veetids, Apothecon)	75
Nitroglycerin (Nitro-Bid, MMD)	60
Penicillin G Potassium (Biocraft)	60
Methotrexate (Lederle)	50
Methicillin (Staphcillin, Bristol)	40
Ceftizoxime (Cefizox, Fujisawa)	30
Captopril (Capozide, Squibb)	25–30
Ciprofloxacin (Cipro, Miles)	20–40
Digoxin (Lanoxin, B/W)	20–25
Ampicillin (Omnipen, Wyeth-Ayerst)	20
Amoxicillin (Amoxil, SKB)	20
Metronidazole (Flagyl, Searle)	<20
Mercaptopurine (Purinethol, B/W)	19
Cephradine (Valosef, Squibb)	8–17
Ranitidine (Zantac, Glaxo)	15
Ceftazidime (Tazicef, SKB)	<10
Nicotine (Prostep, Lederle)	<5
Minoxidil (Loniten, Upjohn)	0

[1] Average literature values, based on conditions usually associated with drug therapy.

Any unbound drug is free to leave the blood stream for tissues or cellular sites within the body.

Bound drug is neither exposed to the body's detoxication (metabolism) processes nor is it filtered through the renal glomeruli. Bound drug is therefore referred to as the *inactive* portion in the blood, and unbound drug, with its ability to penetrate cells, is termed the *active* blood portion. The bound portion of drug serves as a drug reservoir or a depot, from which the drug is released as the free form when the level of free drug in the blood no longer is adequate to ensure protein saturation. The free drug may be only slowly released, thereby increasing the duration of the drug's stay in the body. For this reason a drug that is highly protein bound may remain in the body for longer periods of time and require less frequent dosage administration than another drug that may be only slightly protein bound and may remain in the body for only a short period of time. Evidence suggests that the concentration of serum albumin decreases about 20% in the elderly. This may be clinically significant for drugs that bind strongly to albumin, e.g., phenytoin, because if there is less albumin available to bind the drug there will be a corresponding increase of the free drug in the body. Without a downward dosage adjustment in an elderly patient there could be an increase incidence of adverse effects.

A drug's binding to blood proteins may be affected by the simultaneous presence of a second (or more) drug(s). The additional drug(s) may result in drug effects or durations of drug action quite dissimilar to that found when each is administered alone. Salicylates, for instance, have the effect of decreasing the binding capacity of thyroxin, the thyroid hormone, to proteins. Phenylbutazone is an example of a drug that competitively displaces several other drugs from serum binding sites, including other antiinflammatory drugs, oral anticoagulants, oral antidiabetics, and sulfonamides. Through this action, the displaced drugs become less protein bound and their activity (and toxicity) may be increased. The intensity of a drug's pharmacologic response is related to the ratio of the bound drug *versus* free, active drug, and the therapeutic index of the drug. Warfarin, an anticoagulant is 97% bound to plasma protein leaving 3% in free form to exert its effect. If a second drug, such as naproxen, which is strongly bound to plasma proteins is administered and results in only 90% of the warfarin being bound, this means that 10% of warfarin is now in the free form. Thus, the blood level of the free warfarin (3 to 10%) has tripled and could result in serious toxicity. The displacement of drugs from plasma protein sites is typical in the elderly who normally are maintained on numerous medicines. Coupled with the aforementioned decrease in serum protein through the aging process the addition of a highly protein-bound drug to an elderly patient's existing treatment regimen could pose significant problems if the patient is not monitored carefully for signs of toxicity.

In the same manner as they are bound to blood proteins, drugs may become bound to specific components of certain cells. Thus drugs are not distributed uniformly among all cells of the body, but rather tend to pass from the blood into the fluid bathing the tissues and may accumulate in certain cells according to their permeability capabilities and chemical and physical affinities. This affinity for certain body sites influences their action, for they may be brought into contact with reactive tissues (their *receptor sites*) or deposited in places where they may be inactive. Many drugs, because of their affinity for and solubility in lipids, are found to be deposited in fatty body tissue, thereby creating a storage place or drug reservoir from which they are slowly released to other tissues.

Drug Metabolism (Biotransformation)

Although some drugs are excreted from the body in their original form, many drugs undergo biotransformation prior to excretion. Biotransformation is a term used to indicate the chemical changes that occur with drugs within the body as they are metabolized and altered by various biochemical mechanisms. Generally, the biotransformation of a drug results in its conversion to one or more compounds that are more water soluble, more ionized, less capable of binding to proteins of the plasma and tissues, less capable of being stored in fat tissue, and less able to penetrate cell membranes, and thereby less active pharmacologically. Because of its new characteristics, a drug so transformed is rendered less toxic and is more readily excreted. It is for this reason that the process of biotransformation is also commonly referred to as the "detoxification" or "inactivation" process. (However, sometimes the metabolites are more active than the parent compound; see *prodrugs,* following.)

The exact metabolic processes (pathways) by which drugs are transformed represent an active area of biomedical research. Much work has been done with the processes of animal degradation of drugs and in many instances the biotransformation in the animal is thought to parallel that in man. There are four principal chemical reactions involved in the metabolism of drugs: oxidation, reduction, hydrolysis, and conjugation. Most oxidation reactions are catalyzed by enzymes (oxidases) bound to the endoplasmic reticulum, a tubular system within liver cells; only a small fraction of drugs are metabolized by reduction, through the action of reductases, present in the gut and liver; esterases in the liver participate in the hydrolytic breakdown of drugs containing ester groups as well as amides; glucuronide conjugation is the most common pathway for drug metabolism, through combination of the drug with glucuronic acid, forming ionized compounds that are easily eliminated.[8] Other metabolic processes, including methylation and acylation conjugation reactions, occur with certain drugs to foster elimination.

In recent years, much interest has been shown in the metabolites of drug biotransformation. It is known that certain metabolites may be as active or even more active pharmacologically than the original compound. Occasionally an active drug may be converted into an active metabolite, which must be excreted as such or undergo further biotransformation to an inactive metabolite, e.g., amitriptyline to nortriptyline. In other instances of drug therapy, an inactive parent compound, referred to as a *prodrug,* may be converted to an active therapeutic agent by chemical transformation in the body. An example is the prodrug enalapril (Vasotec), which after oral administration is hydrolyzed to enalaprilat, an active angiotensin-converting enzyme (ACE) inhibitor used in the treatment of hypertension. Enalaprilat itself is poorly absorbed when taken orally (and thus the prodrug) but may be administered intravenously in aqueous solution. The use of these active metabolites as "original" drugs represents a new area of drug investigation and a vast reservoir of potential therapeutic agents.

Several examples of biotransformations occurring within the body are as follows:

(1) Acetaminophen (active) $\xrightarrow{\text{conjugation}}$ Acetaminophen glucuronide (inactive)

(2) Amoxapine (active) $\xrightarrow{\text{oxidation}}$ 8-hydroxy-amoxapine (inactive)

(3) Procainamide (active) $\xrightarrow{\text{hydrolysis}}$ p-Aminobenzoic acid (inactive)

(4) Nitroglycerin (active) $\xrightarrow{\text{reduction}}$ 1-2 and 1-3 dinitroglycerol (active)

Some parent compounds undergo full, partial, or no biotransformation following administration. Lisinopril (Zestril), for example, does not undergo metabolism and is excreted unchanged in the urine. On the other hand, verapamil (Calan) metabolizes to at least 12 metabolites, the most prevalent of which is norverapamil. Norverapamil has 20% of the cardiovascular activity of the parent compound. Diltiazem (Cardizem) is partially metabolized (about 20%) to desacetyldiltiazem, which has 10–20% the coronary vasodilator activity of the parent compound. Indomethacin (Indocin) is metabolized in part to desmethyl, desbenzoyl, and desmethyldesbenzoyl metabolites. Propoxyphene napsylate (Darvon N) is metabolized to norpropoxyphene, which has less central nervous system depressant action than the parent compound but greater local anesthetic effects. The majority of metabolic transformations takes place in the liver, with some drugs as diltiazem and verapamil undergoing extensive first-pass effects. Other drugs, such as terazosin (Hytrin), undergo minimal first-pass metabolism effects. The excretion of both drug and metabolites takes place primarily, but to varying degrees, via the urine and feces. For example, indomethacin and its metabolites are excreted primarily (60%) in the urine, with the remainder in the feces, whereas terazosin and its metabolites are excreted largely (60%) through the feces, and the remainder in the urine.

It is important to mention that several factors influence drug metabolism. For example, there are marked differences between *species* in pathways of hepatic metabolism of a given drug. Species differences make it extremely difficult to extrapolate from one species to another, e.g., laboratory animals to humans. Furthermore, there are many examples of *interindividual variations* in hepatic metabolism of drugs within one species. Genetic factors are involved in the determination of the basal activity of the drug-metabolizing enzyme systems. Thus, there can be marked intersubject variation in the rate at which certain individuals metabolically handle drugs. Because of this variation, a physician must individualize therapy to maximize the chances for a constructive therapeutic outcome with minimal toxicity. Studies in humans have demonstrated that these differences have occurred within the cytochrome P-450 genes codes for a family of isoenzymes responsible to drug metabolism.

Age of the patient is another significant factor that influences drug metabolism. Although pharmacokinetic calculations have not been able to develop a specific correlative relationship with age, it is known, for example, that the ability to metabolize drugs decreases at the extremes of the age scale, i.e., elderly, neonate. Liver blood flow is reduced by aging at about 1% per year beginning around age 30.[9] This decreased blood flow to the liver reduces the capacity for hepatic drug metabolism and elimination. For example, the half-life of chlordiazepoxide increases from about 6 hours at age 20 to about 36 hours at age 80. Further, an immature hepatic system disallows the effective metabolism of drugs by the newborn or premature infant. As mentioned earlier, the half-life of theophylline ranges between 14 to 58 hours in the premature infant to 2.5 to 5 hours in young children between the ages of 1 to 4 whose liver enzyme systems are mature.

Diet has also been demonstrated to modify the metabolism of some drugs. For example, the conversion of an asthmatic patient from a high to a low protein diet will increase the half-life of theophylline. It has also been demonstrated that the production of polycyclic hydrocarbons by the charcoal broiling of beef enhances the hepatic metabolism and shortens the plasma half-life of theophylline. It is conceivable that this effect could also occur with drugs that are metabolized in similar fashion to theophylline. Diet type, e.g., starvation, certain vegetables (brussels sprouts, cabbage, broccoli), has been shown to influence the metabolism of certain drugs. Lastly, it is important to mention that exposure to other drugs or chemicals, e.g., pesticides, alcohol, nicotine, and the presence of disease states, e.g., hepatitis, have all demonstrated an influence on the drug metabolism and consequently the pharmacokinetic profile of certain drugs.

Excretion of Drugs

The excretion of drugs and their metabolites terminates their activity and presence in the body. They may be eliminated by various routes, with the kidney playing the dominant role by eliminating drugs via the urine. Drug excretion with the feces is also important, especially for drugs that are poorly absorbed and remain in the gastrointestinal tract after oral administration. Exit through the bile is significant only when the drug's reabsorption from the gastrointestinal tract is minimal. The lungs provide the exit for many volatile drugs through the expired breath. The sweat glands, saliva, and milk play only minor roles in drug elimination. However, it should be recognized that if a drug gains access to the milk of a mother during lactation, it could easily exert its drug effects in the nursing infant. Examples of drugs that do enter breast milk and may be passed on to nursing infants include theophylline, penicillin, reserpine, codeine, meperidine, barbiturates, diltiazem, and thiazide diuretics. It is generally good practice for the mother to abstain from taking medication during the period of time she is nursing her infant. If she must take medication, she should abide by a dosage regimen and nursing schedule that permit her own therapy yet ensure the safety of her child. Not all drugs gain entrance into the milk; nevertheless, caution is advisable. Manufacturers' package inserts contain product-specific information (usually in the "Precautions" section) on drug migration into breast milk.

The unnecessary use of medications during the early stages of pregnancy is likewise restricted by physicians, because certain drugs are known to have the ability to cross the placental barrier and gain entrance to the tissues and blood of the fetus. Among the many drugs known to do so after administration to an expectant mother are all of the anesthetic gases, many barbiturates, sulfonamides, salicylates, and a number of other potent agents like quinine, meperidine, and morphine, the latter two drugs being narcotic analgesics with great addiction liabilities. In fact, it is not unusual for a newborn infant to be born an addict due to the narcotic addiction of its mother and the passage of the narcotic drugs across the placental barrier.

The kidney, as the main organ for the elimination of drugs from the body, must be functioning adequately if drugs are to be efficiently eliminated. For instance, elimination of digoxin occurs largely through the kidney according to first-order kinetics; that is, the quantity of digoxin eliminated at any time is proportional to the total body content. Renal excretion of digoxin is proportional to the glomerular filtration rate which when normal results in a digoxin half-life that may range from 1.5 to 2.0 days. When the glomerular filtration rate becomes impaired or disrupted, however, as in an anuric patient, the elimination rate decreases. Consequently, the half-life of digoxin may be between 4 to 6 days. Because of this prolongation of digoxin's half-life, the dosage of the drug must be decreased or the dosage interval prolonged. Otherwise, the patient will experience digoxin toxicity. The degree of impairment can be estimated by measurements of glomerular filtration rates, most often by creatinine clearance determination. Usually, however, this is not feasible and the patient's serum creatinine value is used within appropriate pharmacokinetic equations to help determine a drug's dosage regimen.

Some drugs may be reabsorbed from the renal tubule even after having been sent there for excretion. Because the rate of reabsorption is proportional to the concentration of drug in unionized form, it is possible to modify this rate by adjusting the pH of the urine. By acidifying the urine, as with the oral administration of ammonium chloride, or by alkalinizing it, as with the administration of sodium bicarbonate, one can increase or decrease the ionization of the drug and thereby alter its prospect of being reabsorbed. Alkalinization of the urine has been shown to enhance the urinary excretion of weak acids such as salicylates, sulfonamides, and phenobarbital. The opposite effect can be achieved by acidifying the urine. Thus, the duration of a drug's stay within the body may be markedly altered by changing the pH of the urine.

The urinary excretion of drugs may also be retarded by the concurrent administration of agents capable of inhibiting their tubular secretion. A well-known example is the use of probenecid to inhibit the tubular secretion of various types of penicillin, thereby reducing the frequency of dosage administrations usually necessary to maintain adequate therapeutic blood levels of the antibiotic drug. In this particular instance, the elevation of penicillin blood levels, by whatever route the antibiotic is administered, to twofold and even fourfold levels has been demonstrated by adjuvant therapy with probenecid. The effects are completely reversible upon withdrawal of the probenecid from concomitant therapy.

The fecal excretion of drugs appears to lag behind the rate of urinary excretion partly because a day or so elapses before the feces reach the rectum. It should be easily seen that drugs administered orally for local activity within the gastrointestinal trace and not absorbed will be eliminated completely via the feces. Unless a drug is particularly irritating to the gastrointestinal tract, there is generally no urgency in removing unabsorbable drugs from the system by means other than the normal defecation process. Some drugs that are only partially absorbed after oral administration will naturally be partly eliminated through the rectum.

Pharmacokinetic Principles

This section introduces the concept of pharmacokinetics and how it interrelates the various processes that take place when one administers a drug to a patient, i.e., absorption, distribution, metabolism, excretion. It is not intended to be comprehensive, and thus for further information about the subject the reader is referred to other appropriate literature sources.

A problem encountered when one needs to determine a more accurate dosage of a drug or a more meaningful interpretation of a biologic response to a dose is the inability to determine the drug concentration at the active site in the body. Consequently, to solve this dilemma, the concept of compartmental analysis is used within the discipline of pharmacokinetics in an attempt to quantitatively define what has become of the drug as a function of time from the moment it is administered until it is no longer in the body. Pharmacokinetic analysis utilizes mathematical models to simplify or simulate the disposition of the drug in the body. The idea is to begin with a simple model and then modify as necessary. The principal assumption is that the human body may be represented by one or more *compartments* or pools in which a drug resides in a dynamic state for a short period of time. A compartment is a hypothetical space bound by an unspecified membrane across which drugs are transferred (Fig. 3–13). The transfer of drugs into and out of this compartment is indicated by arrows that point in the direction of drug movement into or out of the compartment. The rate at which a drug is transferred throughout the system is designated by a symbol that usually represents an exponential rate constant. Typically, the letter K or k with numerical or alphanumerical subscripts is utilized.

There are several assumptions associated with modeling of drug behavior once in the body. It is assumed that the volume of each compartment remains constant. Thus, an equation that describes the time course of the amount of drug in the compartment can be converted to an equation that depicts the time course of the drug concentration in the compartment by dividing both sides of the equation by the volume of the compartment. Secondly, it is assumed that once a drug enters the compartment it is instantaneously and uniformly distributed throughout the entire compartment. Thus, it is assumed that a sampling of any one portion of the compartment will yield the drug concentration of the entire compartment.

In compartment models it is assumed that drug passes freely into and out of compartments. Thus, these compartmental systems are known as "open" systems. Typically, the process of drug transport between compartments follows

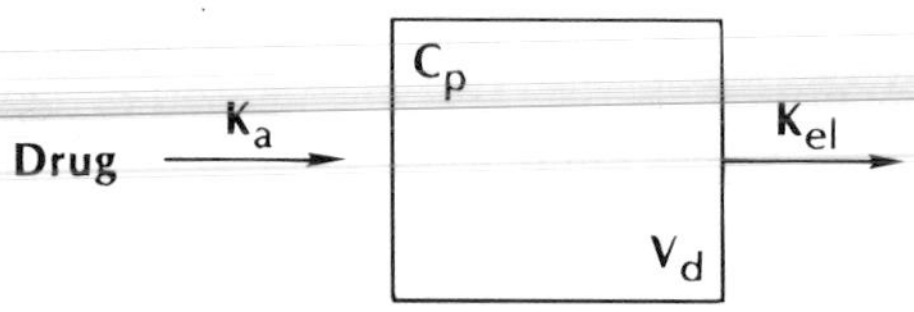

Where:
C_p is the drug concentration in plasma
V_d is the volume of the compartment or volume of distribution

Fig. 3–13. *Schematic of a one-compartment system.*

first-order kinetics, herein a constant fraction of drug present is eliminated per unit time, and can be described by ordinary differential equations. In these linear systems the time constants that describe the rate at which the plasma or blood concentration curve of a drug decays are independent of the dose of the drug, the volume of distribution of the drug and the route of administration.

The simplest pharmacokinetic model is the single compartment *open-model system* (Fig. 3–13). This model depicts the body as one compartment characterized by a certain volume of distribution (V_d) that remains constant. Each drug has its own distinct volume of distribution and this can be influenced by certain patient factors, e.g., age, disease state status. In this scheme a drug can be instantaneously introduced into the compartment, i.e., rapid intravenous administration, or gradually, e.g., oral administration. In the former example it is assumed that the drug distributes immediately to tissues with instantaneous attainment of equilibrium. In the latter example, the drug is absorbed at a certain rate and is characterized by the rate constant K_a. Lastly, the drug is eliminated from the compartment at a certain rate that is characterized by a rate constant K_{el}.

It is relevant at this point to consider the *volume of distribution*, V_d. The volume of distribution is a proportionality constant and is a term that refers to the volume into which the total amount of drug in the body would have to be uniformly distributed to provide the concentration of drug actually measured, e.g., in plasma, in blood. This term can be misleading because it does not represent a specific body fluid or volume. It is influenced by the plasma-protein binding and tissue binding characteristics of a drug. These then influence the distribution of the drug between plasma water, extracellular fluid, intracellular fluid and total body water. Further, because a drug can partition between fat and water according to its unique partition coefficient, this can also influence the volume of distribution. Because of these phenomena, pharmacokineticists find it convenient to describe a drug distribution in terms of compartment models.

To determine the rate of drug transfer into and out of the compartment, plasma, serum, or blood samples are drawn at predetermined times after the drug is administered and analyzed for drug concentration. Once a sufficient number of experimental data points is determined, these are plotted on semi-logarithmic paper and an attempt is made to fit the experimental points with the smoothest curve to fit these points. Figure 3–14 depicts the plasma concentration *versus* time profile for a hypothetical drug following rapid intravenous injection of a bolus dose of the drug with instantaneous distribution. For drugs whose distribution follows first-order, one-compartment pharmacokinetics, a plot of the logarithm of the concentration of drug in the plasma (or blood) versus time will yield a straight line. The equation that describes the plasma decay curve is:

$$C_p = C_p^0 \, e^{-K_{el}t} \qquad \text{(Equation 3–1)}$$

where K_{el} is the first-order rate of elimination of the drug from the body, C_p is the concentration

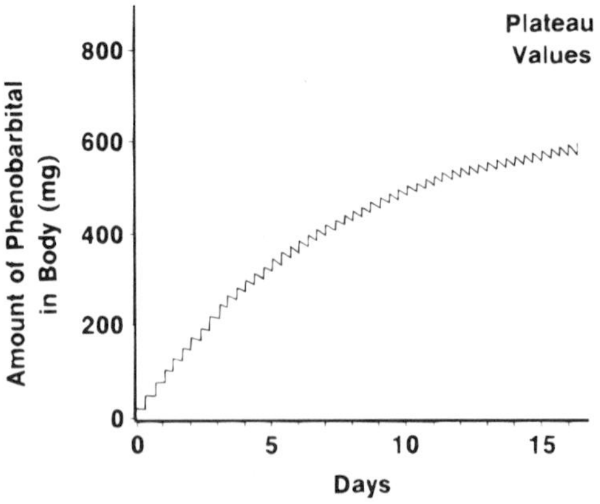

Fig. 3–14. *Semilogarithmic plot of the plasma concentration-time data. (From Rowland, M., and Tozer, T.N.:* Clinical Pharmacokinetics. *2nd Ed., Philadelphia, Lea & Febiger, 1989.)*

of the drug at a time equal to t, and C_p^0 is the concentration of drug at time equal to zero, when all the drug administered has been absorbed but none has been removed from the body through elimination mechanisms, e.g., metabolism, renal excretion. The apparent first-order rate of elimination, K_{el}, is usually the sum of the rate constants of a number of individual processes, e.g., metabolic transformation, renal excretion.

For the purpose of pharmacokinetic calculation it is simpler to convert Equation 3–1 to natural logs:

$$\text{Ln } C_p = \text{Ln } C_p^0 - K_{el}\,(t) \qquad \text{(Equation 3–2)}$$

and then to log base_{10}:

$$\text{Log } C_p = \text{Log } C_p^0 - K_{el}\,(t)/2.303 \qquad \text{(Equation 3–3)}$$

Equation 3–3 is then thought of in terms of the Y-intercept form:

$$Y = b + m\,X$$

$$\text{Log } C_p = \text{Log } C_p^0 - K_{el}/2.303\,(t)$$

and interpreted as such in the semi-logarithmic plot illustrated in Figure 3–14. Most drugs administered orally can be adequately described using a one-compartment model, whereas drugs administered by rapid intravenous infusion are usually best described by a two-compartment or three-compartment model system.

Assuming that a drug's volume of distribution, V_d, is constant within this system, the total amount of drug in the body (Q_b) can be calculated from the following equation:

$$Q_b = [C_p^0]\,[V_d] \qquad \text{(Equation 3–4)}$$

Usually, C_p^0 is determined by extrapolating the drug-concentration time plot back to time zero.

In this simple one-compartment system it is assumed that the administered drug is confined to the plasma (or blood) and then excreted. Drugs that exhibit this behavior will have small volumes of distribution. For example, a drug such as warfarin which is extensively bound to plasma albumin will have a volume of distribution equivalent to that of plasma water, about 2.8 liters in an average 70 kg adult. Some drugs, however, will initially be distributed at somewhat different rates in various fluids and tissues. Consequently, these drugs' kinetic behavior can best be illustrated by considering an expansion of the one-compartment system to the *two-compartment model* (Fig. 3–15).

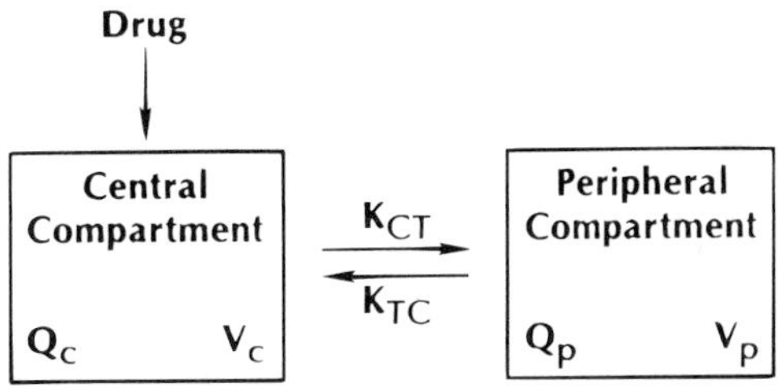

Where:
Q_C = Quantity of drug in central compartment
V_C = Volume of the central compartment
Q_P = Quantity of drug in peripheral compartment
V_P = Volume of the peripheral compartment

Fig. 3–15. *Schematic of a two-compartment system.*

In the two-compartment system, a drug enters into and is instantaneously distributed throughout the central compartment. Its subsequent distribution into the second or peripheral compartment is slower. For simplicity, on the basis of blood perfusion and tissue-plasma partition coefficients for a given drug, various tissues and organs are considered together and given the designation as central compartment or peripheral compartment. The central compartment is usually considered to include the blood, the extracellular space, and organs with good blood perfusion, e.g., lungs, liver, kidneys, heart. The peripheral compartment is usually constituted by those tissues and organs which are poorly perfused by blood, e.g., skin, bones, fat.

Figure 3–16 depicts the plasma-drug concentration versus time plot for a rapidly administered intravenous dose of a hypothetical drug which exhibits kinetic behavior exemplifying a two-compartment system. Note the initial steep decline of the plasma drug concentration curve. This typifies the distribution of the drug from the central compartment to the peripheral compartment. During this phase the drug concentration in the plasma will decrease more rapidly than in the post-distributive phase, i.e., elimination phase. Whether or not this distributive

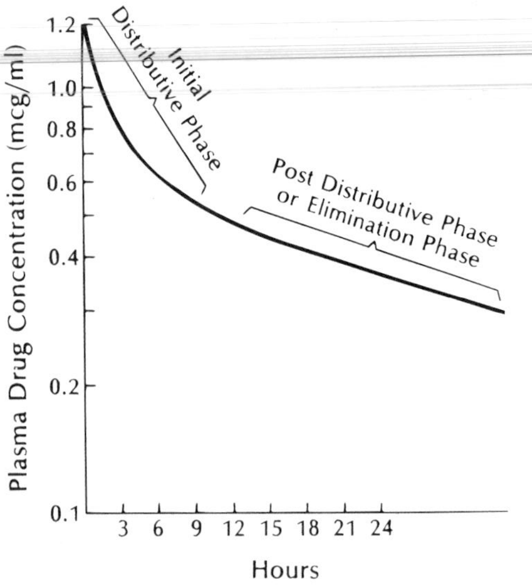

Fig. 3–16. *A semilogarithmic plasma concentration versus time plot of an intravenously administered drug that follows first order, two-compartment pharmacokinetics.*

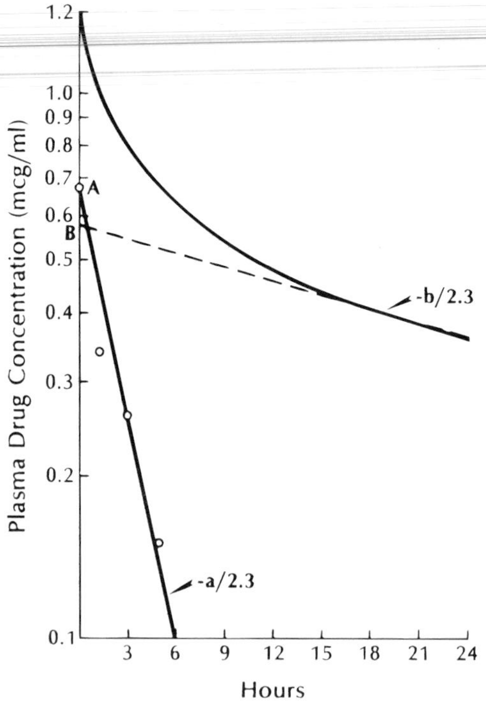

Fig. 3–17. *The logarithm of the drug concentration in plasma plotted versus time (solid line) after intravenous administration of a drug whose disposition can be described by a two-compartment model.*

phase is apparent will depend upon the timing of the plasma samples, particularly in the time immediately following administration. A distributive phase can be very short, a few minutes, or last for hours and even days.

A semi-logarithmic plot of the plasma concentration versus time after rapid intravenous injection of a drug which is best described by a two-compartment model system can often be resolved into two linear components. This procedure can be performed by the method of residuals (or feathering), Figure 3–17. In this procedure, a straight line is fitted through the tail of the original curve and extrapolated back to the Y-axis (the value obtained is B). A plot is then made of the absolute difference values of the original curve and the resultant extrapolated straight line. The slope of the feathered line ($-a/2.303$) and the extrapolated line ($-b/2.303$) and the intercepts, A and B, are determined. Then the following equation is constructed that describes a two-compartment system:

$$C_p = Ae^{-at} + Be^{-bt} \qquad \text{(Equation 3–5)}$$

This is a bi-exponential equation which describes the two-compartment system.

In this scheme, the slope of the line, i.e., $-a/2.303$, obtained from feathering yields the distributive rate of the drug. The slope of the terminal linear phase or elimination phase, i.e., $-b/2.303$, describes the rate of loss of the drug from the body, and usually is considered to be a reflection of the metabolic processes and renal elimination from the body. Appropriate pharmacokinetic formulas allow the clinician to calculate the various volumes of distribution and rates of distribution and elimination for drugs whose pharmacokinetic behavior is exemplified by the two-compartment system.

Half-Life

The half-life ($T_{1/2}$) of a drug describes the time required for a drug's blood or plasma concentration to decrease by one half. This fall in drug concentration is a reflection of metabolic processes and/or excretion, e.g., renal, fecal. The biological half-life of a drug in the blood may be determined graphically off of a pharmacokinetic plot of a drug's blood-concentration time plot, typically after intravenous administration to a sample population. The amount of time required for the concentration of the drug to decrease by one half is considered its half-life. The half-life can also be mathematically determined. Recall Equation 3–3 and rearrange the equation as follows:

$$\frac{K_{el}\,t}{2.303} = \text{Log } C_p^0 - \text{Log } C_p$$

$$= \text{Log } \frac{C_p^0}{C_p} \quad \text{(Equation 3–6)}$$

Then, if it assumed that C_p is equal to one-half of C_p^0, the equation will become:

$$\frac{K_{el}\,t}{2.303} = \text{Log } \frac{C_p^0}{0.5\,C_p^0} = \text{Log } 2 \quad \text{(Equation 3–7)}$$

Thus,

$$t_{1/2} = \frac{2.303 \text{ Log } 2}{K_{el}} = \frac{0.693}{K_{el}} \quad \text{(Equation 3–8)}$$

If this latter equation is rearranged, the half-life finds utility in the determination of drug elimination from the body, provided of course that the drug follows first-order kinetics. Rearranging the prior equation:

$$K_{el} = \frac{0.693}{t_{1/2}} \quad \text{(Equation 3–9)}$$

Elimination rate constants are reported in $time^{-1}$, e.g., $minutes^{-1}$, $hours^{-1}$. Thus, an elimination constant of a drug is 0.3 hr^1 indicates that 30% of the drug is eliminated per hour.

The half-life varies widely between drugs; for some drugs it may be a few minutes, whereas for other drugs it may be hours or even days (Table 3–10). Data on a drug's biologic half-life are useful in determining the most appropriate dosage regimen to achieve and maintain the desired blood level of drug. Such determinations usually result in such recommended dosage schedules for a drug, as the drug to be taken every 4 hours, 6 hours, 8 hours, etc. Although these types of recommendations generally suit the requirements of most patients, they do not suit all patients. The most exceptional patients are those with reduced or impaired ability to metabolize or excrete drugs. These patients, generally suffering from liver dysfunction or kidney disease, retain the administered drug in the blood or tissues for extended periods of time due to their decreased ability to eliminate the drug. The resulting extended biologic half-life of the drug generally necessitates an individualized dosage regimen calling for less frequent drug administration than that called for in patients with normal processes of drug elimination, or a maintenance of the usual dosage schedule, but a decrease in the amount of drug administered.

Table 3–10. Some Elimination Half-Life Values

Drug Substance/Product	*Elimination Half-Life** ($t_{1/2}$)
Acetaminophen (Tylenol, McNeil)	1–4 hours
Amoxicillin (Amoxil, SKB)	1 hour
Butabarbital Sodium (Butisol Sodium, Wallace)	100 hours
Cimetidine (Tagamet, SKB)	2 hours
Digitoxin (Crystodigin, Lilly)	7–9 days
Digoxin (Lanoxin, Burroughs Wellcome)	1.5–2 days
Diltiazem (Cardizem, MMD)	2.5 hours
Ibuprofen (Motrin, Upjohn)	1.8–2 hours
Indomethacin (Indocin, Merck)	4.5 hours
Lithium Carbonate (Eskalith, SKB)	24 hours
Nitroglycerin (Tridil, DuPont)	3 minutes†
Phenytoin Sodium (Dilantin, Parke-Davis)	7–29 hours
Pentobarbital Sodium (Nembutal Sodium, Abbott)	15–50 hours
Propoxyphene (Darvon, Lilly)	6–12 hours
Propranolol HCl (Inderal, Wyeth-Ayerst)	4 hours
Ranitidine HCl (Zantac, Glaxo)	2.5–3 hours
Theophylline (Theo-Dur, Key)	3–15 hours
Tobramycin Sulfate (Nebcin, Lilly)	2 hours
Tolbutamide (Orinase, Upjohn)	4.5–6.5 hours

* Mean, average, or value ranges, taken from product information found in *Physicians' Desk Reference*, 48th ed., 1994, Medical Economics Data, Montvale, New Jersey. Half-life values may vary depending upon patient characteristics (age, liver or renal function, smoking habits, etc.), dose levels administered, and routes of administration.

† After intravenous infusion; nitroglycerin is rapidly metabolized to dinitrates and mononitrates.

The drug digoxin presents a good example of a drug having a half-life which is affected by the patient's pathologic condition. Digoxin is eliminated in the urine. Renal excretion of digoxin is proportional to glomerular filtration rate. In subjects with normal renal function, digoxin has a half-life of 1.5 to 2.0 days. In anuric patients (absence of urine formation), the half-life may be prolonged to 4 to 6 days. Theophylline also demonstrates differing half-lives dependent upon certain patient populations. In premature infants with immature liver enzyme systems in the cytochrome P-450 family, the half-life of theophylline ranges from 14 to 58 hours, whereas in young children between the ages of 1 to 4 whose liver enzyme systems are more mature the theophylline half-life ranges between 2 to 5.5 hours. In adult nonsmokers, the half-life ranges from 6.1 to 12.8 hours, whereas in adult smokers the average half-life of theophylline is 4.3 hours. The increase in theophylline clearance from the body among smokers is believed to be due to an induction of the hepatic metabolism of theophylline. The half-life of theophylline is decreased and total body clearance is enhanced to such a degree in smokers that these individuals may actually require a 50 to 100% increase in theophylline dosage to produce effective therapeutic results. Between 3 months and 2 years may actually be required to normalize the effect of smoking on theophylline metabolism in the body once the patient stops smoking. Because theophylline is metabolized in the liver, the half-life of theophylline will be extended in liver disease. For example, in one study 9 patients with decompensated cirrhosis, the average theophylline half-life was 32 hours.

The half-life of a drug in the blood stream may also be affected by a change in the extent to which it is bound to blood protein or cellular components. Such a change in a drug's binding pattern may be brought about by the administration of a second drug having a greater affinity than the first drug for the same binding sites. The result is the displacement of the first drug from these sites by the second drug and the sudden availability of free (unbound) drug which may pass from the blood stream to other body sites, including those concerned with its elimination. It should be noted that the displacement of one drug from its binding sites by another is generally viewed as an undesired event, since the amount of free drug resulting is greater than the level normally achieved during single drug therapy and may result in untoward drug effects.

Concept of Clearance

The three main mechanisms by which a drug is removed or cleared from the body include (1) the hepatic metabolism, i.e., hepatic clearance, Cl_h, of a drug to either an active or inactive metabolite, (2) the renal excretion, i.e., renal clearance, Cl_r, of a drug unchanged in the urine, and (3) elimination of the drug into the bile and subsequently into the intestines for excretion in feces. An alternate way to express this removal or elimination from the body is to use total body clearance (Cl_B), which is defined as the fraction of the total volume of distribution that can be cleared per unit time. Because most drugs when administered will undergo one or more of these processes, the total body clearance, Cl_B, of a drug is the sum of these clearances, usually hepatic, Cl_h and renal clearances Cl_r. Clearance via the bile and feces is usually not significant for most drugs.

These processes of elimination within the body work together and consequently a drug that is eliminated by renal excretion and hepatic biotransformation will have an overall rate of elimination. K_{el}, that is the sum of the renal excretion, k_u, and hepatic biotransformation, k_m. In the one compartment model described earlier, total body clearance is the product of the volume of distribution, V_d, and the overall rate of elimination, k_{el} (Equation 3–10):

$$Cl_B = V_d \times k_{el} \qquad \text{(Equation 3–10)}$$

But, recall that k_{el} equals $0.693/t_{1/2}$. If this is substituted into Equation 3–10, and one solves for the half-life, $t_{1/2}$, the following equation is obtained:

$$t_{1/2} = \frac{0.693\ V_d}{Cl_B} \qquad \text{(Equation 3–11)}$$

Recall that total body clearance is a function of one or more processes, thus if a drug were eliminated from the body through hepatic biotransformation and renal clearance, Equation 3–11 becomes:

$$t_{1/2} = \frac{0.693\ V_d}{Cl_h + Cl_r} \qquad \text{(Equation 3–12)}$$

Thus, a drug's half-life is directly proportional to the volume of distribution and inversely proportional to the total body clearance which is comprised of hepatic and renal clearances. Illustratively, if one considers infants and children who exhibit larger volumes of distribution and have lower clearance values, drugs will usually have greater half-lives than that exhibited in adults.

A decrease in the hepatic or renal clearances will prolong the half-life of a drug. This typically occurs for example in renal failure, and consequently, if one can estimate the percentage decrease in excretion due to renal failure one can use Equation 3–12 to calculate the new half-life of the drug in the patient. Thus, an adjusted dosage regimen can then be calculated to decrease the chance of drug toxicity.

Dosage Regimen Considerations

In the previous chapter those factors that can influence the dosage of a drug were mentioned. The question of how much drug and how often to administer it for a desired therapeutic effect is not easily attainable. Basically, there are two approaches to the development of dosage regimens. The first is the *empirical approach,* which involves the administration of a drug in a certain quantity, noting the therapeutic response and then modifying the dosage of drug and the dosing interval accordingly. Unfortunately, experience with the administration of a drug usually starts with the first patient, and eventually a sufficient number of patients receive the drug so that a fairly accurate prediction can be made. Besides the desired therapeutic effect, consideration must also involve the occurrence and severity of side effects. Empirical therapy is usually employed when the drug concentration in serum or plasma does not reflect the concentration of drug at the receptor site in the body, or the pharmacodynamic effect of the drug is not related (or correlated) with the receptor site drug concentration. Empirical therapy, for example, is utilized for many anticancer drugs that demonstrate effects long after they have been excreted from the body. It is difficult to relate the serum level of these drugs with the desired therapeutic effect.

The second approach to the development of a dosage regimen is through the use of pharmacokinetics or the *kinetic approach.* This approach is based on the assumption that the therapeutic and toxic effects of a drug are related to the amount of drug in the body or to the plasma (or serum) concentration of drug at the receptor site. Through careful pharmacokinetic evaluation of a drug's absorption, distribution, metabolism and excretion in the body from a single dose, the levels of drug attained from multiple dosing can be estimated. One can then determine the appropriateness of a dosage regimen to achieve a desired therapeutic concentration of drug in the body

Table 3–11. Factors That Determine a Dosage Regimen*

Activity-Toxicity	*Pharmacokinetics*
Minimum therapeutic dose	Absorption
Toxic dose	Distribution
Therapeutic index	Metabolism
Side effects	Excretion
Dose-response relationships	

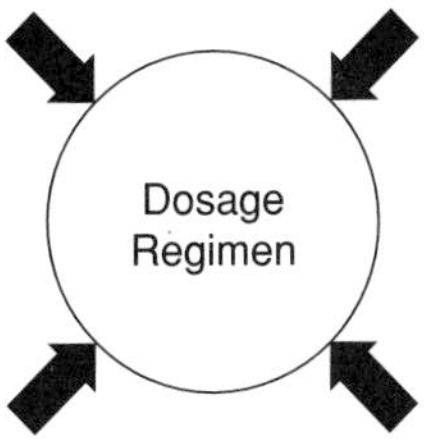

Clinical Factors		*Other Factors*
Clinical State of Patient	*Management of Therapy*	
Age, weight, urine pH	Multiple drug therapy	Tolerance-dependence
Condition being treated	Convenience of regimen	Pharmacogenetics-idiosyncrasy
Existence of other disease states	Compliance of patient	Drug interactions

* From Rowland, M. and Tozer, T.N.: *Clinical Pharmacokinetics.* 2nd Ed., Philadelphia, Lea & Febiger, 1989.

and evaluate the regimen based upon therapeutic response.

When one considers the development of a dosage regimen, pharmacokinetics is but one of a number of factors that should be considered. Table 3–11 illustrates a number of these. Certainly an important factor is the inherent activity, i.e., pharmacodynamics, and toxicity, i.e., toxicology of the drug. A second consideration is the pharmacokinetics of the drug, which are influenced by the dosage form in which the drug is administered to the patient, e.g., biopharmaceutical considerations. The third factor focuses upon the patient to whom the drug will be given and encompasses the clinical state of the patient and how the patient will be managed. Lastly, atypical factors may influence the dosage regimen. Collectively, all of these factors influence the dosage regimen.

The dosage regimen of a drug may simply involve the administration of a drug once for its desired therapeutic effect, e.g., pinworm medication, or encompass the administration of drug for a specific time through multiple doses. In the latter instance, the objective of pharmacokinetic dosing is to design a dosage regimen that will continually maintain a drug's therapeutic serum or plasma concentration within the drug's therapeutic index, i.e., above the minimum effective concentration but below the minimum toxic level.

Frequently drugs are administered between 1 to 4 times per day, most often in a fixed dose, e.g., 75 mg 3 times daily after meals. As mentioned earlier, after a drug is administered its level within the body varies because of the influence of all of the processes, e.g., absorption, distribution, metabolism and excretion. A drug will accumulate in the body when the dosing interval is less than the time needed for the body to eliminate a single dose. For example, Figure 3–18 illustrates the plasma concentration for a drug given by intravenous administration and oral administration. The 50 mg dose of this drug was given at a dosing interval of 8 hours. The drug has an elimination half-life of 12 hours. As one can see with continued dosing the drug concentration reaches a *steady state* or *plateau* concentration. At this limit the amount of drug lost per interval is replenished when the drug is dosed again. Consequently the concentration of drug in the plasma or serum fluctuates between a minimum concentration and a maximum concentration. Thus for certain patient types it is optimal to target dosing so that the plateau concentration resides within the therapeutic index of a drug to maintain a minimum effective concentration of drug. For example, the asthmatic patient maintained on theophylline must have a serum concentration between 10 and 20 μg/mL. Otherwise the patient may be susceptible to an asthma attack. Thus, when dosing the asthmatic patient it is preferable to give theophylline around the clock 4 times daily to sustain levels at least above

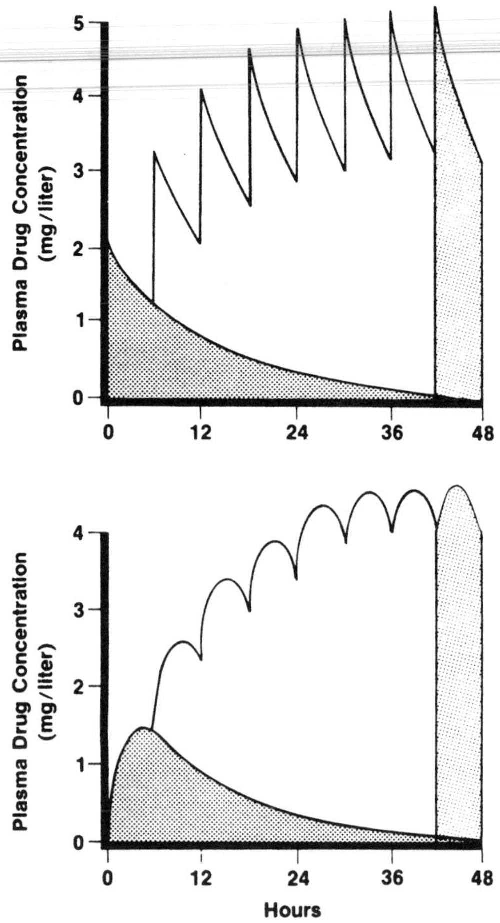

Fig. 3–18. *Plasma concentration of a drug given intravenously (top) and orally (bottom) on a fixed dose of 50 mg and fixed dosing interval of 8 hours. The half-life is 12 hours. Note that the area under the plasma concentration-time curve during a dosing interval at steady state is equal to the total area under the curve for a single dose. The fluctuation of the concentration is diminished when given orally (half-life of absorption is 1.4 hours) but the average steady-state concentration is the same as that after intravenous administration, since F = 1. (From Rowland, M. and Tozer, T.N.:* Clinical Pharmacokinetics, *Lea & Febiger, 1989.)*

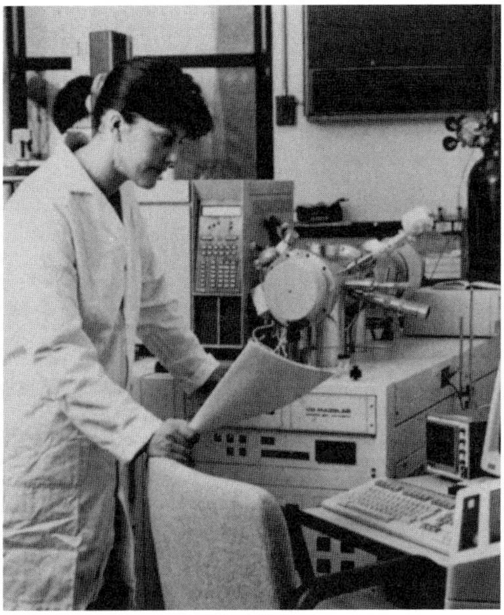

Fig. 3–19. *Computerized gas chromatography mass spectrometry used in bioanalytical studies. Consists of Hewlett Packard Gas Chromatograph (Model 5890 A) and VG Mass Spectrometer (Model UG 12-250). (Courtesy of Elan Corporation, plc.)*

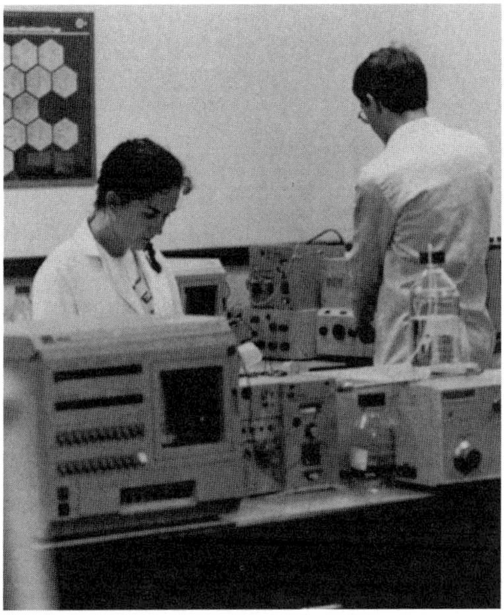

Fig. 3–20. *Assay of biological fluids using Waters HPLC (High Performance Liquid Chromatography) system consisting of (from left to right) Autosampler (Model 712 Wisp), Pump (Model M-45), Shimadzu Fluorescence Detector (Model RF-535). (Courtesy of Elan Corporation, plc.)*

the minimum effective concentration. If on the other hand this medicine is only administered every 4 hours during the waking hours, it is possible that the minimum concentration will fall below effective levels between the at-bedtime dose and the next morning dose. Consequently, the patient may awaken in the middle of the night and exhibit an asthma attack.

Patients can be monitored pharmacokinetically through appropriate plasma, serum or blood samples, and many hospital pharmacies have implemented pharmacokinetic dosing services. The intent is to maximize drug efficacy, minimize drug toxicity and keep health care costs at a minimum. Thus, for example, complications associated with overdose are controlled or drug interactions that are known to occur, e.g., smoking-theophylline, can be accommodated. In these services, for example, once the physician prescribes a certain amount of drug and monitors the clinical response, it is the clinical pharmacist who coordinates the appropriate sample time to determine drug concentration in the appropriate body fluid. After the level of drug is attained, it is the clinical pharmacist who interprets the result, and consults with the physician regarding subsequent dosages.

Pharmacokinetic research has demonstrated that the determination of a patient's dosage regimen depends on numerous factors and daily dose formulas exist for a number of drugs that must be administered on a routine maintenance schedule, e.g., digoxin, procainamide, theophylline. For certain drugs such as digoxin, which are not highly lipid soluble, it is preferable to use a patient's lean body weight (LBW) rather than total body weight (TBW) to provide a better estimate of the patient's volume of distribution. Alternatively, even though pharmacokinetic dosing formulas may exist, one must be cognizant that patient factors may be more relevant. For example, with the geriatric patient it is advisable to begin drug therapy with the lowest possible dose and increase the dosage as necessary in small increments to optimize the patient's clinical response. Then the patient should be monitored for drug efficacy and reevaluated periodically.

Examples of bioanalytical research laboratories are shown in Figures 3–19 and 3–20.

References

1. Cogburn, J.N., Donovan, M.G., and Schasteen: A Model of Human Small Intestinal Absorptive Cells. 1. Transport Barrier. *Pharm. Res., 8*:210–216, 1991.

2. Christensen, F.N. et al.: The Use of Gamma Scintigraphy to Follow the Gastrointestinal Transit of Pharmaceutical Formulations. *J. Phar. Pharmacol. 37:* 91–95 (1985).
3. Coupe, A.J., Davis, S.S., and Wilding, I.R.: Variation in Gastrointestinal Transit of Pharmaceutical Dosage Forms in Healthy Subjects. *Pharm. Res. 8:* 360–364 (1991).
4. Poole, J.: *Curr. Therapeut. Res., 10:*292–303, 1968.
5. *Code of Federal Regulations,* Title 21, Part 320—Bioavailability and Bioequivalence Requirements.
6. Chodos, D.J., and DiSanto, A.R.: *Basics of Bioavailability.* The Upjohn Company, Kalamazoo, MI, 1973.
7. *FDA Drug Bulletin, 16,* No. 2, 1986, pp 14–15.
8. Smith, H.J.: Process of Drug Handling by the Body. *Introduction to the Principles of Drug Design,* 2nd ed., Buttersworth & Co., London, 1988.
9. Cooper, J.W.: Monitoring of Drugs and Hepatic Status. *Clinical Consult, 10,* No. 6, 1991.

4

Dosage Form Design: General Considerations, Pharmaceutic Ingredients, and Current Good Manufacturing Practice

DRUG SUBSTANCES are seldom administered alone, but rather as part of a formulation in combination with one or more nonmedical agents that serve varied and specialized pharmaceutical functions. Through selective use of these nonmedicinal agents, referred to as *pharmaceutic ingredients,* dosage forms of various types result. The pharmaceutic ingredients solubilize, suspend, thicken, dilute, emulsify, stabilize, preserve, color, flavor, and fashion medicinal agents into efficacious and appealing dosage forms. Each type of dosage form is unique in its physical and pharmaceutical characteristics. These varied preparations provide the manufacturing pharmacist with the challenges of formulation and the physician with the choice of drug and drug delivery system to prescribe. The general area of study concerned with the formulation, manufacture, stability, and effectiveness of pharmaceutical dosage forms is termed *pharmaceutics.*

The proper design and formulation of a dosage form requires consideration of the physical, chemical and biological characteristics of all of the drug substances and pharmaceutic ingredients to be used in fabricating the product. The drug and pharmaceutic materials utilized must be compatible with one another to produce a drug product that is stable, efficacious, attractive, easy to administer and safe. The product should be manufactured under appropriate measures of quality control and packaged in containers that contribute to product stability. The product should be labeled to promote correct use and be stored under conditions that contribute to maximum shelf life.

Methods for the preparation of specific types of dosage forms and drug delivery systems are described in subsequent chapters. This chapter presents some general considerations regarding pharmaceutic ingredients, drug product formulation, and standards for good manufacturing practice.

The Need for Dosage Forms

The potent nature and low dosage of most of the drugs in use today precludes any expectation that the general public could safely obtain the appropriate dose of a drug from the bulk material. The vast majority of drug substances are administered in milligram quantities, much too small to be weighed on anything but a sensitive laboratory balance. For instance, how could the layman accurately obtain the 325 mg or 5 gr of aspirin found in the common aspirin tablet from a bulk supply of aspirin? He couldn't. Yet, compared with many other drugs, the dose of aspirin is formidable (Table 4–1). For example, the dose of ethinyl estradiol, 0.05 mg, is 1/6500 the amount of aspirin in an aspirin tablet. To put it another way, 6500 ethinyl estradiol tablets, each containing 0.05 mg of drug, could be made from an amount of ethinyl estradiol equal to the amount of aspirin in just one 325 mg aspirin tablet. When the dose of the drug is minute, as that for ethinyl estradiol, solid dosage forms such as tablets and capsules must be prepared with fillers or diluents so that the size of the resultant dosage unit is large enough to pick up with the fingertips.

Besides providing the mechanism for the safe and convenient delivery of accurate dosage, dosage forms are needed for additional reasons:

1. For the protection of a drug substance from the destructive influences of atmospheric oxygen or humidity (e.g., coated tablets, sealed ampuls).
2. For the protection of a drug substance from the destructive influence of gastric acid after oral administration (e.g., enteric-coated tablets).

Table 4–1. Examples of Some Drugs with Relatively Low Usual Doses

Drug	*Usual Dose, mg*	*Category*
Lithium Carbonate	300	Antidepressant
Ferrous Sulfate	300	Hematinic
Cimetidine	300	Antiulcer
Ibuprofen	300	Antiinflammatory
Amoxicillin	250	Antibacterial
Erythromycin	250	Antibacterial
Nitrofurantoin	100	Antibacterial (urinary)
Propoxyphene HCl	65	Analgesic
Thyroid	60	Thyroid
Hydrochlorothiazide	50	Diuretic
Codeine Phosphate	30	Analgesic
Phenobarbital	30	Sedative
Chlorpromazine HCl	25	Tranquilizer
Diphenhydramine HCl	25	Antihistaminic
Morphine Sulfate	10	Narcotic analgesic
Prednisolone	5	Adrenocortical steroid
Chlorpheniramine Maleate	4	Antihistaminic
Colchicine	0.5	Gout suppressant
Nitroglycerin	0.4	Antianginal
Digoxin	0.25	Cardiotonic (maintenance)
Levothyroxine	0.1	Thyroid
Ethinyl Estradiol	0.05	Estrogen

3. To conceal the bitter, salty, or offensive taste or odor of a drug substance (e.g., capsules, coated tablets, flavored syrups).
4. To provide liquid preparations of substances that are either insoluble or unstable in the desired vehicle (e.g., suspensions).
5. To provide clear liquid dosage forms of substances (e.g., syrups, solutions).
6. To provide time-controlled drug action (e.g., various controlled-release tablets, capsules, and suspensions).
7. To provide optimal drug action from topical administration sites (e.g., ointments, creams, transdermal patches, ophthalmic, ear, and nasal preparations).
8. To provide for the insertion of a drug into one of the body's orifices (e.g., rectal or vaginal suppositories).
9. To provide for the placement of drugs directly into the bloodstream or into body tissues (e.g., injections).
10. To provide for optimal drug action through inhalation therapy (e.g., inhalants and inhalation aerosols).

General Considerations in Dosage Form Design

Before formulating a drug substance into a dosage form, it is important to predetermine the desired product type insofar as possible in order to establish the framework for product development activities. Then, various initial formulations of the product are developed and examined for desired features (e.g., drug release profile, bioavailability, clinical effectiveness) and for pilot plant studies and production scale-up. The formulation that best meets the goals for the product is selected and represents its *master formula.* Each batch of product subsequently prepared must meet the specifications established in the master formula.

There are many different forms into which a medicinal agent may be placed for the convenient and efficacious treatment of disease (Table 3–6). Most commonly, a pharmaceutical manufacturer prepares a drug substance in several dosage forms and strengths for the efficacious and convenient treatment of disease (Fig. 4–1). Before a medicinal agent is formulated into one or more dosage forms, among the factors considered are such therapeutic matters as: the nature of the illness, the manner in which it is generally treated, locally or through systemic action, and the age and anticipated condition of the patient.

If the medication is intended for systemic use and oral administration is desired, tablets and/or capsules are generally prepared. These dosage units are easily handled by the patient and are most convenient in the self-administration of medication. If a drug substance has application in an emergency situation in which the patient may be comatose or unable to take oral medication, an injectable form of the medication may also be prepared. Many other examples of therapeutic situations affecting dosage form design could be cited, including the preparation of agents for motion sickness, nausea, and vomiting into tablets and skin patches for prevention and suppositories and injections for treatment.

The age of the intended patient also plays a role in dosage form design. For infants and children under 5 years of age, pharmaceutical liquids rather than solid dosage forms are preferred for oral administration. These liquids, which are generally flavored aqueous solutions, syrups or

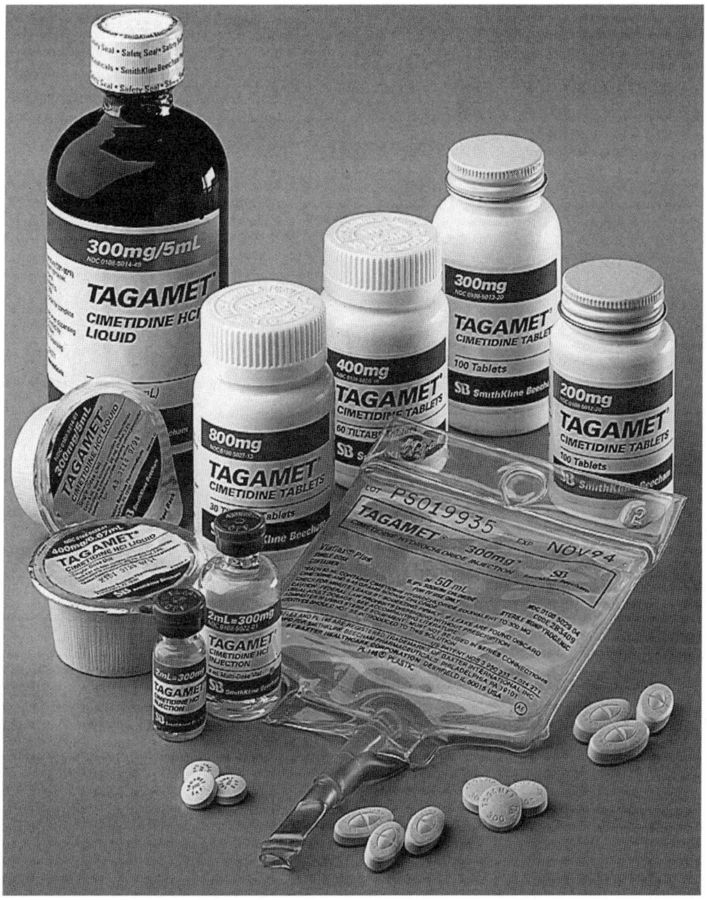

Fig. 4–1. *Examples of varied dosage forms of a drug substance marketed by a pharmaceutical manufacturer to meet the special requirements of the patient. (Courtesy of SmithKline Beecham)*

suspensions, are usually administered directly into the infant's or child's mouth by drop, spoon, or oral dispenser (Fig. 4–2) or incorporated into the child's food. A single liquid pediatric preparation may be used for infants and children of all ages, with the dose of the drug varied by the volume administered. When an infant is in the throes of a vomiting crisis, is gagging, has a productive cough, or is simply rebellious, there may be some question as how much of the medicine administered is actually swallowed and how much is expectorated. In such instances, injections may be required. Infant size rectal suppositories may also be employed although drug absorption from the rectum is often erratic.

During childhood and even in adult years, a person may have difficulty swallowing solid dosage forms, especially uncoated tablets. For this reason, some medications are formulated as chewable tablets that can be broken up in the mouth before swallowing. Many of these tablets are comparable in texture to an after-dinner mint and break down into a pleasant tasting, creamy material. Capsules have been found by many to be more easily swallowed than whole tablets. If a capsule is allowed to become moist in the mouth before swallowing, it becomes slippery and slides down the throat more readily with a glass of water. In instances in which a person has difficulty swallowing a capsule, the contents may be emptied into a spoon, mixed with jam, honey, or other similar food to mask the taste of the medication and swallowed. Some older persons have difficulty in swallowing and thus tablets and capsules are frequently avoided. Medications intended for the elderly are commonly for-

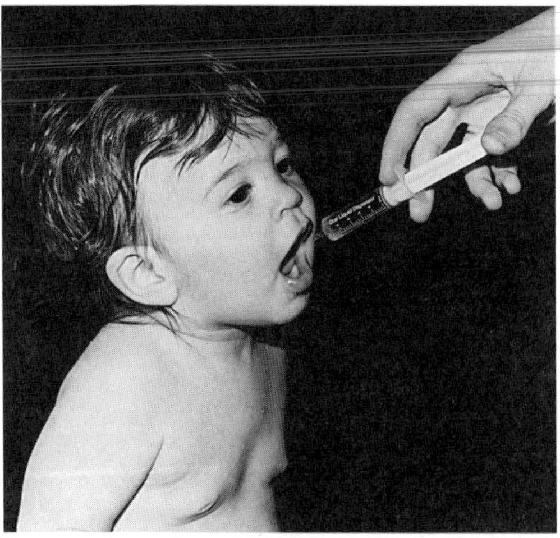

Fig. 4–2. *"Pee Dee Dose" brand of oral liquid dispenser used to administer measured volumes of liquid medication to youngsters. (Courtesy of Baxa Corporation)*

mulated into oral liquids or may be extemporaneously prepared into an oral liquid by the pharmacist.

Many patients, particularly the elderly, take multiple medications daily. The more distinctive the size, shape, and color of solid dosage forms, the easier is the proper identification of the medications. Frequent errors in taking medications among the elderly occur because of their multiple drug therapy and reduced eyesight. Dosage forms that allow reduced frequency of administration without sacrifice of efficiency are particularly advantageous.

In dealing with the problem of formulating a drug substance into a proper dosage form, research pharmacists employ knowledge that has been gained through experience with other chemically similar drugs and through the proper utilization of the disciplines of the physical, chemical, and biologic and pharmaceutical sciences. The early stages of any new formulation involves studies to collect basic information on the physical and chemical characteristics of the drug substance to be prepared into pharmaceutical dosage forms. These basic studies comprise the *preformulation* work needed before actual product formulation begins.

Preformulation Studies

Before the formulation of a drug substance into a dosage it is essential that it be chemically and physically characterized. The following *preformulation studies,*[1] and others, provide the type of information needed to define the nature of the drug substance. This information then provides the framework for the drug's combination with pharmaceutic ingredients in the fabrication of a dosage form.

Physical Description

It is important to have an understanding of the physical description of a drug substance prior to dosage form development. The majority of drug substances in use today occur as solid materials. Most of them are pure chemical compounds of either crystalline or amorphous constitution. The purity of the chemical substance is essential for its identification as well as for the evaluation of its chemical, physical, and biologic properties. *One parameter in determining chemical purity is melting point depression, the physical pharmacy concept of which is summarized in the accompanying Physical Pharmacy Capsule.* Liquid drugs are used to a much lesser extent than solid drugs; gases, even less frequently.

Among the few liquid medicinal agents in use today are the following:

Amyl nitrite, vasodilator by inhalation
Castor oil, cathartic
Clofibrate, antihyperlipidemic
Dimercaprol, antidote for arsenic, gold, and mercury poisoning
Dimethylsulfoxide, analgesic in interstitial cystitis
Ethchlorvynol, hypnotic
Glycerin, cathartic in suppository form
Mineral oil, cathartic
Nitroglycerin (as tablets), anti-anginal
Paraldehyde, sedative-hypnotic
Paramethadione, anticonvulsant
Prochlorperazine, tranquilizer and antiemetic
Propylhexedrine, vasoconstrictor by nasal inhalation
Undecylenic acid, fungistatic agent

Liquid drugs pose an interesting problem in the design of dosage forms or drug delivery systems. Many of the liquids are volatile substances and as such must be physically sealed from the atmosphere to prevent their loss. Amyl nitrite, for example, is a clear yellowish liquid that is volatile even at low temperatures and is also highly flammable. It is maintained for medicinal purposes in small sealed glass cylinders wrapped with gauze or another suitable material. When amyl nitrite is administered, the glass is broken between the fingertips and the liquid

Melting Point Depression

The *melting point,* or *freezing point,* of a pure crystalline solid is defined as that temperature where the pure liquid and solid exist in equilibrium. This characteristic can be used as an indicator of purity of chemical substances (a pure substance would ordinarily be characterized by a very sharp melting peak).

The *latent heat of fusion* is the quantity of heat absorbed when 1 g of a solid melts; the molar heat of fusion (ΔH_f) is the quantity of heat absorbed when 1 mole of a solid melts. High-melting-point substances have high heats of fusion and low-melting-point substances have low heats of fusion. These characteristics are related to the types of bonding in the specific substance. For example, ionic materials have high heats of fusion (NaCl melts at 801°C with a heat of fusion of 124 cal/G) and those with weaker van der Waals forces have low heats of fusion (paraffin melts at 52°C with a heat of fusion of 35.1 cal/g). Ice, with weaker hydrogen bonding, has a melting point of 0°C and a heat of fusion of 80 cal/G.

The addition of a second component to a pure compound (A), resulting in a mixture, will result in a melting point that is lower than that of the pure compound. The degree to which the melting point is lowered is proportional to the mole fraction (N_A) of the second component that is added. This can be expressed as:

$$\Delta T = \frac{2.303\ RTT_0}{\Delta H_f} \log N_A$$

where ΔH_F is the molar heat of fusion,
T is the absolute equilibrium temperature,
T_0 is the melting point of pure A, and
R is the gas constant.

Two things are noteworthy in contributing to the extent of melting-point lowering.

1. Evident from this relationship is the inverse proportion between the melting point and the heat of fusion. When a second ingredient is added to a compound with a low molar heat of fusion, a large lowering of the melting point is observed; substances with a high molar heat of fusion will show little change in melting point with the addition of a second component.
2. The extent of lowering of the melting point is also related to the melting point itself. Compounds with low melting points are affected to a greater extent than compounds with high melting points upon the addition of a second component (i.e., low-melting-point compounds will result in a greater lowering of the melting point than those with high melting points).

wets the gauze covering, producing vapors that are inhaled by the patient requiring vasodilation. Propylhexedrine provides another example of a volatile liquid drug that must be contained in a closed system to maintain its presence. This drug is used as a nasal inhalant for its vasoconstrictor action. A cylindrical roll of fibrous material is impregnated with propylhexedrine, and the saturated cylinder is placed in a suitable, generally plastic, sealed nasal inhaler. The inhaler's cap must be securely tightened each time it is used. Even then, the inhaler maintains its effectiveness for only a limited period of time due to the volatilization of the drug.

Another problem associated with liquid drugs is that those intended for oral administration cannot generally be formulated into tablet form, the most popular form of oral medication, without undertaking chemical modification of the drug. An exception to this is the liquid drug nitroglycerin, which is formulated into sublingual tablets that disintegrate within seconds after placement under the tongue. However, because the drug is volatile, it has a tendency to escape from the tablets during storage and it is critical that the tablets be stored in tightly sealed glass containers. For the most part, when a liquid drug is to be administered orally and a solid dosage form is desired, two approaches are used. First, the liquid substance may be sealed in a soft gelatin capsule. Paramethadione (Paradione) and ethchlorvynol (Placidyl) are examples of liquid drugs commercially available in capsule form. Secondly, the liquid drug may be developed into a solid ester or salt form that will be suitable for tableting or drug encapsulating. For instance, scopolamine hydrobromide is a solid salt of the liquid drug scopolamine and is easily produced into tablets.

For certain liquid drugs, especially those employed orally in large doses or applied topically, their liquid nature may be of some advantage in therapy. For example, 15-mL doses of mineral oil may be administered conveniently as such. Also, the liquid nature of undecylenic acid certainly does not hinder but rather enhances its use topically in the treatment of fungus infections of the skin. However, for the most part, solid materials are preferred by pharmacists in formulation work because of their ease of preparation into tablets and capsules.

Formulation and stability difficulties arise less frequently with solid dosage forms than with liquid pharmaceutical preparations, and for this reason many new drugs first reach the market as tablets or dry-filled capsules. Later, when the pharmaceutical problems are resolved, a liquid form of the same drug may be marketed. This procedure, when practiced, is doubly advantageous, because for the most part physicians and patients alike prefer small, generally tasteless, accurately dosed tablets or capsules to the analogous liquid forms. Therefore, marketing a drug in solid form first is more practical for the manufacturer and also suits the majority of patients. It is estimated that tablets and capsules comprise the dosage form dispensed 70% of the time by community pharmacists, with tablets dispensed twice as frequently as capsules.

Microscopic Examination

Microscopic examination of the raw drug substance is an important step in preformulation work. It gives an indication of particle size and particle size range of the raw material as well as the crystal structure. Photomicrographs of the initial and subsequent batch lots of the drug substance can provide important information should problems arise in formulation processing attributable to changes in particle or crystal characteristics of the drug.

Particle Size

Certain physical and chemical properties of drug substances are affected by the particle size distribution, including drug dissolution rate, bioavailability, content uniformity, taste, texture, color, and stability. In addition, properties such as flow characteristics and sedimentation rates, among others, are also important factors related to particle size. It is essential to establish as early as possible how the particle size of the drug substance may affect formulation and product efficacy. Of special interest is the effect of particle size on the drug's absorption. Particle size has been shown to significantly influence the oral absorption profiles of certain drugs as griseofulvin, nitrofurantoin, spironolactone, and procaine penicillin.

Satisfactory content uniformity in solid dosage forms depends to a large degree on particle size and the equal distribution of the active ingredient throughout the formulation.

There are several methods available to evaluate particle size and distribution including sieving or screening, microscopy, sedimentation, and stream scanning. For powders in the range of approximately 44 microns and greater, sieving or screening is the most widely used method of size analysis. The difficulty with using this method early in the preformulation program is the requirement of a relatively large sample size. The main advantage of the sieve method is simplicity, both in technique and equipment requirements. Optical microscopy is frequently the first step in the determination of particle size and shape for the new drug substance. This is usually a qualitative assessment since quantitation by the microscope technique is tedious and time consuming. A key element in utilizing the microscope for particle size determination is preparation of the slide. It must be representative of the bulk of the material and be properly suspended and thoroughly dispersed in a suitable liquid phase. In order to do a quantitative particle size evaluation a minimum of 1000 of the particles should be counted.

Sedimentation techniques utilize the relationship between rate of fall of particles and their size. Techniques utilizing devices that continuously collect a settling suspension are used. These methods share the disadvantage of the microscope technique in that it is tedious to obtain the data. Also, proper dispersion, consistent sampling, temperature control, and other experimental variables must be carefully controlled in order to obtain consistent and reliable results.

Stream scanning is a valuable method for determining particle size distribution of powdered drug substances. This technique utilizes a fluid suspension of particles which pass the sensing zone where individual particles are sized, counted, and tabulated. Sensing units may be based on light scattering or transmission, as well as conductance. Two popular units in the pharmaceutical industry for this purpose are the Coulter Counter and Hiac Counter. Both units electronically size, count, and tabulate the individual particles that pass through the sensing zone. This technique has obvious advantages in that data can be generated in a relatively short time with reasonable accuracy. Thousands of particles can be counted in seconds and used to determine the size distribution curve. All stream scanning units convert the particles to effective diameter, and therefore, have the shortcoming of not providing information relative to particle shape. Nevertheless, stream scanning methods are powerful tools and can be used for evaluation of such parameters as crystal growth in suspension formulations.

Particle size is discussed further in the next chapter.

Partition Coefficient and Dissociation Constant

As discussed in the previous chapter, in order to produce a biological response, the drug molecule must first cross a biological membrane. The biological membrane acts as a lipid barrier to most drugs and permits the absorption of lipid soluble substances by passive diffusion while lipid insoluble substances can diffuse across the barrier only with considerable difficulty, if at all. The interrelationship of the dissociation constant, lipid solubility, and pH at the absorption site and absorption characteristics of various drugs are the basis of the pH-partition theory.

The oil/water partition coefficient is a measure of a molecule's lipophilic character; that is, its preference for the hydrophilic or lipophilic phase.

The partition coefficient should be considered in developing a drug substance into a dosage form. The partition coefficient (P) represents the ratio of the drug distribution in a two-phase system of organic solvent and aqueous phase. Using octanol-water as an example, it is defined as:

$$P = \frac{[\text{Conc. of drug in octanol}]}{[\text{Conc. of drug in water}]}$$

P is dependent on the drug concentration only if the drug molecules have a tendency to associate in solution. For an ionizable drug, the following equation is applicable:

$$P = \frac{[\text{Conc. of drug in octanol}]}{(1 - \alpha)[\text{Conc. of drug in water}]}$$

where α equals the degree of ionization.

A summary of the concepts of solubility and distribution phenomena is found in accompanying Physical Pharmacy Capsules.

The determination of the degree of ionization or pKa value of the drug substance is an important physical-chemical characteristic relative to evaluation of possible effects on absorption from various sites of administration.

Dissociation constant or pKa is usually determined by potentiometric titration.

Polymorphism

An important factor on formulation is the crystal or amorphous form of the drug substance. Polymorphic forms usually exhibit different physical-chemical properties including melting point and solubility. The occurrence of polymorphic forms with drugs is relatively common and it has been estimated that polymorphism is exhibited by at least one-third of all organic compounds.

In addition to the polymorphic forms in which compounds may exist, they also can occur in non-crystalline or amorphous forms. The energy required for a molecule of drug to escape from a crystal is much greater than required to escape from an amorphous powder. Therefore, the amorphous form of a compound is always more soluble than a corresponding crystal form.

Evaluation of crystal structure, polymorphism, and solvate form is an important preformulation activity. The changes in crystal characteristics can influence bioavailability, chemical and physical stability, and have important implications in dosage form process functions. For example, it can be a significant factor relating to the tableting processes due to flow and compaction behaviors, among others.

Various techniques are used in determining crystal properties. The most widely used methods are hot stage microscopy, thermal analysis, infrared spectroscopy, and x-ray diffraction.

Solubility

An important physical-chemical property of a drug substance is solubility, especially aqueous system solubility. A drug must possess some aqueous solubility for therapeutic efficacy. In

Solubility and Distribution Phenomena

If a solute is added to a mixture of two immiscible liquids, it will distribute between the two phases and reach an equilibrium at a constant temperature. The distribution of the solute (unaggregated and undissociated) between the two immiscible layers can be described as:

$$K = C_U/C_L$$

where K is the distribution constant or partition constant,
C_U is the concentration of the drug in the upper phase, and
C_L is the concentration of the drug in the lower phase.

This information can be effectively used in the:

1. extraction of crude drugs,
2. recovery of antibiotics from fermentation broths,
3. recovery of biotechnology-derived drugs from bacterial cultures,
4. extraction of drugs from biologic fluids for therapeutic drug monitoring,
5. absorption of drugs from dosage forms (ointments, suppositories, transdermal patches),
6. study of the distribution of flavoring oil between oil and water phases of emulsions, and
7. in other applications.

The basic relationship given above can be used to calculate the quantity of drug extracted from, or remaining behind in, a given layer and to calculate the number of extractions required to remove a drug from a mixture.

The concentration of drug found in the upper layer (U) of two immiscible layers is given by:

$$U = Kr/(Kr + 1)$$

where K is the distribution partition constant, and
r is V_u/V_l, or the ratio of the volume of upper and lower phases.

The concentration of drug remaining in the lower layer (L) is given by:

$$L = 1/(Kr + 1)$$

If the lower phase is successively re-extracted with *n* equal volumes of the upper layer, each upper (U_n) contains the following fraction of the drug:

$$U_n = Kr/(Kr + 1)^n$$

where U_n is the fraction contained in the *n*th extraction, and
n is the *n*th successive volume.

The fraction of solute remaining in the lower layer (L_n) is given by:

$$L_n = 1/(kr + 1)^n$$

More efficient extractions are obtained using successive small volumes of the extraction solvent (as compared to single larger volumes). This can be calculated as follows when the same volume of extracting solvent is used, but in divided portions. For example, the fraction L_n remaining after the *n*th extraction is given by:

$$L_n = \frac{1}{\left(\frac{Kr}{n} + 1\right)^n}$$

EXAMPLE 1

At 25°C and at pH 6.8, the K for a second generation cephalosporin is 0.7 between equal volumes of butanol and the fermentation broth. Calculate the U, L, and L_n (using the same volume divided into fourths).

$U = 0.7/(0.7 + 1) = 0.41$ The fraction of drug extracted into the upper layer
$L = 1/(0.7 + 1) = 0.59$ The fraction of drug remaining in the lower layer

The total of the fractions in the U and L = 0.41 + 0.59 = 1.

Solubility and Distribution Phenomena (Continued)

If the fermentation broth is extracted with four successive extractions accomplished by dividing the quantity of butanol used into fourths, the quantity of drug remaining after the fourth extraction is

$$L_{4th} = \frac{1}{\left(\frac{0.7 \times 1}{4} + 1\right)^4} = 0.525$$

From this, the quantity remaining after a single volume, single extraction is 0.59, but when the single volume is divided into fourths and four successive extractions are done, the quantity remaining is 0.525; therefore, more was extracted using divided portions of the extracting solvent.

Inherent in this procedure is the selection of appropriate extraction solvents, drug stability, use of salting-out additives, and environmental concerns.

The Phase Rule

A phase diagram, or temperature-composition diagram, represents the melting point as a function of composition of two or three component systems. The figure is an example of such a representation for a two-component mixture. This phase diagram is of a two-component mixture in which the components are completely miscible in the molten state and no solid

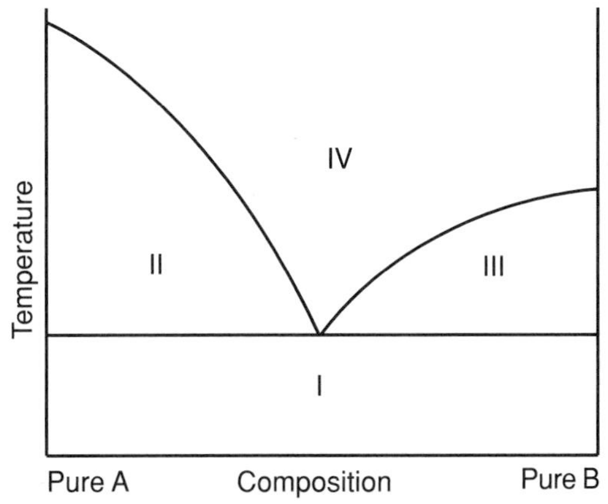

solution or addition compound is formed in the solid state. As is evident, starting from the extremes of either pure component A or pure component B, as the second component is added, the melting point of the pure component decreases. There is a point on this phase diagram at which a minimum melting point occurs (i.e., the eutectic point). As is evident, there are four regions, or phases, in this diagram, representing the following:

I. Solid A + Solid B
II. Solid A + Melt
III. Solid B + Melt
IV. Melt

The Phase Rule (Continued)

Each phase is a homogenous part of the system, physically separated by distinct boundaries. A description of the conditions under which these phases can exist is called the *Phase Rule,* which can be presented as:

$$F = C - P + X$$

where F is the number of degrees of freedom,
C is the number of components,
P is the number of phases, and
X is a variable dependent upon selected considerations of the phase diagram (1,2 or 3).

"C" describes the minimum number of chemical components that need to be specified to define the phases present. The F is the number of independent variables that must be specified to define the complete system (e.g., temperature, pressure, concentration).

EXAMPLE 1

In a mixture of menthol and thymol, a phase diagram similar to that illustrated can be obtained. To describe the number of degrees of freedom in the part of the graph moving from the curved line starting at pure A, progressing downward to the eutectic point, and then following an increasing melting point to pure B, it is evident from this presentation that either temperature or composition will describe this system, since it is assumed in this instance that pressure is constant. Therefore, the number of degrees of freedom to describe this portion of the phase diagram is given by:

$$F = 2 - 2 + 1 = 1$$

In other words, along this line, either temperature or composition will describe the system.

EXAMPLE 2

When in the area of a single phase of the diagram, such as the melt (IV), the system can be described as:

$$F = 2 - 1 + 1 = 2$$

In this portion of the phase diagram, it is apparent that two factors, temperature and composition, can be varied without a change in the number of phases in the system.

EXAMPLE 3

At the eutectic point,

$$F = 2 - 3 + 1 = 0$$

and any change in the concentration or temperature may cause a disappearance of one of the two solid phases or the liquid phase.

Phase diagrams are valuable in interpreting interactions between two or more components, relating not only to melting point depression and possible liquefaction at room temperature but also the formation of solid solutions, coprecipitates, and other solid-state interactions.

order for a drug to enter the systemic circulation to exert a therapeutic effect, it must first be in solution. Relatively insoluble compounds often exhibit incomplete or erratic absorption. If the solubility of the drug substance is less than desirable, consideration must be given to improve its solubility. The methods to accomplish this will depend on the chemical nature of the drug and the type of drug product under consideration. The chemical modification of the drug into salt or ester forms is a technique frequently used to obtain more soluble compounds. Another technique, if the drug is to be formulated into a liquid product, involves the adjustment of the pH of the solvent in which the drug is to be dissolved to enhance solubility. However, there are many drug substances for which pH adjustment is not an effective means of improving solubility. Weak acidic or basic drugs may require extremes in pH that are outside accepted physiologic limits or may cause stability problems with formulation ingredients. Adjustment of pH usually has little effect on the solubility of non-electrolytes. In many cases, it is desirable to utilize co-solvents or other techniques such as complexation, micronization, or solid dispersion to improve aqueous solubility.

A drug's solubility is usually determined by the equilibrium solubility method, by which an excess of the drug is placed in a solvent and shaken at a constant temperature over a prolonged period of time until equilibrium is obtained. Chemical analysis of the drug content in solution is performed to determine degree of solubility.

Dissolution

As discussed in the previous chapter, variations in the biological activity of a drug substance may be brought about by the rate at which it becomes available to the organism. In many instances, dissolution rate, or the time it takes for the drug to dissolve in the fluids at the absorption site, is the rate-limiting step in the absorption process. This is true for drugs administered orally in solid forms such as tablets, capsules or suspensions, as well as drugs administered intramuscularly in the form of pellets or suspensions. When the dissolution rate is the rate-limiting step, anything which affects it will also affect absorption. Consequently, dissolution rate can affect the onset, intensity, and duration of response, and control the overall bioavailability of the drug from the dosage form, as discussed in the previous chapter.

The dissolution rate of drugs may be increased by decreasing the drug's particle size. It may also be increased by increasing its solubility in the diffusion layer. The most effective means of obtaining higher dissolution rates is to use a highly water soluble salt of the parent substance. Although a soluble salt of a weak acid will subsequently precipitate as the free acid in the bulk phase of an acidic solution, such as gastric fluid, it will do so in the form of fine particles with a large surface area.

The dissolution rates of chemical compounds are generally determined by two methods: the constant surface method which provides the intrinsic dissolution rate of the agent, and particulate dissolution in which a suspension of the agent is added to a fixed amount of solvent without exact control of surface area.

The constant surface method utilizes a compressed disc of known area. This method eliminates surface area and surface electrical charges as dissolution variables. The dissolution rate obtained by this method is termed the *intrinsic dissolution rate,* and is characteristic of each solid compound and a given solvent under the fixed experimental conditions. The value is generally expressed as milligrams dissolved per minute centimeters squared ($mg/min/cm^2$). It has been suggested that this value is useful in predicting probable absorption problems due to dissolution rate. In particulate dissolution, a weighed amount of powdered sample is added to the dissolution medium in a constant agitation system. This method is frequently used to study the influence of particle size, surface area, and excipients upon the active agent. Occasionally, an inverse relationship of particle size to dissolution is noted due to the surface properties of the drug. In these instances, surface charge and/or agglomeration results in the reduced particle size form of the drug presenting a lower effective surface area to the solvent due to incomplete wetting or agglomeration.

Early formulation studies should include the effects of pharmaceutic ingredients on the dissolution characteristics of the drug substance.

Membrane Permeability

Modern preformulation studies include an early assessment of passage of drug molecules across biological membranes.

Data obtained from the basic physical-chemical studies, specifically, pKa, solubility, and dissolution rate provide an indication of absorption expectations.

To enhance these data, a technique utilizing the "everted intestinal sac" may be used in evaluating absorption characteristics of drug substances. In this method, a piece of intestine is removed from an intact animal, everted, filled with a solution of the drug substance, and the degree and rate of passage of the drug through the membrane sac is determined. Through this method, both passive and active transport can be evaluated.

In the latter stages of preformulation testing or early formulation studies, animals and man must be studied to assess the absorption efficiency, pharmacokinetic parameters and to establish possible *in vitro/in vivo* correlation for dissolution and bioavailability.

Drug Stability

One of the most important activities of preformulation work is the evaluation of the physical and chemical stability of the pure drug substance. It is essential that these initial studies be conducted using drug samples of known purity. The presence of impurities can lead to erroneous conclusions in such evaluations. Stability studies conducted in the preformulation phase include solid state stability of the drug alone, solution phase stability, and stability in the presence of expected excipients.

Initial investigation begins through knowledge of the drug's chemical structure which allows the preformulation scientist to anticipate the possible degradation reactions.

Chemical instability of medicinal agents may take many forms, because the drugs in use today are of such diverse chemical constitution. Chemically, drug substances are alcohols, phenols, aldehydes, ketones, esters, ethers, acids, salts, alkaloids, glycosides, and others, each with reactive chemical groups having different susceptibilities toward chemical instability. Chemically, the most frequently encountered destructive processes are hydrolysis and oxidation.

Hydrolysis is a solvolysis process in which (drug) molecules interact with water molecules to yield breakdown products of different chemical constitution. For example, aspirin or acetylsalicylic acid combines with a water molecule and hydrolyzes into one molecule of salicylic acid and one molecule of acetic acid:

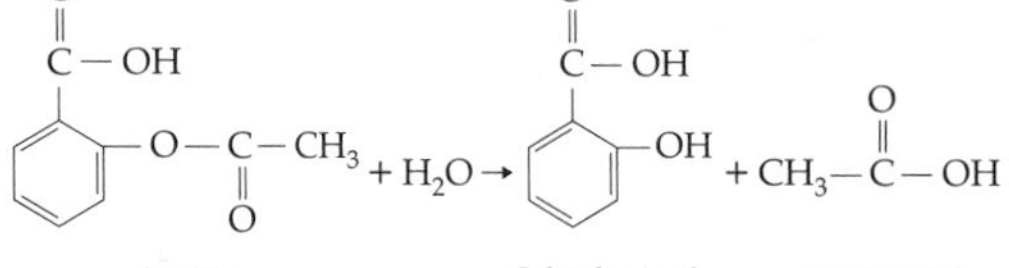

The process of hydrolysis is probably the most important single cause of drug decomposition mainly because a great number of medicinal agents are esters or contain such other groupings as substituted amides, lactones, and lactams, which are susceptible to the hydrolytic process.

Another destructive process is oxidation. The oxidative process is destructive to many drug types, including aldehydes, alcohols, phenols, sugars, alkaloids, and unsaturated fats and oils.

Chemically, oxidation involves the loss of electrons from an atom or a molecule. Each electron lost is accepted by some other atom or molecule, thereby accomplishing the reduction of the recipient. In inorganic chemistry, oxidation is accompanied by an increase in the positive valence of an element—for example, ferrous (+2) oxidizing to ferric (+3). In organic chemistry, oxidation is frequently considered synonymous with the loss of hydrogen (dehydrogenation) from a molecule. The oxidative process frequently involves free chemical radicals, which are molecules or atoms containing one or more unpaired electrons, as molecular (atmospheric) oxygen (•O—O•) and free hydroxyl (•OH). These radicals tend to take electrons from other chemicals, thereby oxidizing the donor. Many of the oxidative changes in pharmaceutical preparations have the character of autoxidations. Autoxidations occur spontaneously under the initial influence of atmospheric oxygen and proceed slowly at first and then more rapidly as the process continues. The process has been described as a type of chain reaction commencing by the union of oxygen with the drug molecule and continuing with a free radical of this oxidized molecule participating in the destruction of other drug molecules and so forth.

In drug product formulation work, steps are taken to reduce or prevent the occurrence of drug substance deterioration due to hydrolysis, oxidation, and other processes. These techniques are discussed in a later section.

Pharmaceutic Ingredients

In order to prepare a drug substance into a final dosage form, pharmaceutic ingredients are required. For example, in the preparation of pharmaceutic solutions, one or more *solvents* are utilized to dissolve the drug substance, *preservatives* may be added to prevent microbial growth, *stabilizers* may be used to prevent drug decomposition, and *colorants* and *flavorants* added to enhance product appeal. In the preparation of tablets, *diluents* or *fillers* are commonly added to increase the bulk of the formulation, *binders* to cause the adhesion of the powdered drug and pharmaceutic substances, *antiadherents* or *lubricants* to assist the smooth tableting process, *disintegrating agents* to promote tablet break-up after administration, and coatings to improve stability, control disintegration, or to enhance appearance. Ointments, creams, and suppositories achieve their characteristic features due to the pharmaceutic *bases* which are utilized. Thus, for each dosage form, the pharmaceutic ingredients establish the primary features of the product, and contribute to the physical form, texture, stability, taste and overall appearance.

Table 4–2 presents the principal categories of pharmaceutic ingredients, with examples of some of the official and commercial agents currently used. Additional discussion of many of the pharmaceutic ingredients may be found in the chapters where they are most relevant; for example, pharmaceutic materials used in tablet and capsule formulation are discussed in Chapter 5, *Peroral Solids, Capsules, Tablets, and Controlled-Release Dosage Forms.*

The reader should also be aware of the *Hand-*

Table 4–2. Examples of Pharmaceutic Ingredients

Ingredient Type	*Definition*	*Examples*
Acidifying Agent	Used in liquid preparations to provide acidic medium for product stability.	acetic acid citric acid fumaric acid hydrochloric acid nitric acid
Alkalinizing Agent	Used in liquid preparations to provide alkaline medium for product stability.	ammonia solution ammonium carbonate diethanolamine monoethanolamine potassium hydroxide sodium borate sodium carbonate sodium hydroxide triethanolamine trolamine
Adsorbent	An agent capable of holding other molecules onto its surface by physical or chemical (chemisorption) means.	powdered cellulose activated charcoal
Aerosol Propellant	An agent responsible for developing the pressure within an aerosol container and expelling the product when the valve is opened.	carbon dioxide dichlorodifluoromethane dichlorotetrafluoroethane trichloromonofluoromethane
Air Displacement	An agent which is employed to displace air in a hermetically sealed container to enhance product stability.	nitrogen
Antifungal Preservative	Used in liquid and semi-solid preparations to prevent the growth of fungi. The effectiveness of the parabens is usually enhanced when they are used in combination.	benzoic acid butylparaben ethylparaben methylparaben propylparaben sodium benzoate sodium propionate
Antimicrobial Preservative	Used in liquid and semi-solid preparations to prevent the growth of microorganisms.	benzalkonium chloride benzethonium chloride benzyl alcohol cetylpyridinium chloride chlorobutanol phenol phenylethyl alcohol phenylmercuric nitrate thimerosal

Table 4–2. Continued

Ingredient Type	*Definition*	*Examples*
Antioxidant	An agent which inhibits oxidation and thus is used to prevent the deterioration of preparations by the oxidative process.	ascorbic acid ascorbyl palmitate butylated hydroxyanisole butylated hydroxytoluene hypophophorous acid monothioglycerol propyl gallate sodium ascorbate sodium bisulfite sodium formaldehyde sulfoxylate sodium metabisulfite
Buffering Agent	Used to resist change in pH upon dilution or addition of acid or alkali.	potassium metaphosphate potassium phosphate, monobasic sodium acetate sodium citrate anhydrous and dihydrate
Chelating Agent	A substance that forms stable, water soluble complexes (chelates) with metals. Chelating agents are used in some liquid pharmaceuticals as stabilizers to complex heavy metals which might promote instability. In such use they are also called *sequestering* agents.	edetate disodium edetic acid
Colorant	Used to impart color to liquid and solid (e.g., tablets and capsules) pharmaceutical preparations.	FD&C Red No. 3 FD&C Red No. 20 FD&C Yellow No. 6 FD&C Blue No. 2 D&C Green No. 5 D&C Orange No. 5 D&C Red No. 8 caramel ferric oxide, red
Clarifying Agent	Used as a filtering aid because of adsorbent qualities.	bentonite
Emulsifying Agent	Used to promote and maintain the dispersion of finely subdivided particles of a liquid in a vehicle in which it is immiscible. The end product may be a liquid emulsion or semisolid emulsion (e.g., a cream).	acacia cetomacrogol cetyl alcohol glyceryl monostearate sorbitan monooleate polyoxyethylene 50 stearate
Encapsulating Agent	Used to form thin shells for the purpose of enclosing a drug substance or drug formulation for ease of administration.	gelatin cellulose acetate phthalate
Flavorant	Used to impart a pleasant flavor and often odor to a pharmaceutical preparation. In addition to the natural flavorants listed, many synthetic flavorants are also used.	anise oil cinnamon oil cocoa menthol orange oil peppermint oil vanillin

Table 4–2. Continued

Ingredient Type	*Definition*	*Examples*
Humectant	Used to prevent the drying out of preparations—particularly ointments and creams—due to the agent's ability to retain moisture.	glycerin propylene glycol sorbitol
Levigating Agent	A liquid used as an intervening agent to reduce the particle size of a drug powder by grinding together, usually in a mortar.	mineral oil glycerin
Ointment Base	The semisolid vehicle into which drug substances may be incorporated in preparing medicated ointments.	lanolin hydrophilic ointment polyethylene glycol ointment petrolatum hydrophilic petrolatum white ointment yellow ointment rose water ointment
Plasticizer	Used as a component of film-coating solutions to enhance the spread of the coat over tablets, beads, and granules.	diethyl phthalate glycerin
Solvent	An agent used to dissolve another pharmaceutic substance or a drug in the preparation of a solution. The solvent may be aqueous or nonaqueous (e.g., oleaginous). Cosolvents, such as water and alcohol (hydroalcoholic) and water and glycerin, may be used when needed. Solvents rendered sterile are used in certain preparations (e.g., injections).	alcohol corn oil cottonseed oil glycerin isopropyl alcohol mineral oil oleic acid peanut oil purified water water for injection sterile water for injection sterile water for irrigation
Stiffening Agent	Used to increase the thickness or hardness of a pharmaceutical preparation, usually an ointment.	cetyl alcohol cetyl esters wax microcrystalline wax paraffin stearyl alcohol white wax yellow wax
Suppository Base	Used as a vehicle into which drug substances are incorporated in the preparation of suppositories.	cocoa butter polyethylene glycols (mixtures)
Surfactant (surface active agent)	Substances which absorb to surfaces or interfaces to reduce surface or interfacial tension. May be used as wetting agents, detergents or emulsifying agents.	benzalkonium chloride nonoxynol 10 oxtoxynol 9 polysorbate 80 sodium lauryl sulfate sorbitan monopalmitate

Table 4–2. Continued

Ingredient Type	*Definition*	*Examples*
Suspending Agent	A viscosity increasing agent used to reduce the rate of sedimentation of (drug) particles dispersed throughout a vehicle in which they are not soluble. The resultant suspensions may be formulated for use orally, parenterally, ophthalmically, topically, or by other routes.	agar bentonite carbomer (e.g., Carbopol) carboxymethylcellulose sodium hydroxyethyl cellulose hydroxypropyl cellulose hydroxypropyl methylcellulose kaolin methylcellulose tragacanth veegum
Sweetening Agent	Used to impart sweetness to a preparation.	aspartame dextrose glycerin mannitol saccharin sodium sorbitol sucrose
Tablet Antiadherents	Agents which prevent the sticking of tablet formulation ingredients to punches and dies in a tableting machine during production.	magnesium stearate talc
Tablet Binders	Substances used to cause adhesion of powder particles in tablet granulations.	acacia alginic acid carboxymethylcellulose sodium compressible sugar (e.g., Nu-Tab) ethylcellulose gelatin liquid glucose methylcellulose povidone pregelatinized starch
Tablet and Capsule Diluent	Inert substances used as fillers to create the desired bulk, flow properties, and compression characteristics in the preparation of tablets and capsules.	dibasic calcium phosphate kaolin lactose mannitol microcrystalline cellulose powdered cellulose precipitated calcium carbonate sorbitol starch

Table 4–2. Continued

Ingredient Type	*Definition*	*Examples*
Tablet Coating Agent	Used to coat a formed tablet for the purpose of protecting against drug decomposition by atmospheric oxygen or humidity, to provide a desired release pattern for the drug substance after administration, to mask the taste or odor of the drug substance, or for aesthetic purposes. The coating may be of various types, including sugar-coating, film coating, or enteric coating. Sugar coating is water-based and results in a thickened covering around a formed tablet. Sugar-coated tablets generally start to break up in the stomach. A film coat is a thin cover around a formed tablet or bead. Unless it is an enteric coat, the film coat will dissolve in the stomach. An enteric-coated tablet or bead will pass through the stomach and break up in the intestines. Some coatings that are water-insoluble (e.g., ethylcellulose) may be used to coat tablets and beads to slow the release of drug as they pass through the gastrointestinal tract.	*sugar coating:* liquid glucose sucrose *film coating:* hydroxyethyl cellulose hydroxypropyl cellulose hydroxypropyl methylcellulose methylcellulose (e.g., Methocel) ethylcellulose (e.g., Ethocel) *enteric coating:* cellulose acetate phthalate shellac (35% in alcohol, "pharmaceutical glaze")
Tablet Direct Compression Excipient	Used in direct compression tablet formulations.	dibasic calcium phosphate (e.g., Ditab)
Tablet Disintegrant	Used in solid dosage forms to promote the disruption of the solid mass into smaller particles which are more readily dispersed or dissolved.	alginic acid carboxymethylcellulose calcium microcrystalline cellulose (e.g., Avicel) polacrilin potassium (e.g., Amberlite) sodium alginate sodium starch glycollate starch
Tablet Glidant	Agents used in tablet and capsule formulations to improve the flow properties of the powder mixture.	colloidal silica cornstarch talc
Tablet Lubricant	Substances used in tablet formulations to reduce friction during tablet compression.	calcium stearate magnesium stearate mineral oil stearic acid zinc stearate
Tablet/Capsule Opaquant	Used to render a capsule or a tablet coating opaque. May be used alone or in combination with a colorant.	titanium dioxide
Tablet Polishing Agent	Used to impart an attractive sheen to coated tablets.	carnauba wax white wax

Table 4–2. Continued

Ingredient Type	*Definition*	*Examples*
Tonicity Agent	Used to render a solution similar in osmotic characteristics to physiologic fluids. Ophthalmic, parenteral, and irrigation fluids are examples of preparations in which tonicity is a consideration.	dextrose sodium chloride
Vehicle	A carrying agent for a drug substance. They are used in formulating a variety of liquid dosage for oral and parenteral administration. Generally, oral liquids are aqueous preparations (as syrups) or hydroalcoholic (as elixirs). Parenteral solutions for intravenous use are aqueous, whereas intramuscular injections may be aqueous or oleaginous.	*Flavored/Sweetened* Acacia Syrup Aromatic Syrup Aromatic Elixir Cherry Syrup Cocoa Syrup Orange Syrup Syrup *Oleaginous* Corn Oil Mineral Oil Peanut Oil Sesame Oil *Sterile* Bacteriostatic Sodium Chloride Injection Bacteriostatic Water for Injection
Viscosity Increasing Agent	Used to change the consistency of a preparation to render it more resistant to flow. Used in suspensions to deter sedimentation, in ophthalmic solutions to enhance contact time (e.g., methylcellulose), to thicken topical creams, etc.	alginic acid bentonite carbomer carboxymethylcellulose sodium methylcellulose povidone sodium alginate tragacanth

book of Pharmaceutical Excipients,[2] which presents monographs on about 150 excipients used in pharmaceutical dosage form preparation. Included in each monograph is such information as: nonproprietary, chemical, and commercial names; empirical and chemical formulas and molecular weight; pharmaceutic specifications and chemical and physical properties; incompatibilities and interactions with other excipients and drug substances; regulatory status; and applications in pharmaceutic formulation or technology.

There is great interest nowadays in the international "harmonization" of standards applicable to pharmaceutical excipients. This is due to the fact that the pharmaceutical industry is multinational, with major companies having facilities in more than a single country, with products sold in markets worldwide, and with regulatory approval for these products generally required in each individual country. Standards for each drug substance and excipient used in pharmaceuticals are contained in pharmacopeias—or, for new agents, in an application for regulatory approval by the FDA or another nation's governing authority. The four pharmacopeias with the largest international use are the *United States Pharmacopeia/National Formulary* (USP/NF), *British Pharmacopeia* (BP), *European Pharmacopeia* (EP), and the *Japanese Pharmacopeia* (JP). Uniform standards for excipients in these and other pharmacopeias would facilitate production efficiency, enable the marketing of a single formulation of a product internationally, and enhance regulatory approval of pharmaceutical products worldwide. The goal of harmonization is an ongoing effort undertaken by corporate representatives and international regulatory authorities.

Drug Product Stability

As indicated previously, many pharmaceutic ingredients may be utilized in preparing the desired dosage form of a drug substance. Some of these agents may be used to achieve the desired physical and chemical characteristics of the product or to enhance its appearance, odor, and taste. Other substances may be used to increase the stability of the drug substance, particularly against the hydrolytic and oxidative processes. In each instance, the added pharmaceutic ingredient must be compatible with and must not detract from the stability of the drug substance in the particular dosage form prepared.

There are several approaches to the stabilization of pharmaceutical preparations containing drugs subject to deterioration by hydrolysis. Perhaps the most obvious is the reduction, or better yet, the elimination of water from the pharmaceutical system. Even solid dosage forms containing water-labile drugs must be protected from the humidity of the atmosphere. This may be accomplished by applying a waterproof protective coating over tablets or by enclosing and maintaining the drug in tightly closed containers. It is not unusual to detect hydrolyzed aspirin by noticing an odor of acetic acid upon opening a bottle of aspirin tablets. In liquid preparations, water can frequently be replaced or reduced in the formulation through the use of substitute liquids such as glycerin, propylene glycol, and alcohol. In certain injectable products, anhydrous vegetable oils may be used as the drug's solvent to reduce the chance of hydrolytic decomposition.

Decomposition by hydrolysis may be prevented for other drugs to be administered in liquid form by suspending them in a non-aqueous vehicle rather than by dissolving them in an aqueous solvent. In still other instances, particularly for certain unstable antibiotic drugs, when an aqueous preparation is desired, the drug may be supplied to the pharmacist in a dry form for *reconstitution* by adding a specified volume of purified water just before dispensing. The dry powder supplied commercially is actually a mixture of the antibiotic, suspending agents, flavorants, and colorants, which, when reconstituted by the pharmacist, remains a stable suspension or solution of the drug for the time period in which the preparation is normally consumed. Storage under refrigeration is advisable for most preparations considered unstable due to hydrolytic causes. Together with temperature, pH is a major determinant in the stability of a drug prone to hydrolytic decomposition. The hydrolysis of most drugs is dependent upon the relative concentrations of the hydroxyl and hydronium ions, and a pH at which each drug is optimally stable can be easily determined. For most hydrolyzable drugs the pH of optimum stability is on the acid side, somewhere between pH 5 and 6. Therefore, through judicious use of buffering agents, the stability of otherwise unstable compounds can be increased.

Pharmaceutically, the oxidation of a susceptible drug substance is most likely to occur when it is maintained in other than the dry state in the presence of oxygen, exposed to light, or combined in formulation with other chemical agents without proper regard to their influence on the oxidation process. The oxidation of a chemical in a pharmaceutical preparation is usually attendant with an alteration in the color of that preparation. It may also result in precipitation or a change in the usual odor of a preparation.

The oxidative process is diverted, and the stability of the drug is preserved by agents called *antioxidants*, which react with one or more compounds in the drug to prevent progress of the chain reaction. In general, antioxidants act by providing electrons and easily available hydrogen atoms that are accepted more readily by the free radicals than are those of the drug being protected. Various antioxidants are employed in pharmacy. Among those more frequently used in aqueous preparations are sodium sulfite (Na_2SO_3), sodium bisulfite ($NaHSO_3$), hypophosphorous acid (H_3PO_2), and ascorbic acid. In oleaginous (oily or unctuous) preparations, alphatocopherol, butylhydroxyanisole, and ascorbyl palmitate find application.

In June 1987, FDA labeling regulations went into effect requiring a warning about possible allergic-type reactions, including anaphylaxis in the package insert for prescription drugs to which sulfites have been added to the final dosage form. Sulfites are used as preservatives in many injectable drugs, such as antibiotics and local anesthetics. Some inhalants and ophthalmic preparations also contain sulfites, but relatively few oral drugs contain these chemicals. The purpose of the regulation is to protect the estimated 0.2% of the population who suffer allergic reactions from the chemicals. Many of the sulfite-sensitive persons suffer from asthma or other allergic conditions. Previous to the regulations dealing with prescription medication, the FDA issued regulations for the use of sulfites in food. Asthmatics and other patients who may be sulfite-sensitive should be reminded to read the labels of packaged foods and medications to check for the presence of these agents.

The most frequent symptom of a sulfite reaction is difficulty breathing. Other symptoms include diarrhea, nausea and vomiting, abdominal pain and cramps, dizziness, wheezing, hives, itching, local swelling, rash, difficulty swallowing, headache, fainting, change in body temperature, chest pain, change in heart rate, unconsciousness and coma. Symptoms usually occur within minutes of ingesting or taking sulfited foods or drug products.

Sulfiting agents covered by the regulations are potassium bisulfite, potassium metabisulfite, sodium bisulfite, sodium metabisulfite, sodium sulfite and sulfur dioxide.

The labeling of drugs to which sulfites have been added to the final dosage form must contain the following statement in the "Warnings" section of the labeling:

"Contains (name of the sulfite), a sulfite that may cause allergic-type reactions including anaphylactic symptoms and life-threatening or less severe asthmatic episodes in certain susceptible people. The overall prevalence of sulfite sensitivity in the general population is unknown and probably low. Sulfite sensitivity is seen more frequently in asthmatic than nonasthmatic people."

Sulfite-containing epinephrine for injection for use in allergic emergencies must contain the following statement:

"Epinephrine is the preferred treatment for serious allergic or emergency situations even though this product contains (name of sulfite), a sulfite that may in other products cause allergic-type reactions including anaphylactic symptoms or life-threatening or less severe asthmatic episodes in certain susceptible persons. The alternatives to using epinephrine in a life-threatening situation may not be satisfactory. The presence of a sulfite(s) in this product should not deter the administration of the drug for treatment of serious allergic or other emergency situations."

The FDA permits the use of sulfites in prescription products, with the proper labeling, because there are no generally suitable substitutes for sulfites to maintain potency in certain medications.

The proper use of antioxidants involves their specific application only after appropriate biomedical and pharmaceutical studies. In certain instances other pharmaceutical additives have been found to inactivate a given antioxidant when used in the same formulation. In other cases certain antioxidants have been found to react chemically with the drugs they were intended to stabilize, without a noticeable change in the appearance of the preparation.

Because the stability of oxidizable drugs may be adversely affected by oxygen, certain pharmaceuticals may require an oxygen-free atmosphere during their preparation and storage. Oxygen may be present in pharmaceutical liquids in the airspace within the container or may be dissolved in the liquid vehicle. To avoid these exposures, oxygen-sensitive drugs may be prepared in the dry state and they, as well as liquid preparations, may be packaged in sealed containers with the air replaced by an inert gas such as nitrogen. This is common practice in the commercial production of vials and ampuls of easily oxidizable preparations intended for parenteral use.

Trace metals originating in the drug, solvent, container, or stopper are a constant source of difficulty in preparing stable solutions of oxidizable drugs. The rate of formation of color in epinephrine solutions, for instance, is greatly increased by the presence of ferric, ferrous, cupric, and chromic ions. Great care must be taken to eliminate these trace metals from labile preparations by thorough purification of the source of the contaminant or by chemically complexing or binding the metal through the use of specialized agents that make it chemically unavailable for participation in the oxidative process. These agents are referred to as *chelating agents* and are exemplified by calcium disodium edetate and ethylenediamine tetra-acetic acid (EDTA).

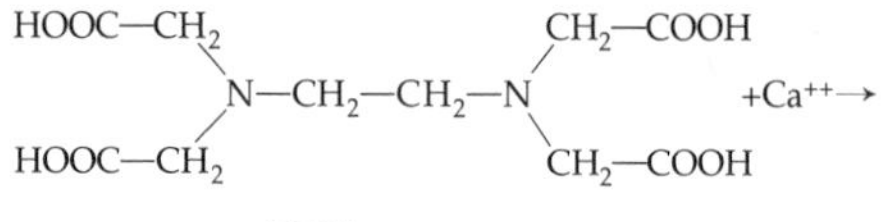

EDTA

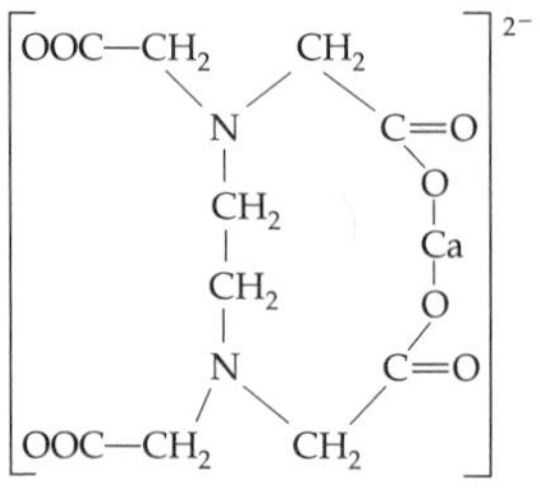

Proposed calcium complex of EDTA

Light can also act as a catalyst to oxidation reactions. As a photocatalyst, light waves trans-

Table 4–3. Examples of Some Official Drugs and Preparations Especially Subject to Chemical or Physical Deterioration

Preparation	*Category*	*Monograph or Label Warning*
Epinephrine Bitartrate Ophthalmic Solution, USP Epinephrine Inhalation Solution, USP Epinephrine Injection, USP Epinephrine Nasal Solution, USP Epinephrine Ophthalmic Solution, USP	Adrenergic	Do not use the inhalation, injection, nasal or ophthalmic solution if it is brown or contains a precipitate.
Isoproterenol Sulfate Inhalation, Solution, USP Isoproterenol Inhalation Solution, USP	Adrenergic (bronchodilator)	Do not use the inhalation or injection if it is pink to brown in color or contains a precipitate.
Nitroglycerin Tablets, USP	Antianginal	To prevent loss of potency, keep these tablets in the original container or in a supplemental nitroglycerin container specifically labeled as being suitable for nitroglycerin tablets.
Paraldehyde, USP	Hypnotic	Paraldehyde is subject to oxidation to form acetic acid.

fer their energy (photon) to drug molecules, making the latter more reactive through increased energy capability. As a precaution against the acceleration of the oxidative process, sensitive preparations are packaged in light-resistant or opaque containers.

Since most drug degradations proceed more rapidly with an advanced temperature, it is also advisable to maintain oxidizable drugs in a cool place. Another factor that could affect the stability of an oxidizable drug in solution is the pH of the preparation. Each drug must be maintained in solution at the pH most favorable to its stability. This, in fact, varies from preparation to preparation and must be determined on an individual basis for the drug in question.

Statements in the USP, as those in Table 4–3, warn of the oxidative decomposition of drugs and preparations. In some instances the specific agent to employ as a stabilizer is mentioned in the monograph, and in others the term "suitable stabilizer" is used. An example in which a particular agent is designated for use is in the monograph for Potassium Iodide Oral Solution, USP. Potassium iodide in solution is prone to photocatalyzed oxidation and the release of free iodine with a resultant brown discoloration of the solution. The use of light-resistant containers is essential to its stability. As a further precaution against decomposition if the solution is not to be used within a short time, the USP recommends the addition of 0.5 mg of sodium thiosulfate for each gram of potassium iodide in the preparation. In the event free iodine is released during storage, the sodium thiosulfate converts it to colorless and soluble sodium iodide:

$$I_2 + 2Na_2S_2O_3 \rightarrow 2\ NaI + Na_2S_4O_6$$

In summary, for easily oxidizable drugs, the formulation pharmacist may stabilize the respective preparations by the selective exclusion from the system of oxygen, oxidizing agents, trace metals, light, heat, and other chemical catalysts to the oxidation process. Antioxidants, chelating agents, and buffering agents may be added to create and maintain a favorable pH.

In addition to oxidation and hydrolysis, other destructive processes such as polymerization, chemical decarboxylation, and deamination may occur in pharmaceutical preparations. However, these processes occur less frequently and are peculiar to only small groups of chemical substances. Drug polymerization involves a reaction between two or more identical molecules with resultant formation of a new and generally larger molecule. Formaldehyde is an example of a drug capable of polymerization. In solution it may polymerize to paraformaldehyde $(CH_2O)_n$, a slowly soluble white crystalline substance that may cause the solution to become cloudy. The formation of paraformaldehyde is enhanced by cool storage temperatures, especially in solutions with high concentrations of formaldehyde. The official formaldehyde solution contains approximately 37% formaldehyde and according to the USP should be stored at temperatures not below 15°C (59°F). If the solution becomes cloudy upon standing in a cool place, it generally may be cleared by gentle warming. Formaldehyde is prepared by the limited oxidation of methanol (methyl alcohol), and the USP permits a residual amount of this material to remain in the final product, since it has the ability to retard the formation of paraformaldehyde. Formaldehyde solution must be maintained in tight containers because oxidation of the formaldehyde yields formic acid.

$$\underset{\text{methanol}}{CH_3OH} \xrightarrow{(O)} \underset{\text{formaldehyde}}{HCHO} \xrightarrow{(O)} \underset{\text{formic acid}}{HCOOH}$$

Other organic drug molecules may be degraded through processes in which one or more of their active chemical groups are removed. These processes may involve various catalysts, including light and enzymes. Decarboxylation and deamination are examples of such processes, with the former involving the decomposition of an organic acid (R•COOH) and the consequent release of carbon dioxide gas and the latter involving the removal of the nitrogen-containing group from an organic amine. For example, insulin, a protein, deteriorates rapidly in acid solutions, due to extensive deamination.[3] Thus, most preparations of insulin are neutralized to reduce its rate of decomposition.

Stability Testing

Drug instability in pharmaceutical formulations may be detected in some instances by a change in the physical appearance, color, odor, taste or texture of the formulation whereas in other instances chemical changes may occur which are not self-evident and may only be ascertained through chemical analysis. Scientific data pertaining to the stability of a formulation leads to the prediction of the expected shelf-life of the proposed product and, when necessary, to the redesign of the drug (e.g. into more stable salt or ester form) and to the reformulation of the dosage form. Obviously the *rate* or speed at which drug degradation occurs in a formulation is of prime importance. The study of the rate of chemical change and the way in which it is influenced by such factors as the concentration of the drug or reactant, the solvent employed, the conditions of temperature and pressure, and the presence of other chemical agents in the formulation is termed *reaction kinetics*.

In general a kinetic study begins by measuring the concentration of the drug being examined at given time intervals under a specific set of conditions including temperature, pH, ionic strength, light intensity, and drug concentration. The measurement of the drug's concentration at the various time intervals reveals the stability or instability of the drug under the specified conditions with the passage of time. From this starting point, each of the original conditions may be varied on an individual basis to determine the influence that such changes make on the drug's stability. For example, the pH of the solution may be changed, whereas the temperature, light intensity, and original drug concentration remain as they were in the original or baseline experiment.

The rate of a drug's degradation often follows first-order kinetics, with the rate of degradation being directly proportional to the concentration of drug. As degradation procedes, the concentration (C) of drug (d) decreases with time (t), as expressed by $-dC/dt = kC$, with the negative sign indicating a decrease in drug concentration. The rate constant, k, has the dimension of reciprocal time; that is, if k is 0.001 hr^{-1}, then 0.1% of the drug degradates each hour. The integrated form of the equation, $\log C = -kt/2.3 + \log C_0$, is often more easily interpreted, where C_0 is the initial drug concentration and C is the drug concentration at time t.[4]

The data collected may be presented graphically, by plotting the drug concentration as a function of time. From the experimental data, the reaction rate may be determined and a rate constant calculated. The rate constant describes the rate at which a drug is degrading under the conditions of the experiment and may be expressed as for example "2.6 mg/day," "0.1%/hour," or "0.155 g/liter/day."

The data also may be utilized in determining the experimental half-life of the drug. The *half-*

life of a drug is defined as the time required for the drug to degrade to one-half of its original concentration. The half-life of a drug is expressed as its $t_{1/2}$ or t_{50}. Other expressions of drug remaining with reference to the original concentration may be used, as t_{90} and t_{95} indicating the drug remaining is 90 and 95% respectively of the original concentration. Half-life, $t_{1/2} = 0.693/k$, as explained on page 93.

The use of *exaggerated* conditions of temperature, humidity, light, and others, to test the stability of drug formulations is termed *accelerated stability testing*. Accelerated temperature stability studies, for example, may be conducted for six months at 40°C with 75% relative humidity. If a significant change occurs in the drug/drug product under these conditions, lesser temperature and humidity may be used, such as 30°C and 60% relative humidity. The use of short-term accelerated studies is for the purpose of determining the most stable of the proposed formulations for a drug product. In *stress testing*, temperature elevations, in 10° increments higher than used in accelerated studies, are employed until chemical or physical degradation. Once the most stable formulation is ascertained, its long-term stability is predicted from the data generated from continuing stability studies. Depending upon the types and severity of conditions employed, it is not unusual to maintain samples under exaggerated conditions of both temperature and varying humidity for periods of 6 to 12 months. Such studies lead to the prediction of shelf-life for a drug product.

In addition to the accelerated stability studies, drug products are also subjected to long-term stability studies under the usual conditions of transport and storage expected during product distribution. In conducting these studies, the different climatic zones, nationally and internationally, to which the product may be subjected must be borne in mind, and expected variances in conditions of temperature and humidity included in the study design. Geographic regions of the world are defined by climatic zones: zone I, "temperate"; zone II, "subtropical"; zone III, "hot and dry"; and zone IV, "hot and humid." A given drug product may encounter more than a single zone of temperature/humidity variations during its production and shelf-life. Further, it may be warehoused, transported, placed on a pharmacy's shelf, and subsequently in the patient's medicine cabinet, over a varying time course and at a wide range of temperature and humidity. In general, however, the long-term (12 months minimum) testing of new drug entities is conducted at 25° C ± 2° C and at a relative humidity of 60% ± 5%. Samples maintained under these conditions may be retained for periods of 5 years or longer during which time they are observed for physical signs of deterioration and chemically assayed. These studies, considered with the accelerated stability studies previously performed, then lead to a more precise determination of drug product stability, actual shelf-life, and the possible extension of expiration dating.

When chemical degradation products are detected, the FDA requires the manufacturer to report their chemical identities, including structures, mechanism of formation, physical and chemical properties, procedures for isolation and purification, specifications and directions for determination at levels expected to be present in the pharmaceutical product, and the pharmacologic action and biologic significance, if any, to their presence.

In addition, signs of degradation of the specific dosage forms must be observed and reported. For the various dosage forms, this includes the following.[5]

Tablets: appearance, friability, hardness, color, odor, moisture content, and dissolution.

Capsules: strength, moisture, color, appearance, shape, brittleness, and dissolution.

Oral solutions and suspensions: appearance, strength, pH, color, odor, redispersibility (suspensions), and clarity (solutions).

Oral powders: appearance, strength, color, odor, moisture.

Metered-dose inhalation aerosols: strength, delivered dose per actuation, number of metered doses, color, particle-size distribution, loss of propellant, pressure, valve corrosion, spray pattern, absence of pathogenic microorganisms.

Topical nonmetered aerosols: appearance, odor, pressure, weight loss, net weight dispensed, delivery rate, and spray pattern.

Topical creams, ointments, lotions, solutions, and gels: appearance, color, homogeneity, odor, pH, resuspendibility (lotions), consistency, particle-size distribution, strength, weight loss.

Ophthalmic preparations: appearance, color, consistency, pH, clarity (solutions), particle size and resuspendibility (suspen-

Stability, Kinetics, and Shelf-Life

Stability is defined as the extent to which a product retains, within specified limits, and throughout its period of storage and use (i.e., its shelf-life), the same properties and characteristics that it possessed at the time of its manufacture.

There are five types of stability of concern to pharmacists:

1. *Chemical.* Each active ingredient retains its chemical integrity and labeled potency, within the specified limits.
2. *Physical.* The original physical properties, including appearance, palatability, uniformity, dissolution and suspendability are retained.
3. *Microbiologic.* Sterility or resistance to microbial growth is retained according to the specified requirements. Antimicrobial agents that are present retain effectiveness within specified limits.
4. *Therapeutic.* The therapeutic effect remains unchanged.
5. *Toxicologic.* No significant increase in toxicity occurs.

Chemical stability is important for selecting storage conditions (temperature, light, humidity), selecting the proper container for dispensing (glass vs. plastic, clear vs. amber or opaque, cap liners) and for anticipating interactions when mixing drugs and dosage forms. Stability and expiration dating are based on reaction kinetics, i.e., the study of the rate of chemical change and the way this rate is influenced by conditions of concentration of reactants, products, and other chemical species that may be present, and by factors such as solvent, pressure, and temperature.

In considering chemical stability of a pharmaceutical, one must know the reaction order and reaction rate. The reaction order may be the overall order (the sum of the exponents of the concentration terms of the rate expression), or the order with respect to each reactant (the exponent of the individual concentration term in the rate expression). The reaction rate expression is a description of the drug concentration with respect to time. Most commonly, zero-order and first-order reactions are encountered in pharmacy.

Zero Order

If the loss of drug is independent of the concentration of the reactants and constant with respect to time (i.e., 1 mg/mL/hour), the rate is called zero order. The mathematical expression is:

$$\frac{-dC}{dt} = k_0$$

where k_0 is the zero-order rate constant [concentration(C)/time(t)].

The integrated, and more useful form of the equation, is:

$$C = -k_0 t + C_0$$

where C_0 is the initial concentration of the drug.

EXAMPLE 1

A drug suspension (125 mg/mL) decays by zero-order kinetics with a reaction rate constant of 0.5 mg/mL/hour. What is the concentration of intact drug remaining after 3 days (72 hours)?

$$C = -(0.5 \text{ mg/mL/hr})\ (72 \text{ hr}) + 125 \text{ mg/mL}$$
$$C = 89 \text{ mg/mL}$$

EXAMPLE 2

How long will it take for the suspension to reach 90% of its original concentration?

$$90\% \times 125 \text{ mg/mL} = 112.5 \text{ mg/mL}$$

$$t = \frac{C - C_0}{-k_0} = \frac{112.5 \text{ mg/mL} - 125 \text{ mg/mL}}{-0.5 \text{ mg/mL/hr}} = 25 \text{ hours}$$

Drug suspensions are examples of pharmaceuticals that ordinarily follow zero-order kinetics for degradation.

Stability, Kinetics, and Shelf-Life (Continued)

FIRST ORDER

If the loss of drug is directly proportional to the concentration remaining with respect to time, it is called a first-order reaction and has the units of reciprocal time, i.e., time^{-1}. The mathematical expression is:

$$\frac{-dC}{dt} = kC$$

where C is the concentration of intact drug remaining, t is time, $(-dC/dt)$ is the rate at which the intact drug degrades, and k is the specific reaction rate constant.

The integrated and more useful form of the equation is:

$$\log C = \frac{-kt}{2.303} + \log C_0$$

where C_0 is the initial concentration of the drug.

In natural log form, the equation is:

$$\ln C = -kt + \ln C_0$$

EXAMPLE 3

An ophthalmic solution of a mydriatic drug, present at a 5 mg/mL concentration, exhibits first-order degradation with a rate of 0.0005/day. How much drug will remain after 120 days?

$$\ln C = -(0.0005/\text{day})\ (120) + \ln\ (5\ \text{mg/mL})$$
$$\ln C = -0.06 + 1.609$$
$$\ln C = 1.549$$
$$C = 4.71\ \text{mg/mL}$$

EXAMPLE 4

In the above example, how long will it take for the drug to degrade to 90% of its original concentration?

$$90\%\ \text{of}\ 5\ \text{mg/mL} = 4.5\ \text{mg/mL}$$
$$\ln 4.5\ \text{mg/mL} = -(0.0005/\text{day})t + \ln\ (5\ \text{mg/mL})$$
$$t = \frac{\ln 4.5\ \text{mg/mL} - \ln 5\ \text{mg/mL}}{-0.0005/\text{day}}$$
$$t = 210\ \text{days}$$

Stability projections for shelf-life (t_{90}) (i.e., the time required for 10% of the drug to degrade with 90% of the intact drug remaining, are commonly based upon the Arrhenius equation:

$$\log \frac{k_2}{k_1} = \frac{Ea\ (t_2 - T_1)}{2.3\ RT_1T_2}$$

which relates the reaction rate constants (k) to temperatures (T) with the gas constant (R) and the energy of activation (Ea).

The relationship of the reaction rate constants at two different temperatures provides the energy of activation for the degradation. By performing the reactions at elevated temperatures, instead of allowing the process to proceed very slowly at room temperature, the Ea can be calculated and a k value for room temperature determined by using the Arrhenius equation.

EXAMPLE 5

The degradation of a new cancer drug follows first-order kinetics and has first-order degradation rate constants of 0.0001/hr at 60°C and 0.0009 at 80°C. What is its Ea?

$$\log \frac{(0.0009)}{(0.0001)} = \frac{EA\ (353 - 333)}{(2.3)(1.987)(353)(333)}$$
$$Ea = 25{,}651\ \text{kcal/mol}$$

Stability, Kinetics, and Shelf-Life (Continued)

The Q_{10} method of shelf-life estimation allows the pharmacist quickly to calculate estimates of shelf-life for a product that may have been stored or is going to be stored under a different set of conditions. The Q_{10} approach, based on Ea, is independent of reaction order and is described as:

$$Q_{10} = e^{\{(Ea/R)[(1/T+10) - (1/T)]\}}$$

where Ea is the energy of activation,
R is the gas constant, and
T is the absolute temperature.

In usable terms, Q_{10} is the ratio of two different reaction rate constants, and is defined as:

$$Q_{10} = \frac{K_{(T+10)}}{K_T}$$

Q values of 2, 3 and 4 are commonly used and relate to the energies of activations of the reactions for temperatures around room temperature (25°C). For example, a Q value of 2 corresponds to an Ea (kcal/mol) of 12.2, a Q value of 3 corresponds to an Ea of 19.4, and a Q value of 4 corresponds to an Ea of 24.5.

Reasonable estimates can often be made using the value of 3.

The equation to use for Q_{10} shelf-life estimates is:

$$t_{90}(T_2) = \frac{t_{90}(T_1)}{Q_{10}^{(\Delta T/10)}}$$

where $t_{90}T_2$ is the estimated shelf-life,
$t_{90}T_1$ is the given shelf-life at a given temperature, and
ΔT is the difference in the temperatures T_1 and T_2.

As is evident from this relationship, an increase in ΔT will decrease the shelf-life and a decrease in ΔT will increase shelf-life. This is the same as saying that storing at a warmer temperature will shorten the life of the drug and storing at a cooler temperature will increase the life of the drug.

EXAMPLE 6

An antibiotic solution has a shelf-life of 48 hours in the refrigerator (5°C). What is its estimated shelf-life at room temperature (25°C)?

Using a Q value of 3, we set up the relationship as follows.

$$t_{90}(T_2) = \frac{t_{90}(T_1)}{Q_{10}^{(\Delta T/10)}} = \frac{48}{3^{[(25-5)/10]}} = \frac{48}{3^2} = 5.33 \text{ hours}$$

EXAMPLE 7

An opthalmic solution has a shelf-life of 6 hours at room temperature (25°C). What would be the estimated shelf-life if stored in a refrigerator (5°C)? (*Note:* Since the temperature is decreasing, ΔT will be negative.)

$$t_{90}(T_2) = \frac{6}{3^{[(5-25)/10]}} = \frac{6}{3^{-2}} = 6 \times 3^2 = 54 \text{ hours}$$

Pharmacists should keep in mind that these are estimates, and actual energies of activation can be often be obtained from the literature for more exact calculations.

sions, creams, ointments), strength, and sterility.

Small-volume parenterals: strength, appearance, color, particulate matter, dispersibility (suspensions), pH, sterility, pyrogenicity, and closure integrity.

Large-volume parenterals: strength, appearance, color, clarity, particulate matter, pH, volume and extractables (when plastic containers are used), sterility, pyrogenicity, and closure integrity.

Suppositories: strength, softening range, appearance, and dissolution.

Emulsions: appearance (as phase separation), color, odor, pH, viscosity, and strength.

Controlled-release membrane drug delivery systems: seal strength of the drug reservoir, decomposition products, membrane integrity, drug strength, and drug release rate.

Under usual circumstances, most manufactured products require a shelf-life of 2 or more years to ensure their stability at the time of patient consumption. Commercial products must bear an appropriate expiration date. This date identifies the time during which the product may be expected to maintain its potency and remain stable under the designated storage conditions. The expiration date limits the time during which the product may be dispensed by the pharmacist or used by the patient.

A summary of the concepts of drug stability, kinetics, and shelf-life is found in the preceding Physical Pharmacy Capsule.

Prescriptions requiring extemporaneous compounding by the pharmacist generally do not require the extended shelf-life that commercially manufactured and distributed products do because they are intended to be utilized immediately upon their receipt by the patient and used only during the immediate course of the prescribed treatment. However, these compounded prescriptions must remain stable and efficacious during the course of their use and the compounding pharmacist must employ formulative components and techniques which will result in a stable product. Thus, in the instance where an oral liquid preparation is made from an existing tablet or capsule formulation, the pharmacist should make up only at most a few days supply. Further, he must also dispense the medication in a container conductive to stability and use and must advise the patient of the proper method of use and conditions of storage of the medication.

In years past pharmacists were confronted primarily with innocuous, topical prescriptions that required extemporaneous formulation. However, in recent years there has been a need to compound other drug delivery systems as well, e.g., progesterone vaginal suppositories, oral suspensions, from existing tablets or capsules. When presented with a prescription that requires extemporaneous compounding, the pharmacist is confronted with a difficult situation because the potency and the stability of these prescriptions is a serious matter. Occasionally, the results of compatibility and stability studies on such prescriptions are published in scientific and professional journals. These are very useful; however, there are also prescriptions for which stability and compatability information is not readily available. In these instances it behooves the pharmacist to at least contact the drug manufacturer of the active ingredient(s) to solicit stability information. Alternatively, the pharmacist should use one's own personal network of professional associates to secure compounding procedure information. This latter approach by a group of hospital pharmacists lead to the eventual publication of the book titled, *Handbook of Extemporaneous Formulations,* by the American Society of Hospital Pharmacists. Finally, when compounding on the basis of extrapolated or less than concrete information it is best for the pharmacist to keep the formulation simple and not to shortcut but use the necessary pharmaceutical adjuvants to prepare the prescription.

Preservation Against Microbial Contamination

In addition to the stabilization of pharmaceutical preparations against chemical and physical degradation due to changed environmental conditions within a formulation, certain liquid and semisolid preparations also must be preserved against microbial contamination. Although some types of pharmaceutical products like ophthalmic and injectable preparations are sterilized by physical methods (autoclaving for 20 minutes at 15 pounds pressure and 120°C, dry heat at 170°C for 1 hour, or by bacterial filtration) during their manufacture, many of them additionally require the presence of an antimicrobial preservative to maintain their aseptic condition throughout the period of their storage and use. Other types of preparations that are not sterilized during their preparation but are particularly susceptible to microbial growth because of the nature of their ingredients, are protected by the addition of an antimicrobial preservative. Preparations that provide excellent growth media for microbes are most aqueous preparations, especially syrups, emulsions, suspensions, and some semisolid preparations, particularly creams. Certain hydroalcoholic and most alcoholic preparations may not require the addition of a chemical preservative when the alcoholic content is sufficient to prevent microbial growth. Generally, 15% alcohol will prevent microbial growth in acid media and 18% in alkaline media. Most alcohol-containing pharmaceuticals such as elixirs, spirits, and tinctures are self-sterilizing and do not require additional preservation. The same would apply to other pharmaceuticals on an individual basis, which by virtue of their vehicles or other formulative agents, may not permit the growth of microorganisms.

Selection of Preservatives

When experience or shelf-storage experiments indicate that a preservative is required in a pharmaceutical preparation, its selection is based on many cross considerations including some of the following.

1. The preservative is effective in preventing the growth of the type of microorganisms considered the most likely contaminants of the preparation being formulated.
2. The preservative is soluble enough in water to achieve adequate concentrations in the aqueous phase of a two or more phase system.
3. The proportion of preservative remaining undissociated at the pH of the preparation makes it capable of penetrating the microorganisms and destroying its integrity.
4. The required concentration of the preservative does not affect the safety or comfort of the patient when the pharmaceutical preparation is administered by the usual or intended route; i.e., nonirritating, nonsensitizing, nontoxic.
5. The preservative has adequate stability and will not be reduced in concentration due to chemical decomposition or volatilization during the desired shelf-life of the preparation.
6. The preservative is completely compatible with all other formulative ingredients and does not interfere with them, nor do they interfere with the effectiveness of the preservative agent.
7. The preservative does not adversely affect the preparation's container or the closure.

General Considerations

Pharmaceutical preparations may be contaminated by molds, yeasts, or bacteria, with the latter generally favoring a slightly alkaline medium and the others an acid medium. Although few microorganisms can grow below a pH of 3 or above pH 9, most aqueous pharmaceutical preparations are within the favorable pH range and therefore must be protected against microbial growth. To be effective, a preservative agent must be dissolved in sufficient concentration in the aqueous phase of a preparation. Further, only the undissociated fraction or molecular form of a preservative possesses preservative capability, because the ionized portion is incapable of penetrating the microorganism. Thus the preservative selected must be largely undissociated at the pH of the formulation being prepared. Acidic preservatives like benzoic, boric, and sorbic acids are more undissociated and thus more effective as the medium is made more acid. Conversely, alkaline preservatives are less effective in acid or neutral media and more effective in alkaline media. Thus, it is meaningless to suggest preservative effectiveness at specific concentrations unless the pH of the system is mentioned and the undissociated concentration of the agent is calculated or otherwise determined. Also, if formulative materials interfere with the solubility or availability of the preservative agent, its chemical concentration may be misleading, because it may not be a true measure of the effective concentration. Many incompatible combinations of preservative agents and other pharmaceutical adjuncts have been discovered in recent years, and undoubtedly many more will be uncovered in the future as new preservatives, pharmaceutical adjuncts, and therapeutic agents are combined for the first time. Many of the recognized incompatible combinations that result in preservative inactivation involve macromolecules such as various cellulose derivatives, polyethylene glycols, and natural gums such as tragacanth, which have been shown to attract and hold preservative agents, such as the parabens and phenolic compounds, rendering them unavailable for their preservative function. It is es-

Table 4–4. Probable Modes of Action of Some Preservatives

Preservative	*Probable Modes of Action*
Benzoic acid, boric acid, and p-hydroxybenzoates	Denaturation of proteins
Phenols and chlorinated phenolic compounds	Lytic and denaturation action on cytoplasmic membranes and for chlorinated preservatives, also by oxidation of enzymes
Alcohols	Lytic and denaturation action on membranes
Quaternary compounds	Lytic action on membranes
Mercurials	Denaturation of enzymes by combining with thiol (−SH) groups)

sential for the research pharmacist to examine all formulative ingredients as one affects the other to assure himself that each agent is free to do the job for which it was included in the formulation. In addition, the preservative must not interact with a container such as a metal ointment tube or a plastic medication bottle or with an enclosure such as a rubber or plastic cap or liner. Such an interaction could result in the decomposition of the preservative or the container closure, or, both, with resultant product decomposition and contamination. Appropriate tests should be devised and conducted to insure against this type of preservative interaction.

Mode of Action for Preservatives

Preservatives interfere with microbial growth, multiplication, and metabolism through one or more of the following mechanisms:

1. modification of cell membrane permeability and leakage of cell constituents (partial lysis)
2. lysis and cytoplasmic leakage
3. irreversible coagulation of cytoplasmic constituents (e.g., protein precipitation)
4. inhibition of cellular metabolism as through interference with enzyme systems or inhibition of cell wall synthesis
5. oxidation of cellular constituents
6. hydrolysis

A few of the commonly used pharmaceutical preservatives and their probable modes of action are presented in Table 4–4.

Preservative Utilization

Suitable substances may be added to a pharmaceutical preparation to enhance its permanency or usefulness. Such additives are suitable only if they are nontoxic and harmless in the amounts administered and do not interfere with the therapeutic efficacy or tests or assays of the preparation. Certain intravenous preparations given in large volumes as blood replenishers or as nutrients are not permitted to contain bacteriostatic additives, because the amounts required to preserve such large volumes would constitute a health hazard when administered to the patient. Thus preparations like Dextrose Injection, USP, and others commonly given as fluid and nutrient replenishers by intravenous injections in amounts of 500 to 1000 mL may not contain antibacterial preservatives. On the other hand, injectable preparations given in small volumes—for example, Morphine Sulfate Injection, USP, which provides a therapeutic amount of morphine sulfate in approximately a 1-mL volume—can be preserved with a suitable preservative without the danger of coadministering an excessive amount of the preservative to the patient.

Examples of the preservatives and their concentrations commonly employed in pharmaceutical preparations are: benzoic acid (0.1 to 0.2%), sodium benzoate (0.1 to 0.2%), alcohol (15 to 20%), phenylmercuric nitrate and acetate (0.002 to 0.01%), phenol (0.1 to 0.5%), cresol (0.1 to 0.5%), chlorobutanol (0.5%), benzalkonium chloride (0.002 to 0.01%), and combinations of methylparaben and propylparaben (0.1 to 0.2%), the latter being especially good against fungus. The required proportion would vary with the factors of pH, dissociation, and others already indicated as well with the presence of other formulative ingredients with inherent preservative capabilities that contribute to the preservation of the preparation and require less additional preservation assistance.

For each type of preparation to be preserved, the research pharmacist must consider the influence of the preservative on the comfort of the patient. For instance, it is apparent that a preservative in an ophthalmic preparation would have to have an extremely low degree of irritant qualities, which is characteristic of chlorobutanol, benzalkonium chloride, and phenylmercuric nitrate, frequently used preservatives in ophthalmic preparations. In all instances, the preserved preparation must be biologically tested to determine its safety and efficacy and shelf-tested to determine its stability for the intended shelf life of the product.

Appearance and Palatability

Although most drug substances in use today are unpalatable and unattractive in their natural state, modern pharmaceutical preparations present them to the patient as colorful, flavorful formulations attractive to the sight, smell, and taste. These qualities, which are the rule rather than the exception, have virtually eliminated the natural reluctance of many patients to take medications because of disagreeable odor or taste. In fact, the inherent attractiveness of today's pharmaceuticals has caused them to acquire the dubious distinction of being a source of accidental poisonings in the home, particularly among children who are lured by their organoleptic appeal.

There is some psychologic basis to drug therapy, and the odor, taste, and color of a pharmaceutical preparation can play a part. An appropriate drug will have its most beneficial effect when it is accepted and taken properly by the patient. The proper combination of flavor, fragrance, and color in a pharmaceutical product contributes to its acceptance.

Flavoring and Sweetening Pharmaceuticals

The flavoring of pharmaceuticals applies primarily to liquid dosage forms intended for oral administration. The 10,000 taste buds, found on the tongue, roof of the mouth, cheeks, and throat, have 60–100 receptor cells each.[6] These receptor cells interact with molecules dissolved in the saliva and produce a positive or negative taste sensation. Medication in liquid form obviously comes into immediate and direct contact with these taste buds. By the addition of flavoring agents to liquid medication, the disagreeable taste of drugs may be successfully masked. Drugs placed in capsules or prepared as coated tablets may be easily swallowed with avoidance of contact between the drug and the taste buds. Tablets containing drugs that are not especially distasteful may remain uncoated and unflavored. Swallowing them with water usually is sufficient to avoid undesirable drug taste sensations. However, tablets of the chewable type as certain antacid and vitamin products, which are intended for mastication in the mouth, usually *are* sweetened and flavored to receive better patient acceptance.

The flavor sensation of a food or pharmaceutical is actually a complex blend of taste and smell with lesser influences of texture, temperature, and even sight. In flavor formulating a pharmaceutical product, the pharmacist must give consideration to the color, odor, texture, and taste of the preparation. It would be incongruous, for example, to color a liquid pharmaceutical red, give it a banana taste, and a mint odor. The color of a pharmaceutical must have a psychogenic balance with the taste, and the odor must also enhance that taste. Odor greatly affects the flavor of a preparation or foodstuff. If one's sense of smell is impaired, as during a head cold, the usual flavor sensation of food is similarly diminished.

The medicinal chemist and the formulation pharmacist are well acquainted with the taste characteristic of certain chemical types of drugs and strive to mask effectively the unwanted taste through the appropriate use of flavoring agents. Although there are no dependable rules for unerringly predicting the taste sensation of a drug based upon its chemical constitution, experience permits the presentation of several observations. For instance, although we recognize and assume the salty taste of sodium chloride, the formulation pharmacist knows that all salts are not salty, but that their taste is a function of both the cation and anion. Whereas salty tastes are evoked by sodium, potassium, and ammonium chlorides and by sodium bromide, potassium and ammonium bromides elicit simultaneous bitter and salty sensations, and potassium iodide and magnesium sulfate (epsom salt) are predominantly bitter. In general, low molecular weight salts are salty, and higher molecular weight salts are bitter. With organic compounds, an increase in the number of hydroxyl groups (—OH) seems to increase the sweetness of the compound. Sucrose, which has eight hydroxyl groups, is sweeter than glycerin, another pharmaceutical sweetener, which has but three hydroxyl groups. In general, the organic esters, alcohols, and aldehydes are pleasant to the taste, and since many of them are volatile, they also contribute to the odor and thus the flavor of preparations in which they are used. Many nitrogen-containing compounds are extremely bitter, especially the plant alkaloids (as quinine), but certain other nitrogen-containing compounds are extremely sweet (as aspartame). The medicinal chemist recognizes that even the most simple structural change in an organic compound can alter its taste. D-glucose is sweet, but L-glucose has a slightly salty taste; saccharin is very sweet, but N-methyl-saccharin is tasteless.[7]

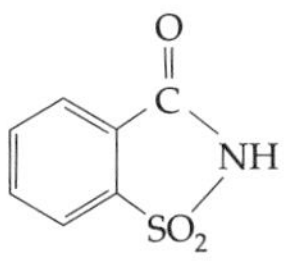

Saccharin
(Very sweet)

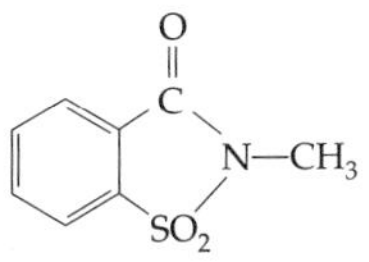

N-Methylsaccharin
(Tasteless)

Thus, the predictability of the taste characteristics of a new drug is only speculative. However, it is soon learned, and the formulation pharmacist is then put to the task of increasing the drug's palatability in the environment of other formulative agents. The selection of an appropriate flavoring agent depends upon several factors, but primarily upon the taste of the drug substance itself. Certain flavoring materials have been found through experience to be more effective than others in masking or disguising the particular bitter, salty, sour, or otherwise undesirable taste of medicinal agents. Although individuals' tastes and flavor preferences differ, cocoa-flavored vehicles are considered effective for masking the taste of bitter drugs. Fruit or citrus flavors are frequently used to combat sour or acid tasting drugs, and cinnamon, orange, raspberry, and other flavors have been successfully employed to make preparations of salty drugs more palatable.

The age of the intended patient should also be considered in the selection of the flavoring agent, because certain age groups seem to prefer certain flavors. Children prefer sweet, candy-like preparations with fruity flavors, but adults seem to prefer less sweet preparations with a tart rather than a fruit flavor.

In addition to sucrose, a number of artificial sweetening agents have been utilized in foods and pharmaceuticals over the years. Some of these, as aspartame, saccharin and cyclamate, have faced challenges over their safety by the FDA and restrictions to their use and sale; in fact, the cyclamates were banned from use in the United States by the FDA in 1969.

The introduction of diet soft drinks in the 1950s provided the spark for the widespread use of artificial sweeteners today. Besides dieters, diabetics are regular users of artificial sweeteners. Over the years, each of the artificial sweeteners has undergone long periods of review and debate. Critical to the evaluation of food additives are issues of metabolism and toxicity. For example, almost none of the saccharin a person consumes is metabolized; it is excreted by the kidneys virtually unchanged. Cyclamate, on the other hand, is metabolized, or processed, in the digestive tract, and its byproducts are excreted by the kidneys. Aspartame breaks down in the body into three basic components: the amino acids phenylalanine and aspartic acid, and methanol. These three components, which also occur naturally in various foods, are in turn metabolized through regular pathways in the body. Because of its metabolism to phenylalanine, the use of aspartame by phenylketonurics is discouraged and diet foods and drinks must bear an appropriate label warning indicating that the particular foodstuff not be consumed by such individuals. Persons with phenylketonuria (PKU) cannot metabolize phenylalanine adequately, resulting in an increase in the serum levels of the amino acid (hyperphenylalaninemia). This can result in mental retardation, and also can affect the fetus of a pregnant woman who has the disorder.

Passage in 1958 of the Food Additives Amendment to the Food, Drug, and Cosmetic Act produced a major change in how food additives are regulated by the federal government. For one thing, no new food additive may be used if animal feeding studies or other appropriate tests showed that it caused cancer. This is the now-famous Delaney Clause. The *amount* of the substance one would have to consume to induce cancer is not of significance under the Delaney Clause.

Another critical feature of the 1958 amendment, however, was that it did not apply to additives that were generally recognized by experts as safe for their intended uses. Saccharin, cyclamate and a long list of other substances were being used in foods before the amendment's passage and were considered "generally recognized as safe"—or what is known today as GRAS. Aspartame, on the other hand, became the first artificial sweetener to fall under the 1958 amendment's requirement for premarketing proof of safety because the first petition to FDA for its approval was filed in 1973. In 1968, the Committee on Food Protection of the National Academy of Sciences issued an interim report on the safety of non-nutritive sweeteners, including saccharin. In the early 1970s, FDA began a major review of hundreds of food additives on the GRAS list to determine whether more current studies still justified their safe status. In 1972, with new studies under way, FDA decided to take saccharin off the GRAS and establish interim limits that would permit its continued use until additional studies were completed. (Previous studies indicated that male and female rats fed doses of saccharin developed a significant incidence of bladder tumors.) In November 1977, Congress passed the Saccharin Study and Labeling Act, which permitted saccharin's continued availability while mandating that warning labels be used to advise consumers that saccharin caused cancer in animals. The law also directed FDA to arrange further studies of carcinogens and toxic substances in foods.

Cyclamate was introduced into beverages and foods in the 1950s and dominated the artificial sweetener market in the 1960s. After much controversy regarding the substance's safety, the FDA issued a final ruling in 1980 stating that the agent's safety has not been demonstrated. Since that date, scientific studies have continued in order to conclusively support or refute the basis for the FDA decision. At question is the agent's possible carcinogenicity and its possible effects in causing genetic damage and testicular atrophy. The student is referred to the indicated references for a review of the recent history of sweeteners including: saccharin, cyclamate, fructose, polyalcohols, sucrose, and aspartame.[8–11]

Acesulfame potassium, a nonnutritive sweetener first discovered in 1967, was approved in 1992 by the FDA. It had been used previously in a number of other countries. The substance, structurally similar to saccharin, is 130 times as sweet as sucrose and is excreted unchanged in the urine. Acesulfame is more stable than aspartame at elevated temperatures and was approved by the FDA initially for use in candy, chewing gum, confectionery, and instant coffees and teas.

Table 4–5 compares three of the most used sweeteners in the food and drug industry.

Most large pharmaceutical manufacturers have special laboratories for the taste-testing of proposed formulations of their products. Panels of employees or interested community participants become involved in evaluating the various formulations and their assessments become the basis for the firm's flavoring decisions.

In flavoring liquid pharmaceutical products, the flavoring agent is added to the solvent or vehicle-component of the formulation in which it is most soluble or miscible. That is, water soluble flavorants are added to the aqueous component of a formulation and poorly water-soluble flavorants are added to the alcoholic or other nonaqueous solvent component of the formulation. In a hydroalcoholic or other multi-solvent system, care must be exercised to maintain the flavorant in solution. This is accomplished by maintaining a sufficient level of solvent in which the flavorant is soluble.

Coloring Pharmaceuticals

Coloring agents are used in pharmaceutical preparations for purposes of esthetics. A distinction should be made between agents that have inherent color and those agents which are employed as colorants. Certain agents—sulfur (yel-

Table 4–5. Comparison of Sweeteners

	Sucrose	*Saccharin*	*Aspartame*
Source:	sugar cane; sugar beet	chemical synthesis; phthalic anhydride, a petroleum product	chemical synthesis; methyl ester dipeptide of phenylalanine and aspartic acid
Relative Sweetness:	1	300	180–200
Bitterness:	none	moderate/strong	none
Aftertaste:	none	moderate/strong; sometimes metallic or bitter	none
Calories	4/g	0	4/g
Acid Stability:	good	excellent	fair
Heat Stability:	good	excellent	poor

low), cupric sulfate (blue), ferrous sulfate (bluish green), and red mercuric iodide (vivid red)—have inherent color and are not thought of as pharmaceutical colorants in the usual sense of the term.

Although most pharmaceutical colorants in use today are of synthetic origin, a few are obtained from natural mineral and plant sources. For example, red ferric oxide is mixed in small proportions with zinc oxide powder to prepare calamine, giving the latter its characteristic pink color, which is intended to match the skin tone upon application.

The synthetic coloring agents used in pharmaceutical products were first prepared in the middle of the 19th century from principles of coal tar. Coal tar *(pix carbonis)*, a thick, black, viscid liquid, is a by-product in the destructive distillation of coal. Its composition is extremely complex, and many of its constituents may be separated by fractional distillation. Among the products obtained are anthracene, benzene, naphtha, creosote, phenol, and pitch. About 90% of the total dyes used in the products FDA regulates are synthesized from a single, colorless derivative of benzene, called aniline. These aniline dyes are also known as synthetic organic dyes or as "coal tar" dyes since aniline was originally obtained from bituminous coal. Aniline dyes today come mainly from petroleum.

Many coal-tar dyes were originally used indiscriminately in foods and beverages to enhance their appeal without regard to their toxic potential. It was only after careful scrutiny that some dyes were found to be hazardous to health due to either their own chemical nature or the impurities they carried. As more dyestuffs became available, it became apparent that some expert guidance and regulation was needed to insure the safety of the public. After passage of the Food and Drug Act in 1906, the United States Department of Agriculture established regulations by which a few colorants were *permitted* or *certified* for use in certain products. Today, the use of color additives in foods, drugs, and cosmetics is regulated by the Food and Drug Administration through the provisions of the Federal Food, Drug, and Cosmetic Act of 1938, as amended in 1960 with the Color Additive Amendments. Lists of color additives *exempt* from certification and those *subject* to certification are codified into law and regulated by the FDA.[12] Certified color additives are classified according to their approved use: (a) FD&C color additives, which may be used in foods, drugs, and cosmetics; (b) D&C color additives, some of which are approved for use in drugs, some in cosmetics, and some in medical devices; and (c) external D&C color additives, the use of which is restricted to external parts of the body, not including the lips or any other body surface covered by mucous membrane. Within each certification category there is a variety of basic colors and shades for coloring pharmaceuticals. One may select from a variety of FD&C, D&C, and External D&C reds, yellows, oranges, greens, blues, and violets. By selective combinations of the colorants one can create distinctive colors (Table 4–6).

As a part of the National Toxicology Program of the Department of Health and Human Services, various substances, including color addi-

Table 4–6. Examples of Color Formulations*

Shade/Color	*FD&C Dye*	*% of Blend*
Orange	Yellow #6	100
	or	
	Yellow #5	95
	Red #40	5
Cherry	Red #40	100
	or	
	Red #40	99
	Blue #1	1
Strawberry	Red #40	100
	or	
	Red #40	95
	Red #3	5
Lemon	Yellow #5	100
Lime	Yellow #5	95
	Blue #1	5
Grape	Red #40	80
	Blue #1	20
Raspberry	Red #3	75
	Yellow #6	20
	Blue #1	5
Butterscotch	Yellow #5	74
	Red #40	24
	Blue #1	2
Chocolate	Red #40	52
	Yellow #5	40
	Blue #1	8
Caramel	Yellow #5	64
	Red #3	21
	Yellow #6	9
	Blue #1	6
Cinnamon	Yellow #5	60
	Red #40	35
	Blue #1	5

* From literature of Warner-Jenkinson Co., St. Louis, Mo.

tives, are studied for their toxicology and carcinogenesis. For color additives, the study protocols usually call for a two-year study in which groups of male and female mice and rats are fed diets containing various quantities of the colorant. The nonsurviving and surviving animals are examined for evidence of long-term toxicity and carcinogenesis. Five categories of evidence of carcinogenic activity are used in reporting observations: (1) "clear evidence" of carcinogenic activity; (2) "some evidence"; (3) "equivocal evidence," indicating uncertainty; (4) "no evidence," indicating no observable effect; and (5) "inadequate study," for studies that cannot be evaluated because of major flaws incurred.

The certification status of the colorants is continuously reviewed, and changes are made in the list of certified colors in accordance with toxicologic findings. These changes may involve (1) the withdrawal of certification, (2) the transfer of a colorant from one certification category to another, or (3) the addition of new colors to the list. Before gaining certification, a color additive must be demonstrated to be safe. In the case of pharmaceutical preparations, color additives, like all additives, must not interfere with the therapeutic efficacy of the product in which they are used nor may they interfere with the prescribed assay procedure for that preparation.

In the 1970s, concern and scientific questioning of the safety of some color additives heightened. A color that drew particular attention was FD&C Red No. 2, because of its extensive use in foods, drugs and cosmetics. Researchers in Russia had reported that this color, also known as amaranth, caused cancer in rats. Although the FDA was never able to determine the purity of the amaranth tested in Russia, these reports led to FDA investigations and a series of tests that eventually resulted in withdrawal of FD&C Red No. 2 from the FDA certified list in 1976 because its sponsors were unable to prove safety. That year, the Agency also terminated approval for use of FD&C Red No. 4 in maraschino cherries and ingested drugs because of unresolved safety questions. FD&C Red No. 4 is now permitted only in externally applied drugs and cosmetics.

The dye FD&C Yellow No. 5 (also known as tartrazine) can cause many people to have allergic-type reactions. People who are allergic to aspirin will also likely be allergic to this dye. As a result, the FDA requires the listing of this dye by name on the labels of foods (e.g., butter, cheese, ice cream) and ingested drugs containing the substance.

A colorant becomes an integral part of a pharmaceutical formulation, and its exact quantitative amount must be reproducible each time the formulation is prepared, or else the preparation would have a different appearance from batch to batch. This requires a high degree of pharmaceutical skill, for the amount of colorant generally added to liquid preparations ranges between 0.0005 and 0.001% depending upon the colorant and the depth of color desired. Because of their color potency, dyes generally are added to pharmaceutical preparations in the form of diluted solutions rather than as concentrated dry powders. This permits greater accuracy in measurement and more consistent color production.

In addition to liquid dyes in the coloring of pharmaceuticals, *lake pigments* may also be used. Whereas a chemical material exhibits coloring power or tinctorial strength when *dissolved,* pigment is an insoluble material which colors by dispersion. An FD&C lake is a pigment consisting of a substratum of alumina hydrate on which the dye is absorbed or precipitated. Having aluminum hydroxide as the substrate, the lakes are insoluble in nearly all solvents. FD&C lakes are subject to certification and must be made from dyes which have been previously certified. Lakes do not have a specified dye content and range from 10 to 40% pure dye. By their very nature, lakes are suitable for coloring products in which the moisture levels are low.

Lakes are commonly utilized in the form of fine dispersons or suspensions when coloring pharmaceuticals. The pigment particles may range in size from less than 1 μm up to 30 μm. The finer the particle, the less chance there would be for color speckling to occur in the finished product. Blends of various lake pigments may be used to achieve a variety of colors and different vehicles may be employed to disperse the colorants, as glycerin, propylene glycol, and sucrose-based syrup.

In the preparation of capsules, various colored empty gelatin capsule shells may be used to hold the powdered drug mixture. Many commercial capsules are prepared with capsule bodies of one color and a different colored capsule cap, resulting in a two-colored capsule. This makes certain commercial products even more readily identifiable than solid colored capsules. For powdered drugs dispensed as such or compressed into tablets, a generally larger proportion of dye is required (about 0.1%) to achieve the desired hue than with liquid preparations.

Both dyes and lakes have application in the coloring of sugar-coated tablets, film-coated tablets, direct-compression tablets, pharmaceutical suspensions and other dosage forms.[13] Traditionally, sugar-coated tablets have been colored with syrup solutions containing varying amounts of the water-soluble dyes, starting with very dilute solutions, working up to concentrated color syrup solutions. As many as 30 to 60 coats are not uncommon. Using the FD&C lakes, fewer color coats are used. Appealing tablets have been made with as few as 8 to 12 coats using lakes dispersed in syrup. Water-soluble dyes in aqueous vehicles or lakes dispersed in organic solvents may be effectively sprayed on tablets to achieve attractive film coatings. There is continued interest today in chewable tablets, due to the availability of many direct-compression materials such as dextrose, sucrose, mannitol, sorbitol, and spray-dried lactose. The direct-compression colored chewable tablets may be prepared utilizing 1 pound of lake per 1000 pounds of tablet mix. For aqueous suspensions, FD&C water-soluble colors or lakes may be satisfactory. In non-aqueous suspensions, FD&C lakes are necessary. The lakes, added either to the aqueous or non-aqueous phase, generally at a level of 1 pound of color per 1000 pounds of suspension, require homogenizing or mechanical blending to achieve uniform coloring.

For the most part, ointments, suppositories, and ophthalmic and parenteral products assume the color of their ingredients and do not contain color additives. Should a dye lose the certification status it held when a product was first formulated, manufactured, and marketed, the manufacturer must, within a reasonable length of time, reformulate, using only color additives certified at the new date of manufacture.

In addition to esthetics and the certification status of a dye, a formulation pharmacist must select the dyes to be used in a particular formula on the basis of the physical and chemical properties of the dyes available. Of prime importance is the solubility of a prospective dye in the vehicle to be used for a liquid formulation or in a solvent to be employed during a pharmaceutical process, as when the dye is sprayed on a batch of tablets. In general, most dyes are broadly grouped into those that are water-soluble and those that are oil-soluble; few, if any, dyes are both. Usually, a water-soluble dye is also adequately soluble in commonly used pharmaceutical liquids like glycerin, alcohol, and glycol ethers. Oil-soluble dyes may also be soluble to some extent in these solvents, as well as in liquid petrolatum (mineral oil), fatty acids, fixed oils, and waxes. It should be remembered that a great deal of solubility is not required, since the concentration of dye in a given preparation is rather minimal.

Another important consideration when selecting a dye for use in a liquid pharmaceutical is the pH and pH stability of the preparation to be colored. Dyes can change color with a change in pH, and a dye must be selected for a product so that any anticipated pH change will not alter the color during the usual shelf-life. The dye also must be chemically stable in the presence of the other formulative ingredients and must not interfere with the stability of the other agents. To maintain their original colors, FD&C dyes must be protected from oxidizing agents, reducing agents (especially metals as iron, aluminum, zinc and tin), strong acids and alkalis, and excessive heating. Dyes must also be reasonably photostable; that is, they must not change color when exposed to light of anticipated intensities and wavelengths under the usual conditions of shelf storage. Certain medicinal agents, particularly those prepared in liquid form, must be protected from light to maintain their chemical stability and their therapeutic effectiveness. These preparations are generally maintained and dispensed in dark amber or opaque containers. For solid dosage forms of photolabile drugs, a colored or opaque capsule shell may actually enhance the drug's stability by shielding out light rays.

Packaging, Labeling, and Storage of Pharmaceuticals

The proper packaging, labeling, and storage of pharmaceutical products are essential in maintaining product stability and efficacious use. Proper labeling of manufactured products and dispensed prescriptions is also vital to the appropriate use of medication. Standards for the packaging, labeling and storage of pharmaceutical products have been established by the USP and NF, the Food and Drug Administration, the Consumer Product Safety Commission, and state regulatory agencies, as Boards of Pharmacy, to ensure their safe and effective use.

Containers

Standards for the packaging of pharmaceuticals by manufacturers are contained in the Current Good Manufacturing Practice section of Code of Federal Regulations,[14] in the *United States Pharmacopeia/National Formulary,*[15] and in the FDA's *Guideline for Submitting Documentation for Packaging for Human Drugs and Biologics.*[16] When submitting a drug application to the FDA for approval, including INDs, NDAs, and ANDAs, the manufacturer must include all relevant specifications for the packaging of the product. During the initial stages of clinical use, as during Phases 1 and 2, the packaging must be shown to be effective in providing adequate drug stability. As the studies advance to Phase 3, additional information must be developed on the chemical, physical, and biologic characteristics of, and the test methods used for, the container, closure, and other component parts of the drug package system to assure their suitability in fulfilling the requirements for an approved application.

Different specifications are required for parenteral, nonparenteral, pressurized, and bulk containers, and for those made of glass, plastic, and metal. In each instance, the package and closure system must be shown to be effective for the particular product for which it is intended. Depending upon the intended use and type of container, among the tests performed are: physicochemical tests; light-transmission tests for glass or plastic; drug compatibility, including leaching and/or migration tests; vapor-transmission test for plastics; moisture barrier tests; toxicity studies for plastics; valve, actuator, metered-dose, particle size, spray characteristics, and leak testing for aerosols; sterility and permeation tests for parenteral containers; and drug stability for all packaging.

Compendial terms applying to *types of containers* and *conditions of storage* have defined meanings. According to the USP, a *container* is the device that holds a drug and is, or may be, in direct contact with the drug. The *immediate container* is that which is in direct contact with the drug at all times. The *closure* is part of the container. The container, including the closure, should be clean and dry prior to its being filled with the drug. The container must not interact physically or chemically with the drug to alter its strength, quality, or purity beyond the official requirements.

Containers may be classified according to their ability to protect their contents from external conditions. The minimally acceptable container is termed a *well-closed container.* It protects the contents from extraneous solids and from loss of the drug under ordinary conditions of handling, shipment, storage, and distribution. A *tight container* protects the contents from contamination by extraneous liquids, solids, or vapors, from loss of the drug, and from efflorescence, deliquescence, or evaporation under the usual conditions of handling, shipment, storage, and distribution. A tight container is capable of reclosure to its original capability after being opened. A *hermetic container* is impervious to air or any other gas under the ordinary or customary conditions of handling, shipment, storage, and distribution. Hermetic containers which are sterile are generally used to hold pharmaceutical preparations intended for injection or parenteral administration. These containers may be *single-dose containers* in which the quantity of sterile drug contained is intended as a single dose and which once opened cannot be resealed with assurance that sterility has been maintained. These containers include fusion-sealed ampuls, prefilled syringes, disposable syringes and cartridges. A *multiple-dose container* is a hermetic container which permits withdrawal of successive portions of the contents without changing the strength or endangering the quality or purity of the remaining portion. These containers are commonly referred to as vials. Examples of single-dose and multiple-dose products are shown in Figure 4–3.

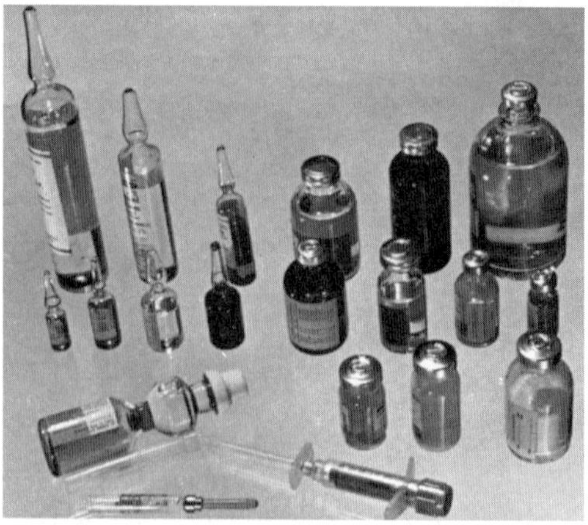

Fig. 4–3. *Examples of injectable products packaged in single-dose (ampuls) and multiple-dose (vials) containers and in unit-dose syringes.*

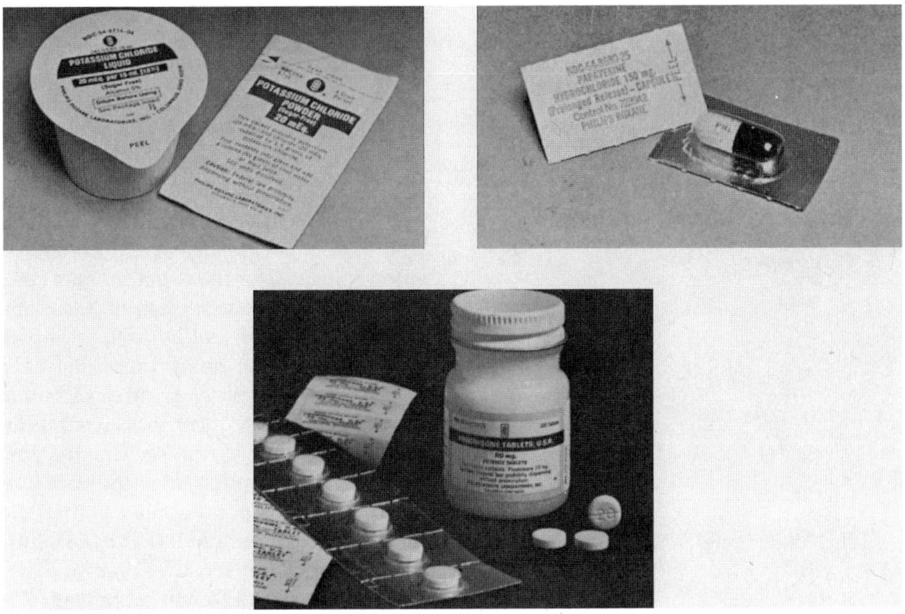

Fig. 4–4. *Examples of multiple-unit and single-unit packaging, including patient cup, unit dose of powder, blister packaging of single capsule, and strip packaging of tablets. (Courtesy of Philips Roxane Laboratories.)*

Dosage forms, as tablets, capsules, and oral liquids, may be packaged in *single-unit* or *multiple-unit* containers. A single-unit container is one that is designed to hold a quantity of drug intended for administration as a single dose promptly after the container is opened. Multiple unit containers contain more than a single unit or dose of the medication. Examples of single-unit and multiple-unit packages are shown in Figure 4–4. A single-use package is termed a *unit-dose* package at the time a prescribing physician orders that particular amount of the drug for a specific patient. The single-unit packaging of drugs may be performed on a large scale by the industrial manufacturer or distributor or on a smaller in-house scale by the pharmacy actually dispensing the medication. In each instance, the single-unit package is appropriately labeled with the product identity, quality and/or strength, name of manufacturer, and lot number of product to insure the positive identification of the medication. Although single-unit packaging has particular usefulness in institutional settings as hospitals and extended care facilities it is not limited to such. Many outpatients find single-unit packages a convenient and sanitary means of maintaining and utilizing their medication. Among the advantages cited for single-unit packaging and unit-dose dispensing are the following: positive identification of each dosage unit after it leaves the pharmacy or nursing station and the consequent reduction of medication errors, reduced contamination of the drug by virtue of its protective wrapping, reduced preparation and dispensing time, greater ease of inventory control in the pharmacy or nursing station, and elimination of waste through better medication management with less discarded medication.

Most hospitals with unit-dose systems use strip packaging equipment for the packaging of oral solids (Fig. 4–5). Such equipment seals solid dosage forms into four-sided pouches and imprints dose identification on each package at the same time. The equipment can be adjusted to produce individual single-cut packages or perforated strips or rolls of singly packaged dosage units. The packaging materials may be paper, foil, plastics or cellophane, alone or in combination. Some drugs must be packaged in foil-to-foil wrappings to prevent the deteriorating effects of light or the permeation of moisture. The packaging of solid dosage forms in clear plastic blister wells is another popular method of single-unit packaging. Oral liquids are generally single-unit dispensed in paper, plastic, or foil cups, or pre-

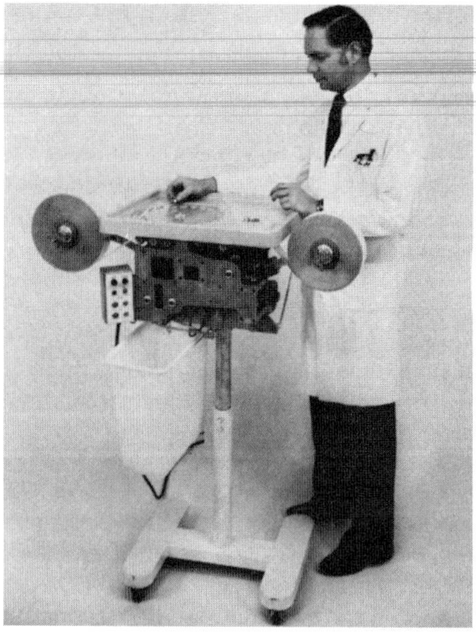

Fig. 4–5. *Strip packaging equipment capable of producing 50 packages per minute. Seals solid dosage units in a variety of wrapping materials and labels each package simultaneously. (Courtesy of Packaging Machinery Associates.)*

packaged and dispensed in glass containers having threaded caps or crimped aluminum caps (Fig. 4–6). A number of hospital pharmacies package oral liquids for pediatric use in disposable plastic syringes with rubber tips on the orifice for closure. In these instances the nursing staff must be fully aware of the novel packaging and special labeling used to indicate "not for injection." Medications which *are* used for injection may also be prepackaged in syringes for direct administration to the patient. However, great care must be exercised in the preparation and packaging of parenteral products and appropriate laboratory tests performed to insure their sterility and stability. Other dosage forms, as suppositories, powders, ointments, creams, and ophthalmic solutions, are also commonly found in single-unit packages provided by large manufacturers. However, the relatively infrequent use of these dosage forms in a given hospital, extended care facility, or community pharmacy does not generally justify the expense of purchasing the specialized packaging machinery necessary for the small-scale packaging of these forms.

Some pharmaceutical manufacturers are now placing some of their pharmaceutical products in *unit-of-use* packaging. This is packaging in which an amount of drug product to be used during the usual course of a patient's treatment, or an otherwise commonly prescribed amount of that drug, is packaged in a container and requires only labeling before dispensing. For example, the antibiotic tetracycline is frequently prescribed to be taken 4 times a day for 10 days. Unit-of-use packaging would contain 40 capsules, sufficient for the usual course of treatment. For long-term treatment, as in the case of treating hypertension with antihypertensive drugs, the dosage forms may be packaged in quantities to last the patient a given number of months.

Many pharmaceutical products require *light-resistant containers* to protect them from photochemical deterioration. In most instances a container made of a good quality of amber glass or plastic will reduce light transmission sufficiently to protect the light-sensitive pharmaceutical. The types of containers shown in Figure 4–7 are used for this purpose. In some instances containers rendered opaque by special coatings are employed. Opaque plastic containers are becoming increasingly popular in the packaging of phar-

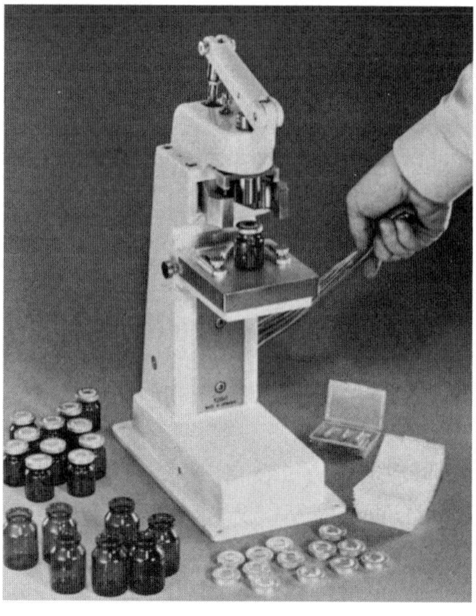

Fig. 4–6. *Components of Owens-Illinois' UNI-PAK System, including amber vials for oral liquids, aluminum closures, capper, and plastic hinged boxes for blister packaged solid dosage forms. Approximately 2,000 vials may be sealed per hour using the capper shown. (Courtesy of Owens-Illinois.)*

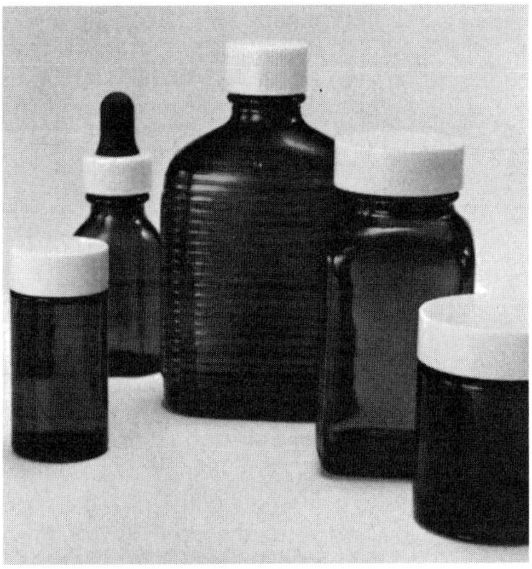

Fig. 4–7. *Examples of light-protective amber prescription containers for, from left to right: small numbers of solid dosage forms, as tablets and capsules; liquid preparations administered by drops; liquid preparations; powders, or large numbers of solid dosage forms; and semisolid preparations, such as ointments and pastes. (Courtesy of Armstrong Cork Company.)*

maceutical products. Outer wrappings or cartons can also be used to protect light-sensitive pharmaceuticals.

It is generally good practice for the pharmacist to dispense medication to his patients in the same type and quality of container as that used by the manufacturer of the product. In some instances the original container may be used by the pharmacist in dispensing the medication.

The official compendia provide tests and standards for glass and plastic containers with respect to their ability to prevent the transmission of light. Containers intended to provide protection from light or those offered as "light-resistant" containers must meet prescribed compendia standards which define the acceptable limits of light transmission at any wavelength of light between 290 and 450 nm.

The glass used in packaging pharmaceuticals is classified into four categories, depending upon the chemical constitution of the glass and its ability to resist deterioration. Table 4–7 presents the chemical make-up of the various glasses; types I, II, and III are intended for parenteral products and type NP is intended for nonparenteral products and those intended for oral or topical use. Each type is tested according to its resistance to

Table 4–7. Constitution of Official Glass Types

Type	*General Description*
I	Highly resistant, borosilicate glass
II	Treated soda-lime glass
III	Soda-lime glass
NP	General purpose soda-lime glass

water attack. The degree of attack is determined by the amount of alkali released from the glass under the test conditions specified. Obviously the leaching of alkali from the glass into a pharmaceutical solution or preparation placed in the container could alter the pH and thus the stability of the product. Pharmaceutical manufacturers must select and utilize containers which do not adversely affect the composition or stability of their products. Type I is the most resistant glass of the four categories.

The interest and widespread use of plastic containers in the pharmaceutical industry has been generated by a number of factors including: (1) the advantage of plastic over glass containers in lightness of weight and resistance to impact and thus lower transportation costs and losses due to container damage; (2) the versatility in container design and in consumer acceptance afforded by plastics; (3) the interest and convenience in utilizing low and medium density polyethylene in the formation of squeeze bottles which serve a dual function of both package and applicator for preparations as ophthalmics, nasal solutions, and lotions; and (4) the advent of newer techniques in drug distribution, dispensing, and inventory control particularly in hospitals which required the development of packaging as the strip package, blister package, and plastic disposable syringe for unit-dose delivery.

Today a wide variety of dosage forms may be found packaged in plastic. The modern compact-type container used for oral contraceptives, which contains sufficient tablets for a monthly cycle of administration and permits the scheduled removal of one tablet at a time, is a prime example of the contemporary packaging with plastics (Fig. 4–8). Plastic bags for intravenous fluids, plastic ointment tubes, plastic film protected suppositories and plastic tablet and capsule vials are other examples of the widespread use of plastics in pharmaceutical packaging.

The term "plastic" does not apply to a single type of material but rather to a vast number of existing and possible materials. For example, the

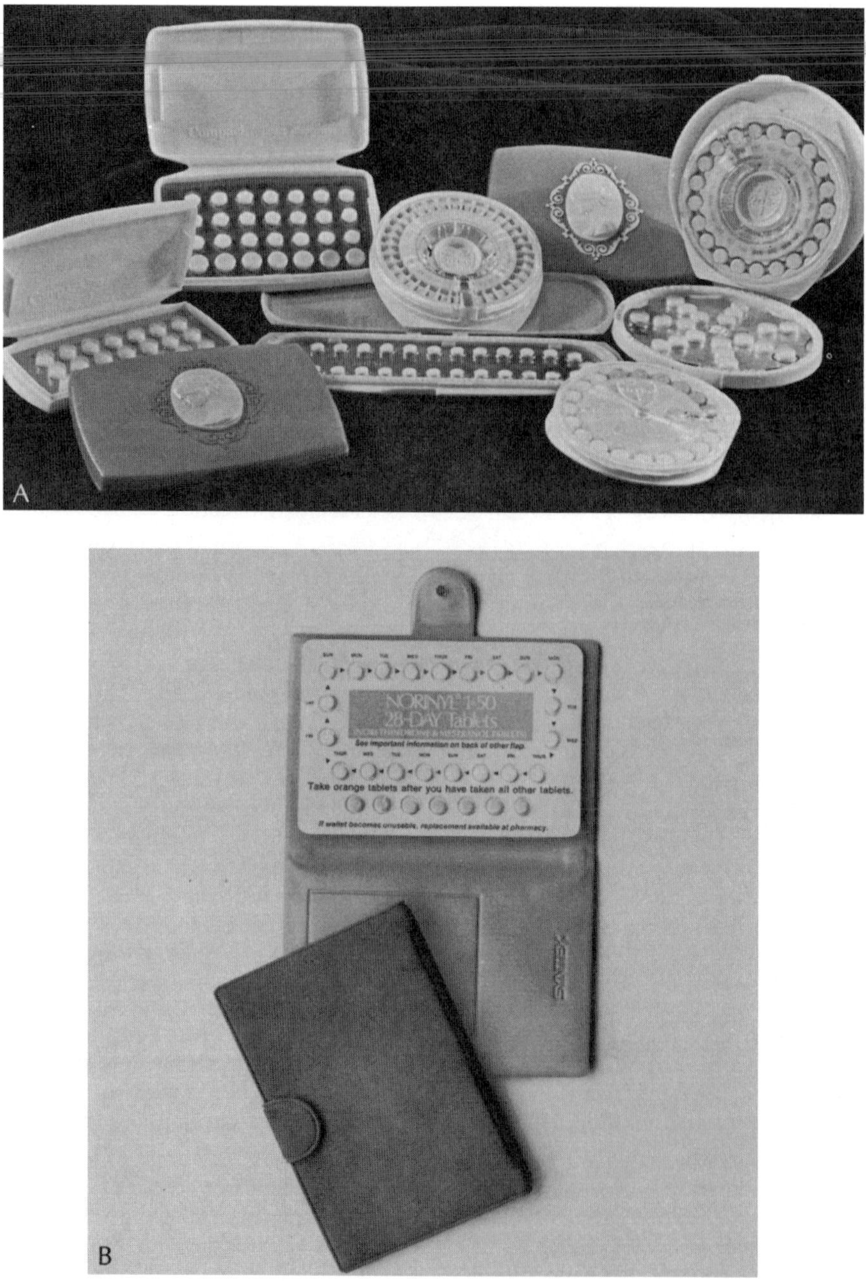

Fig. 4–8. *A and B. Examples of plastic packaging used for oral contraceptive products. (B) The "Wallette" dispenser allows an easy to follow format. (Courtesy of Syntex Laboratories.)*

addition of methyl groups to every other carbon atom in the polymer chains of polyethylene will give polypropylene a material which can be effectively autoclaved, whereas polyethylene cannot. If a chlorine atom is added to every other carbon in the polyethylene polymer, polyvinyl chloride is produced. This material is rigid and has good clarity making it a useful material in certain packaging situations. It is used widely for the blister packaging of tablets and capsules.

However, it does have a significant drawback for packaging medical devices (e.g., syringes) since it is unsuitable for gamma sterilization, a method that is increasingly chosen over ethylene oxide sterilization. The placement of other functional groups on the main chain of polyethylene or added to other types of polymers can give a variety of alterations to the final plastic material. In addition, added agents may be employed to alter the properties of the plastic. These agents include plasticizers, stabilizers, antioxidants, fillers, antistatic agents, antimold agents, colorants, and others.

Among the problems encountered with the use of plastics in packaging are (1) permeability of the containers to atmospheric gases and to moisture vapor; (2) leaching of the constituents of the container to the internal contents; (3) sorption of drugs from the contents to the container; (4) transmission of light through the container; and (5) alteration of the container upon storage.

True *permeability* is considered a process of solution and diffusion, with the penetrant initially dissolving in the plastic material on one side and diffusing through to the other side. Permeability should be contrasted with *porosity*, which is a condition in which minute holes or cracks are present in the plastic and through which gas or moisture vapor may move directly.

The permeability of a plastic is a function of several factors including the nature of the polymer itself, the amounts and types of plasticizers, fillers, lubricants, pigments and other additives used, the pressure conditions, and the temperature. Generally, increases in the temperature, pressure, and the use of additives to the polymer tend to increase the permeability of the plastic. In general, glass containers are less permeable than plastic containers. The closure plays as important a role in protecting pharmaceuticals as does the primary container. A tightly fitting closure can often be the difference between a protected or an unprotected drug product.

The movement of moisture vapor or gas, especially oxygen, through a pharmaceutical container can pose one of the greatest threats to the stability of a pharmaceutical product. In the presence of moisture, powders may tend to cake and solid dosage forms may lose their color or physical integrity. A host of pharmaceutical adjuncts, especially those used in tablet formulations, as diluents, binders, and disintegrating agents, are affected by moisture. The majority of these adjuncts are carbohydrates, starches, and natural or synthetic gums, and because of their hygroscopicity they hold moisture and may even serve as nutrient media for the growth of microorganisms. Many of the tablet disintegrating agents fulfill their pharmaceutical function by swelling in an aqueous media, and, if exposed to high moisture vapor upon storage, the disintegrants may prematurely swell, and cause the tablets to become deformed. Further, many medicinal agents, as aspirin, some barbiturates, and vitamins, are quite prone to hydrolytic decomposition and dosage forms of these agents must be especially guarded against moisture penetration. Nitroglycerin is especially prone to moisture and the sublingual tablets must be dispensed to the patient in its original glass container. Under proper storage conditions nitroglycerin sublingual tablets are stable for 2 years; however, once the original container is opened the patient must be advised to discard any unused tablets 6 months after the original bottle is opened.

Drug substances which exhibit oxidation propensity may undergo a greater degree of degradation when packaged in plastic as compared to glass. In glass, the void space is filled with air which is in a confined space and presents only a limited amount of oxygen to the drug contents. On the other hand, a drug packaged in a gas permeable plastic container may be constantly exposed to oxygen due to the replenished supply entering the container.

Liquid pharmaceutical products packaged in plastic which is permeable to the contents tend to lose molecules of solute (drug) or solvent (vehicle) outward toward the container. Such permeation can drastically alter the concentration of the drug in the pharmaceutical product thereby affecting its efficacy.

Leaching is a term used to describe the release or movement of components of a container into the contents. Compounds leached from plastic containers are generally the polymer additives as the plasticizers, stabilizers, or antioxidants. The leaching of these additives occurs predominantly when liquid or semi-solid dosage forms are packaged in plastic. Little leaching occurs when tablets or capsules are packaged in plastic.

Leaching may be influenced by temperature, excessive agitation of the filled container, and by the solubilizing effect of the contents on one or more of the polymer additives. The leaching of polymer additives from plastic containers of fluids intended for intravenous administration is an especially worrisome problem because the additive is injected along with the medication. The toxicologic effect of any leached additive is of prime concern and is presently an important area of investigation. Soft-walled plastic containers of polyvinyl chloride are frequently used to package various intravenous solutions as well as blood for transfusion. Leached material, whether dissolved in the contents or present as minute particles, poses a health hazard to the patient and sufficient studies should be performed on the leaching characteristics of each plastic material prior to its use in packaging a given pharmaceutical product.

Sorption is a term used to indicate the binding of molecules to polymer materials. Both *adsorption* and *absorption* may be considered within this term. Sorption occurs through chemical or physical means, or both, with the phenomena related to the chemical structure of the solute molecules and the physical and chemical properties of the polymer. Generally, the unionized species of a solute has a greater tendency to be bound than does the ionized species. Because the degree of ionization of a solute may be affected by the pH of the solution in which it is contained, the pH of a pharmaceutical solution may influence the sorption tendency of a particular solute. Further, the pH of a solution may affect the chemical nature of a plastic container in such a way to either increase or decrease the active bonding sites available to the solute molecules. Plastic materials with polar groups are particularly prone to the sorption process. Because the process of sorption is dependent upon the penetration or diffusion of a solute into the plastic, the pharmaceutical vehicle or solvent for the solute also plays a major role in the sorption process. Certain solvents may alter the plastic and increase its permeability to solute.

The process of sorption may be initiated by the adsorption of a solute to the inner surface of a plastic container. After the saturation of the surface, the solute may then diffuse into the plastic, perhaps with the assistance of the pharmaceutical solvent or vehicle, to be absorbed and bound to sites within the plastic. The sorption of a drug component from a pharmaceutical solution would naturally reduce the concentration of that agent in the solution and render the product unreliable as to potency and unacceptable for use. The sorption of antimicrobial preservatives or stabilizers from a pharmaceutical product would likewise render the product unsuitable for use. Even the sorption of colorants and flavorants which would alter a preparation's color stability and taste would be unacceptable to a pharmaceutical manufacturer. Thus, each formulative ingredient must be examined in the proposed plastic packaging to ascertain its tendency for sorption and to insure the continued stability and potency of a product during its anticipated shelf life. Active ingredients also can adsorb onto plastic. For example, insulin adsorption onto plastic intravenous infusion sets has been reported to be as high as 80% of a dose.

Insofar as the ability of plastic containers to protect pharmaceutical products from destructive light transmission, clear and uncolored plastic containers behave in much the same manner as clear and uncolored glass containers in allowing such transmissions. Agents termed UV-absorbers may be added to the plastic to decrease the transmission of these short ultraviolet rays and thus may be used to protect light-sensitive drugs.

Deformations, softening, hardening, and other physical changes in plastic containers have been observed. These changes may result from the permeation or sorption of the contents into the container changing its chemical or physical makeup. They may also result from the leaching of a component of the container into the contents, or from changes in temperature or physical stress placed upon the container in handling, shipping or storage.

The everchanging field of plastic technology will continue to yield innovative and effective materials for the packaging of pharmaceuticals in the future and eliminate the aforementioned problems. Today's so-called "superplastics" can be produced to withstand continuous temperatures of greater than 300°F, and possess a tensile strength of 10,000 pounds per square inch (compared to 32,000 psi for brass). Plastics are being produced that are stronger than steel, and employed in such products as bullet-proof vests. There are more than 4000 major polymers on the market today, with hundreds added each year with greater features and application. Plastics prepared by *coextrusion*, using barrier layers, and formed into sheets offer unique, strong, and flexible containers for the present and future. These plastic containers (exemplified by the potato chip bag) can be prepared to shield out light, oxygen, and moisture, a feature also particularly attractive to the packaging of pharmaceuticals.

In conclusion, each pharmaceutical preparation must be considered separately with respect to packaging and type of container selected. The container must be suited to the prolonged stability of the pharmaceutical preparation and must be conducive to the safe and effective utilization by the patient. A good guideline for the practicing pharmacist is to utilize the original or the same type of container in which the drug product was supplied by the manufacturer. For prescribed mixtures of drugs, especially liquid preparations and products containing volatile substances, a tightly closed, light-resistant glass container is usually the most protective container to use.

Safety Closures

To reduce the occurrence of accidental poisonings through the ingestion of drugs and other household chemicals, the Poison Prevention Packaging Act was passed into law in 1970. The responsibility for the administration and enforcement of the Act, originally with the Food and Drug Administration, was transferred to the Consumer Product Safety Commission in 1973 when this agency was created through the enactment of the Consumer Product Safety Act. The initial regulations called for the use of "childproof" closures for aspirin products and certain household chemical products shown to have a significant potential for causing accidental poisoning in youngsters. As the technical capability in producing effective closures was developed, the regulations were extended to include the use of such safety closures in the packaging of both legend and over-the-counter medications. Presently, all legend drugs intended for oral use must be dispensed by the pharmacist to the patient in containers having safety closures unless the prescribing physician or the patient specifically requests otherwise or unless the product has been made specifically exempt from the requirement.

The manufacturer or packager of an over-the-counter drug product may provide a single-size noncomplying (not child-safe) package of the product provided it bears conspicuous labeling stating "This package for households without young children" or, if the package is small, stating, "Package not child-resistant," and provided the manufacturer also supplies the substance in complying packages.

Examples of commonly used safety closures in dispensing medication are presented in Figures 4–9 and 4–10.

A child-resistant (CR) container is defined as

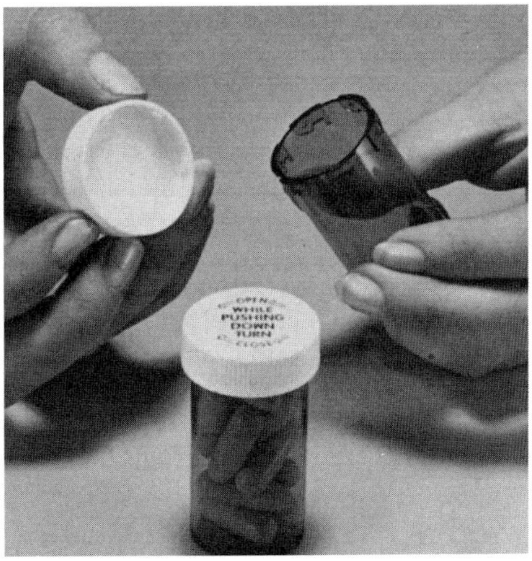

Fig. 4–9. *Example of child-resistant safety closure on a prescription container. (Courtesy of Brockway Prescription Products)*

one that is difficult for most children under 5 years of age to open or to obtain a harmful amount of the contents. It is not necessarily packaging that *all* children under 5 years of age cannot open. Further, the packaging should not be difficult for normal adults to open. A testing procedure has been designed by the Consumer Product Safety Commission to evaluate the effectiveness of such containers. The procedure is outlined in the USP.[17]

The Consumer Product Safety Commission may propose the exemption of certain drugs and drug products from the safety closure regulation based on toxicologic data or on practical considerations. For instance, certain cardiac drugs, as sublingual tablets of nitroglycerin, are exempt from the regulations because of the importance to the welfare of the patient for direct and immediate access to his medication. Exemptions are also permitted in the case of over-the-counter medications for one package size or specially marked package to be available to consumers for whom safety closures might be unnecessary or too difficult to manipulate. These consumers would include childless persons, arthritic patients, and the debilitated.

Drugs which are utilized or dispensed in inpatient institutions, as hospitals, nursing homes, and extended care facilities, need not be dispensed with safety closures unless they are intended for patients who are leaving the confines of the institution (outpatients).

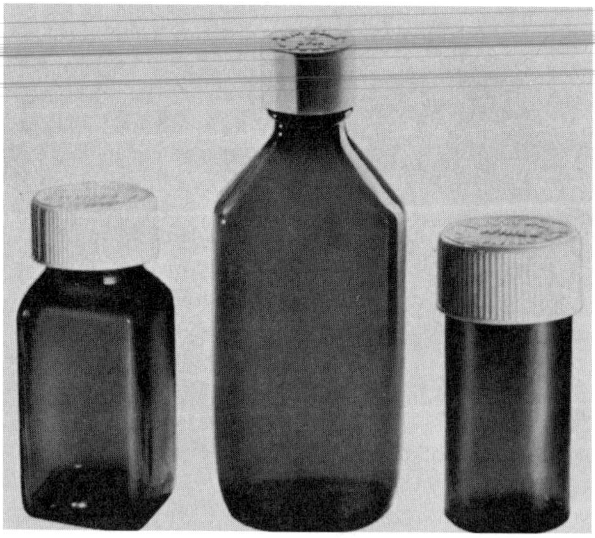

Fig. 4–10. *Child-resistant prescription containers. (Courtesy of Kerr Glass Manufacturing Corporation.)*

Tamper-Resistant or Tamper-Evident Packaging

On November 5, 1982, the Food and Drug Administration published regulations on tamper-resistant packaging in the *Federal Register.* These regulations were promulgated following the criminal tampering with over-the-counter drug products earlier in that year resulting in consumer illness and deaths. In the primary incident, cyanide surreptitiously had been placed in acetaminophen capsules in commercial packages for consumer purchase.

The regulations required tamper-resistant packaging for all over-the-counter drugs, with the exception of dermatologics, dentrifices, and insulin. In addition to these exempt product categories, a manufacturer or drug packer may request an exemption for a specific product by filing with the FDA a "Request for Exemption from Tamper Resistant Rule." The petition is required to contain specific information on the drug product, the reasons the requirement is unnecessary or cannot be achieved, and alternative steps the petitioner has taken, or may take, to reduce the likelihood of malicious adulteration to the product.

A tamper-resistant or tamper-evident package is defined as "one having indicators or barriers to entry which, if breached or missing, can reasonably be expected to provide visible evidence to consumers that tampering has occurred."[14] Exempt from the regulations are products distributed to hospitals, nursing homes, and health care clinics "that are not distributed in a manner that affords the general public access to them while they are held for sale."

The fact that *tamper-resistant* packaging is not *tamper-proof* was demonstrated by a second episode of criminal tampering with over-the-counter products resulting in death in early 1986. Once again, the primary incident involved the placement of cyanide in acetaminophen capsules, except this time, the capsules were apparently triple sealed in containers with foil coverings over the bottle mouths, stretch seals over the bottle caps, and glued end-flaps of the outer packaging cartons. Immediately following this occurrence, the manufacturer recalled all of the product from the marketplace and replaced the encapsulated product with a tableted product considered much more difficult to adulterate. In 1994, the FDA proposed that all over-the-counter products sold as two-piece, hard gelatin capsules be sealed so as to make malicious tampering evident. The agency also proposed a change in regulatory agency terminology from "tamper-resistant" to "tamper-evident."

Even with the safeguards in effect, the possibility of drug product tampering requires the pharmacist and consumer to remain constantly vigilant for signs of product entry.

Pharmaceutical manufacturers have the op-

Table 4–8. Tamper-Resistant Packaging Examples

Package Type	*Tamper Protection*
Film Wrappers	Film wrapped and sealed around product and/or product containers; the film must be cut or torn to remove product.
Blister/Strip Packs	Individually sealed dosage units; removal requires tearing or breaking individual compartment.
Bubble Packs	Product and container sealed in plastic, usually mounted on/in display card; plastic must be cut or broken open to remove product.
Shrink Seals/Bands	Bands or wrappers which are shrunk by heat or drying to conform to cap and containers must be torn to open.
Foil, Paper, or Plastic Pouches	Sealed individual packets; must be torn to reach product.
Bottle Seals	Paper or foil sealed to mouth of a container under cap; must be torn or broken to reach product.
Tape Seals	Paper or foil sealed over carton flap or bottle cap; must be torn or broken to reach product.
Breakable Caps	Plastic or metal "tearaway" caps over container; must be broken to remove.
Sealed Tubes	Seal over mouth of tube; must be punctured to reach product.
Sealed Cartons	Carton flaps are sealed; carton cannot be opened without damage.
Aerosol Containers	Tamper-resistant by design.

tion of determining the type of tamper-resistant packaging to utilize. Table 4–8 presents some examples of tamper-resistant packaging.

Compliance Packaging

Many patients are not compliant with the prescribed schedule for the taking of their medications. There are many factors associated with such noncompliance: a misunderstanding of the dosing schedule; confusion due to the taking of multiple medications; forgetfulness; or a feeling of well-being, with the premature discontinuance of medication.

To assist patients in taking their medications on schedule, manufacturers and pharmacists have devised numerous educational techniques, reminder aids, compliance packages, and devices.[18] The oral contraceptive compact-type plastic package, shown in Figure 4–8, was among the earliest product packages developed within the pharmaceutical industry to support patient adherence to a required dosing schedule. Since then, additional manufacturer-provided, unit-of-use packaging has been developed to help simplify complicated dosing schedules. For prescriptions dispensed in traditional containers (as capsule vials), pharmacists may provide individualized calendar medication schedules or commercially available devices for the daily or weekly scheduling of dosage units. These techniques and devices are particularly useful for patients taking multiple medications.

Labeling

The labeling of all drug products distributed in the United States must meet the specific labeling requirements as set forth in the federal regulations. These labeling requirements apply not only to proprietary products sold over-the-counter, but also to prescription drugs distributed to various health practitioners for ultimate dispensing to the patient. The labeling regulations are changed from time to time to meet the changing informational needs of the health professional and the patient. The federal labeling requirements for drug products may be further enhanced by state and local drug laws. The contents of the label that the pharmacist affixes to dispensed medication is another topic, but it too is subject to specific requirements of the federal, state, and local regulations.

According to federal regulations, drug labeling includes not only the labels placed on the immediate container and packaging, but also the package inserts accompanying the product as well as all company literature and advertising or promotional material pertaining to the drug product. This includes such things as brochures, booklets, mailing pieces, file cards, bulletins, price lists, catalogs, sound recordings, film strips, motion-picture films, lantern slides, exhibits, displays, literature reprints and any other material containing product information provided by the manufacturer or distributor.

The essential information on a prescription-only drug is generally provided to the health professional through the product's *package insert.* This insert must provide *full disclosure;* that is, it must contain a full and balanced presentation of the positive as well as the negative aspects of the drug product to enable the prescriber to utilize the drug most safely and effectively.

Drug Package Insert

As described more fully in Chapter 2, included in the prescription drug package insert is the following information:

1. Description of the product, including proprietary and non-proprietary names of the drugs present
2. Clinical pharmacology
3. Indications and usage
4. Contraindications
5. Warnings
6. Precautions
7. Adverse reactions
8. Drug abuse and dependence potential
9. Overdosage signs and treatment
10. Dosage and administration
11. Dosage forms, strengths and package sizes supplied

Among other information, it is important for the package insert to provide any special guidance needed for the use of the medication during pregnancy and when breastfeeding an infant, since many drugs are capable of affecting a fetus or infant through the mother. Today there is also emphasis on the different dosage and/or effects of a drug in women vs. men, in the elderly, and in pediatric patients. Research efforts are ongoing to obtain additional information on the effects of specific drugs in these patient groups and to include such information in professional labeling.

Drug manufacturers and distributors are occasionally required to mail important information to physicians, pharmacists, and others responsible for patient care. The mailings must be in distinctively marked envelopes. When the information concerns a significant hazard to health, the statement shall be in 36-point Gothic Bold type, stating:

IMPORTANT
DRUG
WARNING

A recent example for Vincristine Sulfate for Injection, USP warned that the drug could be "FATAL IF GIVEN INTRATHECALLY" and should be "FOR INTRAVENOUS USE ONLY." The warning was in response to several deaths from improper administration of the injection through the spinal sheath and into the spinal cord. Other similar manufacturer's letters of alert in similar bold type are used for "IMPORTANT PRESCRIBING INFORMATION" to advise of important changes in drug product labeling, and "IMPORTANT CORRECTION OF DRUG INFORMATION," when the information concerns a correction of prescription drug advertising or labeling.

Manufacturer's Label

Included among the information usually appearing on the manufacturer's or distributor's label affixed to the container of Legend drugs are the following:

1. The nonproprietary name(s) of the drug(s) present and the proprietary trademark name of the product if one is used.
2. The name and address of the manufacturer or distributor of the product.
3. A quantitative statement of the amount of each drug present per unit of weight, volume, or dosage unit, whichever is most appropriate.
4. The pharmaceutical type of dosage form constituting the product.
5. The net amount of drug product contained in the package, in units of weight, volume or number of dosage units, as is appropriate.
6. The Federal Legend: "Caution—Federal law prohibits dispensing without prescription," or a similar statement.
7. The usual dose of the product including special dosage guidelines for children or for other patients under certain conditions, when appropriate.
8. A label reference to see the accompanying package insert or other product literature for additional information.

9. Special storage instructions, when applicable.
10. The National Drug Code identification number for the product.
11. The manufacturer's control number identifying the batch or lot of the drug.
12. An expiration date.
13. For controlled drug substances, the DEA symbol "C" together with the schedule assigned (e.g. III). The statement: "Warning—May be habit forming" may appear also.

Prescription Label

When filling a prescription, the pharmacist is required by the federal Food, Drug and Cosmetic Act to include the following information on the label of the dispensed medication:

1. The name and address of the pharmacy
2. The serial number of the prescription
3. The date of the prescription or the date of its filling or refilling (state law often determines which date is to be used)
4. The name of the prescriber
5. The name of the patient
6. Directions for use, including precautions, if any, as indicated on the prescription

In addition to the above, state laws may require additional information as:

7. The address of the patient
8. The initials or name of the dispensing pharmacist
9. The telephone number of the pharmacy
10. The drug name, strength and manufacturer's lot or control number
11. The expiration date of the drug, if any
12. The name of the manufacturer or distributor

OTC Labeling

The label on the container of products sold over-the-counter without prescription usually contains much of the same type of product information as the prescription-only items with the exception of the Federal Legend and the DEA symbol. However, to advance the safe and proper use of over-the-counter medications, additional patient-oriented information is included in the labeling, including the following:

1. Product name and statement of identity, e.g., liquid antacid, listing of active ingredients and net quantity of contents.
2. Statements of all conditions, purposes, or uses for which the drug is intended or commonly used. Also included are conditions against which the drug is contraindicated or to be used only with professional supervision.
3. Directions for use—quantity of dose, including usual quantities for each of the uses for which it is intended and the usual quantities for persons of different ages and physical conditions, if pertinent.
4. Dosage instructions—frequency of administration, if used internally, or application, if used externally, and time of administration or application, with respect to meals, onset of symptoms or other time factors.
5. Warnings—maximum duration of administration or application prior to consulting a physician, and anticipated side effects of the drug's action which might be experienced by the user.
6. Cautionary statements—storage in a safe place out of the reach of children, appropriate instructions in the event of accidental overdosage, sodium content, etc.
7. Drug interaction precautions—heighten patient awareness of other medicines that could interfere with or enhance the effect of the OTC drug.
8. Route of administration or application.
9. Preparation for use—shaking, dilution, adjustment of temperature, or other manipulations or processes.
10. Declaration of presence of the dye Yellow No. 5 (to alert persons hypersensitive to this agent) and alcohol.
11. If the medication is to be taken internally, the label must contain the statement: "As with any drug, if you are pregnant or nursing a baby, seek the advice of a health professional before using this product."

As noted above, over-the-counter package labeling must include appropriate warning statements whenever the medication is such that indiscriminate use may lead to serious medical complications or mask a condition more serious than that for which the medication was intended. For example, the use of laxatives is a dangerous practice when symptoms of appendicitis are present and can result in an intensification of the problem and even a rupturing of the appendix. For this reason the following statement is required by law to appear on laxative preparations:

"Warning: Do not use when abdominal pain, nausea, or vomiting is present. Frequent or prolonged use of this preparation may result in dependence on laxatives."

The seriousness of a cough may be underestimated by a patient if a proprietary cough syrup temporarily relieves the cough; however, coughing is a symptom of many serious conditions requiring specific treatment. Cough remedies sold over-the-counter must therefore bear the following warning statement:

WARNING. A persistent cough may be a sign of a serious condition. If cough persists for more than 1 week, tends to recur, or is accompanied by a fever, rash, or persistent headache, consult a doctor.

These are but two examples of the statements required on various types of proprietary products. The statements themselves and the types of preparations requiring them are written into the law and are available through the government literature. The labels of drugs sold directly to the layman should recommend their use against only those conditions that have been shown scientifically to be treated effectively by the drug. Serious conditions that cannot be diagnosed or successfully treated by the layman should not be mentioned in the labeling, nor should it contain any false or misleading statement. The label must be perfectly clear in meaning and this will become even more important in the future. Trends indicate that in future years more legend drugs will become available for over the counter purchase. Thus, the importance of labeling of these products for consumer use in understandable terms cannot be overemphasized.

As a part of the FDA's Current Good Manufacturing Practice (CGMP) Regulations of 1978, as revised in 1983, all over-the-counter drug products are required to bear expiration dates.

Storage

To insure the stability of a pharmaceutical preparation for the period of its intended shelf life, the product must be stored under proper conditions. The labeling of each product includes the desired conditions of storage. The terms generally employed in such labeling have meanings defined by the official compendia:[19]

Cold—Any temperature not exceeding 8°C (46°F). A *refrigerator* is a cold place in which the temperature is maintained thermostatically between 2° and 8°C (36° and 46°F). A *freezer* is a cold place in which the temperature is maintained thermostatically between −10° and −20°C (14° and −4°F).
Cool—Any temperature between 8° and 15°C (46° and 59°F). An article for which storage in a cool place is directed may, alternatively be stored in a refrigerator unless otherwise specified in the individual monograph.
Room Temperature—The temperature prevailing in a working area. A *controlled room temperature* encompasses the usual working environment of 20°C to 25°C (68°F to 77°F) but also allows for temperature variations between 15°C and 30°C (59°F and 86°F) that may be experienced in pharmacies, hospitals, and drug warehouses.
Warm—Any temperature between 30° and 40°C (86° and 104°F).
Excessive Heat—Any temperature above 40°C (104°F).
Protection from Freezing—Where in addition to the risk of breakage of the container, freezing subjects a product to loss of strength or potency, or to destructive alteration of the dosage form, the container label bears an appropriate instruction to protect the product from freezing.

When no specific storage or limitations are provided, it is understood that the storage conditions include protection from moisture, freezing, and excessive heat.

Standards for Current Good Manufacturing Practice

To insure high standards for drug product quality, the Food and Drug Administration enforces compliance with the requirements of its Current Good Manufacturing Practice (CGMP or GMP) regulations. The first GMP regulations were promulgated in 1963 under one of the provisions of the Kefauver-Harris Drug Amendments of 1962. They were revised in 1978 and have been updated periodically. A topical outline of these regulations is presented in Table 4–9 and summarized in the sections that follow. A more detailed presentation of CGMP regulations may be found in the *Code of Federal Regulations*[14] and in the *United States Pharmacopeia*.[15] The CGMP regulations establish standards for all aspects of pharmaceutical manufacture in the United States, and also apply to foreign suppliers and manufacturers of bulk components and finished pharmaceutical products that are imported, distributed, or sold in this country. The Food and Drug Administration has a program for the CGMP inspection of the facilities of domestic, as well as foreign, suppliers and manu-

Table 4–9. Topical Outline of Current Good Manufacturing Practice Regulations[1]

A. General Provisions
   1. Scope.
   2. Definitions.
B. Organization and Personnel
   1. Responsibilities of quality control unit.
   2. Personnel qualifications.
   3. Personnel responsibilities.
   4. Consultants.
C. Buildings and Facilities
   1. Design and construction features.
   2. Lighting.
   3. Ventilation, air filtration, air heating and cooling.
   4. Plumbing.
   5. Sewage and refuse.
   6. Washing and toilet facilities.
   7. Sanitation.
   8. Maintenance.
D. Equipment
   1. Equipment design, size, and location.
   2. Equipment construction.
   3. Equipment cleaning and maintenance.
   4. Automatic, mechanical, and electronic equipment.
   5. Filters.
E. Control of Components and Drug Product Containers and Closures
   1. General requirements.
   2. Receipt and storage of untested components, drug product containers, and closures.
   3. Testing and approval or rejection of components, drug product containers, and closures.
   4. Use of approved components, drug product containers, and closures.
   5. Retesting of approved components, drug product containers, and closures.
   6. Rejected components, drug product containers, and closures.
   7. Drug product containers and closures.
F. Production and Process Controls
   1. Written procedures; deviations.
   2. Charge-in of components.
   3. Calculation of yield.
   4. Equipment identification.
   5. Sampling and testing of in-process materials and drug products.
   6. Time limitations on production.
   7. Control of microbiological contamination.
   8. Reprocessing.
G. Packaging and Labeling Control
   1. Materials examination and usage criteria.
   2. Labeling issuance.
   3. Packaging and labeling operations.
   4. Tamper-resistant packaging requirements for over-the-counter human drug products.
   5. Drug product inspection.
   6. Expiration dating.
H. Holding and Distribution
   1. Warehousing procedures.
   2. Distribution procedures.
I. Laboratory Controls
   1. General requirements.
   2. Testing and release for distribution.
   3. Stability testing.
   4. Special testing requirements.
   5. Reserve samples.
   6. Laboratory animals.
   7. Penicillin contamination.
J. Records and Reports
   1. General requirements.
   2. Equipment cleaning and use log.
   3. Component, drug product container, closure, and labeling records.
   4. Master production and control records.
   5. Batch production and control records.
   6. Production record review.
   7. Laboratory records.
   8. Distribution records.
   9. Complaint files.
K. Returned and Salvaged Drug Products
   1. Returned drug products.
   2. Drug product salvaging

[1] Code of Federal Regulations, *21*, part 211, revised April 1, 1993.

facturers who export to the United States. Compliance with CGMP standards is our best assurance that the products dispensed by the pharmacist to the patient are of appropriate and uniform high quality.

General Provisions—Scope and Definitions

The regulations in 21 CFR, Part 211 contain the minimum good manufacturing practice requirements for the preparation of finished pharmaceutical products for administration to humans or animals. Additional regulations for the preparation of biologic products,[20] medical devices,[21] and medicated articles[22] are required as applicable.

Common terms used in manufacturing-practice standards and in process validation are defined as follows:

Component—any material used in the manufacture of a drug product, including those which may not be present in the finished product.
Batch—a specific quantity of a drug of uniform speci-

fied quality produced according to a single manufacturing order during the same cycle of manufacture.
Lot—a batch or any portion of a batch having uniform specified quality and a distinctive identifying "lot number."
Lot Number, Control Number, or Batch Number—any distinctive combination of letters, numbers or symbols from which the complete history of the manufacture, processing, packaging, holding, and distribution of a batch or lot of a drug product may be determined.
Active Ingredient—any component which is intended to furnish pharmacological activity or other direct effect in the diagnosis, cure, mitigation, treatment or prevention of disease or to affect the structure or function of the body of man or other animals.
Inactive Ingredient—any component other than the active ingredients in a drug product.
Drug Product—a finished dosage form that contains an active drug ingredient generally, but not necessarily, in association with inactive ingredients. The term may also include a dosage form that does not contain an active ingredient intended to be used as a placebo.
Master Record—records containing the formulation, specifications, manufacturing procedures, quality assurance requirements, and labeling of a finished product.
Verified—signed by a second individual or recorded by automated equipment.
Quarantined—an area that is marked, designated, or set aside for the holding of incoming components prior to acceptance examination.
Reprocessing—the activity whereby the finished product or any of its components is recycled through all or part of the manufacturing process.
Quality Control—the regulatory process through which industry measures actual quality performance, compares it with standards, and acts on the difference.
Batchwise Control—the use of validated in-process sampling and testing methods in such a way that results prove the process has done what it purports to do for the specific batch concerned, assuming control parameters have been appropriately respected.
Quality Assurance—the activity of providing, to all concerned, the evidence needed to establish confidence that the activities relating to quality are being performed adequately.
Quality Audit—a documented activity performed in accordance with established procedures on a planned and periodic basis to verify compliance with the procedures to assure quality.
Validation—establishing documented evidence that a system does what it purports to do (e.g., equipment, software, controls).
Process Validation—establishing documented evidence that a process does what it purports to do (e.g., sterilization).
Validation Protocol—a prospective experimental plan that, when executed, is intended to produce documented evidence that the system has been validated.
Validation Task Report—a scientific report of the results derived from executing a validation protocol.
Prospective Validation—establishing documented evidence that a system does what it purports to do based on a preplanned protocol.
Concurrent Processes Validation—establishing documented evidence that a process does what it purports to do based on information generated during actual implementation of the process.
Retrospective Validation—establishing documented evidence that a system does what it purports to do based on review and analysis of historic information.
Revalidation—repetition of the validation process or a specific portion of it.
Worst Case—the highest or lowest value of a given control parameter actually evaluated in a validation exercise.
Proven Acceptable Range (PAR)—all values of a given control parameter that fall between proven high and low worst-case conditions.
Compliance—determination through inspection of the extent to which a manufacturer is complying with prescribed regulations, standards, and practices.
Certification—documented testimony by qualified authorities that a system qualification, calibration, validation, or revalidation has been performed appropriately and that the results are acceptable.

Although not a part of the subject matter of this textbook, the reader should be aware that the FDA has developed Good Manufacturing Practice regulations for medical devices and has proposed CGMP regulations for large volume parenterals. Included in the list of critical medical devices are: airways, catheters, dialyzers, cardiac pacemakers, prosthetics, infusion pumps, respirators, valves, and ventilators.[8]

Organization and Personnel

This section of the regulations deals with the responsibilities of the quality control unit, employees, and consultants.

The regulations require that a quality control unit have the authority and responsibility for all functions that may affect product quality. This includes accepting or rejecting product components, product specifications, finished products, packaging, and labeling. Adequate laboratory facilities shall be provided, written procedures followed, and all records maintained.

All personnel engaged in the manufacture, processing, packing, or holding of a drug product, including those in supervisory positions, are required to have the education, training, and/or experience needed to fulfill the assigned responsibility. Appropriate programs of skill development, continuing education and training, and performance evaluations are essential in maintaining quality assurance. Any consultants advising on scientific and technical matters should possess requisite qualifications for the tasks.

Buildings and Facilities

As outlined in Table 4–9, the regulations in this section include the design, structural features, and functional aspects of buildings and facilities. Each building's structure, space, design, and placement of equipment must be such to enable thorough cleaning, inspection, and safe and effective use for the designated operations. Proper considerations must be given to such factors as water quality standards; security; materials used for floors, walls, and ceilings; segregated areas for raw materials subject to quality control approval; weighing and measuring rooms; sterile areas for ophthalmic and parenteral products; flammable materials storage areas; finished products storage, etc.; control of heat, humidity, light, temperature, and ventilation; waste handling; employee facilities and safety procedures in compliance with the Occupational Safety and Health Administration (OSHA) regulations; and procedures and practices of personal sanitation.

All work in the manufacture, processing, packing, or holding of a pharmaceutical product must be logged in, supervisor-inspected, and signed off. Similarly, a log of building maintenance must be kept to document this component of the regulations.

Equipment

Each piece of equipment must be of appropriate design and size, and suitably located to facilitate operations for its intended use, cleaning, and maintenance. The equipment's surfaces and parts must not interact with the processes or product's components so as to alter the purity, strength, or quality.

Standard operating procedures (SOPs) must be written and followed for the proper use, maintenance, and cleaning of each piece of equipment, and appropriate logs and records must be kept. Automated equipment and computers utilized in the processes must be routinely calibrated, maintained, and validated for accuracy.

Control of Components, Containers, and Closures

Written procedures are required to be maintained and followed describing the receipt, identification, storage, handling, sampling, testing, and approval or rejection of drug-product components (active and inactive ingredients), drug-product containers, and closures.

Bulk pharmaceutical chemicals, containers, and closures must meet the exact physical and chemical specifications established with the supplier at the time of ordering.

When product components are received from a supplier, each lot must be logged in with the purchase order number, date of receipt, bill of lading, name and vital information on the supplier, supplier's stock or control number, and quantity received. The component is assigned a control number, identifying both the component and the intended product. Raw materials are quarantined until they are verified, through careful qualitative and quantitative analysis, as meeting the required specifications. Only then are they approved and released by the quality control unit for use in product manufacture. The assigned control number follows the component throughout production so it can be traced if necessary.

Production and Process Controls

Written procedures are required for production and process controls to assure that the drug products have the correct identity, strength, quality, and purity. These procedures must be followed in the execution of the various control and production functions for quality assurance. Any deviation from the written procedures must be recorded and justified. In most instances, a system of time and date recording by the operator and supervisor sign-off is applied to each key operation. When operations are controlled by automated equipment, such equipment must be validated regularly for precision.

All product ingredients, equipment used, and drums or other containers of bulk finished product must be distinctively identified by labeling as to content or status (e.g., clean equipment scheduled for tablet production) at all times.

In-process samples are taken from production batches periodically for product control. In-process controls are of two general types: (a) those performed by production personnel at the time of operation to assure that the machinery is producing output within preestablished control limits (e.g., tablet size, hardness), and (b) those performed by the quality control laboratory personnel to assure compliance to all product specifications (e.g., tablet content, dissolution) and batch-to-batch consistency. Product found out-of-standard sometimes may be reprocessed for subsequent use. However, in this, as in all instances, procedures must be performed according to established protocol, all materials must be accounted for, all specifications met, and all records meticulously maintained.

Packaging and Labeling Control

Written procedures are required for the receipt, identification, storage, handling, sampling and testing, and issuance of labeling and packaging materials. All materials must be withheld for use in the packaging and labeling of product until approved and released by the quality control unit. Control procedures must be followed and records maintained for the issuance and use of product labeling. Quantities issued, used, and returned must be reconciled and discrepancies investigated. Before labeling operations commence, the labeling facilities must be inspected to assure that all drug products and labels have been removed from the previous operations. During, and at the conclusion of, an operation the products are examined for assurance of correct labeling and packaging. All of these procedures are essential to avoid label mixups and the mislabeling of products. All records of inspections and controls must be documented in the batch production records.

Labels must meet the legal requirements for content, as outlined in Chapter 2 and earlier in this chapter. Each label shall contain expiration dating and the production batch or lot number to facilitate product identification. Special packaging requirements may apply in certain instances (e.g., tamper-resistant packaging for OTC products).

Holding and Distribution

Written procedures must be established and followed for the holding and distribution of product. Finished pharmaceuticals must be quarantined in storage until released by the quality control unit. Products must be stored and shipped under conditions that do not affect product quality. Ordinarily, the oldest approved stock is distributed first. A distribution control system must be in place through which the distributed point of each lot of drug product may be readily determined, to facilitate its recall if necessary.

Laboratory Controls

This section contains requirements for the establishment of, and conformance to, written specifications, standards, sampling plans, test procedures, and other laboratory control mechanisms. The specifications apply to each batch of drug product and include provisions for sample size, test intervals, sample storage, stability testing, and special testing requirements for certain dosage forms, such as parenterals, ophthalmics, controlled-release products, and radioactive pharmaceuticals. Reserve samples must be retained for distributed products for specified periods of time depending upon their category. In general, reserve samples must be maintained for 3 to 6 months after the expiration date of the last lot of the drug product. Reserve samples of drug products used to conduct bioavailability or bioequivalence studies must be retained for 5 years. This is intended to help ensure the FDA's ability to investigate bioequivalence between generic drugs and the pioneer products. For certain OTC products that are exempt from expiration dating, reserve samples must be maintained for 3 years after distribution of the last lot of the production.

Records and Reports

Production, control, and distribution records are required to be maintained for at least a year following the expiration date of a product batch. This includes equipment cleaning and maintenance logs, specifications and lot numbers of product components, including raw materials and product containers/closures, and label records. Complete master production and control records for each production batch must be maintained, including the name and strength of the product, dosage form, quantitative amounts of components and dosage units, complete manufacturing and control procedures, specifications, special notations, equipment used, in-process controls, sampling and laboratory methods used and assay results, calibration of instrumentation, distribution records, and dated and employee-identified records documenting that each step in the production, control, packaging, labeling, and distribution of the product was accomplished and approved by the quality control unit. Depending upon the operation, the operator's and/or supervisor's full signatures, initials, or other written or electronic identification codes are required.

Records of written and oral complaints regarding a drug product (e.g., product failure, adverse drug experience) must also be maintained, along with information regarding the internal disposition of each complaint. All records must be made available at the time of inspection by FDA officials.

Returned and Salvaged Drug Products

Returned drug products (as from wholesalers) must be identified by lot number and product quality determined through appropriate testing. Drug products that meet specifications may be salvaged or reprocessed. Those that do not, as well as those that have been subjected to improper storage conditions (e.g., extremes in temperature) shall not be returned to the marketplace. Records for all returned products must be maintained, and must include the date and reasons for the return; quantity and lot number of product returned; procedures employed for holding, testing, and reprocessing the product; and the product's disposition.

Manufacturing vs. Compounding

The FDA's CGMP regulations apply to a community or institutional pharmacy only if it is engaged in the manufacture, repackaging, or relabeling of drugs and drug products beyond the usual conduct of dispensing. Pharmacies which do engage in such activities must register with the FDA as a manufacturer or distributor and be subject to FDA inspection at regular intervals. These pharmacies would also be bound to the standards of Current Good Manufacturing Practice. Examples of pharmacies engaged in such activities include: hospital pharmacies that repackage drug products for their own use as well as the use of other hospitals; chain pharmacies that repackage and relabel bulk quantities of products from the manufacturer's original containers for distribution to individual pharmacies within the chain; and similar repackaging and relabeling activities conducted by individual pharmacists or pharmacies for distribution to other pharmacies or retailers.

Recently, professional and regulatory attention has been directed toward differentiating between pharmaceutical *manufacturing* and *compounding* as practiced by community pharmacists.[23–24] In general, pharmaceutical manufacturing involves the large-scale production of drugs or drug products for distribution and sale, whereas compounding involves the professional preparation of prescriptions for specific patients as a part of the traditional practice of pharmacy.

It is well recognized that community pharmacists, as a part of their traditional professional practice roles, are called upon to extemporaneously compound prescriptions, requiring the weighing, measuring, and admixture of ingredients. Prescriptions requiring compounding are ordered when in the judgment of the prescriber, in consultation with the pharmacist, there is no prefabricated commercial product available to meet a particular patient's medication requirements. In these instances, the pharmacist applies his pharmaceutical expertise by combining bulk active and inactive ingredients, or by modifying the strength or form of an existing commercial product. For instance, the pharmacist may utilize adult-strength prefabricated tablets or capsules to prepare an otherwise-unavailable syrup or suspension of the drug that is suitable for pediatric use.

By tradition, compounding (in contrast to manufacturing) also occurs when a pharmacist *anticipates* the receipt of multiple prescriptions for the same formula, based on an established prescriber-patient-pharmacy relationship, and prepares a larger, but limited, quantity of the formula ahead of time for use in filling those prescriptions.[24]

In these compounding functions, pharmacists and pharmacies operate under the licenses issued and regulations promulgated by state Boards of Pharmacy and also in accord with the applicable requirements of the Federal Food, Drug, and Cosmetic Act, as pertaining to unapproved new drugs, drug adulteration, drug misbranding, and so forth.

Pharmaceutical manufacturing includes the preparation, production, processing, packaging or repackaging, distribution, and/or promotion of a drug/drug product for wholesale or retail sale outside the bounds of traditional pharmacy practice. It involves the large-scale production and distribution of products as a *supplier function* rather than as a practitioner function. Manufacturers of pharmaceuticals must be licensed under the requirements of the jurisdictional state Board of Pharmacy *and* must meet all of the applicable requirements of the Federal Food, Drug, and Cosmetic Act. As noted above, this would include compliance with the regulations of the Food and Drug Administration which apply to manufacturers, as registration as a manufacturer; regular facilities inspection; conformance with the drug listing requirement; establishment and documented procedures for quality assurance and quality control; and, compliance with Current Good Manufacturing Practice.

Thus, depending upon a pharmacy's scope of practice and scale of activity, it may require both licensure as a pharmacy and registration as a pharmaceutical manufacturing facility.

Pharmaceutical compounding and manufacturing require careful considerations including: the selection of active and nonactive ingredients that meet specified high standards of quality (as USP/NF) and are chemically, physically, and therapeutically compatible; utilization of the most appropriate compounding or manufacturing processes and equipment; consideration of drug bioavailability; application of measures of quality control and quality assurance; and assessment of product stability, storage requirements, shelf-life, and labeling. Pharmacists may draw upon many texts (including this one), reference books (the *United States Pharmacopeia/National Formulary* and *Remington's Pharmaceutical Sciences*[25]), the National Association of Boards of Pharmacy's (NABP) *Good Compounding Practices (GCPs)* guidelines, and scientific and professional papers and articles[26–30] to provide needed guidance. It is not unusual today for pharmacists to be called upon to compound special ointments, vaginal and rectal suppositories, oral solutions and suspensions, parenteral admixtures, and other dosage forms. The active drug substance may be obtained as bulk powder, if available, or from commercial tablets, capsules, or injections.

Computerization in the Pharmaceutical Industry

Computers play an important role in the pharmaceutical industry. They are used extensively for administrative and business functions as well as in plant operations such as production scheduling, in-process manufacturing and quality control, packaging, and labeling. In addition, there is a growing emphasis toward the networking of computers in the production and quality control areas within companies, to fully integrate laboratory information and manufacturing operations into sophisticated management systems. These integrated systems support compliance with Good Manufacturing Practice regulations, process validation, resource management, and cost control. Figure 4–11 represents an example of computer use in the pharmaceutical industry for the management of plant operations.

In addition to computers, robotic devices increasingly are being employed to replace manual operations in production lines, analytical sam-

Fig. 4–11. *Example of computer use in the pharmaceutical industry. The machine shown is an Allen Bradley, Advisor 2+ operator interface. This allows the plant operator to communicate with the main programmable logical controller (PLC). The advisor 2+ gives a constant real-time update of the process on a series of screens and allows an operator to perform preprogrammed operations at the push of a button. (Courtesy of Elan Corporation, plc.)*

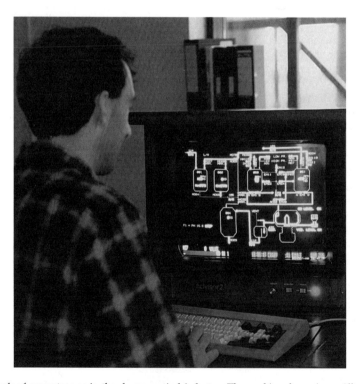

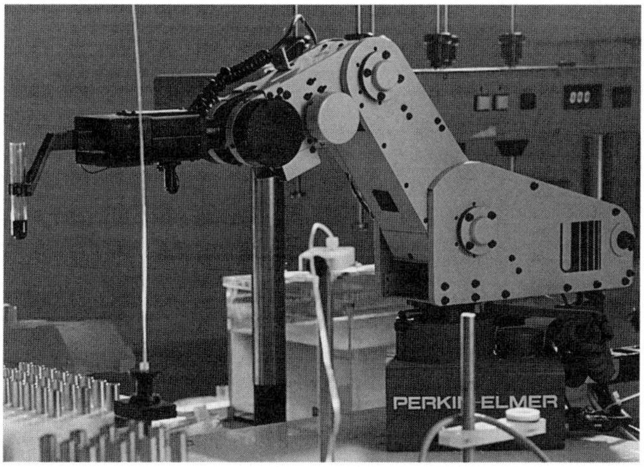

Fig. 4–12. *Robotics in laboratory use. Perkin-Elmer Robotic Arm and Perkin-Elmer Lambda 1a UV/VIS Spectrophotometer. (Courtesy of Elan Corporation, plc.)*

pling, and packaging. Figure 4–12 presents an example of the use of robotics in laboratory use. Laboratory robotics provides automation in such areas as sample preparation and handling, wet chemistry procedures, laboratory process control, and instrumental analysis.[31] Pharmaceutical applications include automated product handling in production lines and in procedures as sampling and analysis, tablet content uniformity, and dissolution testing.

Among the advantages cited for computer use and automation within the pharmaceutical industry are:[32–33]

- increased productivity reducing labor
- improved process and product quality
- reduction in operator error and levels of product rejections
- increased process yields (as from chemical synthesis of drug compounds)
- enhanced repeatability of processes
- improved operator protection due to less "hands on" activity
- automated diagnostic and alarm actions alerting of possible mechanical malfunction, process decontrol or product defect
- assist in process and product validation efforts
- assist in bookkeeping efforts
- assist in scheduling efficacy
- reduced cost per product unit

Movement toward Paperless Electronic Records

There is an effort underway by the FDA and the pharmaceutical industry to replace the traditional use of paper with electronic systems to record, transmit, and maintain needed documentation. This includes records developed by industry to support applications for drug product approvals—e.g., computer assisted new drug applications (CANDAs)—and FDA inspections for CGMP compliance.

Among the regulatory and legal issues involved in the effort toward a paperless system are the authenticity, integrity, and security of electronic records, and the electronic means of replacing conventional handwritten signatures and initials, as required on reports and documents to identify individuals having functional responsibility and operational authority.

References

1. Poole, J.W.: *Preformulation.* FMC Corporation, 1982.
2. *Handbook of Pharmaceutical Excipients.* American Pharmaceutical Association, Washington, DC, 1986.
3. Brange, J., Langkjaer, L., Havelund, S., and Vølund, A.: Chemical Stability of Insulin. Hydrolytic Degradation During Storage of Pharmaceutical Preparations. *Pharm. Res, 9*:715–726, 1992.
4. Parrott, E.L.: Stability of Pharmaceuticals. *J. Am. Pharm. Assoc., NS6*:73–76, 1966.
5. *Guideline for Submitting Documentation for the Stability of Human Drugs and Biologics,* Food and Drug Administration, Rockville, MD, 1987.
6. Lewis, R.: When Smell and Taste Go Awry. *FDA Consumer 25*:29–33, 1991.
7. Hornstein, I., and Teranishi, R.: The Chemistry of Flavor. *Chem. Eng. News, 45*:92–108, 1967.
8. Murphy, D.H.: A Practical Compendium on Sweetening Agents. *Amer. Pharm., NS23*:32–37, 1983.

9. Jacknowitz, A.I.: Artificial Sweeteners: How Safe Are They? *U.S. Pharmacist, 13:*28–31, 1988.
10. Krueger, R.J., Topolewski, M., and Havican, S.: In Search of the Ideal Sweetener. *Pharmacy Times,* 72–77, July 1991.
11. Lecos, C.W.: Sweetness Minus Calories = Controversy. *FDA Consumer, 19:*18–23, 1985.
12. *Code of Federal Regulations,* Title 21, Parts 70–82.
13. Colorants for Drug Tablets and Capsules. *Drug and Cosmetic Industry, 133*(2):44, 1983.
14. *Code of Federal Regulations,* Title 21, Parts 210–211.
15. *The United States Pharmacopeia 23/National Formulary 18,* The United States Pharmacopeial Convention, Rockville, MD, 1995.
16. *Guideline for Submitting Documentation for Packaging of Human Drugs and Biologics.* Food and Drug Administration, Rockville, MD, 1987.
17. *The United States Pharmacopeia XXII/National Formulary XVII,* The United States Pharmacopeial Convention, Rockville, MD, 1990, 1686–1687.
18. Smith, D.L.: Compliance Packaging: A Patient Education Tool. *Amer. Pharm., NS29:*42–53, 1989.
19. *The United States Pharmacopeia 23/National Formulary 18.* The United States Pharmacopeial Convention, Rockville, MD, 1995, 11.
20. *Code of Federal Regulations,* Title 21, Parts 600–680.
21. *Code of Federal Regulations,* Title 21, Part 820.
22. *Code of Federal Regulations,* Title 21, Part 226.
23. *Manufacture, Distribution, and Promotion of Adulterated, Misbranded, or Unapproved New Drugs for Human Use by State-Licensed Pharmacies—FDA Compliance Policy Guide.* Food and Drug Administration, 1992.
24. Resolution: Pharmacy Compounding and the Manufacturing of Drugs. National Association of Boards of Pharmacy, 1992.
25. *Remington's Pharmaceutical Sciences,* 19th ed., Easton, PA, Mack Publishing Co., 1995.
26. Allen, L.V., Jr.: Extemporaneous Compounding in the 1990's. *U.S. Pharmacist, 14:*58–64, 1989.
27. Allen, L.V., Jr.: Vehicles for Liquid Oral Dosage Forms. *U.S. Pharmacist, 16:*72–76, 1991.
28. Crawford, S.Y., and Dombrowski, S.R.: Extemporaneous Compounding Activities and the Associated Informational Needs of Pharmacists. *Am. J. Hosp. Pharm., 48:*1205–1210, 1991.
29. Wiest, D.B., Garner, S.S., Pagacz, L.R., and Zeigler, V.: Stability of Flecainide Acetate in an Extemporaneously Compounded Oral Suspension. *Am. J. Hosp. Pharm., 49:*1467–1470, 1992.
30. *Guidelines on Compounding of Nonsterile Products in Pharmacies.* Amer. Society Hospital Pharm., Bethesda, MD, 1993.
31. *Laboratory Robotics Handbook,* Zymark Corp., Hopkinton, MA, 1988.
32. Fraade, D.J.: An Overview and Case Histories of Computer Applications in a Pharmaceutical Industry. *Proceedings, Eighth International Good Manufacturing Practices Conference,* The University of Georgia, Athens, 1984.
33. Comstock, T.A.: Computer Utilization in GMP Regulated Manufacturing. *Proceedings, Seventeenth International Good Manufacturing Practice Conference.* The University of Georgia, Athens, 1993.

5

Peroral Solids, Capsules, Tablets, and Controlled-Release Dosage Forms

WHEN MEDICATIONS are to be administered orally in dry form, capsules and tablets are most frequently used. They are effective and provide the patient with convenience of handling, identification, and administration. From a pharmaceutic standpoint, solid dosage forms are generally more stable than are their liquid counterparts and thus are preferred for poorly stable drugs. Dry powders are taken orally (usually after mixing in water) to a much lesser extent than are capsules and tablets, but are preferred by some patients who are unable to swallow the solid dosage forms. However, most medicated powders are utilized as external applications to the skin. While the use of powders *per se* in therapeutics is limited, the use of powders in dosage form preparation is extensive. Most of the medicinal substances in use today occur in crystalline or powdered form and are blended with other powdered materials, as inert fillers and disintegrants, prior to fabrication into solid dosage forms. Powdered drugs are also frequently added to ointments, pastes, suppositories, and other dosage forms during their preparation. Similarly, granules, which are agglomerates of powdered materials prepared into larger free flowing particles, are utilized chiefly in the preparation of tablets and in dry preparations intended to be reconstituted to liquid forms prior to use by the addition of the appropriate vehicle.

Powders

As a pharmaceutical preparation, a *powder* (Latin, *pulvis*) is a mixture of finely divided drugs and/or chemicals in dry form. This should be differentiated from the general use of the term "powder" or "powdered" which is commonly used to describe the physical state of a single chemical substance or a single drug.

A powder may be a finely subdivided preparation, a coarsely comminuted product, or a product of intermediate particle size. It may be prepared from a naturally occurring dried vegetable drug, or it may be a physical admixture of two or more powdered pure chemical agents present in definite proportions. Powders may contain small proportions of liquids dispersed thoroughly and uniformly over the solid components of the mixture, or the powder may be composed entirely of solid materials.

Some powders are intended to be used internally; others, externally. Certain powders are dispensed by the pharmacist to the patient in bulk quantities; others, in divided, individually packaged portions, depending primarily on the use, dose, or potency of the powder.

The disadvantages of powders as a dosage form include the potential for patient misunderstanding of the correct method of use, the undesirability of taking bitter or unpleasant tasting drugs in this manner, the difficulty of protecting from decomposition powders containing hygroscopic, deliquescent, or aromatic materials, and the manufacturing expense required in the preparation of uniform individually wrapped doses of powders. To be of high efficacy, the powder must be a homogeneous blend of all of the components and must be of the most advantageous particle size. As noted earlier (Chapter 3), the particle size of a drug not only contributes to its rate of solubility in a glass of water or within the stomach or intestine, but also may influence its biologic availability.

Particle Size and Analysis

The particles of pharmaceutical powders may be very coarse, of the dimensions of about 10,000 microns or 10 mm, or they may be extremely fine, approaching colloidal dimensions of 1 micron or less. In order to standardize the particle size of a given powder, the USP employs descriptive terms such as "Very Coarse, Coarse, Moderately Coarse, Fine, and Very Fine," which are related to the proportion of powder that is capable of passing through the openings of standardized sieves of varying dimensions in a specified time

Table 5–1. Opening of Standard Sieves*

Sieve Number	*Sieve Opening*
2	9.5 mm
3.5	5.6 mm
4	4.75 mm
8	2.36 mm
10	2.00 mm
20	850 μm
30	600 μm
40	425 μm
50	300 μm
60	250 μm
70	212 μm
80	180 μm
100	150 μm
120	125 μm
200	75 μm
230	63 μm
270	53 μm
325	45 μm
400	38 μm

* Adapted from USP23-NF18.

period under shaking, generally in a *mechanical sieve shaker*. Table 5–1 presents the Standard Sieve Numbers and the sieve openings in each, expressed in millimeters and in micrometers. Sieves for such pharmaceutical testing and measurement are generally made of wire cloth woven from brass, bronze, or other suitable wire. They are not coated or plated.

Powders of vegetable and animal drugs are officially defined as follows:[1]

Very Coarse (or a No. 8) powder—All particles pass through a No. 8 sieve and not more than 20% through a No. 60 sieve.

Coarse (or a No. 20) powder—All particles pass through a No. 20 sieve and not more than 40% through a No. 60 sieve.

Moderately Coarse (or a No. 40) powder—All particles pass through a No. 40 sieve and not more than 40% through a No. 80 sieve.

Fine (or a No. 60) powder—All particles pass through a No. 60 sieve and not more than 40% through a No. 100 sieve.

Very Fine (or a No. 80) powder—All particles pass through a No. 80 sieve. There is no limit as to greater fineness.

The powder fineness for chemicals is defined as follows. It should be noted that there is no "Very Coarse" category.

Coarse (or a No. 20) powder—All particles pass through a No. 20 sieve and not more than 60% through a No. 40 sieve.

Moderately Coarse (or a No. 40) powder—All particles pass through a No. 40 sieve and not more than 60% through a No. 60 sieve.

Fine (or a No. 80) powder—All particles pass through a No. 80 sieve. There is no limit as to greater fineness.

Very Fine (or a No. 120) powder—All particles pass through a No. 120 sieve. There is no limit as to greater fineness.

Granules typically fall within the range of 4- to 12-sieve size, although granulations of powders prepared in the 12- to 20-sieve range are not uncommon when used in tablet making.

The purpose of particle size analysis in pharmacy is to obtain quantitative data on the size, distribution, and shapes of drug and nondrug components to be used in pharmaceutical formulations. There may be substantial differences in particle size, crystalline type, and amorphous shape within and between substances. Particle size can influence a variety of important factors:

- *Dissolution rate* of particles intended to dissolve;
- *Suspendability* of particles intended to remain undissolved but uniformly dispersed in a liquid vehicle (e.g., fine dispersions have particles of from approximately 0.5 to 10 micrometers or μm);
- *Uniform distribution* of a drug substance in a powder mixture or solid dosage form;[2]
- *Penetrability* of particles intended to be inhaled to reach a desired location within the respiratory tract (e.g., 1–5 micrometers) for deposition deep in the respiratory tract);[3] and the
- *Nongrittiness* of solid particles in dermal ointments, creams, and ophthalmic preparations (e.g., fine powders may be 50–100 micrometers in size).

A number of methods exist for the determination of particle size, including the following:

- *Sieving*, in which particles are passed by mechanical shaking through a series of sieves of known and successively smaller size and the determination of the proportion of powder passing through or being withheld on each sieve (range: from about 50 to 3360 micrometers, depending upon sieve sizes).[4]
- *Microscopy*, in which the particles are sized through the use of a calibrated grid background or other measuring device (range: 0.2 to 100 micrometers).[5,6]

Micromeritics

Micromeritics is the science of small particles; a *particle* is any unit of matter having defined physical dimensions. It is important to study particles because the majority of drug dosage forms are solids; solids are not "static" systems—the physical state of particles can be altered by physical manipulation and particle characteristics can alter therapeutic effectiveness.

Micromeritics includes a number of characteristics including particle size, particle size distribution, particle shape, angle of repose, porosity, true volume, bulk volume, apparent density and bulkiness.

PARTICLE SIZE

A number of techniques can be used for determining particle size and particle size distributions. Particle size determinations are complicated by the fact that particles are nonuniform in shape. Only two relatively simple examples will be provided for a detailed calculation of the average particle size of a powder mixture. Other methods will be generally discussed. The techniques utilized will include the microscopic method and the sieving method.

The *microscopic method* can include counting not less than 200 particles in a single plane using a calibrated ocular on a microscope. Given the following data, what is the average diameter of the particles?

Size Group of Counted Particles (μ)	Middle Value μ "d"	No. Particles Per Group "n"	*"nd"*
40–60	50	15	750
60–80	70	25	1750
80–100	90	95	8550
100–120	110	140	15400
120–140	130	80	10400
		Σn = 355	Σnd = 36850

$$d_{av} = \frac{\Sigma\, nd}{\Sigma n} = \frac{36{,}850}{355} = 103.8\ \mu$$

The *sieving method* involves using a set of U.S. Standard sieves in the size range desired. A stack of sieves is arranged in order, the powder placed in the top sieve, the stack shaken, the quantity of powder resting on each sieve weighed, and the following calculation performed.

Sieve No.	*Arithmetic Mean Opening (mm)*	*Weight Retained (G)*	*% Retained*	*% Retained × Mean Opening*
20/40	0.630	15.5	14.3	9.009
40/60	0.335	25.8	23.7	7.939
60/80	0.214	48.3	44.4	9.502
80/100	0.163	15.6	14.3	2.330
100/120	0.137	3.5	3.3	0.452
		108.7	100.0	29.232

$$d_{av} = \frac{\Sigma\,(\%\ \text{retained}) \times (\text{ave size})}{100} = \frac{29.232}{100} = 0.2923\ \text{mm}$$

Another method of particle size determination involves *sedimentation* using the "Andreasen Pipet." The Andreasen pipet is a special cylindrical container designed such that a sample can be removed from the lower portion at selected time intervals. The powder is dispersed in a nonsolvent in the Andreasen Pipet, agitated, and 20 mL samples removed over a period of time. Each 20 mL sample is dried and weighed. Using the following equation, the particle diameters can be calculated.

$$d = \frac{18\, h\eta}{(\rho_i - \rho_e)\, gt}$$

Micromeritics (Continued)

where d is the diameter of the particles,
h is the height of the liquid above the sampling tube orifice,
η is the viscosity of the suspending liquid,
$\rho_i - \rho_e$ is the density difference between the suspending liquid and the particles,
g is the gravitational constant, and
t is the time in seconds.

Other methods of particle size determinations include the *elutriation method, centrifugal method, permeation method, adsorption method, electronic sensing zone (the Coulter Counter), and the light obstruction methods.* The latter includes the use of both standard light and laser methods. In general, the resulting average particle sizes by these techniques can provide average particle size by weight (sieve method, light scattering, sedimentation method), and average particle size by volume (light scattering, electronic sensing zone, light obstruction, air permeation and even the optical microscope).

ANGLE OF REPOSE

The *angle of repose* is a relatively simple technique for estimating the flowability of a powder. It can be easily experimentally determined by allowing a powder to flow through a funnel and fall freely onto a surface. The height and diameter of the resulting cone is measured and, using the following equation, the angle of repose can be calculated.

$$\tan \theta = h/r$$

where h is the height of the powder cone, and
r is the radius of the powder cone.

EXAMPLE 1

A powder was poured through the funnel and resulted in a cone that was 3.3 cm high and 9 cm in diameter. What is the angle of repose?

$$\tan \theta = h/r = 3.3/4.5 = 0.73$$
$$\text{arc tan } 0.73 = 36.25^\circ$$

Powders with low angles of repose will flow freely and powders with high angles of repose will flow poorly. A number of factors, including shape and size, determine the flowability of powders. Spherical particles flow better than needles. Very fine particles do not flow as freely as large particles. In general, particles in the size range of 250–2000 μ flow freely if the shape is amenable. Particles in the size range of 75–250 μ may flow freely or cause problems, depending on shape and other factors. With particles less than 100 μ in size, flow is a problem with most substances.

POROSITY, VOID AND BULK VOLUME

If spheres are used as an example, and the different ways they pack together, two possibilities will be considered. First, the closest packing may include the *rhombus/triangle* packing where angles of 60° and 120° are common. The space between the particles, the void, is about 0.26, resulting in a porosity, as described below, of about 26%. Another packing, called *cubical,* may be considered where the cubes are packed at 90° angles to each other. This results in a void of about 0.47, or a porosity of about 47%. This is the most open type of packing. It should be noted that if particles are not uniform, the smaller particles will slip into the void spaces between the larger particles and decrease the void areas.

Packing and flow is important, as it will impact the size of container required for packaging, the flow of granulations, the efficiency of the filling apparatus during the tabletting and encapsulating process, and for the ease of working with the powders.

A number of characteristics can be used to describe powders, including porosity, true volume, bulk volume, apparent density, true density, and bulkiness.

Micromeritics (Continued)

Porosity is

$$\text{Void} \times 100$$

This value should be determined experimentally by measuring the volume occupied by a selected weight of a powder. This volume is called the V_{bulk}. The true volume, V, of a powder is the space occupied by the powder exclusive of spaces greater than the intramolecular space.

Void can be defined as

$$\frac{V_{bulk} - V}{V_{bulk}}$$

therefore, porosity is

$$\frac{V_{bulk} - V}{V_{bulk}} \times 100$$

The bulk volume is

$$\text{True volume} + \text{Porosity}$$

APPARENT DENSITY, TRUE DENSITY AND BULKINESS

The apparent density, ρ_a, is

$$\frac{\text{Weight of the sample}}{V_{bulk}}$$

The true density, ρ, is

$$\frac{\text{Weight of the sample}}{V}$$

The bulkiness, B, is the reciprocal of the apparent density,

$$B = 1/\rho a$$

EXAMPLE 2

A selected powder has a true density (ρ) of 3.5 g/cc. Experimentally, 2.5 g of the powder measures 40 mL in a cyclindrical graduate. Calculate the true volume, void, porosity, apparent density and bulkiness.

True volume:

$$\begin{aligned} \text{Density} &= \text{Mass (weight)/Volume} \\ \therefore \text{Volume} &= \text{Mass (weight)/Density} \\ &= 2.5\text{ g}/(3.5\text{ g/cc}) = 0.715\text{ cc} \end{aligned}$$

Void:

$$\frac{V_{bulk} - V}{V_{bulk}} = \frac{40\text{ mL} - 0.715\text{ mL}}{40\text{ mL}} = 0.982$$

Porosity:

$$\text{Void} \times 100 = 0.982 \times 100 = 98.2\%$$

Apparent density:

$$(\rho a) = \frac{2.5\text{ g}}{40\text{ mL}} = 0.0625\text{ g/mL}$$

Bulkiness:

$$1/\rho a = \frac{1}{0.0625\text{ (g/mL)}} = 16\text{ mL/g}$$

Powders with a low apparent density and a large bulk volume are "light" powders, and those with a high apparent density and a small bulk volume are "heavy" powders.

- *Sedimentation rate,* in which particle size is determined by measuring the terminal settling velocity of particles through a liquid medium in a gravitational or centrifugal environment (range: 0.8–300 micrometers).[4] Sedimentation rate may be calculated from Stokes' law (page 256).
- *Light energy diffraction,* in which particle size is determined by the reduction in light reaching the sensor as the particle, dispersed in a liquid or gas, passes through the sensing zone (range 0.2–500 micrometers).[3]
- *Laser holography,* in which a pulsed laser is fired through an aerosolized particle spray and photographed in three dimensions with a holographic camera, allowing the particles to be individually imaged and sized (range: 1.4–100 micrometers).[7]
- *Cascade impaction* is based on the principle that a particle, driven by an airstream, will impact on a surface in its path, provided that its inertia is sufficient to overcome the drag force that tends to keep it in the airstream.[8] Particles are separated into various size ranges by successively increasing the velocity of the airstream in which they are carried.

Particle Size Reduction

Comminution, the process of reducing the particle size of a solid substance to a finer state of subdivision, is used to facilitate crude drug extraction, increase the dissolution rates of a drug, aid in the formulation of pharmaceutically acceptable dosage forms, and enhance the absorption of drugs. The reduction in the particle size of a solid is accompanied by a great increase in the specific surface area of that substance. An example of the increase in the number of particles formed and the resulting surface area is as follows.

EXAMPLE

Increase in number of particles

If a powder consists of cubes 1 mm on edge, and it is reduced to particles 10 μ on edge, what is the number of particles produced?

1. 1 mm equals 1000 μ.
2. 1000 μ/10 μ = 100 pieces produced on each edge, i.e., if the cube is sliced into 100 pieces, each 10 μ long, 100 pieces would result.
3. If this is repeated in each of the other two dimensions, i.e., to include the x, y and z axes, then there would be 100 $\times$ 100 $\times$ 100 = 1,000,000 particles produced, each 10 μ on edge, for each original particle 1 mm on edge. This can also be written $[(10^2)^3 = 10^6]$.

Increase in surface area

What is the increase in the surface area of the powder by decreasing the particle size from 1 mm to 10 μ?

1. The 1 mm cube has 6 surfaces, each 1 mm on edge. Each face has a surface area of 1 mm^2. Since there are 6 faces, this is 6 mm^2 surface area for this one particle.
2. Each 10 μ cube has 6 surfaces, each 10 μ on edge. Each face has a surface area of $10 \times 10 = 100\ \mu^2$. Since there are 6 faces, this is $6 \times 100\ \mu^2$, or 600 μ^2 surface area for this one particle. Since there are 10^6 particles that resulted by comminuting the 1 mm cube into smaller cubes, each 10 μ on edge, there would be $600\ \mu^2 \times 10^6$ or $6 \times 10^8\ \mu^2$ surface area now.
3. To get everything in the same units for ease of comparison, we convert the $6 \times 10^8\ \mu^2$ into mm^2 as follows.
4. Since there are 1,000 μ/mm, there must be $1{,}000^2$, or 1,000,000 μ^2/mm^2. This is more appropriately expressed as $10^6\ \mu^2/mm^2$,

$$\frac{6 \times 10^8 \mu^2}{10^6 \mu^2/mm^2} = 6 \times 10^2\ mm^2$$

As is evident here, the surface areas have been increased from 6 mm^2 to 600 mm^2 by the reduction in particle size of cubes 1 mm on edge to cubes 10 μ on edge (i.e., a hundred-fold increase in surface area). This can have a significant increase in the rate of dissolution of a drug product.

The above, and other, methods may be used for the quantitation of particle size and shape. For some materials, a single method may be sufficient; however, a combination of methods is frequently required to provide greater assurance of size and shape parameters.[6] The study of particle size is termed *micromeritics (see preceding Physical Pharmacy Capsule, pages 157–159)*.

Comminution of Drugs

On a small scale, as in the community pharmacy, the pharmacist usually reduces the size of chemical substances *(see preceding Physical Pharmacy Capsule, page 160)* by exposing them to the rigor of the mortar and pestle. A finer grinding action is accomplished in a mortar with a rough surface (as a porcelain mortar) than one with a smooth surface (as a glass mortar). The process of grinding a drug in a mortar to reduce its particle size is termed *trituration*. On a large scale, various types of mills and pulverizers may be used to reduce powder fineness. Figure 5–1 shows one such piece of equipment.

A process termed *levigation* is commonly employed in the reduction of particle size particularly in the small-scale preparation of ointments.

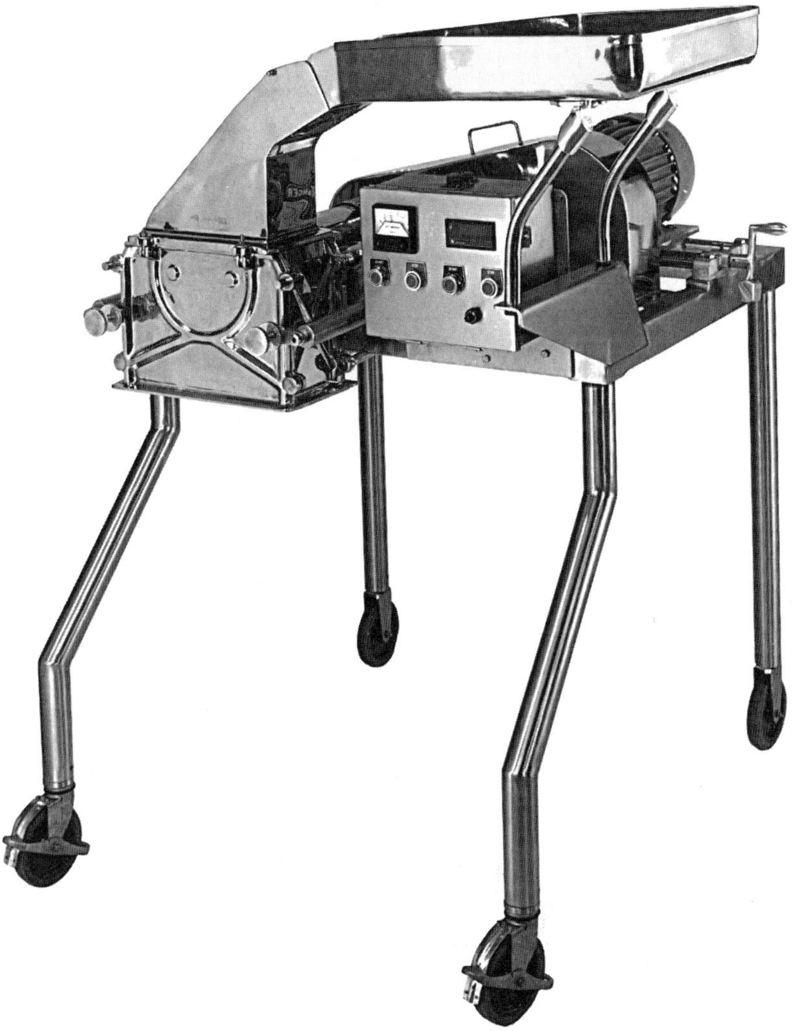

Fig. 5–1. *Model D6-A Fitz®Mill Comminutor used for particle-reduction. Variable motor operating speed and 16 blades permit the low-speed sifting of powders as well as high-speed pulverizing. (Courtesy of The Fitzpatrick Company.)*

This is done to prevent the feeling of grittiness in the preparation due to the solid drug present. In the process, a mortar and pestle or ointment tile is generally used, and a paste is formed of the solid material and a small amount of liquid (the *levigating agent*) in which the solid material is insoluble. The paste is then triturated, effecting a reduction in particle size. The levigated paste may then be added to the ointment base and the mixture made uniform and smooth, usually by rubbing them together with a spatula on the ointment tile. The entire levigation procedure may be performed with the spatula, usually employing a "figure 8" track to incorporate and levigate the materials. Mineral oil and glycerin are commonly used levigating agents.

Blending Powders

When two or more substances are to be combined to form a uniform powder mixture, it is best to reduce the particle size of each individually before weighing and blending. Depending upon the nature of the ingredients, the amount of powder to prepare, and the equipment available, powders may be prepared by *spatulation, trituration, sifting, tumbling* or by *mechanical mixers.*

Spatulation is a method by which small amounts of powders may be blended by the movement of a pharmaceutical spatula through the powders on a sheet of paper or an ointment tile. The method is not generally suitable for large quantities of powders or for powders containing one or more potent substances, because homogeneous blending is not as certain as with other methods. Very little compression or compacting of the powder results from this method. This method is especially suited to the mixing of solid substances that liquify or form *eutectic* mixtures when in close and prolonged contact with one another. This includes phenol, camphor, menthol, thymol, aspirin, phenylsalicylate and similar chemicals. To diminish contact, a powder prepared from such substances is commonly mixed in the presence of an inert diluent such as light magnesium oxide or magnesium carbonate to separate physically the troublesome agents.

Trituration may be employed both to comminute and to mix powders. If comminution is especially desired, a porcelain or a Wedgewood mortar having a rough inner surface is preferred over the generally smooth working surface of the glass mortar. However, for chemicals that may stain the porcelain or Wedgewood surface, a glass mortar may be preferred. Also, if simple admixture is desired without special need for comminution, the glass mortar is usually preferred, because it cleans more readily after use. When potent substances are to be mixed with a large amount of diluent, the *geometric dilution method* is employed to ensure the uniform distribution of the potent drug. The use of this method is especially indicated in instances in which the potent and the nonpotent substances are of the same color and a visible sign of thorough mixing is lacking. By this method, the potent drug is placed upon an approximately equal volume of the diluent in a mortar and the mixture is thoroughly mixed by trituration. Then a second portion of diluent equal in volume to the powder mixture in the mortar is added, and the trituration is repeated. This process is continued by adding equal volumes of diluent to that powder present in the mortar and repeating the mixing until all of the diluent is incorporated.

Powders may also be mixed by passing them through sifters like the type used in the kitchen to sift flour. This process of *sifting* generally results in a light fluffy product. This process is not acceptable for the incorporation of potent drugs into a diluent base.

Another method of mixing powders is *tumbling* the powder enclosed in a large container which rotates generally by a motorized process. Special *powder blenders* have been devised and mix powders by a tumbling motion (Fig. 5–2). Mixing by this process is thorough, although time-consuming. Such blenders are widely employed in industry, as are large volume powder mixers with motorized blades to blend the powder contained in a large mixing vessel.

Use and Packaging of Powders

Depending upon their intended use, powders are packaged and dispensed by pharmacists in two main ways, as *bulk powders* or as *divided powders.* Nowadays, powders are generally supplied pre-packaged by the manufacturer to the community pharmacist for dispensing.

BULK POWDERS. Among the bulk powders commonly dispensed are (a) antacid and laxative powders, which the patient generally takes by mixing the directed amount of powder (usually a teaspoon or so) in a portion of water or other beverage and swallowing; (b) douche powders, generally dissolved in warm water by the patient for vaginal use; (c) medicated or nonmedicated

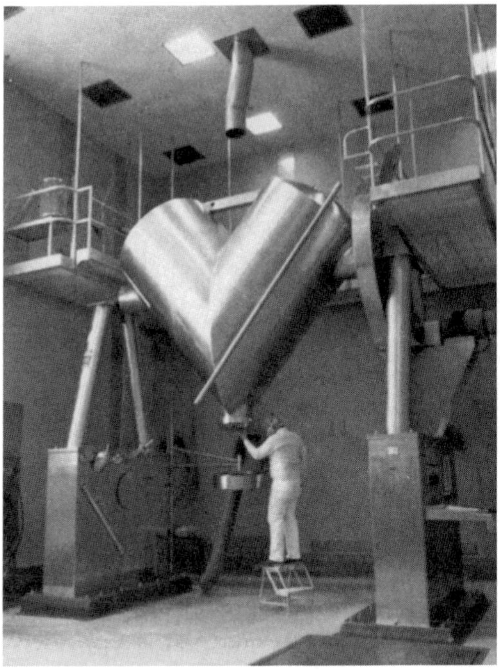

Fig. 5–2. *Industrial size solid state processor or "twin shell" blender used to mix solid particles. (Courtesy of Abbott Laboratories.)*

powders for external application, usually dispensed in sifter cans for convenient application to the skin; (d) dentifrices or dental cleansing powders, used in dental hygiene; (e) denture powders, some used as dentifrices and others as adhesives to hold the dentures in place; and (f) Brewer's Yeast powder containing B-complex vitamins.

Depending upon the intended use of the powder, it may be supplied to the patient in a perforated or sifter-type can or container for external dusting, in an aerosol container for spraying onto the skin, or in a wide-mouthed glass or plastic jar which permits the entrance of a spoon and the easy removal of a spoonful of powder. All powders should be stored in tightly closed containers.

Dispensing powdered drugs in bulk amounts is limited to nonpotent substances. Powders containing potent substances or those that should be administered in controlled dosage are supplied to the patient in divided amounts. Powders supplied to the patient in either bulk or in divided portions that are intended for external use should bear an EXTERNAL USE ONLY or a similar label.

DIVIDED POWDERS. (Latin, *chartulae* (pl.); abbrev: *charts.*) After the powder has been properly mixed (using the geometric dilution method for potent substances), it may be divided into individual units based upon the dose to be administered or the amount to be used at a single time. Each divided portion of powder may be placed on a small piece of paper, which is then folded so as to enclose the medication. Today's community pharmacist infrequently prepares divided powders, although a number of commercially prepared products are available as such, including headache powders, powdered laxatives, and douche powders. The reader is referred to Chapter 14 for a discussion of the preparation of divided powders.

Examples of Official Powders

The following powders have been recently made official in the USP/NF:

Ampicillin Soluble Powder, USP. A dry mixture of the ampicillin and diluents and stabilizing agents used as an anti-infective in veterinary medicine.

Polymyxin B Sulfate and Bacitracin Zinc Topical Powder, USP. Used as a topical anti-infective.

Compound Clioquinol Powder, USP. A mixture of clioquinol, lactic acid, zinc stearate, and lactose, used by vaginal insufflation as an antitrichomonal.

Nystatin Topical Powder, USP. Employed as a topical dusting powder in the treatment of mycotic infections.

Tolnaftate Powder, USP. Used topically in the treatment of fungal infections.

Granules

As indicated previously, granules are prepared agglomerates of smaller particles. They are generally irregularly shaped and behave as single larger particles. They are usually in the 4- to 12-sieve size range although granules of various mesh sizes may be prepared depending upon their application.

Generally, granules are prepared by moistening the desired powder or blended powder mixture and passing the moistened mass through a screen of the mesh size that will produce the desired size granules. The larger particles thus formed are then dried by air or under heat (as the nature of the drug will allow), while they are occasionally moved about on the drying trays to prevent the adhesion of the granules. Granules may also be prepared without the use of moisture by passing compressed masses of powdered material through a granulating machine.

Granules flow well compared to powders. For the purpose of comparison, consider the pouring characteristics of granulated sugar and powdered sugar. Because of their flow properties, granulations are usually made when powder mixtures are intended to be compressed into tablets. The flow characteristics allow the material to flow freely from the hopper or feeding container into the tableting presses. This will be discussed later in this chapter in greater detail.

Granules are generally more stable physically and chemically than are the corresponding powders from which they were prepared. Granules are less likely to cake or harden upon standing than are powders. Because their surface area is less than a comparable volume of powders, granules are usually more stable to the effects of the atmosphere. Because granules are more easily "wetted" by a solvent than are certain powders which tend to float on the solvent's surface, granules are frequently preferred for the making of solutions.

A number of commercial products containing antibiotic drugs which are unstable in aqueous solution are prepared as granules for reconstitution by the pharmacist with purified water just prior to dispensing [e.g. Principen® (ampicillin) for Oral Suspension (Squibb)]. The granules are prepared to contain not only the medicinal agent, but the colorants, flavorants, and other pharmaceutic ingredients. Upon reconstitution, the resultant liquid (solution or suspension) has all of the desired medicinal and pharmaceutic features of a liquid pharmaceutical.

Other types of granular products are prepared and sold commercially including a number which are packaged in bulk and utilized as laxatives. One example of this type of product is Senokot® Granules (Purdue Frederick), which are cocoa-flavored granules containing standardized senna concentrate. The granules are measured by the teaspoon and usually mixed with water upon administration. Effervescent products as Bromo Seltzer® (Warner Lambert) represent another popular type of granulated product. Granulations of effervescent products may be compressed into tablet form. K-Lyte® (Mead Johnson) is an example of a product of this type. Effervescent granules and tablets are placed in a portion of water and taken as the effervescence subsides. Effervescent granulated salts are discussed more fully below.

Effervescent Granulated Salts

Effervescent salts are granules or coarse to very coarse powders containing a medicinal agent in a dry mixture usually composed of sodium bicarbonate, citric acid, and tartaric acid. When added to water, the acids and base react to liberate carbon dioxide, resulting in effervescence. The resulting carbonated solution masks the usually saline or otherwise undesirable taste of the medicinal agent present. By using granules or coarse particles of the mixed powders rather than the ordinary smaller sized particles of these substances, the rate of solution of the substances is decreased upon addition to water, and the otherwise violent reaction and rapid, uncontrollable effervescence is eliminated. Such violent effervescence would likely overflow the glass of water to which it was added with subsequent loss of solution and little residual carbonation of the solution. The methods for the preparation of effervescent salts appear in Chapter 14.

An example of an effervescent salt is Effervescent Sodium Phosphate. It is used as a cathartic and has a usual dose of 10 g. About 2 teaspoonfuls of the granules are added to a glass of water, and the mixture is swallowed as the effervescence subsides. Each 10 g of the granules contain 2 g of exsiccated sodium phosphate, the usual dose of this agent, which is the active component of the effervescent salt.

A summary of the chemistry of effervescent granules may be found in the accompanying Physical Pharmacy Capsule.

Capsules

Capsules are solid dosage forms in which one or more medicinal and/or inert substances are enclosed within a small shell or container generally prepared from a suitable form of gelatin. Depending upon their formulation, the gelatin capsule shells may be hard or soft. The majority of capsules dispensed are intended to be swallowed whole by the patient for the benefit of the medication contained therein. In certain instances the contents of a capsule may be removed from the gelatin shell and employed as

Effervescent Granules

Granules are dosage forms that consist of particles ranging from about 4 to 10 mesh in size (4.76 mm to 2.00 mm), formed by moistening blended powders and passing through a screen or a special granulator. These moist granules are then either air- or oven-dried. A special form of granules can be used to provide a pleasant vehicle for selected drug products, especially those with either a bitter or salty taste. This special formulation is an "effervescent granule" and may consist of mixtures of citric acid and/or tartaric acid and/or sodium biophosphate combined with sodium bicarbonate.

EXAMPLE

Rx	Active Drug	500 mg/5 g tsp
	in effervescent granule qs	120 g

Sig: Dissolve one teaspoonful in one-half glass of cool water and drink. Repeat every 8 hours.

It is desired to dispense this as a granule, where the patient will measure out a teaspoonful (5 g) dose, mix, and administer. Since each dose weighs 5 g and there will be 120 g of the prescription, there will be 24 doses. Each dose contains 0.5 g, which will be 12 g of active drug for the entire prescription. This results in 120 g − 12 g = 108 g of effervescent vehicle that will be required. A good effervescent blend consists of both citric acid and tartaric acid (1:2 ratio), since the former is rather sticky to manipulate and the latter produces a chalky, friable granule. It then becomes necessary to calculate the amount of each ingredient required to prepare 108 g of the granulation.

Citric Acid

$$3\ NaHCO_3 + C_6H_8O_7.H_2O \rightarrow 4\ H_2O + 3CO_2 + Na_3C_6H_5O_7$$

3 × 84   210

One gram of citric acid (MW = 210) reacts with 1.2 g of sodium bicarbonate (MW = 84) as obtained from the following:

$$\frac{1}{210} = \frac{x}{3 \times 84}$$

$$x = 1.2\ g$$

Tartaric Acid

$$2\ NaHCO_3 + C_4H_6O_6 \rightarrow 2\ H_2O + 2CO_2 + Na_2C_4H_4O_6$$

2 × 84   150

Since it is desired to use a 1:2 ratio of critic acid to tartaric acid, two grams of tartaric acid (MW = 150) reacts with 2.24 g of sodium bicarbonate according to the following calculation:

$$\frac{2}{150} = \frac{x}{2 \times 84}$$

$$x = 2.24\ g$$

From the above, it has been calculated that 1.2 g and 2.24 g of sodium bicarbonate is required to react with 1 + 2 g of the citric:tartaric acid combination. Since it is desired to leave a small amount of the acids unreacted to enhance palatability and taste, 2.24 g + 1.2 g = 3.44 g, only 3.4 g of sodium bicarbonate will be utilized. Therefore, the ratio of the effervescent ingredients is 1:2:3.4 for the citric acid:tartaric acid:sodium bicarbonate. Since the prescription requires 108 g of the effervescent mix, the quantity of each ingredient can be calculated as follows:

$$1 + 2 + 3.4 = 6.4$$

$$1/6.4 \times 108\ g = 16.875\ g \text{ Citric acid}$$
$$2/6.4 \times 108\ g = 33.750\ g \text{ Tartaric acid}$$
$$3.4/6.4 \times 108\ g = 57.375\ g \text{ Sodium bicarbonate}$$
$$\text{Total} = 108\ g$$

The prescription will require 12 g of the active drug and 108 g of this effervescent vehicle.

a premeasured medicinal powder. For example, the product THEO-DUR SPRINKLE® (Key Pharmaceuticals) is recommended for use in the latter manner, for children or other patients unable to swallow a tablet or capsule. It is recommended that the contents of the capsule, anhydrous theophylline in sustained release form, be sprinkled on a small amount of soft food immediately prior to ingestion.

It has become somewhat common practice in hospitals and extended care facilities to open capsules or crush tablets to mix with food or drink for ease of swallowing. This should only be done with the concurrence *of the pharmacist* because the release characteristics of the drug from the dosage form could be dramatically altered. Subsequently, the amount of drug and the rate with which the drug is absorbed *could adversely* affect the patient's welfare. These products generally include: enteric coated dosage forms, designed to pass through the stomach intact for absorption in the intestine; extended release dosage forms, designed to provide extended or prolonged release of the medication; and sublingual or buccal tablets, formulated to dissolve under the tongue or in the oral cavity. In many instances, if a patient is unable to swallow a solid dosage form, an alternative product, as an oral liquid, suppository or injection may be employed.

Hard Gelatin Capsules

Hard gelatin capsules are the type used by pharmaceutical manufacturers in the preparation of the majority of their capsule products and by the community pharmacist in the extemporaneous compounding of prescriptions. The basic empty capsule shells are made from a mixture of gelatin, sugar, and water and are clear, colorless, and essentially tasteless. Gelatin, NF, is a product obtained by the partial hydrolysis of collagen obtained from the skin, white connective tissue, and bones of animals. It is found in commerce in the form of a fine powder, a coarse powder, shreds, flakes, or sheets (Fig. 5–3).

Gelatin is stable in air when dry but is subject to microbic decomposition when it becomes moist or when it is maintained in aqueous solution. For this reason, soft gelatin capsules, which contain more moisture than the hard capsules, may be prepared with a preservative agent added to prevent the growth of fungi in the capsule shells. Normally, hard gelatin capsules contain between 13 and 16% of moisture.[9] However, if stored in an environment of high humidity, additional moisture is absorbed by the capsules, and they may become distorted and lose their rigid shape. On the other hand, in an environment of extreme dryness, some of the moisture normally present in the gelatin capsules may be lost, and the capsules may become brittle and may crumble when handled.

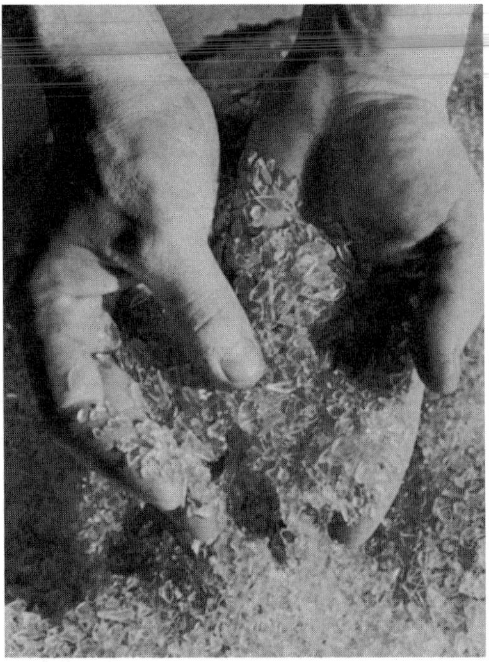

Fig. 5–3. *Pork skin gelatin used as raw material in the manufacture of gelatin capsules. (Courtesy of SmithKline Beecham.)*

Because moisture may be absorbed or released by gelatin capsules, depending upon the environmental conditions, it follows that little physical protection is afforded hygroscopic or deliquescent materials enclosed within a capsule when stored in an area of high humidity. It is not unusual to find capsules of such moisture-affected materials packaged in containers along with a packet of a desiccant material as a precaution against the capsules absorbing atmospheric moisture. With or without such desiccant materials, capsules should be generally stored in areas of low humidity.

Although gelatin is insoluble in cold water, it does soften through the absorption of up to ten times its weight of the water. Some patients prefer to swallow a capsule wetted with water or saliva, because the capsule softens and slides down the throat more readily than does a dry capsule. Gelatin is soluble in hot water, and in warm gastric fluid a gelatin capsule rapidly releases its contents. Gelatin, being a protein, is digested and absorbed.

Hard gelatin capsule shells are manufactured in two sections, the capsule body and a shorter cap. The two parts overlap when joined, with the cap fitting snugly over the open end of the capsule body. The shells are produced by the mechanical dipping of pins or pegs of the desired shape and diameter into a reservoir of the melted gelatin mixture, maintained at a constant temperature to achieve the desired degree of fluidity. The pegs, made of manganese bronze, are affixed to plates, each capable of holding up to about 500 pegs. Each plate is mechanically lowered to the gelatin bath, the pegs being submerged to the desired depth and for the desired period of time to achieve the proper length and thickness of coating. Then the plate and the pegs are slowly lifted from the gelatin bath, and the gelatin on the pegs is gently dried by a flow of temperature and humidity controlled air (see Figs. 5–4 and 5–5A). When dried, each capsule part is trimmed mechanically to the proper length and removed from the pegs, and the capsule bodies and caps are joined together. It is important that the thickness of the gelatin walls be strictly controlled so that the capsule body and cap fit snugly to prevent disengagement. Naturally, the pegs on which the caps are formed are slightly larger in diameter than the pegs on which the bodies are formed, since the caps overlap the bodies. In production, there is a continuous dipping, drying, removing, and joining of capsules as many peg-containing plates are rotated in and out of the gelatin bath.

Several methods of making capsules distinctive are available to the pharmaceutical manufacturer. One way is to color the gelatin used in the preparation of the capsules. Colorants may be used to prepare capsule bodies and caps having the same or different colors. By combining the various capsule parts, beautiful, transparent, and distinctive capsules may be prepared.

Opaque capsules may also be prepared to make a pharmaceutical product distinctive. These capsules are formed by adding an insoluble substance such as titanium dioxide to the gelatin mixture. Colored, opaque capsules may be prepared by using both a colorant and the opaque-producing substance.

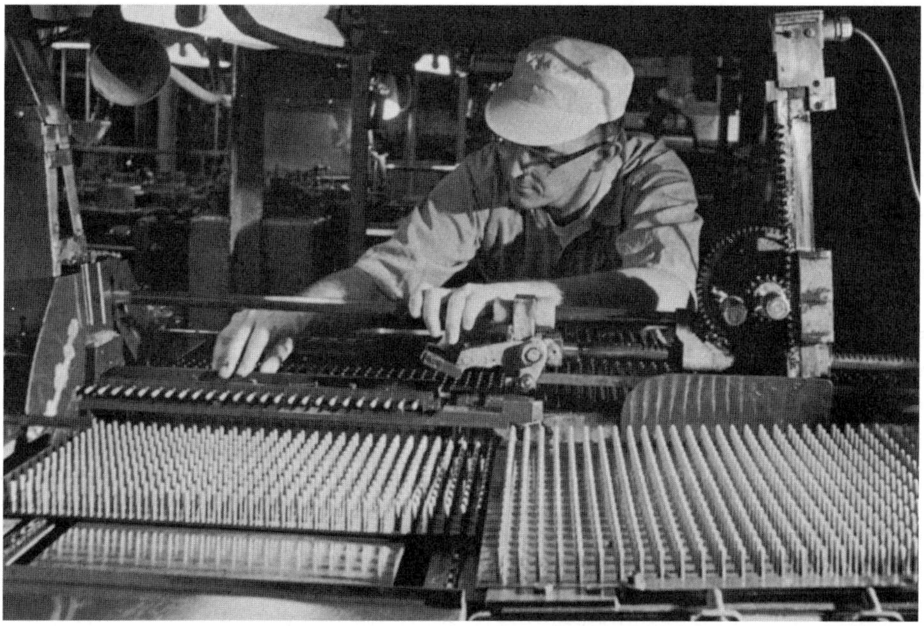

Fig. 5–4. *Body of capsules and their caps are shown as they move through automated capsule-making machine. Each machine is capable of producing 30,000 capsules per hour. It takes a 40-minute cycle to produce a capsule. (Courtesy of SmithKline Beecham.)*

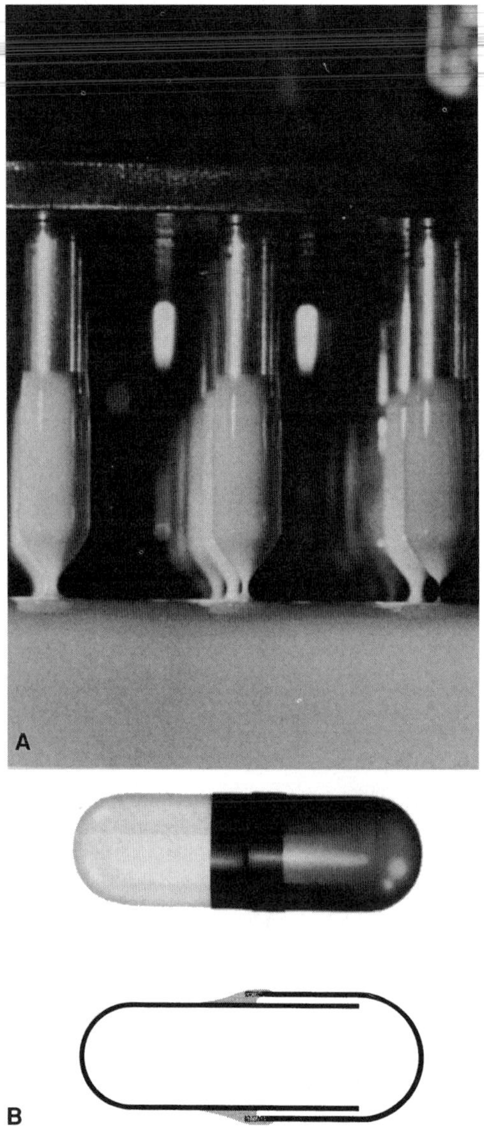

Fig. 5–5. *A, Capsules being dipped for coloring on automated capsule-making equipment. (Courtesy of SmithKline Beecham.) B, Z-Weld's gelatin seal fuses the two capsule halves together to create a one-piece capsule that is tamper-evident. (Courtesy of Raymond Automation Co.)*

A manufacturer may also alter the usually rounded shape of the capsule-making pegs to produce capsule shells of distinctive shapes. By tapering the end of the body-producing peg while leaving the cap-making peg rounded, one manufacturer prepares capsules easily differentiated from those of other manufacturers (Pulvules, Eli Lilly). Another firm produces capsules with the ends of both the bodies and caps highly tapered, but not pointed (Spansule Capsules, Smith, Kline & French). Still another manufacturer makes distinctive and tamper-proof and leakproof capsules by sealing the joint between the two capsule parts with a colored band of gelatin (Kapseals, Parke-Davis). Removal of the band through tampering is evident, as the bands cannot be returned to place without a great deal of trouble and resealing with gelatin. Figure 5–5B depicts a gelatin seal for capsules.

A recent innovation in capsule shell design is the Snap-Fit™, Coni-Snap™, and Coni Snap Supro™ hard gelatin capsules, depicted in Figures 5–6 and 5–7. The original Snap-Fit construction enables the two halves of the capsule shells to be positively joined through locking grooves in the shell walls. The two grooves fit into each other and thus ensure reliable closing of the filled capsule. During the closing process, the capsule body is inserted into the cap. With the high-capacity filling rates of the modern capsule filling

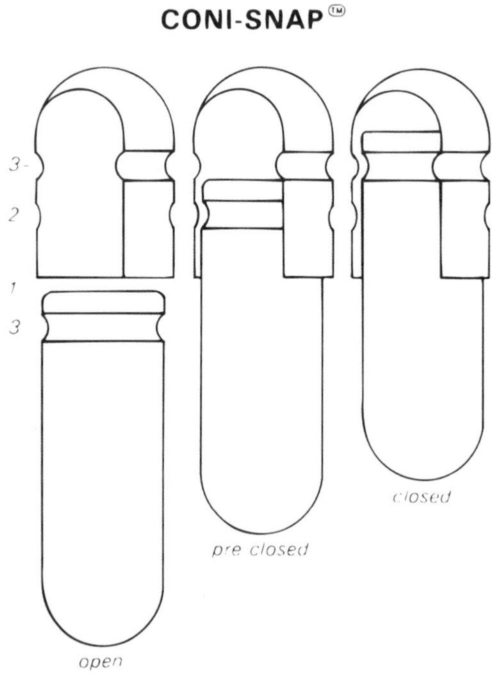

Fig. 5–6. *Line drawings of the CONI-SNAP™ capsule in open, pre-closed, and closed positions. The tapered rims (1) avoid telescoping, the indentations (2) prevent premature opening, and the grooves (3) lock the two capsule parts together after the capsule has been filled. (Courtesy of Capsugel Division, Warner-Lambert Co.)*

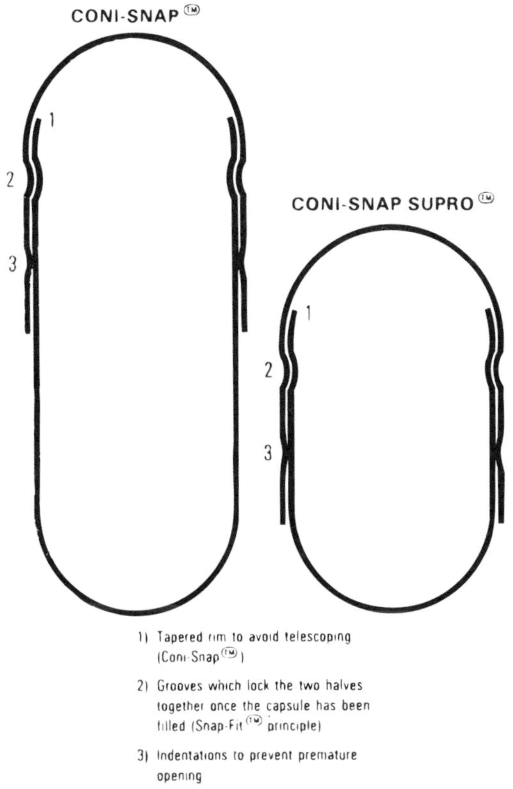
CONI-SNAP(TM)
CONI-SNAP SUPRO(TM)
1
2
3
1) Tapered rim to avoid telescoping (Coni-Snap(TM))
2) Grooves which lock the two halves together once the capsule has been filled (Snap-Fit(TM) principle)
3) Indentations to prevent premature opening

Fig. 5–7. *Line drawings of the CONI-SNAP™ and CONI-SNAP SUPRO™ (on right) capsules. The latter is designed to be smaller and to have the lower portion of the capsule shell concealed except for the rounded end. This makes separation of the two parts more difficult and contributes to capsule integrity. (Courtesy of Capsugel Division, Warner-Lambert Co.)*

machines (over 180,000 capsules per hour), capsule splitting ("telescoping") and/or denting of the capsule shell occurs with the slightest contact between the two capsule-part rims when they are joined. This problem, which exists primarily with straight-walled capsule shells, led to the development of the Coni-Snap capsule, in which the rim of the capsule body is not straight, but tapered slightly (see Fig. 5–7). This reduces the risk of the capsule-rims touching on joining, and essentially eliminates the problem of splitting. In the Coni-Snap Supro capsules, the upper capsule part extends so far over the lower part that only the rounded edge of the latter is visible (Fig. 5–7). Opening of such a filled capsule is difficult because the lower surface offers less gripping surface to pull the two halves apart. This increases the security of the contents and the integrity of

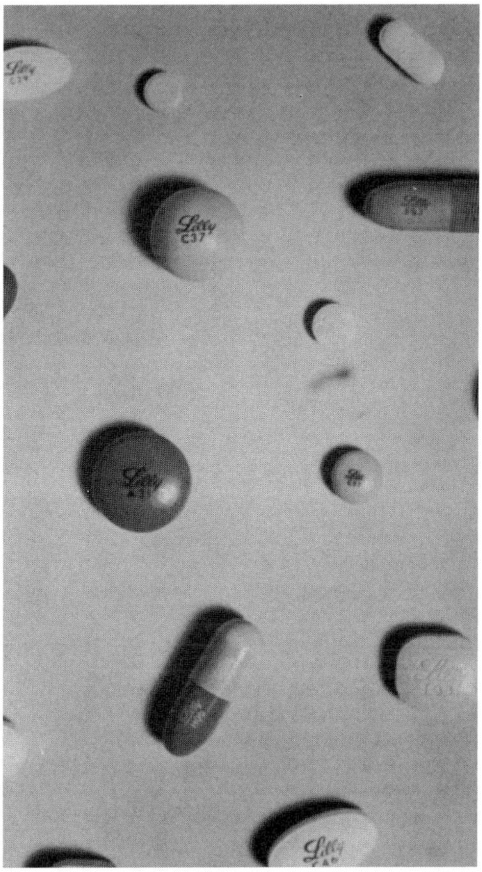

Fig. 5–8. *Examples of tablets and capsules marked with a letter-number code to facilitate identification. (Courtesy of Eli Lilly and Company.)*

the capsule. Capsules may be imprinted with monograms of the manufacturer, the strength of the drug in the capsule, a code designation for product identification, or some other symbol making the product unique and distinguishable from other manufacturers' products (see Fig. 5–8).

Capsule Sizes

Empty gelatin capsules are manufactured in various sizes, varying in length, in diameter, and capacity. The size selected for use is determined by the amount of material to be encapsulated. Since the density and compressibility of a powder or a powder mixture will largely determine to what extent it may be packed into a capsule shell and because these are individual features of the materials themselves, there are no strict rules for predicting the proper capsule size for

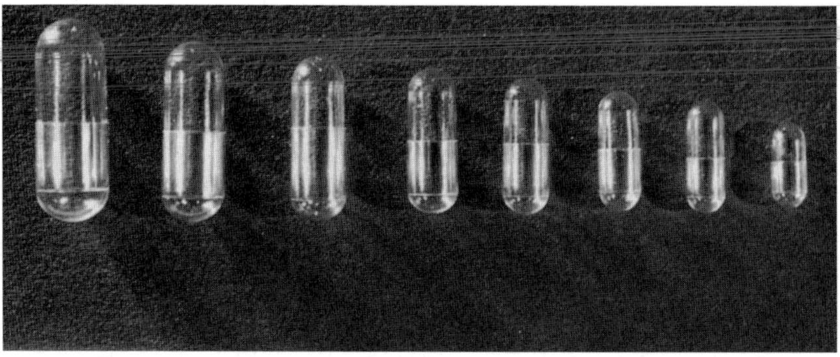

Fig. 5–9. *Actual sizes of hard gelatin capsules. From left to right, sizes 000, 00, 0, 1, 2, 3, 4, and 5.*

a given powder or formulation. However, comparison may be made with powders of well-known features (Table 5–2), and an initial judgment made as to the approximate capsule size to hold a specific amount of material, but the final decision is largely the result of trial. For human use, empty capsules ranging in size from 000, the largest, to 5, the smallest are commercially available, plain or colored (Fig. 5–9). Larger capsules are available for veterinary use.

Hard gelatin capsules permit a wide prescribing latitude by the physician in that the pharmacist may extemporaneously prepare capsules containing a single chemical substance or a combination of drugs at the precise dosage level considered appropriate for the individual patient. This degree of flexibility is an advantage that capsules have as a dosage form over tablets, which are not prepared today in the community pharmacy.

Preparation of Filled Hard Gelatin Capsules

The preparation of filled hard gelatin capsules may be divided into the following steps:

1. Developing and preparing the formulation and selecting the size capsule.
2. Filling the capsule shells.
3. Cleaning and polishing the filled capsules.

Capsule Formulation and Selection of Capsule Size

In developing a capsule formulation, the goal is to prepare a formulation that results in accurate dosage, good bioavailability characteristics, and ease of capsule filling during production.

In dry formulations, the active and inactive components must be blended thoroughly to assure a uniform powder mix for the capsule fill. Preformulation studies are used to determine if the bulk powders may be blended together as such, or if they require reduction of particle size or processing into formed granules.

To achieve uniform drug distribution throughout a powder mix, it is advantageous if the density and particle size of the drug and nondrug components are similar. This is particularly important when a drug of low dosage is blended into a powder mixture.[2] When necessary, particle size may be reduced by *milling*. This is the most common means of reducing particle size and results in particles ranging from about 50 to 1000 micrometers (μm), depending upon the equipment used. Milled powders may be blended effectively for uniform distribution throughout a powder mix when the drug's dosage is 10 mg or greater.[2] For drugs of lower dose or when smaller particles are required, *micronization* is employed. Depending upon the materials and equipment used, micronization produces particles ranging from about 1 to 20 micrometers.

In preparing capsules on an industrial scale using high-speed automated equipment, the powder mix or granules must be free-flowing to allow steady passage of the capsule fill from the hopper, through the encapsulating equipment, and into the capsule shells. The addition of a *glidant* such as fumed silicon dioxide (less than 1%) to the powder mix enhances flow properties.[9]

Generally, hard gelatin capsules are used to encapsulate between about 65 mg and 1 g of powdered material, including drug and any diluent required. As indicated in Table 5–2, the smallest capsule, a No. 5 capsule, is usually capable of holding at least 1 gr or 65 mg of powders

Table 5–2. Approximate Capacity of Empty Gelatin Capsules*

	Capsule Size								
Drug Substance	*000*	*00*	*0*	*1*	*2*	*3*	*4*	*5*	
Quinine Sulfate	650	390	325	227	195	130	97	65	mg
	10	6	5	3½	3	2	1½	1	grains
Sodium Bicarbonate	1430	975	715	510	390	325	260	130	mg
	22	15	11	8	6	5	4	2	grains
Aspirin	1040	650	520	325	260	195	162	97	mg
	16	10	8	5	4	3	2½	1½	grains

* Amount may vary according to the degree of pressure used in filling the capsules.

of the type used in medicine. In order to fill completely a capsule of even the smallest size, a minimum of 65 mg of material is generally required. If the dose of the drug or the amount of drug to be placed in a single capsule is inadequate to fill the volume of the capsule, a diluent is necessary to add the proper degree of bulk to produce the proper fill. When the amount of drug to be administered in a single capsule is large enough to fill a capsule completely, a diluent may not be required. Lactose, microcrystalline cellulose, and pregelatinized starch are common diluents used in capsule filling. In addition to providing bulk, diluents also provide cohesion to the powders, which is beneficial in the transfer of measured portions of the powder blend into capsule shells.[9]

In many instances the amount of drug placed in a single capsule falls within the usual dosage range of that drug, a single capsule being taken as a dose of that particular medication. In other instances, especially when the amount of drug representing a usual dose is too large to place in a single capsule, two or more capsules may be required to provide the desired dose of that particular drug. For many medicinal agents, the initial or first dose may be larger than the subsequent doses, in which case more capsules may be required when drug therapy is initiated than when it is continued. In all instances, the amount of drug to be present in a single capsule is first determined, and the amount of diluent or inert materials, if any, is determined subsequently on the basis of its being needed to add bulk to the formulation, to separate chemically incompatible components of the formulation, or as a lubricant to facilitate the flow of the powder when an automatic capsule filling machine is utilized.

Magnesium stearate is a commonly used lubricant in capsule and tablet making to prevent adhesion and facilitate the flow of the drug-fill into the tableting or encapsulating machinery. Although small amounts of magnesium stearate are generally used (frequently less than 1%), the water-proofing characteristics of this insoluble material can pose a problem to the penetration of the solid dosage form by the gastrointestinal fluids intended to dissolve it. This obstacle to water and fluid penetration can delay the dissolution of the drug and its absorption. The practice of adding surfactants or wetting agents, as sodium lauryl sulfate, in capsule and tablet formulations to facilitate the wetting of the drug substance by the bathing of gastrointestinal fluids is a widely followed procedure in industry. The advantage of adding a wetting agent to capsule formulations of lithium carbonate to enhance dissolution has been demonstrated.[10] Even in instances in which magnesium stearate or some other water-insoluble lubricant is not used in capsule formulation, when the gelatin shell of a capsule dissolves, liquid must displace the air that surrounds the dry powder within the capsule and penetrate the drug before the capsule fill can be dispersed and dissolved. Powders of poorly soluble drugs have a tendency to float on the surface of the fluid and agglomerate to further minimize air-liquid contact and if wetting does not occur readily, dissolution is delayed.

Whether it be the presence of a lubricant, surfactant, or some other pharmaceutic excipient, formulation can influence the bioavailability of a drug substance and can account for differences in drug effects which may be encountered between two capsule products of the same medicinal substance.

Eutectic mixtures of drugs, or mixtures that tend to liquefy, may require a diluent or absorbant such as magnesium carbonate, kaolin, or light magnesium oxide to separate physically the interacting agents and to absorb any liquefied material. Generally, when such materials are used for this purpose, approximately 120 mg of diluent are used for each capsule. Drugs that are chemically incompatible with other drugs of the formulation may be physically separated by the same means. Another method for separating drugs within a capsule is to place one of the interfering substances in a small capsule that is then placed within a larger capsule containing the other formulative components. Instead of the smaller capsule, granules, pellets, or compressed tablets may be used for this purpose.

The use of tablets within capsules is also quite common in the extemporaneous filling of a small number of capsules, each to contain a very small quantity of a potent drug. In these instances, many pharmacists insert a small tablet of the desired strength of the potent drug in each capsule, filling the remaining capsule space with the specified amounts of other required less potent and more conveniently weighed drugs and/or with an inert diluent as is necessary.

Capsules of gelatin are unsuitable for the encapsulation of aqueous liquids, because water softens the gelatin to produce distortion of the capsules. Naturally, this would prompt the loss of the liquid contents of the capsules. However, some liquids such as fixed or volatile oils that do not interfere with the stability of the gelatin shells may be placed in gelatin capsules which then may be sealed to ensure the retention of the liquid. In large scale production, liquids are placed in *soft gelatin* capsules which are sealed during their manufacture. Soft capsules are discussed later in this chapter.

Rather than placing a liquid in a capsule as such, it may be desirable in certain instances to absorb a small amount of liquid by mixing it with an absorbent, inert powder. The powder may then be placed in capsules in the usual manner. If the liquid is volatile, it may be necessary to seal the capsules.

AMOUNT OF FORMULA PREPARED. On a small or large industrial scale, the amount of formula prepared is that amount (drugs and diluents) necessary to fill the desired number of capsules. On an industrial scale this may mean many thousands of capsules. In the community pharmacy an individual prescription may call for the extemporaneous preparation of only six or a dozen capsules. Any slight loss in fill material during the preparation of the (powder) mixture or during the capsule-filling process will not materially affect the preparation of an industrial batch, but on a small scale, as in the filling of a prescription, a slight loss of fill material will likely result in an adequate amount of powder for the last capsule. To ensure enough fill for the last capsule in the extemporaneous compounding of small numbers of capsules, the community pharmacist generally calculates for the preparation of one more capsule than is required. This procedure may not be followed for capsules containing a controlled substance, because the amount of drug used and that called for in the prescription must strictly coincide.

SELECTION OF CAPSULE SIZE. The selection of the capsule size is best done during the development of the formulation, because the amount of any inert materials to be employed is dependent upon the size or capacity of the capsule to be selected. When the formulation of medicinal materials does not require diluent to increase the bulk, the capsule size may be selected after the development and preparation of the formulation. As indicated earlier, for drugs having large doses the amount of medication in a capsule may not necessarily correspond to a full dose of that medication. Smaller capsules may be required in instances in which the drug is to be taken by youngsters or by elderly patients, and more than a single capsule may be required to provide the dose of the drug. In instances in which there is a specific need for a small capsule, the capsule size may be selected first, and the formulation may be based on that capsule size. Depending upon the particular situation and requirements of the intended patient, the capsule size may be determined by the formulation, or the formulation may be altered by the capsule size.

A properly filled capsule should have its body filled with the drug mixture and its cap fully extended down the body so as to enclose the powder in the body. The cap is not used to hold powder but to retain it, and a capsule size should be selected to meet this requirement.

Filling the Capsule Shells

When filling a small number of capsules in the pharmacy, the pharmacist generally uses the "punch" method. In this method the pharmacist takes the precise number of empty capsules to be filled from his stock container. By counting out the capsules as the initial step rather than taking a capsule from stock as each one is filled, the pharmacist guards against filling an erroneous number of capsules and avoids contaminating the stock container of empty capsules with drug particles that may cling to his fingertips. The powder to be encapsulated is placed on a sheet of clean paper or a glass or porcelain plate and with a spatula is formed into a cake having a depth of approximately one-fourth to one-third the length of the capsule body. Then the empty capsule body is held between the thumb and forefinger and "punched" vertically into the powder cake repeatedly until filled. Some pharmacists wear surgical gloves or rubber finger cots to avoid handling the capsules with bare fingers. Because the amount of powder packed into a capsule depends upon the degree of compression, the pharmacist should punch each capsule in the same manner and after capping weigh it to ensure equal and accurate filling. When nonpotent materials are being placed in capsules, the first filled capsule should be weighed (using an empty capsule of the same size on the opposite balance pan to counter the weight of the shell) to assist in the determination of the proper capsule size and degree of compression to be used in filling, and then other capsules should be weighed periodically to check the uniformity of this operation. When potent drugs are being used, each capsule should be weighed after filling to ensure accuracy. Such weighings protect against the uneven filling of capsules and the premature exhaustion or lack of total utilization of the powder mixture. After the body of a capsule has been filled and the cap has been placed on the body, the body is squeezed gently to distribute some powder to the cap end of the capsule to give the product a full appearance. Some pharmacists place a small portion of powder in the cap before placing it on the body. Care must be exercised not to overfill a capsule. The cap should fit completely down on the body.

Granular material that does not lend itself well to the "punch" method of filling capsules may be poured into each capsule individually from the powder paper on which it was first weighed.

Pharmacists that prepare capsules on a regular or somewhat extensive basis may use hand-operated capsule machines. These machines are available in capacities of 24, 96, 100, and 144 capsules. When efficiently operated, they can produce from about 2000 capsules per working day for the smallest machine up to 2000 capsules per hour for the largest (Fig. 5–10).

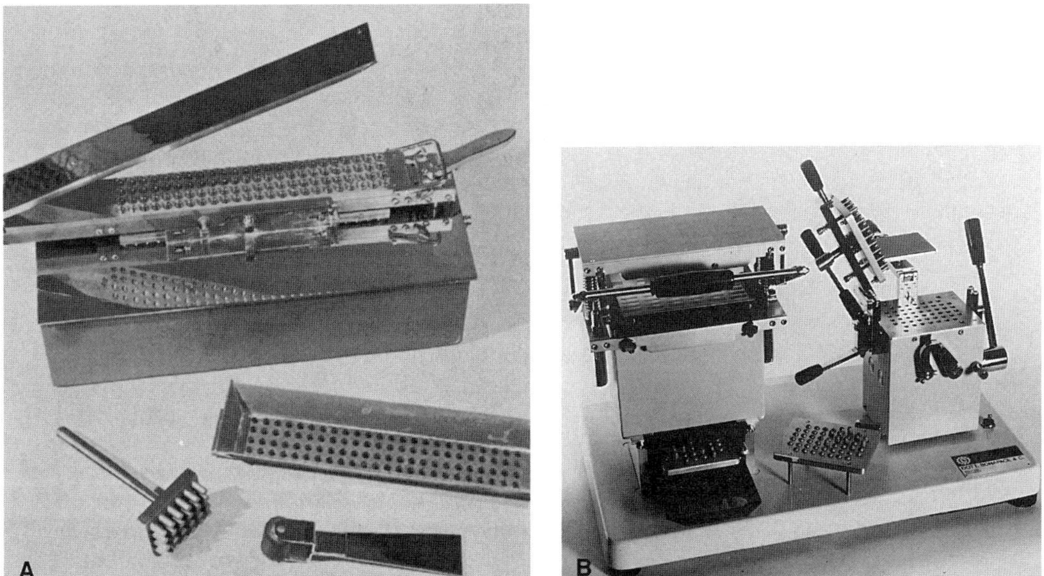

Fig. 5–10. *A, Hand-operated capsule-filling machine. The model shown fills 96 capsules per operation and is made to obtain an hourly production of 1000 capsules. Shown with the basic machine are the tray used to hold the fill over the empty capsules, the spreader and roller used to distribute the fill material in the tray and permit it to enter the capsules uniformly, and the packer used to compact the fill in the capsules. B, A capsule-filling system capable of filling 2000 capsules per hour. Useful for clinical drug trial lots and small scale production. (Courtesy of Scientific Instruments and Technology Corporation.)*

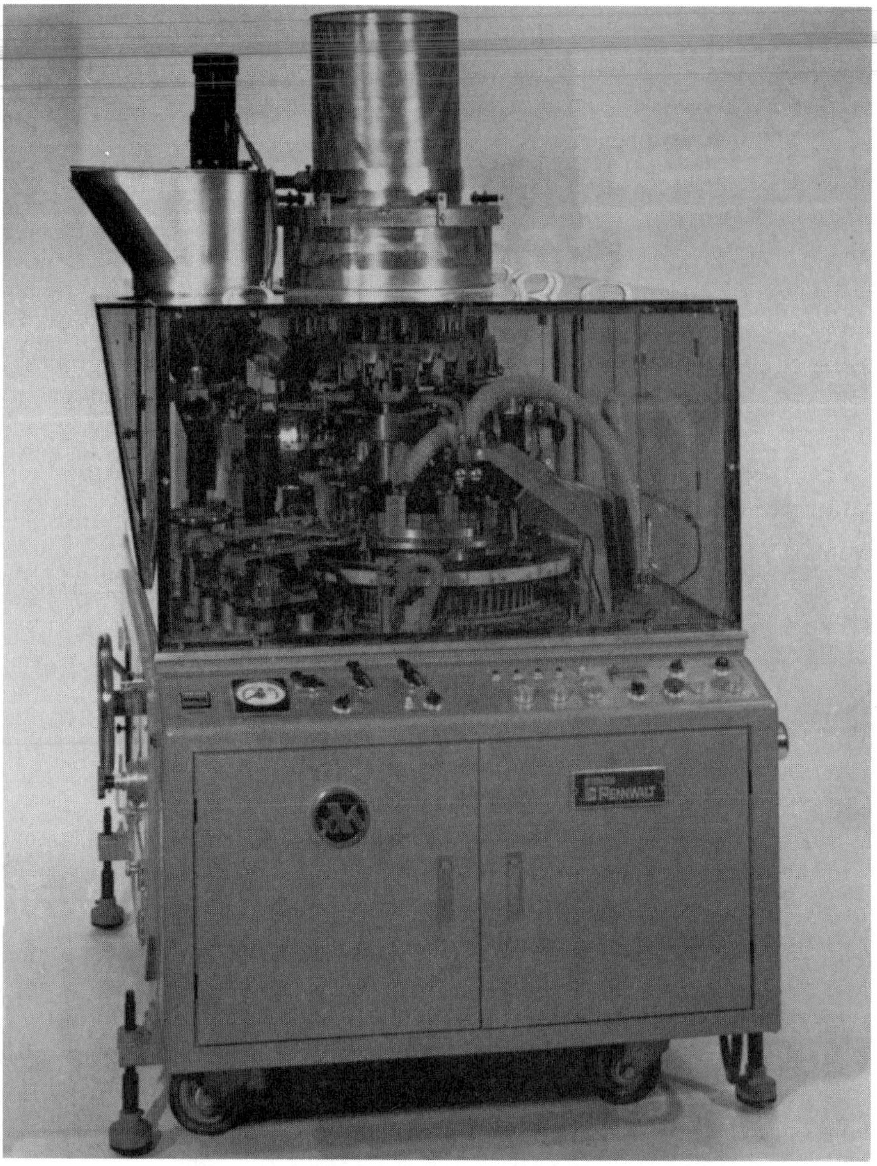

Fig. 5–11. *Osaka Automatic Capsule Filler (Model R-180), capable of filling up to 165,000 capsules per hour. (Courtesy of Sharples-Stokes Div., Stokes-Merrill, Pennwalt Corporation.)*

Machines developed for industrial use can automatically remove the caps from empty capsules, fill the capsules, replace the caps, and clean the outside of the capsules at a rate of up to 165,000 capsules and greater per hour per unit (Fig. 5–11). Most industrial capsule-filling machines are designed to automatically fill the body of the empty capsule with powder and scrape off the excess at the level of fill before capping. Therefore the formulation for each industrially produced capsule must be such that the filled body contains the amount of powder in which the right amount of drug and diluent are present. This may be accomplished with automated equipment (Fig. 5–12) or by taking periodic samples during production and weighing them for total content. Figure 5–13 depicts a process flow diagram for automated capsule filling in which

Fig. 5–12. *Automatic capsule weighing apparatus, Vericap 1800 A Checkweigher, which rejects capsules not having the precise weight. (Courtesy of Elan Corporation)*

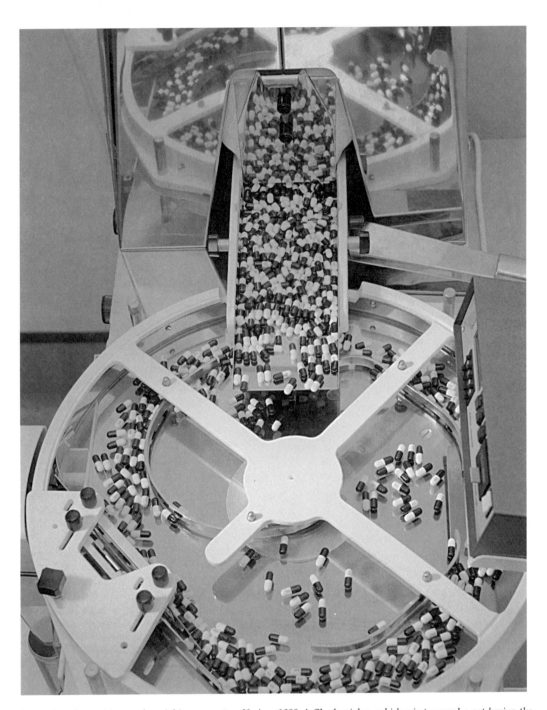

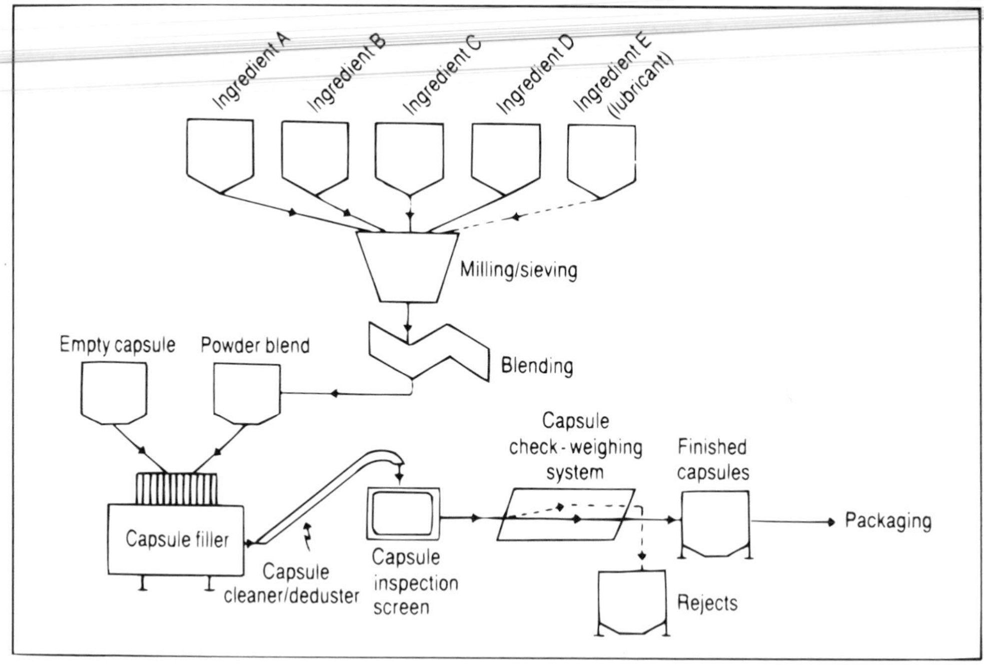

Fig. 5–13. *Process flow diagram for automated capsule filling. (From Yelvig, M.: Principles of process automation for liquid and solid dosage forms. Pharm. Technol., 8:47, 1984.)*

a number of components are blended and placed in capsules.

The USP requires adherence to standards for *content uniformity* and *weight variation* to assure the uniformity of dosage units. These tests are described in the USP23-NF18.[11]

Capsule Sealing

The capsule-tampering incidents of 1982 (refer to p. 142) rekindled industry interest in both tamper-resistant packaging and the protective sealing of capsules, particularly for over-the-counter products. The capsule-sealing process of *banding* (e.g., Kapseals, Parke-Davis; Quali-caps, Elanco) has been utilized for a number of years. In this process, the two capsule parts are sealed with a gelatin or polymer band at the seam of the cap and body. More recently, a tamper-resistant seal on hard gelatin capsules was developed in which the contact areas of the cap and body are wetted with a mixture of water and ethanol and then thermally bonded at 104° to 113°F.[12] Any attempts at the separation of a sealed capsule will result in the capsule's destruction, making tampering evident. Capsule-sealing equipment may be linked with capsule-filling equipment to maintain production levels of up to 150,000 capsules per hour per unit.

Cleaning and Polishing Capsules

Capsules prepared on a small scale or on a large scale may have small amounts of the powder formulation adhering to the outside of the capsules. This powder, which may be bitter or otherwise unpalatable, should be removed before packaging or dispensing to improve the appearance of the capsules and to preserve their quality of being tasteless on administration. On a small scale, capsules may be cleaned individually or in small numbers by rubbing them with a clean gauze or cloth. On a large scale, many capsule-filling machines are affixed with a cleaning vacuum that removes any extraneous material from the capsules as they exit the equipment. Figure 5–14 shows an industrial method of cleaning and polishing hard filled capsules using the Accela-Cota apparatus.

Soft Gelatin Capsules

Soft gelatin capsules are prepared from shells of gelatin to which glycerin or a polyhydric alco-

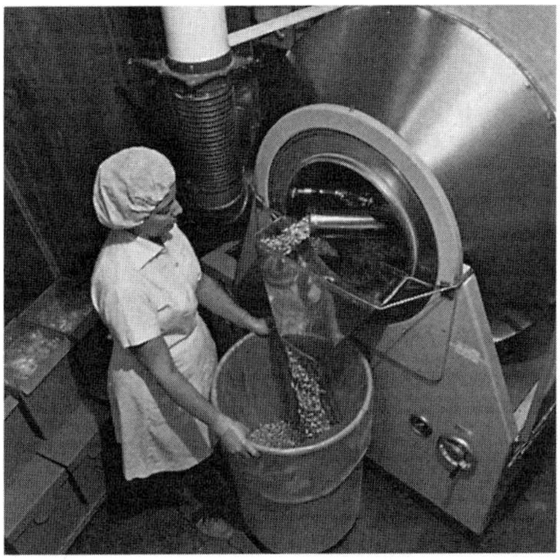

Fig. 5–14. *Cleaning and polishing hard filled capsules using the Accela-Cota apparatus. (Courtesy of Eli Lilly and Company.)*

hol such as sorbitol has been added to render the gelatin elastic or plastic-like. These capsules, which may be oblong, elliptical, or spherical in shape, may be employed to contain liquids, suspensions, pasty materials, or dry powders. Soft gelatin capsules are usually prepared, filled, and sealed in a continuous operation using specialized equipment. Empty soft gelatin capsules may be prepared and hermetically sealed (to prevent the walls from collapsing and adhering to one another) for filling at a later time, but this is not usually performed.

Soft gelatin capsules are useful when it is desirable to seal the medication within the capsule. The capsules are especially important to contain liquid drugs or drug solutions. Also, volatile drug substances or drug materials especially susceptible to deterioration in the presence of air may be better suited to a soft gelatin capsule than to the hard gelatin capsules.

Soft gelatin capsules are handsome and are easily swallowed by the patient. However, they are not easily prepared except on a large scale and then only with specialized equipment (Fig. 5–15).

Preparation of Soft Gelatin Capsules

Soft gelatin capsules may be prepared by the plate process, using a set of molds to form the capsules, or by the more efficient and productive die processes (rotary or reciprocating). By the plate process, a warm sheet of gelatin (plain or colored) is placed on the bottom plate of the mold, and the liquid medication is evenly poured on it. Then a second sheet of the prepared gelatin is carefully laid in place on top of the medication, and the top plate of the mold is put in place. The entire mold is then subjected to a press where pressure is applied to form, fill, and seal the capsules simultaneously. The capsules are then removed and washed with a solvent harmless to the capsules. Highly automated machines have been developed for the preparation of soft capsules by the plate process and are in use today in industry.

However, most industrially produced soft capsules are probably prepared by the rotary die process, a method developed in 1933 by Robert P. Scherer. By this method, liquid gelatin flowing from an overhead tank is formed into two continuous ribbons by the rotary die machine and brought together between twin rotating dies (Fig. 5–16). At the same time, metered fill material is injected between the ribbons precisely at the moment that the dies form pockets of the gelatin ribbons. These pockets of fill-containing gelatin are then sealed by pressure and heat, the capsules then being severed from the ribbon by the same process. The soft gelatin capsules may be manufactured in a number of shapes, including round, oval, oblong, tube-shape, and others. They may also be prepared of single or two-tone color, the latter resulting from the employment of two different colored ribbons of gelatin to form the sides of the capsule. A modern adaptation of this method, the Accogel Capsule Machine developed by Lederle Laboratories, permits the enclosure of dry powder or liquids in soft gelatin capsules. In addition, through the use of an adaptor, the machine is capable of enclosing preformed tablets in a gelatin film.

The reciprocating die process is similar to the rotary process in that ribbons of gelatin are formed and used to encapsulate the fill, but it differs in the actual encapsulating process. The gelatin ribbons are fed between a set of vertical dies that continually open and close to form rows of pockets in the gelatin ribbons. These pockets are filled with the medication and are sealed, shaped, and cut out of the film as they progress through the machinery. As the capsules are cut from the ribbons, they fall into refrigerated tanks which prevent the capsules from adhering to one another and from getting dull.

Fig. 5–15. *Rotary die process equipment. A, Gelatin tank; B, spreader box; C, gelatin ribbon casting drum; D, mineral oil lubricant bath; E, medicine tank; F, filling pump; G, encapsulating mechanism; H, capsule conveyor; I, capsule washer; J, infrared dryer; K, capsule drying tunnel; L, gelatin net receiver. (Courtesy of R.P. Scherer Corporation.)*

Application of Soft Gelatin Capsules

Soft gelatin capsules may be used to contain a variety of liquid and dry fills. Liquids which may be encapsulated into soft gelatin capsules include[13]

1. Water immiscible, volatile and nonvolatile liquids such as vegetable and aromatic oils, aromatic and aliphatic hydrocarbons, chlorinated hydrocarbons, ethers, esters, alcohols, and organic acids.
2. Water miscible, nonvolatile liquids such as polyethylene glycols, and nonionic surface active agents as polysorbate 80.
3. Water miscible and relatively nonvolatile compounds, as propylene glycol and isopropyl alcohol, depending upon factors as concentration used and packaging conditions.

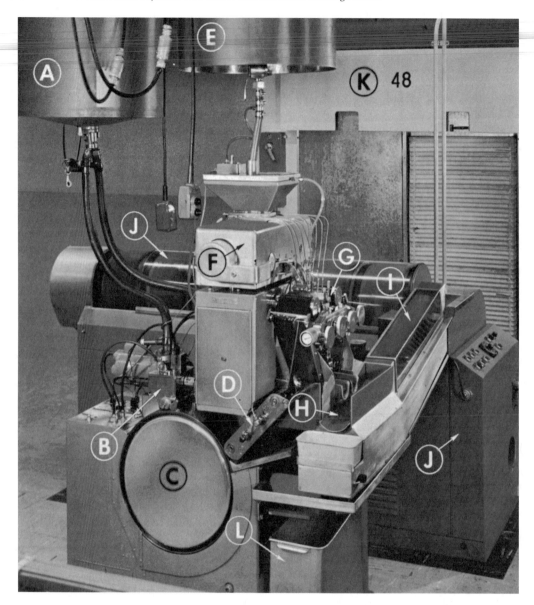

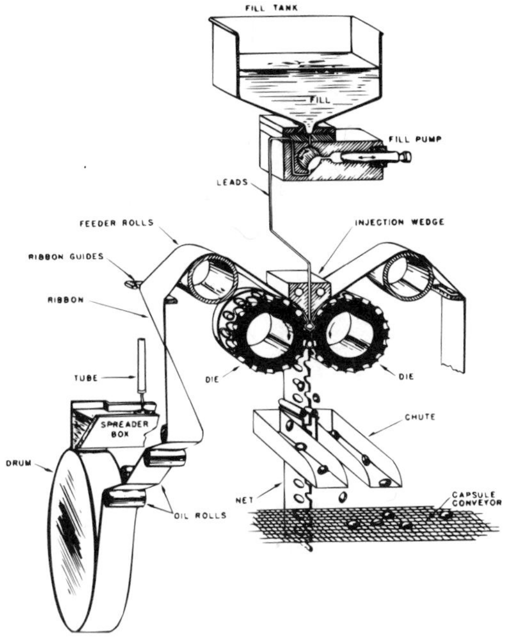

Fig. 5–16. *Schematic drawing of rotary die process. (Courtesy of R.P. Scherer Corporation.)*

Liquids which can easily migrate through the capsule shell cannot be encapsulated into soft gelatin capsules. These materials include: water, above 5%, and low molecular weight water soluble and volatile organic compounds such as alcohols, ketones, acids, amines, and esters.

Solids may be encapsulated into soft gelatin capsules as solutions in one of the suitable liquid solvents, as suspensions, or as dry powders, granules, or pelletized materials.

Among the drugs commercially prepared in soft gelatin capsules are: ethchlorvynol (Placidyl, Abbott), demeclocycline HCl (Declomycin, Lederle), chlortrianisene (TACE, Marion Merrell Dow), digoxin (Lanoxicaps, Burroughs Wellcome), docusate calcium (Surfak, Upjohn), and vitamin E.

Inspecting, Counting, Packaging, and Storing Capsules

Whether capsules are produced on a small or a large scale, they are required to pass not only tests of potency and uniformity but also a visual or electronic inspection to ensure that there are no flaws in the integrity and appearance of the capsules. All capsules produced by the same method should be uniformally colored, uniformly filled, and uniformly shaped. As the pharmacist extemporaneously compounds a prescription for capsules in the community pharmacy, he must take care to prepare uniform capsules. On a large scale, however, the highly productive automatic capsule machines are capable of producing great numbers of capsules simultaneously, and these must be inspected visually or electronically as they are produced. Defective capsules are removed. If the number of capsules removed is excessively high, some production default in the capsule-producing mechanism of the machines is suspected and checked out by machinists.

In the pharmacy, capsules that have been extemporaneously compounded or those taken from a stock package of prefabricated capsules are usually counted by hand, using specially designed counting trays to facilitate the procedure and to ensure the hygienic transfer of the capsules into the final container. One of these trays, the Abbott counting tray, is depicted in Figure 5–17. In using this tray, the pharmacist pours a supply of capsules or tablets from the bulk source onto the clean tray, and using the spatula he counts the desired number of capsules or tablets, sweeping them into the trough as he counts. When the correct number is in the trough, the pharmacist closes the trough cover, picks up the tray, returns the uncounted dosage units to the bulk container by means of the lip at the back of the tray, places the prescription contained at the opening of the trough, and carefully transfers the capsules or tablets into the container. By this method, the capsules or tablets remain untouched by the pharmacist. To prevent contamination of tablets and capsules, the tray must be wiped clean after each counting, as powder tends to get on the tray, especially when uncoated tablets are counted.

On a larger scale, as occurs in some community and hospital pharmacy settings, small automatic counting and container-filling apparatus is becoming increasing popular and useful. Some of these counting machines are shown in Figures 5–18 and 5–19.

On an industrial scale, solid dosage forms may be counted by means of large counting trays. The operator pours the dosage units on a tray containing the desired number of perforations, rotates the tray until each perforation is filled with a capsule or tablet, allows the excess to slide off the tray, and then transfers the counted number

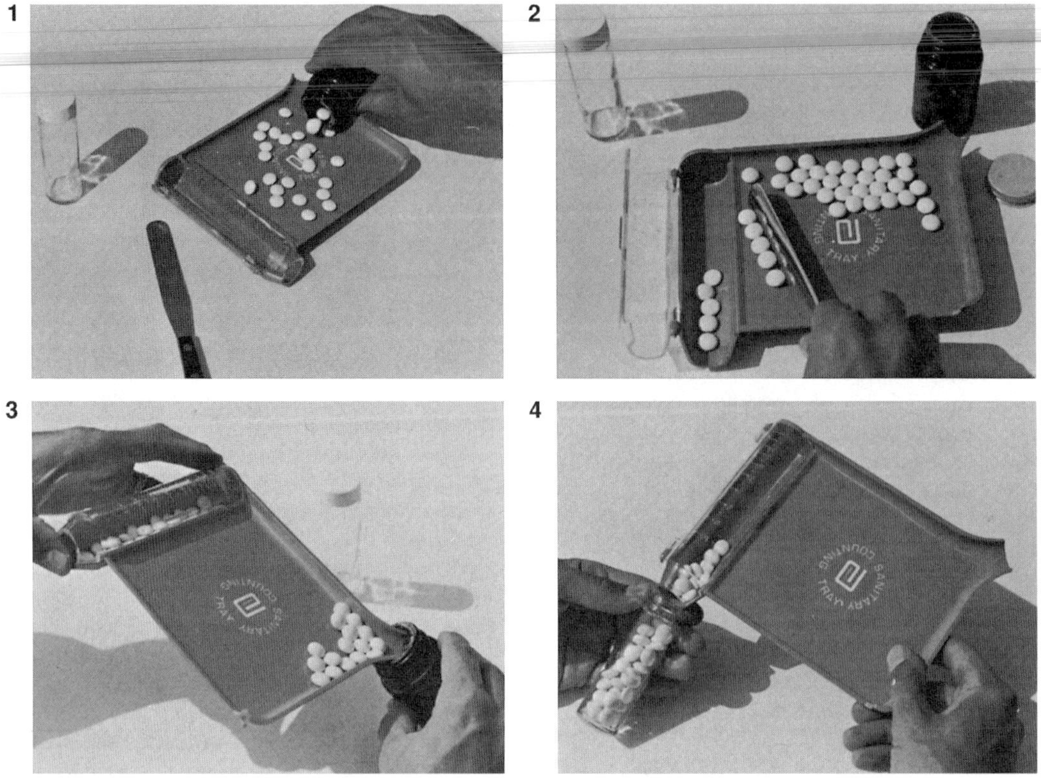

Fig. 5–17. *Steps in the counting of solid dosage units with the Abbott Sanitary Counting Tray: (1) placing units from stock package onto tray, (2) counting and transferring units to trough, (3) returning excess units to stock container, and (4) placing counted units into prescription container.*

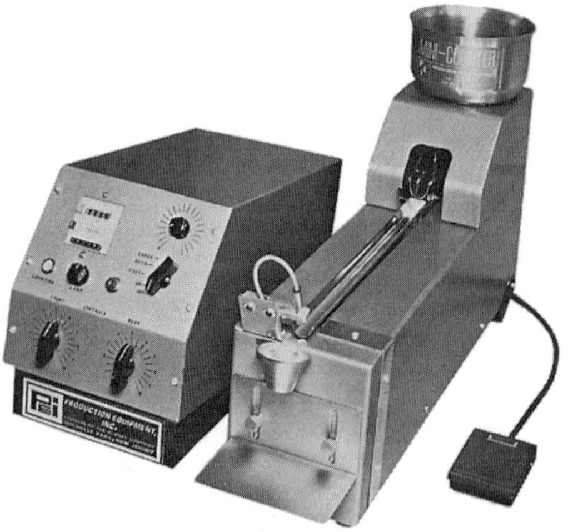

Fig. 5–18. *Mini-Counter II, small automatic tablet and capsule counting and filling apparatus. (Courtesy of Production Equipment Co.)*

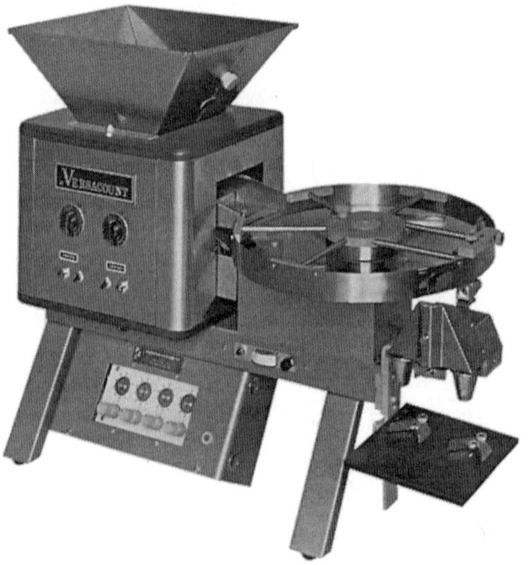

Fig. 5–19. *Versacount Model automatic tablet and capsule counting and filling apparatus. (Courtesy of Production Equipment Co.)*

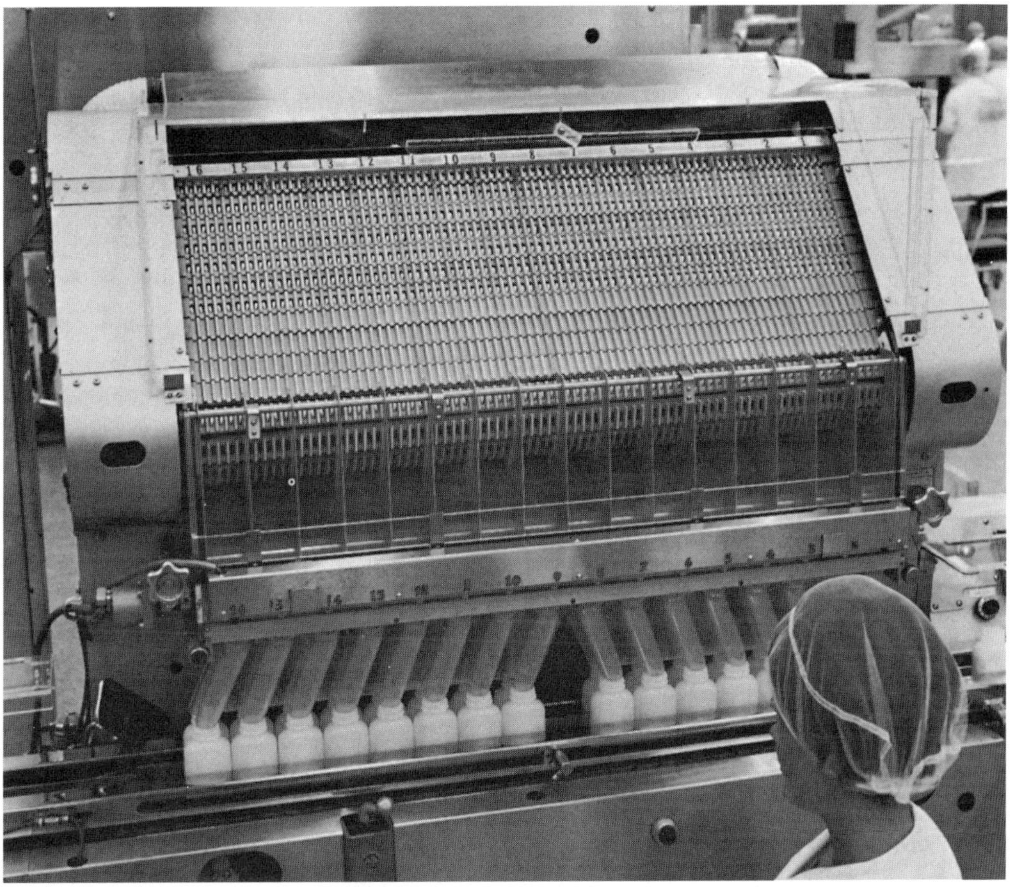

Fig. 5–20. *Large Merrill filling machine that fills 16 bottles with 200 tablets each at one time. A flipper gate in the upper manifold directs the tablets into one row of bottles while the other filled row is evacuated and a new row of bottles moves into place. (Courtesy of The Upjohn Company.)*

from the perforations into the container. This method has largely been replaced by highly automated counting devices that both count and transfer the desired number of dosage units into the containers. Machines have been developed to count and fill a dozen or more containers simultaneously, capping and moving the filled bottles along the production line where they can again be inspected, labeled, and finally packaged into cartons. One of these machines is shown in Figure 5–20.

Capsules are usually packaged in glass or in plastic containers, some containing packets of a desiccant to prevent the absorption of excessive moisture by the capsules. Soft capsules have a greater tendency than do hard capsules to soften and adhere to one another, and they must be maintained in a cool, dry place. In fact, all capsules remain stable longer if maintained tightly sealed in a cool place of low humidity.

The unit dose and strip packaging of solid dosage forms, particularly by pharmacies which service nursing homes and hospitals, provides sanitary handling of the medications, ease of identification, and security in accountability for medications. Typical small scale strip packaging equipment and commercial unit-dose packages of capsules and tablets are presented in Figures 5–21 and 5–22 respectively.

Official Capsules

There are more than a hundred officially recognized medications in capsule form, representing a wide range of therapeutic categories. Examples of these are presented in Table 5–3.

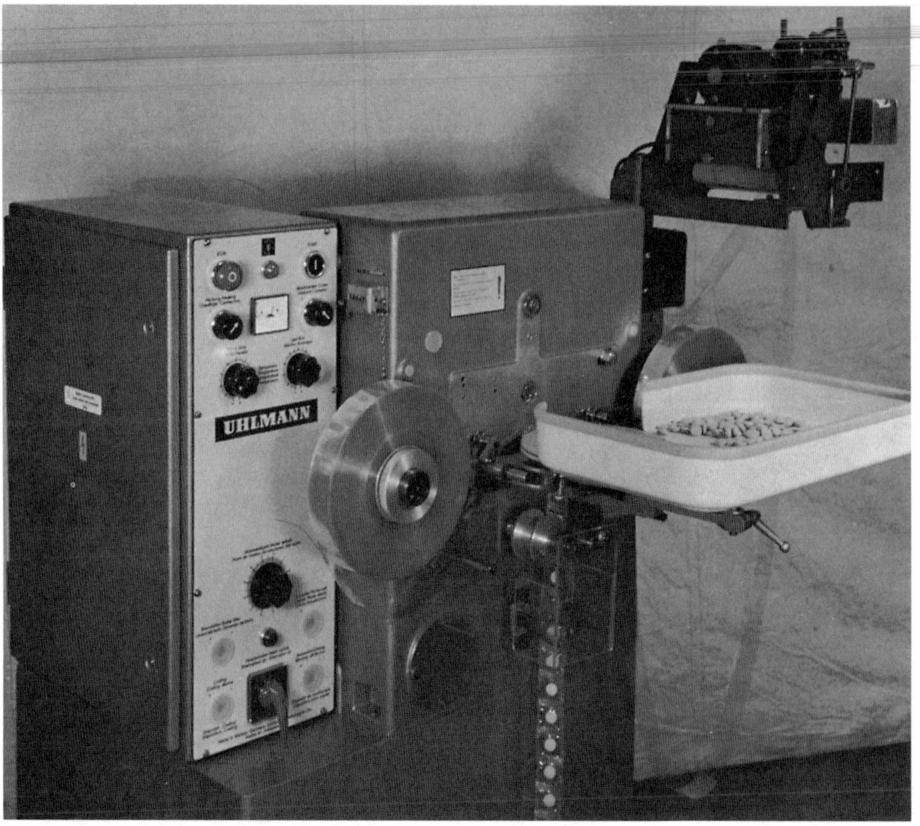

Fig. 5–21. *A strip packager for the unit dose dispensing of solid dosage forms. Drug information is imprinted on each individual package unit. The model shown has a fully automatic cutoff from 1 to 24 dosage units and is especially suited to unit-dose packaging and dispensing in hospitals, dispensaries, nursing homes, and clinics. (Courtesy of Lakso Company, Inc.)*

Specialized Capsule Forms

There are some specialized capsule forms, as those containing drugs to be released in a controlled-release manner. These are discussed later in this chapter.

Tablets

Tablets are solid dosage forms of medicinal substances usually prepared with the aid of suitable pharmaceutical adjuncts. Tablets may vary in size, shape, weight, hardness, thickness, disintegration characteristics, and in other aspects, depending upon the intended use of the tablets and their method of manufacture. The majority of tablets are used in the oral administration of drugs, and many of these tablets are prepared with colorants and coatings of various types. Other tablets such as those intended to be administered sublingually, buccally, or vaginally may not contain the same adjuncts or be prepared to possess the same types of features as tablets for oral administration. Many of the advantages of tablets for the oral administration of drugs have been presented at the outset of this chapter and previously in Chapter 3.

Tablets are prepared primarily by compression. A limited number of tablets are prepared by molding. Compressed tablets are manufactured with tablet machines capable of exerting great pressure in compacting the powdered or granulated tableting material through the use of various shaped punches and dies (Fig. 5–23). The tablet presses are heavy equipment of various capacities selected for use on the basis of the type of tablets to be manufactured and the production rate desired. Molded tablets are prepared by tab-

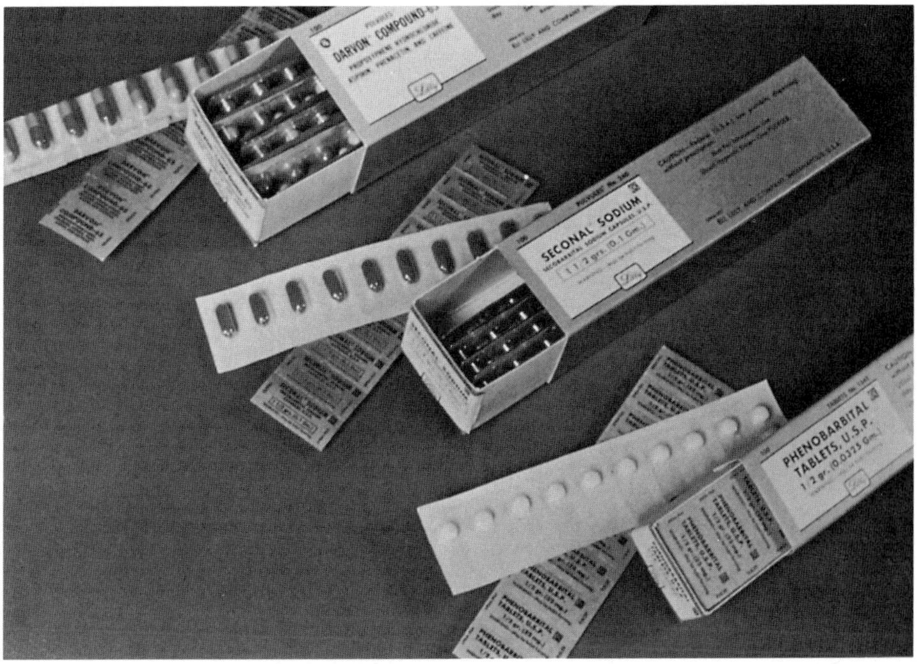

Fig. 5–22. *Example of unit-dose packaging of tablets and capsules. The drug name and other information are imprinted on the backing portion of each unit. (Courtesy of Eli Lilly and Company.)*

Table 5–3. Examples of Some Official Capsules

Official Capsule	*Some Representative Commercial Capsules*	*Capsule Strengths Usually Available*	*Category*
Amoxicillin	Wymox (Wyeth-Ayerst)	250 and 500 mg	Antibacterial
Ampicillin	Amcill (Parke Davis); Polycillin (Apothecon) Omnipen (Wyeth-Ayerst)	250 and 500 mg	Antibacterial
Aspirin	. . .	300 mg	Analgesic
Cephalexin	Keflex (Dista)	250 and 500 mg	Antibacterial
Cloxacillin Sodium	Tegopen (Apothecon)	250 and 500 mg	Antibacterial
Diphenhydramine HCl	Benadryl HCl (Parke Davis)	25 and 50 mg	Antihistaminic
Doxycycline Hyclate	Vibramycin (Pfizer)	50 and 100 mg	Antibacterial
Erythromycin Estolate	Ilosone (Dista)	125 and 250 mg	Antibacterial
Flurazepam HCl	Dalmane (Roche)	15 and 30 mg	Hypnotic
Gemfibrozil	Lopid (Parke-Davis)	300 mg	Antihyperlipidemic
Griseofulvin	Grisactin (Wyeth-Ayerst)	125 and 250 mg	Antifungal
Indomethacin	Indocin (Merck)	25 and 50 mg	Antiinflammatory; antipyretic; analgesic
Levodopa	Dopar (Roberts)	100, 250, and 500 mg	Antiparkinsonian
Loperamide HCl	Imodium (Janssen)	2 mg	Antidiarrheal
Nifedipine	Procardia (Pfizer)	10 and 20 mg	Calcium-channel blocker
Oxazepam	Serax (Wyeth-Ayerst)	10, 15 and 30 mg	Antianxiety
Propoxyphene HCl	Darvon (Lilly)	32 and 65 mg	Analgesic
Rifampin	Rifadin (Marion Merrell Dow)	150 mg	Antiinfective
Secobarbital Sodium	Seconal Sodium (Lilly)	30 mg	Hypnotic; sedative
Tetracycline HCl	Achromycin V (Lederle)	250 and 500 mg	Antibacterial; antiamebic; antirickettsial

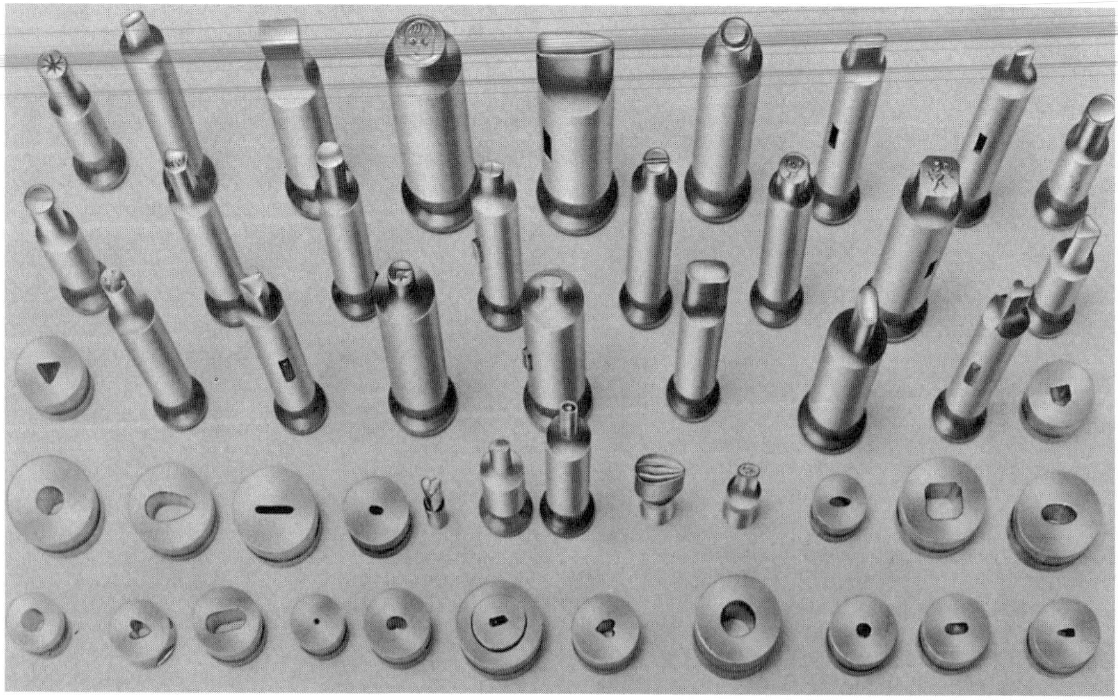

Fig. 5–23. *Various Stokes punches and dies for the production of distinctive tablets. (Courtesy of Stokes Equipment Division, Pennwalt Chemicals Corporation.)*

let machinery or manually by forcing dampened tablet material into a mold from which the formed tablet is then ejected and allowed to dry.

Types of Tablets

The various types of tablets are described as follows, with the abbreviations for the tablet types in parentheses.

COMPRESSED TABLETS **(C.T.).** Compressed tablets, prepared by single compression, occur in various shapes and sizes and usually contain in addition to the medicinal substance(s), a number of pharmaceutical adjuncts including (a) *diluents* or *fillers,* which add the necessary bulk to a formulation to prepare tablets of the desired size; (b) *binders* or *adhesives,* which promote the adhesion of the particles of the formulation, enabling a granulation to be prepared and the maintenance of the integrity of the final tablet; (c) *disintegrators* or *disintegrating agents,* which promote the breakup of the tablets after administration to smaller particles for more ready drug availability; (d) *antiadherents, glidants, lubricants* or *lubricating agents,* which enhance the flow of the tableting material into the tablet dies, prevent the sticking of this material to the punches and dies, and produce tablets having a sheen; and (e) *miscellaneous adjuncts* such as colorants and flavorants. After compression, some compressed tablets may be coated with various materials as described later. Most compressed tablets are employed for the oral administration of drugs, but some may be used for the sublingual, buccal, or vaginal administration of drugs.

MULTIPLE COMPRESSED TABLETS **(M.C.T.).** Multiple compressed tablets are prepared by subjection to more than a single compression. The result may be a multiple-layered tablet or a tablet-within-a-tablet, the inner tablet being the *core* and the outer portion being the *shell* (Fig. 5–24). Layered tablets are prepared by the initial compaction of a portion of fill material in a die and the addition of one or more portions of fill material to the same die, each additional fill being compressed to form a two- or three-layered tablet, depending upon the number of separate fills. Usually each portion of fill material contains a different medicinal agent separated from the others for reasons of incompatibility, for provid-

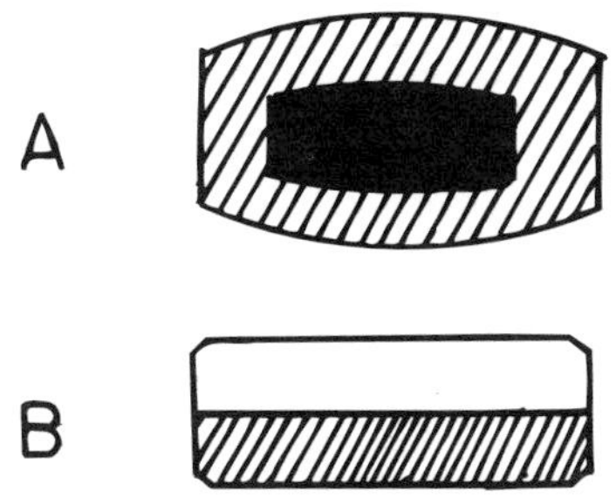

Fig. 5–24. *Diagram of multiple-compressed tablets. A, having a core of one drug and a shell of another, and B, a multiple-layered tablet of two drugs.*

ing drug release in two or more stages, or simply for the unique appearance of a multiple-layered tablet. Generally each portion of fill is colored differently to prepare a multiple-colored as well as a multiple-layered tablet. In the preparation of tablets having another compressed tablet as the inner core, special machines are required to place the preformed tablet precisely within the die for the second compression and the new fill material around the core tablet.

SUGAR-COATED TABLETS (S.C.T.). Compressed tablets may be coated with a colored or an uncolored sugar. The coating is water-soluble and is quickly dissolved after swallowing. It serves the varied purposes of protecting the drug from the air and humidity and providing a taste or a smell barrier to objectional tasting or smelling drugs. Further, it enhances the appearance of many compressed tablets. Disadvantages to sugar-coating tablets are the time and expertise required by the process and the increase in the size and weight of the compressed tablets. Coated tablets may be 50% larger and heavier than the original uncoated tablets.

FILM-COATED TABLETS (F.C.T.). Film-coated tablets are compressed tablets coated with a thin layer of a water-insoluble or water-soluble polymer capable of forming a film over the tablet. The film is generally colored and has the advantage over sugar-coatings in that it is more durable, less bulky, and less time-consuming to apply. The coating ruptures in the gastrointestinal tract.

ENTERIC-COATED TABLETS (E.C.T.). Enteric-coated tablets are tablets with a coating that resists dissolution or disruption in the stomach but not in the intestines, thereby allowing for tablet transit through the stomach in favor of tablet disintegration and drug dissolution and absorption from the intestines. This technique is employed in instances in which the drug substance is destroyed by gastric acid, is irritating to the gastric mucosa, or when by-pass of the stomach enhances drug absorption from the intestines to a significant extent.

BUCCAL OR SUBLINGUAL TABLETS. Buccal or sublingual tablets are generally flat, oval tablets intended to be dissolved in the buccal pouch *(buccal tablets)* or beneath the tongue *(sublingual tablets)* for absorption through the oral mucosa. They are useful in providing for the absorption of drugs that are destroyed by the gastric juice and/or poorly absorbed from the gastrointestinal tract. Tablets intended for buccal administration (as progesterone tablets) are prepared to erode or to dissolve slowly, while those for sublingual use (as nitroglycerin tablets) dissolve very promptly to give rapid drug effects.

CHEWABLE TABLETS. Chewable tablets, which have a smooth, rapid disintegration when chewed or allowed to dissolve in the mouth, yield a creamy base of a specially flavored and colored mannitol. The tablets are especially useful in tablet formulations for children and are commonly employed in the preparation of multiple vitamin tablets. They find other uses in the administration of antacids and antiflatulents. These tablets are prepared by compression.

EFFERVESCENT TABLETS. Effervescent tablets are prepared by compressing granular effervescent salts or other materials having the capacity to release gas when in contact with water. Commercially, alkalinizing-analgesic tablets are frequently made to effervesce to encourage fast disintegration and solution when added to water.

TABLET TRITURATES (T.T.). Tablet triturates are small, usually cylindrical, molded (M.T.T.) or compressed tablets (C.T.T.) containing small amounts of usually potent drugs. Today only a few tablet triturate products are available commercially, with most of these produced by tablet compression. Tablet triturates also may be prepared by molding, a procedure generally reserved for laboratory and small-scale production. Tablet triturates must be readily and completely soluble in water; thus when these tablets are prepared by compression, a minimal amount of pressure is exerted. A combination of sucrose and lactose is usually the diluent, and any water-insoluble material is avoided in the formulation. Some tablet triturates are used for the oral administration of drugs and some for sublingual use (as nitroglycerin tablets). Pharmacists may employ tablet triturates in compounding procedures in the preparation of other solid or liquid dosage forms. For instance, the tablets may be easily inserted into capsules to provide accurate amounts of potent drug substances. They may also be used by pharmacists to fortify liquid preparations, as prescribed, by dissolving the appropriate number of tablets in a small portion of water and then bringing the preparation to the required volume with the liquid medication being fortified.

HYPODERMIC TABLETS **(H.T.).** Hypodermic tablets are tablet triturates originally intended for use by the physician in his extemporaneous preparation of parenteral solutions. The physician dissolved the required number of tablets in a suitable vehicle, attained sterility of the preparation as best he could, and performed the injection. The tablets were intended as a convenience to the physician, since he could carry in his medicine bag a variety of lightweight hypodermic tablets and a suitable vehicle and prepare corresponding injections of the desired strength and volume according to the needs of the individual patients. However, the difficulty in achieving sterility and the current availability of a large number of drugs in injectable form, some in disposable syringes, have eliminated the need for hypodermic tablets.

DISPENSING TABLETS **(D.T.).** Dispensing tablets are no longer in general use. In retrospect, they might better have been termed *compounding tablets,* because they were used by the pharmacist in compounding and not dispensed as such to the patient. The tablets containing relatively large amounts of highly potent drug substances were prepared as a convenience to the pharmacist, enabling him to obtain quickly accurately measured amounts of potent drugs in preparing other solid or liquid dosage forms. The diluent or base of the tablets was usually water-soluble to permit the preparation of clear aqueous solutions. Dispensing tablets were prepared by either molding or compression. Disintegrating agents, water-insoluble lubricants, colorants, flavorants, and coatings were not used in the preparation of dispensing tablets. Primarily because of the potential hazard in the inadvertent dispensing of these tablets to patients, dispensing tablets are not used today. Nowadays, the pharmacist more commonly employs commercially prepared compressed tablets or tablet triturates in the compounding of prescriptions calling for a drug substance unavailable in bulk, but available in these dosage forms.

CONTROLLED RELEASE TABLETS. Controlled release tablets and capsules will be discussed later in this chapter.

Compressed Tablets

Characteristics and Quality

The physical features of compressed tablets are well known to even the layman. Some tablets are round, others oblong, and still others triangular. Some are thick; others are thin. Some tablets have larger diameters than others. Some tablets are flat; others have varying degrees of convexity. Some are *scored* or grooved in halves, thirds, or quadrants to permit the fairly accurate breaking of the tablet for the administration of a partial amount. Scored tablets are generally grooved on a single side (Fig. 5–25). Some tablets are engraved with a symbol of the manufacturer to denote the company, the product, or both. Tablets are produced in different colors to make them further distinctive.

Tablet diameters and shapes are determined by the die and punches used for the compression of the tablet. The less concave the punches, the more flat the resulting tablets; conversely, the more concave the punches, the more convex the resulting tablets (Fig. 5–26). Punches having raised impressions will produce recessed impressions on the tablets; punches having recessed etchings will produce tablets having

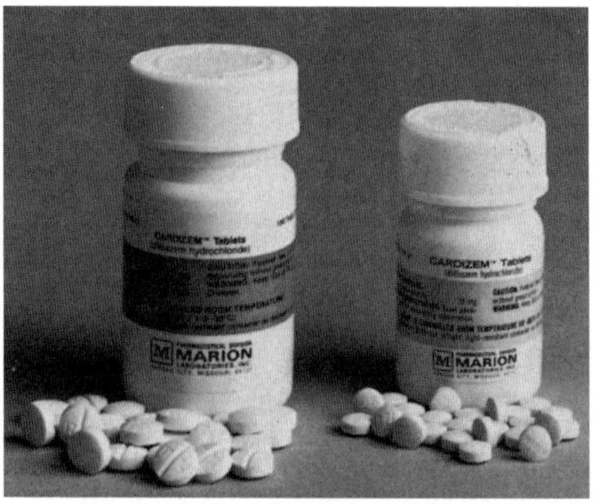

Fig. 5–25. *Packages of a drug product of two different tablet strengths, with one scored for ease of breaking in half. (Courtesy of Marion Laboratories.)*

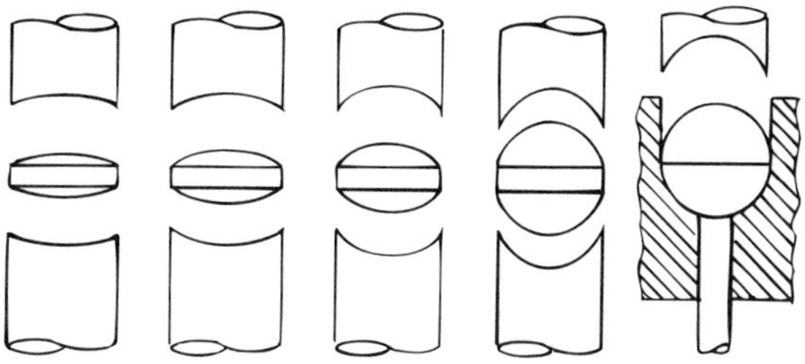

Fig. 5–26. *Contours of the punches determine the shape of the tablets. From left to right, flat face, shallow cup, standard cup, deep cup, and modified ball. (Courtesy of Cherry-Burrell Corporation.)*

raised impression or monograms. Monograms may be placed on one or on both sides of a tablet, depending upon whether monogram-producing lower and/or upper punches are used (Fig. 5–23).

The thickness of a tablet is determined by the amount of fill permitted to enter the die and the amount of pressure applied during compression.

In addition to these apparent features of tablets, pharmacists are aware that tablets must meet other physical specifications that are generally unknown to the layman. These include tablet weight, tablet thickness, tablet hardness, tablet disintegration, content uniformity and drug dissolution. These factors must be controlled within the production of a batch of tablets as well as from production batch to production batch in order to assure not only the outward appearance of the product but also its therapeutic efficacy (Fig. 5–27).

TABLET WEIGHT. The amount of fill placed in the die of a tablet press will determine the weight of the resulting tablet. The volume of fill (granulation or powder) permitted to enter the dies is adjusted with the first few tablets produced to yield tablets of the desired weight and content. Adjustment is necessary, since tablet formulations are based on the weight of the tablets to be prepared. For example, if a tablet is to contain 20 mg of a drug substance and if 10,000 tablets are to be produced, 200 g of that drug are employed in the formula. After the addition of the pharmaceutical additives such as the diluent, disintegrant, lubricant, and binder, the formulation may weigh 2000 g, which means that each tablet must weigh 200 mg in order for 20 mg of drug to be present. Thus, the depth of fill in the tablet die must be adjusted to hold a volume of granulation weighing 200 mg. During a production run, sample tablets are periodically removed for visual inspection and for quality measurement against standards (Fig. 5–28).

The USP contains a weight variation standard to which the official tablets must conform:[11]

Weight Variation

For the determination of dosage-form uniformity by weight variation, select not less than 30 units, and proceed as follows for the dosage form designated. (Note: Specimens other than these test units may be drawn from the same batch for *Assay* determinations.)

UNCOATED TABLETS. Weigh accurately 10 tablets individually, and calculate the average weight. From the result of the *Assay*, obtained as directed in the individual monograph, calculate the content of active ingredient in each of 10 tablets, assuming homogeneous distribution of the active ingredient.

HARD CAPSULES. Weigh accurately 10 capsules individually, taking care to preserve the identity of each capsule. Remove the contents of each capsule by a suitable means. Weigh accurately the emptied shells individually, and calculate for each capsule the net weight of its contents by subtracting the weight of the shell from the respective gross weight. From the results of the *Assay*, obtained as directed in the individual monograph, calculate the content of active ingredient in each of the capsules, assuming homogeneous distribution of the active ingredient.

SOFT CAPSULES. Determine the net weight of the contents of individual capsules as follows: Weigh accurately the 10 intact capsules individually to obtain their gross weights, taking care to preserve the identity of each capsule. Then cut open the capsules by means of a suitable clean, dry cutting instrument such as scissors or a sharp open blade, and remove the contents by washing with a suitable solvent. Allow the occluded solvent to evaporate from the shells at room temperature over a period of about 30 minutes, taking precautions to avoid uptake or loss of moisture. Weigh the individual shells, and calculate the net contents. From the results of the

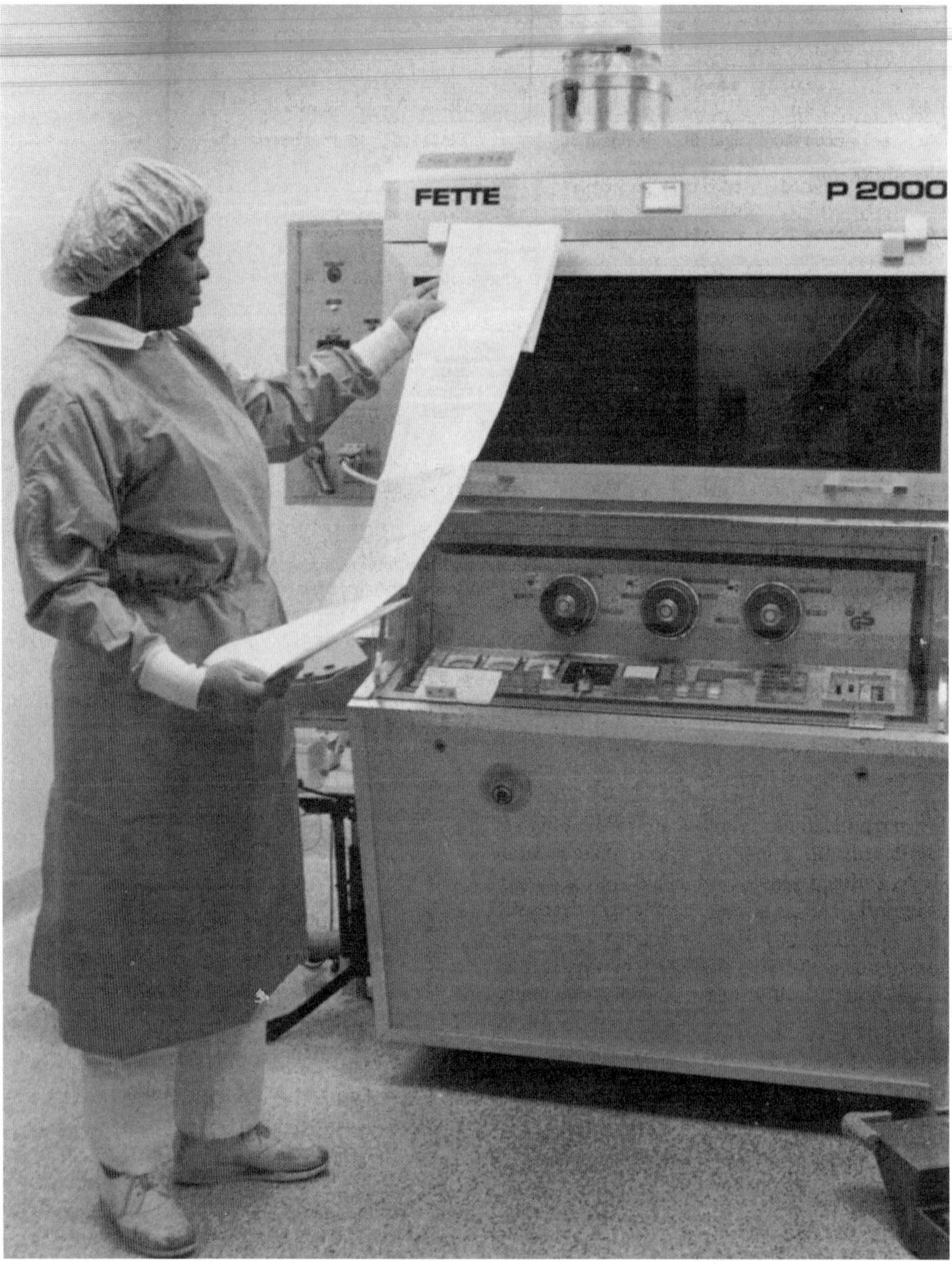

Fig. 5–27. *Quality control in the manufacturing of tablets. (Courtesy of Eli Lilly and Company.)*

Assay, obtained as directed in the individual monograph, calculate the content of active ingredient in each of the capsules, assuming homogeneous distribution of the active ingredient.

Naturally, the dimensions of tablets produced depends not only on the volume and weight of the fill but also on the diameter of the die and upon the pressure applied to the fill on compaction.

TABLET THICKNESS. As indicated above, the thickness desired in a tablet must be coordinated with the volume of fill issued to the die, the di-

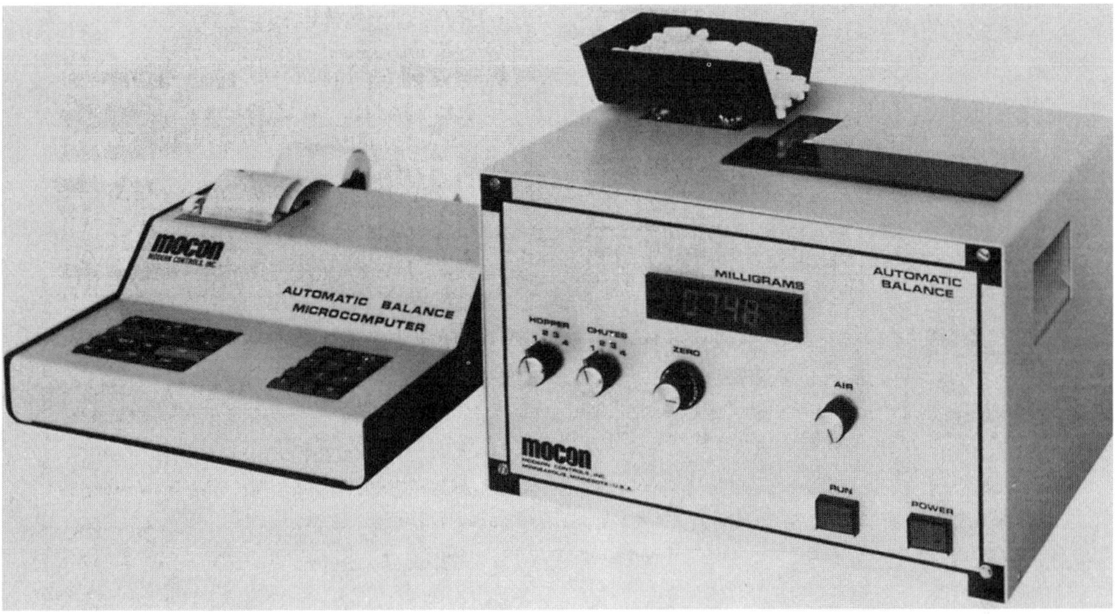

Fig. 5–28. *An automatic balance that weighs product and prints statistics to determine compliance with USP weight variation requirements for tablets. (Courtesy of Mocon Modern Controls, Inc.)*

ameter of the die, and the pressure applied to the fill by the punches. To produce tablets of uniform thickness during production and between productions for the same formulation, care must be exercised to employ the same volume of fill and the same pressure. Tablets are measured with a caliper or gauge during production to make certain of consistent thickness (Figs. 5–29 and 5–30). It should be pointed out that since pressure applied affects not only the thickness of the tablet but also its hardness and since the latter factor is probably the more important of the two, the thickness of a tablet is varied more by the size of the die and the fill permitted than by the pressure. Pressure adjustments are made primarily to control the softness or the hardness of the tablets.

TABLET HARDNESS OR BREAKING STRENGTH. It is not unusual for a tablet press to exert as little as 3000 and as much as 40,000 pounds of force in the production of tablets. Generally, the greater the pressure applied, the harder the tablets, although the characteristics of the granulation also determine the hardness of the tablet. Certain tablets, such as lozenges and buccal tablets that are intended to dissolve slowly, are intentionally made hard; other tablets, such as compressed tablet triturates that are intended to dissolve rap-

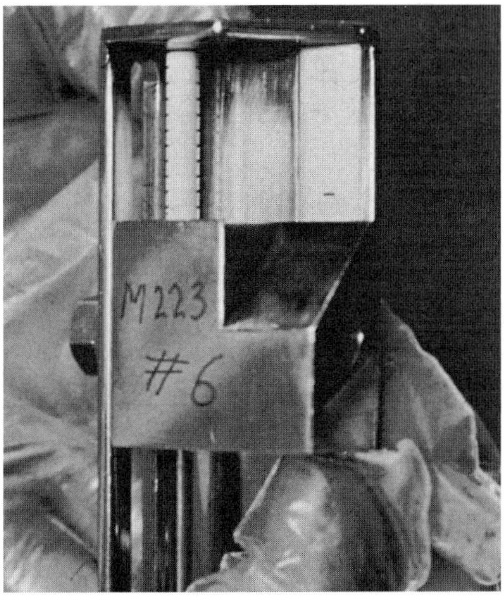

Fig. 5–29. *Tablet gauge used to measure the thickness of tablets. (Courtesy of Eli Lilly and Company.)*

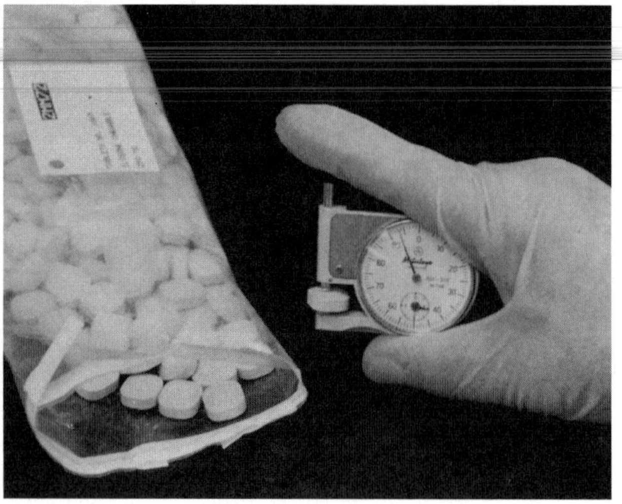

Fig. 5–30. *Tablet thickness gauge. (Courtesy of Eli Lilly and Company.)*

idly, are made soft. In general, tablets should be sufficiently hard to resist breaking during packaging, shipment, and normal handling and yet soft enough to dissolve or disintegrate properly after administered or to be broken between the fingers when a part of a tablet is to be taken.

A number of tablet hardness testers in use today measure the degree of force (in kilograms, pounds, or in arbitrary units) that is required to break a tablet (Figs. 5–31 and 5–32). In the industry, a force of about 4 kilograms is considered to be the minimum permitted for a satisfactory tablet. Hardness determinations are made during production to determine the need for pressure adjustments on the tablet presses.

Another means of determining the hardness of tablets is through the use of a *friabilator*. This apparatus determines the tablet's *friability* (that is, its tendency to crumble), by allowing the tablet to roll and fall within a rotating tumbling apparatus (Fig. 5–33). The tablets are weighed before and after a specified number of rotations, and the loss in weight is determined. Resistance to loss of weight indicates the tablet's ability to withstand abrasion in handling, packaging, and shipment. A maximum weight loss of not more than 1% of the weight of the tablets being tested generally is considered acceptable for most products. Effervescent tablets and chewable tablets normally have individually applied standards.

TABLET DISINTEGRATION. For the medicinal component of a tablet to become fully available for absorption from the gastrointestinal tract, the tablet must first disintegrate and discharge the drug to the body fluids for dissolution. Tablet disintegration is also important for those tablets containing medicinal agents (such as antacids and antidiarrheals) that are not intended to be absorbed but rather to act locally within the gastrointestinal tract. In these instances, tablet disintegration provides drug particles with a greater surface area for localized activity within the body.

All USP tablets must pass the official test for disintegration, which is conducted *in vitro* with a special testing apparatus (Fig. 5–34). Briefly, the apparatus consists of a basket-rack assembly containing 6 open-ended glass tubes held vertically upon a 10-mesh stainless steel wire screen. During testing, a tablet is placed in each of the six tubes of the basket and through the use of a mechanical device, the basket is raised and lowered in the immersion fluid at a frequency of between 29 and 32 cycles per minute, the wire screen always being maintained below the level of the fluid. For uncoated tablets, buccal tablets, and sublingual tablets, water maintained at about 37°C serves as the immersion fluid unless another fluid is specified in the individual monograph. For these tests, complete disintegration of tablets or capsules as "that state in which any residue of the unit, except fragments of insoluble coating or capsule shell, remaining on the screen of the test apparatus is a soft mass having no palpably firm core."[14] Buccal tablets must disintegrate within 4 hours, and the sublingual and other uncoated tablets within the limits of the official monograph, usually 30 minutes but vary-

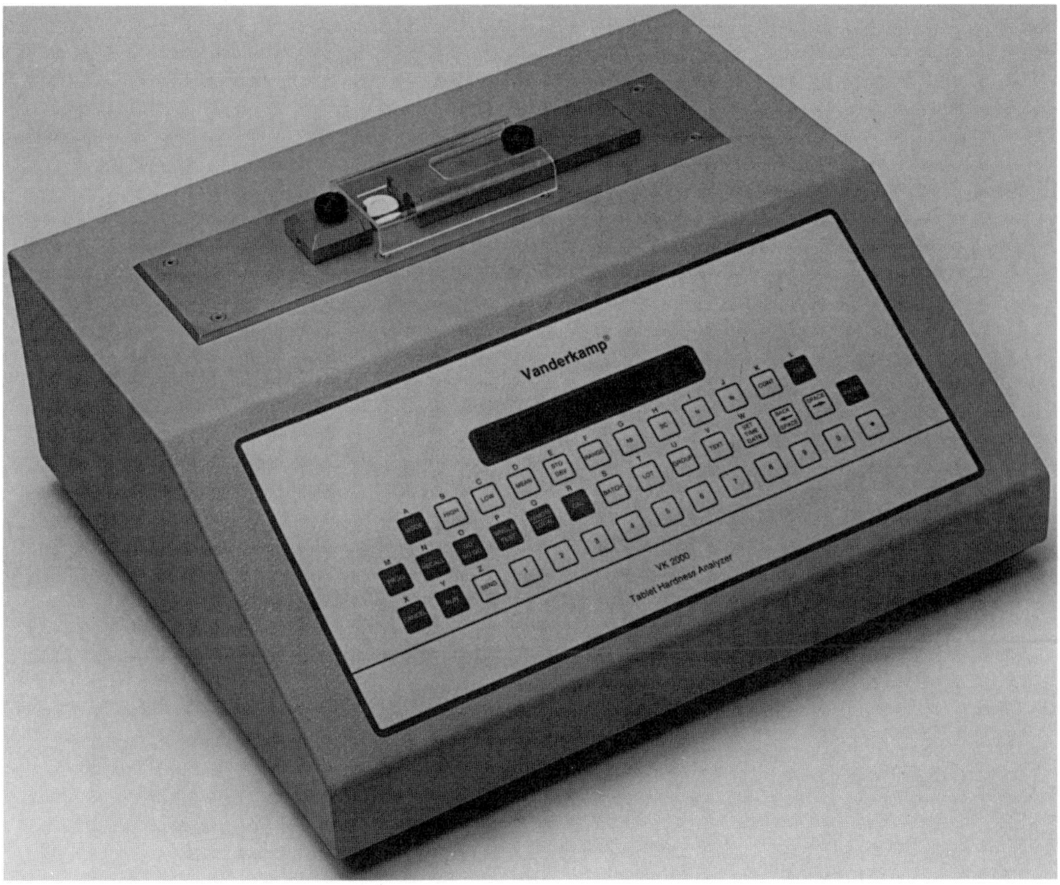

Fig. 5–31. *Programmable tablet hardness analyzer. This unit has the capacity to record lot, group, and batch numbers in up to ten stored programs. It may also be used in a single test mode. (Courtesy of VanKel Industries, Inc.)*

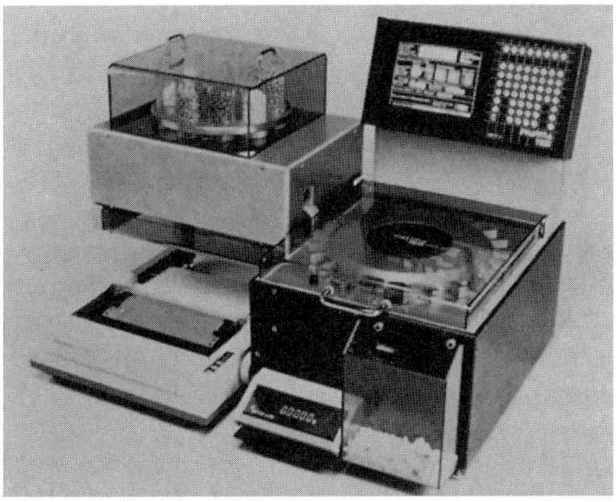

Fig. 5–32. *Automatic weight, hardness, thickness, and tablet diameter test instrument for quality control. Using a microprocessor and monitor for visualization, the instrument can test up to 20 samples at a time. (Courtesy of Scientific Instruments & Technology Corporation.)*

ing from about 2 minutes for Nitroglycerin Tablets, USP, to 30 minutes or longer for other tablets. For plain coated tablets, initial soaking in water at room temperature for 5 minutes is permitted to remove any water-soluble external coating. Then the tablets are immersed in simulated gastric fluid at 37°C for 30 minutes, and if they fail to disintegrate, they are subjected to the test using simulated intestinal fluid also at 37°C for the prescribed period according to the individual monograph. Enteric-coated tablets are similarly tested, except that the tablets are permitted to be tested in the simulated gastric fluid for one hour after which no sign of dissolution or disintegration must be seen. They are then actively immersed in the simulated intestinal fluid for 2 hours or for an individually designated length of time as stated in the monograph during which the tablets should have disintegrated. In each of the above cases, if 1 or 2 of the

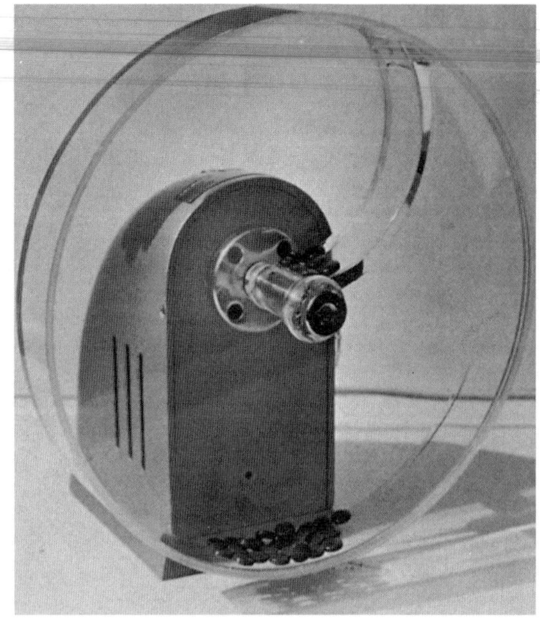

Fig. 5–33. *Erweka tablet testing apparatus for rolling and impact durability. Tablets are weighed and placed in the plexiglass drum in which a curved baffle is mounted. When the motor is activated by setting the timer, the tablets roll and drop. If the free fall within the drum results in the breakage or excessive abrasion of the tablets, they are considered not suited to withstand shipment without being damaged. The motor makes 20 rpm. After the tablets have been tested, they are removed and weighed again. The difference in weight within a given time indicates the rate of abrasion. (Courtesy of Chemical and Pharmaceutical Industry Co., Inc.)*

6 tablets fails to disintegrate completely, tests are repeated on 12 additional tablets, and not less than 16 of the total of 18 tablets tested must disintegrate completely to meet the standard.[12]

TABLET DISSOLUTION. The USP contains a test that determines the dissolution characteristics of a drug present in a solid dosage form. Because drug absorption and physiologic availability are largely dependent upon having the drug in the dissolved state, simple dissolution characteristics are an important property of a satisfactory drug product.

The apparatus for testing the dissolution characteristics of a capsule or tablet dosage form consists of (1) a variable speed stirrer motor, (2) a paddle or a cylindrical stainless steel basket to be affixed to the end of the stirrer shaft, (3) a 1000-mL vessel of glass or other inert, transparent material, fitted with a cover having a center port for the shaft of the stirrer, and three additional ports, two for the removal of samples, and one for the placement of a thermometer, and (4) a suitable water bath to maintain the temperature of the dissolution medium in the vessel (Fig. 5–35). In each test, a volume of the dissolution medium (as stated in the individual monograph) is placed in the vessel and allowed to come to 37°C ± 0.5°C. Then, the single tablet or capsule to be tested is immersed in the vessel or placed in the basket and the stirrer rotated at the speed specified in the monograph. At stated intervals, samples of the medium are withdrawn for chemical analysis of the proportion of drug dissolved.

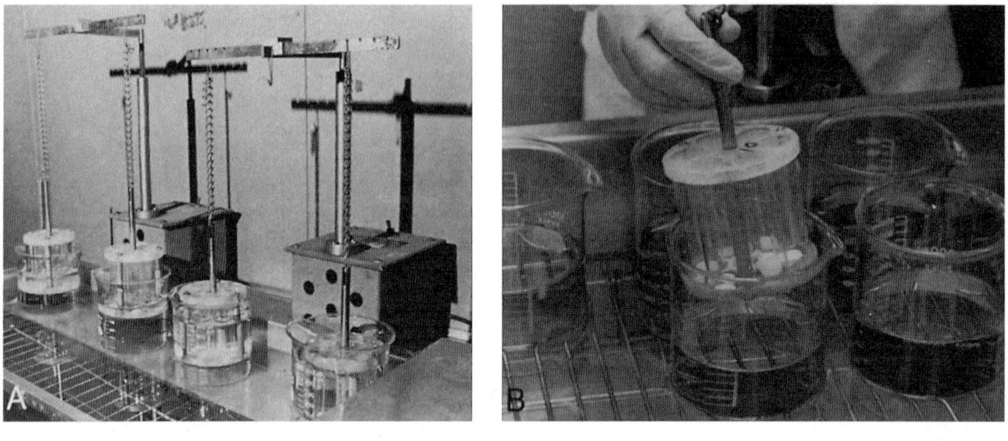

Fig. 5–34. *A, Tablet disintegration testing apparatus. B, Close-up view. (Courtesy of Eli Lilly and Company.)*

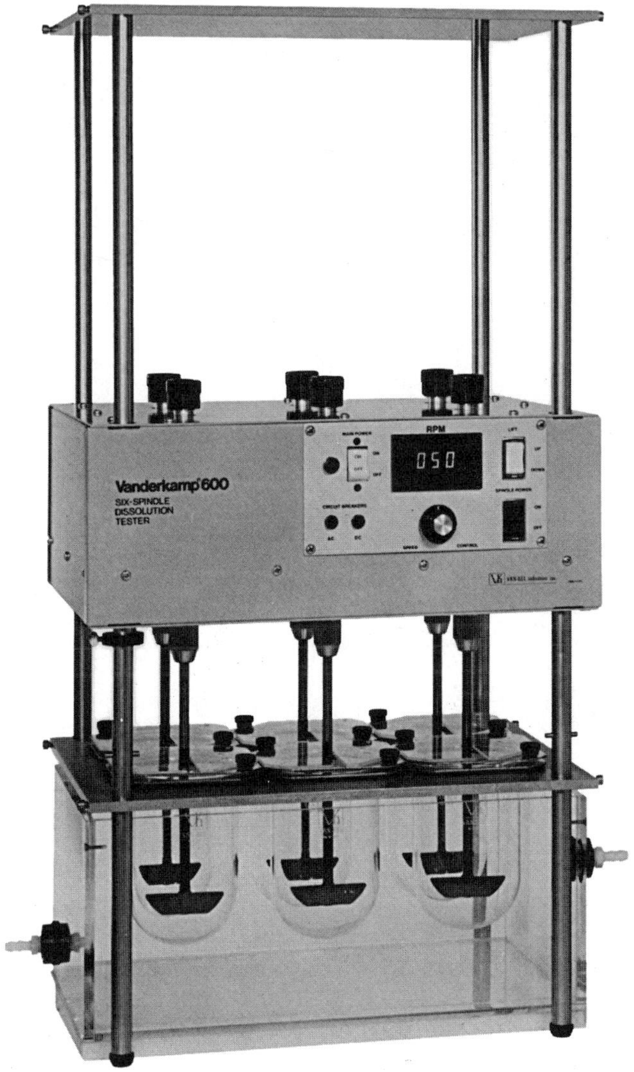

Fig. 5–35. *Solid dosage form dissolution system. (Courtesy of VanKel Industries.)*

The tablet or capsule must meet the monographic requirement for rate of dissolution.

With the increased emphasis on dissolution testing and the determination of the bioavailability of drugs from solid dosage forms has come the introduction of sophisticated systems and laboratories for the testing and analysis of tablet dissolution. One of these laboratories is shown in Figure 5–36.

Methods of Preparation

The three basic methods for the preparation of compressed tablets are the *wet granulation method,* the *dry granulation method,* and *direct compression.* See Figure 5–37 for schematic drawings of each method. In addition to these three basic methods, recent technology has permitted the production of tablet granulations by the *fluid-bed process* (Figs. 5–38 and 5–39). The fluid-bed granulator performs the following three steps with a single piece of equipment: (1) preblending the formulation powder (including the active ingredients, diluents, disintegrants etc.), (2) granulating by means of a suitable liquid binder (e.g., aqueous solutions of acacia, hydroxypropyl cellulose, povidone, etc.), and (3) drying the granulated product to the desired moisture content. In the process, the dry powder mixture is first preblended in the granulating bowl by the fluidizing air. Then, the binding solution is sprayed

Fig. 5–36. *A modern computerized laboratory dedicated to studies of drug dissolution from solid dosage forms. Included are Erweka dissolution baths, Hewlett-Packard computers, and Hewlett-Packard diode assay spectrophotometers. (Courtesy of Elan Corporation, plc.)*

onto the fluidized powder at a specified rate forming the agglomerates of powder, or granules, which are then dried. This process is discussed later in this chapter.

Wet Granulation

Wet granulation is a widely employed method for the production of compressed tablets. The steps required in the preparation of tablets by this method may be separated as follows: (1) weighing and blending the ingredients, (2) preparing the wet granulation, (3) screening the damp mass into pellets or granules, (4) drying, (5) dry screening, (6) lubrication and blending, and (7) tableting by compression.

WEIGHING AND BLENDING. The active ingredient and any filler and disintegrating agent required in the tablet formulation are weighed in amounts required for the preparation of the number of tablets to be produced and are mixed thoroughly, generally in a motor-driven powder blender or mixer. Among the fillers used are lactose, microcrystalline cellulose, starch, powdered sucrose, and calcium phosphate. The selection of the filler is based partly on the experience of the manufacturer in the preparation of other tablets and also on its cost and compatibility with the other formulative ingredients. For example, calcium salts must not be employed as fillers in the preparation of tablets or capsules

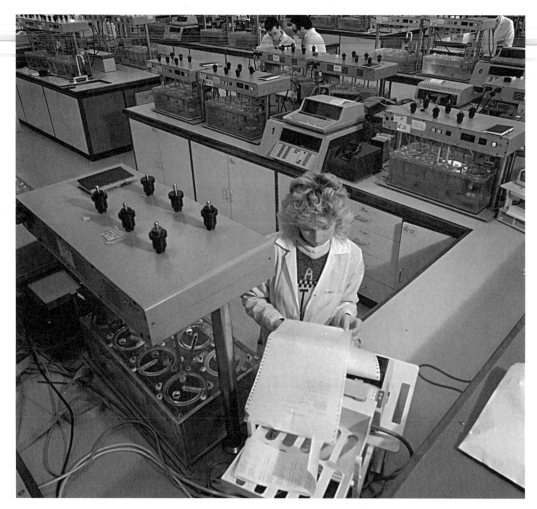

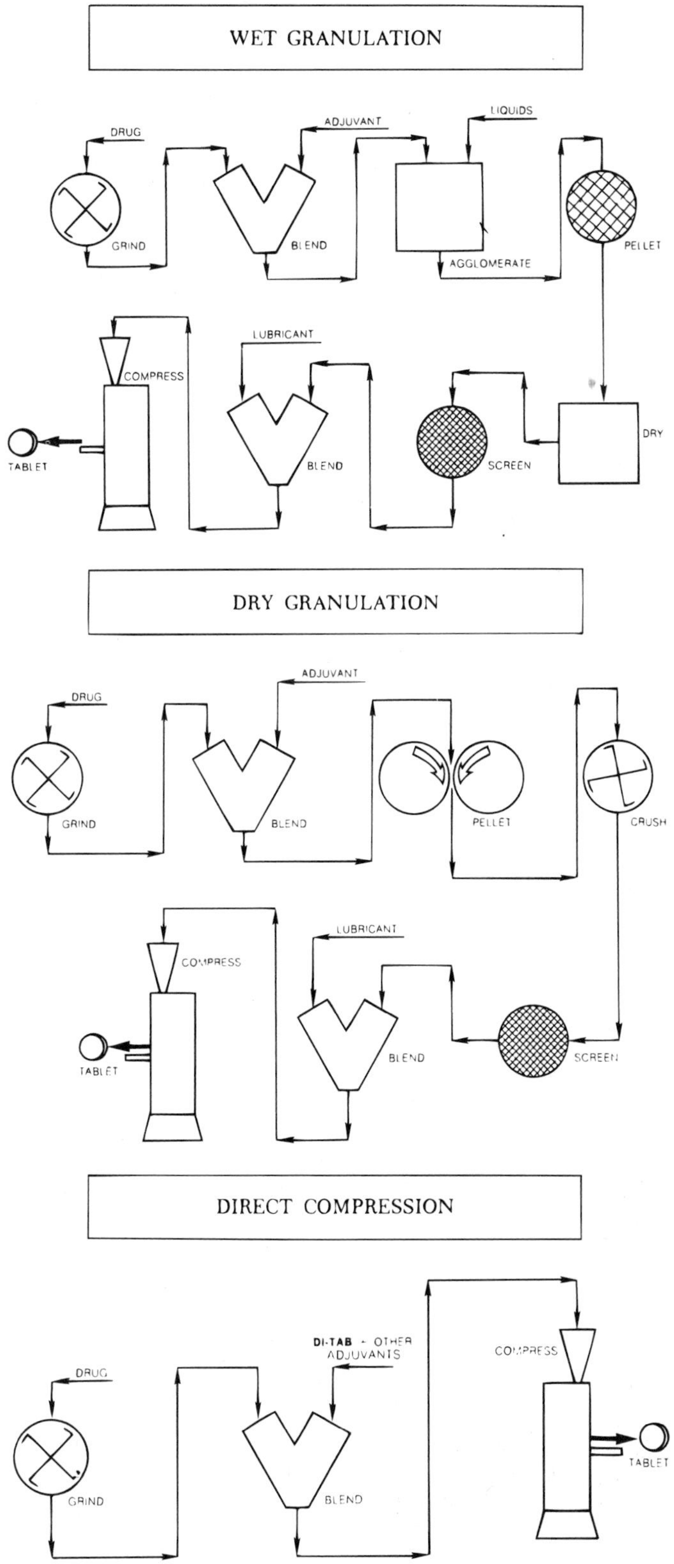

Fig. 5–37. *Schematic drawings of the three main methods for the preparation of tablets: wet granulation (top); dry granulation (center); direct compression (bottom). (Courtesy of Stauffer Chemical Co.)*

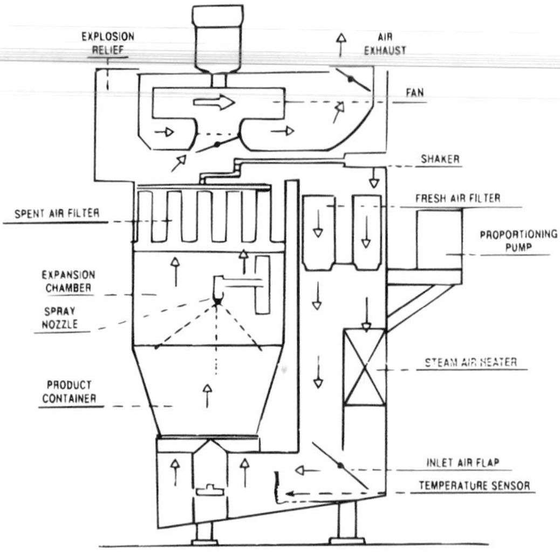

Fig. 5–38. *Cutaway view of a typical fluid bed granulator. (Courtesy of Ashok Y. Gore, Ph.D.* Pharmaceutical Technology, *Astor Publishing Co.).*

of tetracycline antibiotics, because the calcium interferes with the absorption of these drugs from the gastrointestinal tract. Industrially preferred fillers are lactose, because of its solubility and compatibility, and microcrystalline cellulose, because of its compactability, compatibility, and uniformity of supply.[15]

Disintegrating agents include corn and potato starches, starch derivatives such as sodium starch glycolate, croscarmellose, cellulose derivatives as sodium carboxymethylcellulose, polyvinyl polypyrolidone (PVPP), crospovidone, cation-exchange resins, and other materials that swell or expand on exposure to moisture and effect the rupture or breakup of the tablet after it enters the gastrointestinal tract. Industrially preferred tablet disintegrants are croscarmellose and sodium starch glycollate, based on their rapid action.[15] Results of water-sorption studies show that the disintegrants with the highest water uptake are generally the most effective in most tablet systems.[16] Sodium starch glycolate, crospovidone, and the cation exchange resins are particularly effective in the taking up of moisture. In studies of the mechanism of starch as a tablet disintegrant, it has been observed that the rupture of tablet surfaces occurs where agglomerates of starch grains were found and that tablet breakup probably results from the hydration of the hydroxy groups of the starch molecules causing them to move apart.[17] When starch is employed, 5% is usually suitable to promote disintegration, but up to about 20% may be used to promote more rapid tablet disintegration. Ten percent of starch, 5% of sodium starch glycollate, and 2% of croscarmellose are commonly used as tablet disintegrants.[15] The total amount of disintegrant is not always added to the drug-diluent mixture, but a portion (sometimes half of that used) is reserved for later addition, with the lubricant, to the prepared granulation of the drug. This process results in a double disintegration of the tablet—the first from that portion of the disintegrant added last and effecting the breakup of the tablets into small pieces or chunks of tablet and the second disintegration from the initial addition of disintegrant and breaking up the pieces of tablet into fine particles.

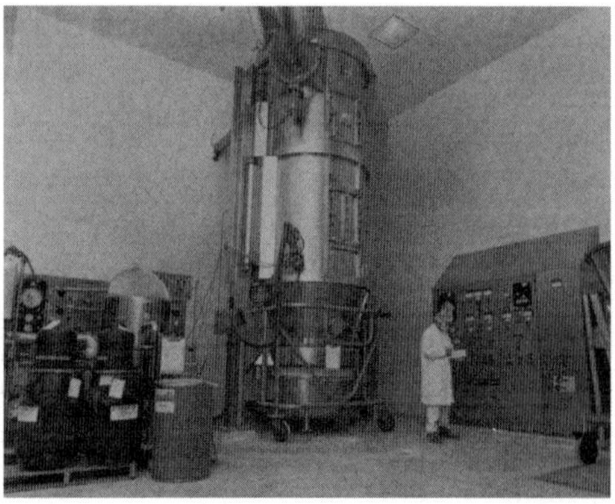

Fig. 5–39. *Example of fluid bed granulator. (Courtesy of Schering Laboratories.)*

Care must be exercised to achieve thorough mixing of the components to insure proper dosage administration as well as the uniform disintegration of all of the tablets produced. Sometimes the blended powders are passed through a sifter or a screen of appropriate fineness to eliminate clumps or compacts of powder.

PREPARING THE WET GRANULATION. For the powder mixture to flow evenly and freely from the hopper (the funnel-like container holding the drug to guide its flow into the machine for tableting) into the dies, it is usually necessary to convert the powder mixture to free-flowing granules called the *granulation.* This is accomplished by adding a liquid binder or an adhesive to the powder mixture, passing the wetted mass through a screen of the desired mesh size, drying the granulation, and then passing through a second screen of smaller mesh to reduce further the size of the granules. The binding agent present in the tablets also contributes to the adhesion of the granules to one another, maintaining the integrity of the tablet after compression. Among the binding agents used are a 10 to 20% aqueous preparation of corn starch, a 25 to 50% solution of glucose, molasses, various natural gums (as acacia), cellulose derivatives (as methylcellulose, carboxymethylcellulose and microcrystalline cellulose), gelatins, and povidone, with the latter preferred by many in industry.[15] If the drug substance is adversely affected by an aqueous binder, the binding agents may be nonaqueous or may be added dry. In general, the binding action is more effective when the adhesive is mixed with the powders in liquid form. The amount of binding agent used is part of the operator's art and is dependent upon the other formulative ingredients. However, an amount that will render the drug mixture moist enough so that the powder is compactible by squeezing in the hand is usually sufficient. Care must be exercised not to overwet or underwet the powder. Overwetting usually results in granules that are too hard for proper tableting; underwetting usually results in the preparation of tablets that are too soft and tend to crumble. If desired, a suitable colorant or flavorant may be added to the binding agent to prepare a colored or flavored granulation.

SCREENING THE DAMP MASS INTO PELLETS OR GRANULES. Generally the wet granulation is pressed through a No. 6- or 8-mesh screen. This may be done by hand or by special granulation equipment (Fig. 5–40), some of which prepares the granulation by extrusion through perforations in the apparatus. After all of the material has been converted into granules, the granulation is spread evenly on large pieces of paper in shallow trays and dried.

DRYING THE GRANULATION. Granules may be dried in special drying ovens that are thermostatically controlled and constantly measure and record time, temperature, and humidity (Fig. 5–41). Among the newer methods of drying in use today is *fluidization* conducted in *fluid bed*

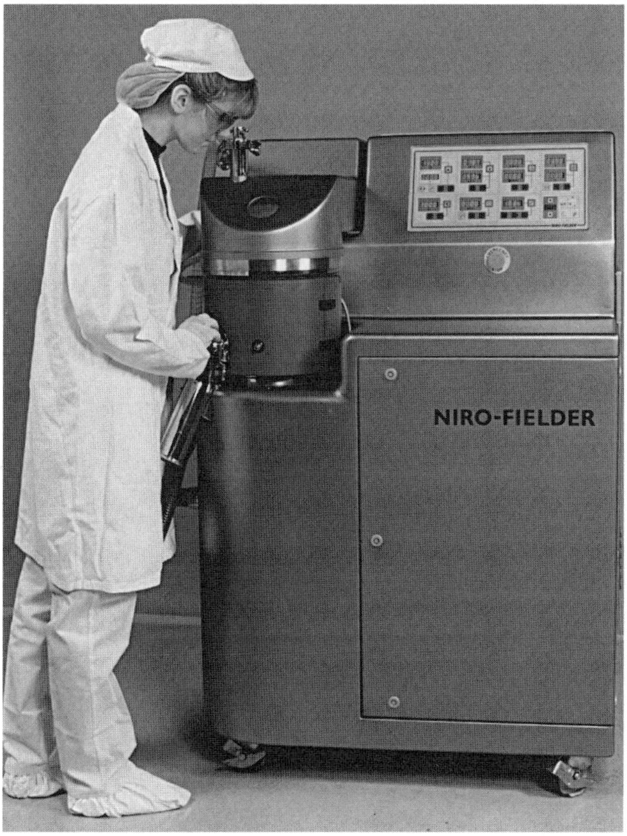

Fig. 5–40. *A laboratory-size vertical-shaft blender-granulator for preparing wet granulations for tablet manufacture. (Courtesy of Niro-Fielder, Inc.)*

Fig. 5–41. *Temperature controlled Casburt Drying Oven used in the preparation of granules and controlled release beads. (Courtesy of Elan Corporation, plc.)*

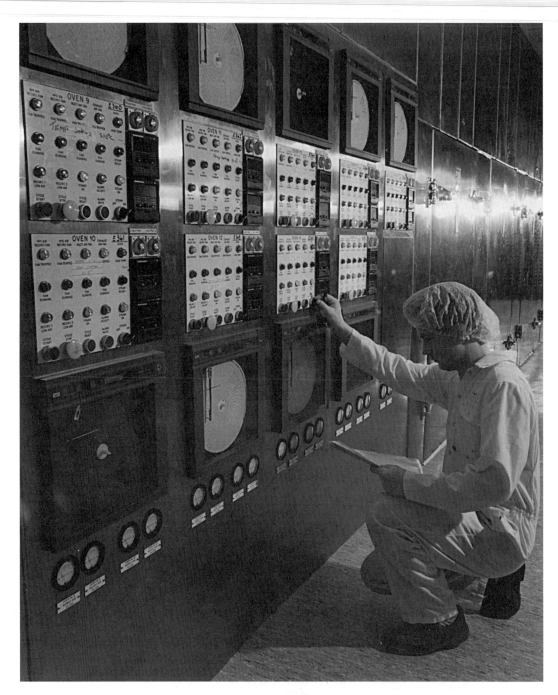

driers (Fig. 5–39). In this method the granules are dried by being suspended and agitated by a stream of warm air. If the effectiveness of the binder is dependent upon the presence of minute amounts of moisture, the granulation is not completely dried. However, an excessive amount of moisture remaining in a granulation is frequently the cause of ruptures occurring to coatings later placed on the compressed tablets.

DRY SCREENING. After drying, the granules are passed through a screen of a smaller mesh than that used to prepare the original granulation. The degree to which the granules are reduced depends upon the size of the punches to be used and the tablets to be produced. The proper selection is based on experience; however, in general, the smaller the tablet to be produced, the smaller are the granules used to produce it. Screens from 12- to 20-mesh size are generally used for this purpose. Sizing of the granules is necessary so that the small die cavity for the production of small tablets may be completely filled by the flowing granulation. The voids or air spaces left by a large granulation in a small die cavity would likely result in the production of tablets of varying evenness.

LUBRICATION. After dry screening, a dry lubricant is generally added to the granulation. So that each granule is covered with lubricant, it may be dusted over the spread-out granulation through a fine mesh screen or blended in a powder mixer. Among the more commonly used lubricants are talc, magnesium stearate, stearic acid, and calcium stearate, but many other agents are occasionally employed. Magnesium stearate is by far the most-used tablet lubricant.[15] One of the reasons cited for the effectiveness of magnesium stearate as a lubricant is its tendency during tablet compression to migrate towards the die wall interface, resulting in a high concentration at the curved tablet surface.[18] The quantity of lubricant used varies from one tableting operation to another and may range from a low of about 0.1% of the weight of the granulation to as much as 5%. Lubricants contribute to the preparation of compressed tablets in several ways; they improve the flow of the granulation in the hopper to the die cavity, they prevent the adhesion of the tablet formulation to the punches and dies during compression, they reduce friction between the tablet and the die wall during the tablet's ejection from the tablet machine, and they give a sheen to the finished tablet.

TABLETING. There are a number of types of tablet presses or tableting machines, each varying in its productivity but similar in its basic operation. That operation is the compression of the tablet granulation within a steel die cavity by the pressure exerted by the movement of two steel punches, a lower punch and an upper punch.

There are single-punch tablet machines, some hand operated and some motor driven, which are capable of producing a single tablet upon completion of each up and down movement of the set of punches. As the lower punch drops, the feed shoe filled with granulation (from the hopper) is positioned over the die cavity which then fills. The feed shoe then retracts, scraping the excessive granulation from the stage and leveling the layer of granulation in the die cavity. The upper punch lowers and compresses the material in the die cavity to form the tablet. The upper punch then retracts, and the lower punch rise to the precise level of the stage, lifting the tablet to be ejected from the stage by the feed shoe which moves over the die cavity once again to repeat the process. The tablet is ejected into a barrel or other suitable container. The first few tablets collected, as well as some tablets prepared during the course of production, are examined for weight variation, hardness, thickness, and disintegration, and the necessary adjustments are made in the volume of fill or the pressure of compression to prepare tablets of the desired quality.

Ordinary rotary tablet machines and high speed rotary tablet machines equipped with multiple punches and dies operate through the continuous rotating movement of the punches and continuous tablet compression (Figs. 5–42

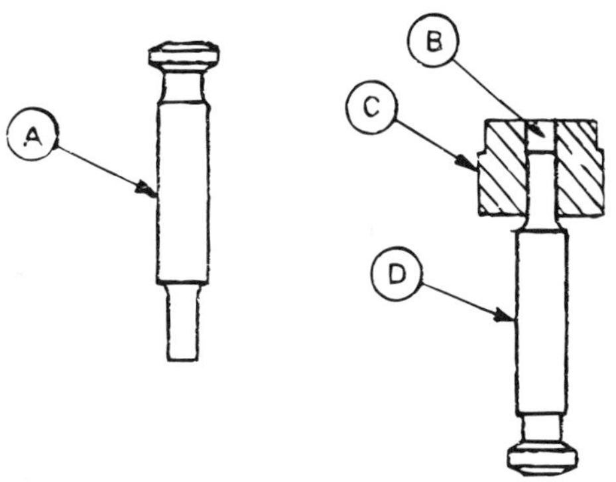

Fig. 5–42. *Punch and die set: (A) upper punch, (B) die cavity, (C) die, and (D) lower punch. (Courtesy of Cherry-Burrell Corporation.)*

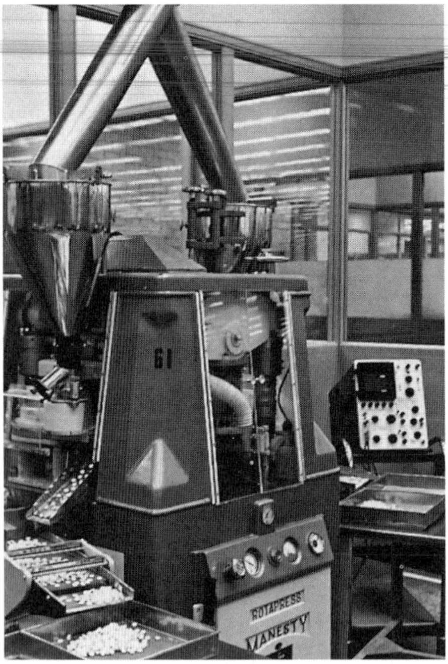

Fig. 5–43. *Manesty Rotapress rotary compression machine making compressed tablets. Tablets leaving the machine run over a tablet duster to screen where they are inspected. Material to be compressed is being fed from overhead hopper through yoke to each of the two compressing machine hoppers. Hardness of tablet is monitored electronically by oscilloscope at the right. (Courtesy of The Upjohn Company.)*

and 5–43). In contrast to the single punch tablet machines generally having a capacity of about 100 tablets per minute, a single rotary press with 16 stations (16 sets of punches and dies) may produce up to 1150 tablets per minute. Double rotary tablet presses with 27, 33, 37, 41, or 49 sets of punches and dies are capable of producing 2 tablets for each die for each complete revolution of the die head because of having two tableting mechanisms. Some of these machines can produce 10,000 and more tablets per minute of operation (Fig. 5–44). For such high speed production, induced die feeders are required (Fig. 5–45). These induced feeders force granulation into the dies by the rotary action of an agitator. This feeding is much more rapid than standard gravity feeding and is necessary for the fast production rates achieved with these tableting machines. A consequence of high-speed production is the increased occurrence of *lamination* (horizontal striations) and tablet *capping,* in which the top of the tablet separates from the whole. The root cause is that the fill material simply does not have enough time to bond after compression. Reduced tableting speed is commonly used to remedy the problem.[19]

As indicated earlier, tablet machines have been developed to form multiple-layered tablets by the multiple feed and multiple compression of fill material within a single die. Also, a layer of material can be compressed onto a tablet core placed strategically and automatically in the die by a special feed apparatus using a special tableting machine.

All-In-One Granulation Methods

Recent technologic advances have allowed the mixing, wetting, agglomeration, and drying of tableting materials in a continuous process, all within a single piece of equipment.

FLUID-BED PROCESS. The *fluid-bed granulator,* depicted in Figure 5–39, performs the following steps within a single piece of equipment: (1) preblending the formulation powder, including active ingredients, fillers, disintegrants, in a bed by fluidized air, (2) granulating by spraying onto the fluidized powder bed, a suitable liquid binder, as an aqueous solution of acacia, hydroxypropyl cellulose, or povidone, and (3) drying the granulated product to the desired moisture content.

MICROWAVE VACUUM PROCESSING. As in the fluid-bed process, the powders to be tableted are mixed, wetted, agglomerated, and dried within the confines of a single piece of equipment (Fig. 5–46). The wet mass is dried by gentle mixing, vacuum, and microwave. The use of the microwave for the drying process reduces the drying time considerably, often by one-fourth. The total-batch production time is usually in the range of 90 minutes. After adding lubricants and screening, the batch is ready for tableting or capsule filling. The typical microwave vacuum process may be adapted to a coating application as well.

Dry Granulation

In the dry granulation method the granulation is formed not by moistening or adding a binding agent to the powdered drug mixture but by compacting large masses of the mixture and subsequently crushing and sizing these pieces into smaller granules (see Fig. 5–37). By this method, either the active ingredient or the diluent must have cohesive properties in order for the large masses to be formed. This method is especially

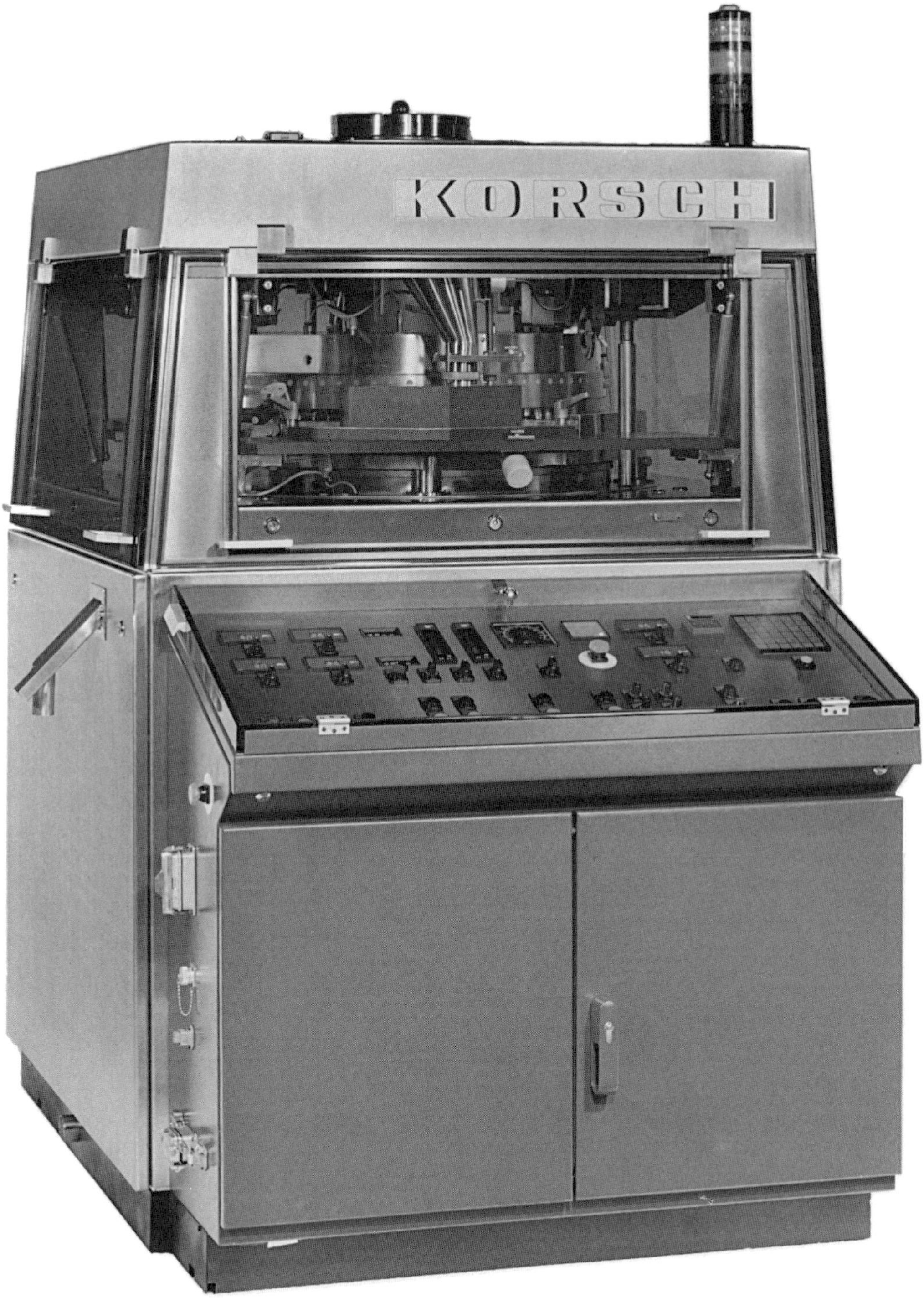

Fig. 5–44. *An example of a high-performance double rotary tablet press. The Korsch Pharmapress® has a maximum output of 1 million tablets per hour but for continuous operation it is generally run to produce 600,000 to 800,000 tablets per hour. (Courtesy of Korsch Tableting, Inc.)*

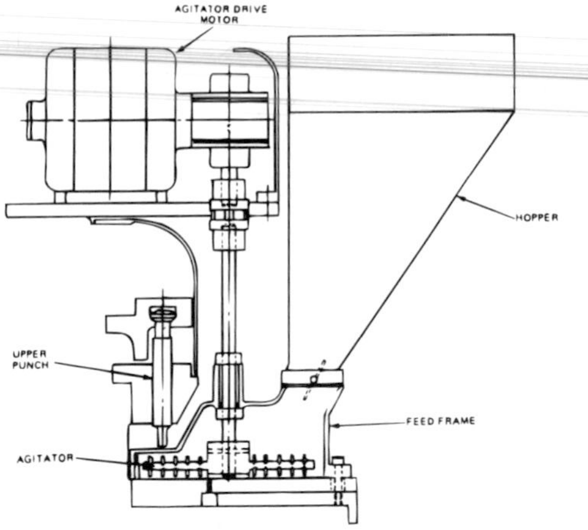

Fig. 5–45. *Induced die feeder. The standard gravity-fed open feed frame can be replaced with an induced die feeder. Using this accessory, granulation is forced into the die by the rotary action of the agitator. (Courtesy of Cherry-Burrell Corporation.)*

applicable to materials that cannot be prepared by the wet granulation method due to their degradation by moisture or to the elevated temperatures required for drying.

After weighing and mixing the ingredients in the same manner as in the wet granulation method, the powder is "slugged" or compressed into large flat tablets or pellets of about 1 inch in diameter. It is possible to do this because the flow of the powder into the slugging machine is facilitated by the large cavity and the tablets need not be of exact size or weight. The slugs must be hard enough to be broken up without producing an excessive amount of powder. The slugs are broken up by hand or by a mill (Fig. 5–47) and passed through a screen of desired mesh for sizing. Lubricant is added in the usual manner, and tablets are prepared by compression. Aspirin, which is hydrolyzed on exposure to moisture, is commonly prepared into tablets after slugging. Instead of the slugging method, compaction mills may be used to increase the density of a powder by pressing it between high-pressure rollers. The densified material is then broken up, sized, and lubricated, and tablets are prepared by compression in the usual manner.

Direct Compression

Some granular chemicals like potassium chloride and methenamine possess free flowing as well as cohesive properties that enable them to be compressed directly in a tablet machine without need of either wet or dry granulation. In past years the number of medicinal substances that could be tableted without prior granulation was quite small. Today the use of special pharmaceutical excipients imparts to certain tablet formulations the required qualities for tablet production by direct compression, and many additional products may now be produced in this manner. In the direct-compression of tablets, the tableting excipients used must be materials with properties of fluidity and compressibility. Tableting excipients having the desired characteristics include: *fillers*—spray-dried lactose, microcrystals of alpha-monohydrate lactose, sucrose-invert sugar-corn starch mixtures (NuTab, Ingredient Technology Corp.), microcrystalline cellulose, and dicalcium phosphate (Di-Tab, Stauffer Chemical Co.); *disintegrating agents*—direct-compression starch (Starch 1500, Colorcon, Inc.), sodium carboxymethyl starch, cross-linked carboxymethylcellulose fibers (Ac-Di-Sol, FMC Corp.), and cross-linked polyvinylpyrrolidone; *lubricants*—magnesium stearate and talc; and *glidants*—fumed silicon dioxide (Cab-O-Sil, Cabot Corp.).[20]

In addition to the use of special excipients, forced or induced feeders which have been developed permit the preparation of certain additional tablets by direct compression because the deaerating action of the feeder on light, bulky powders makes them more dense and permits them to flow evenly and completely into the die cavities under moderate pressure. This deaeration also eliminates air entrapment within the die as the tablets are compressed, thereby reducing a major cause of *capping* (loose at the top like a "cap") or splitting of tablets upon compression.

The capping or splitting of tablets may be caused by a number of factors and is not limited to tablets prepared by direct compression. For instance punches that are not immaculately clean and perfectly smooth may result in capped tablets. Too much pressure on compression can cause capping, as can a granulation which is too soft. Generally there is a portion of "fines" or a fine powder which results when the dry granulation is sized and generally amounts to 10 to 20% of the weight of the granulation and is necessary to properly fill the die cavity. However, an excess of these fines can also lead to capping. When a large quantity of air is trapped in the tablet, a condition called *laminating* results. The tablets appear split and cracked around the sides caused

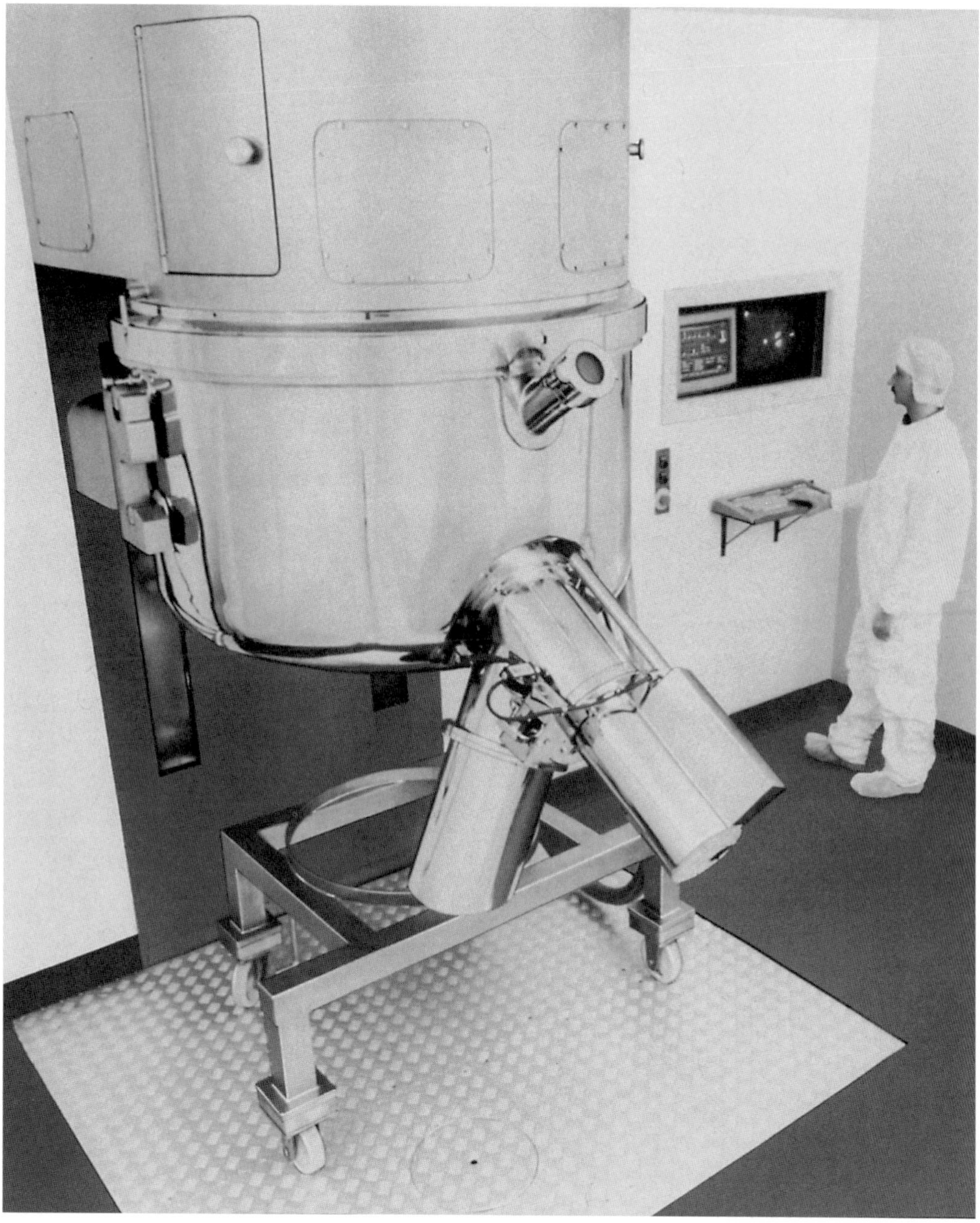

Fig. 5–46. *Microwave vacuum processing in which tableting ingredients are dry mixed, wetted with a binding liquid, and dried by vacuum and microwave within a single piece of equipment. (Courtesy of GEI Processing, Inc.)*

by expansion when the pressure of tableting is released. Figure 5–48 shows tablets which have split. Tablets which have aged (usually beyond the expiration date) may exhibit splitting or other physical deformation.

Tablet Dedusting

To remove traces of loose powder adhering to tablets following compression, the tablets are conveyed directly from the tableting machine to

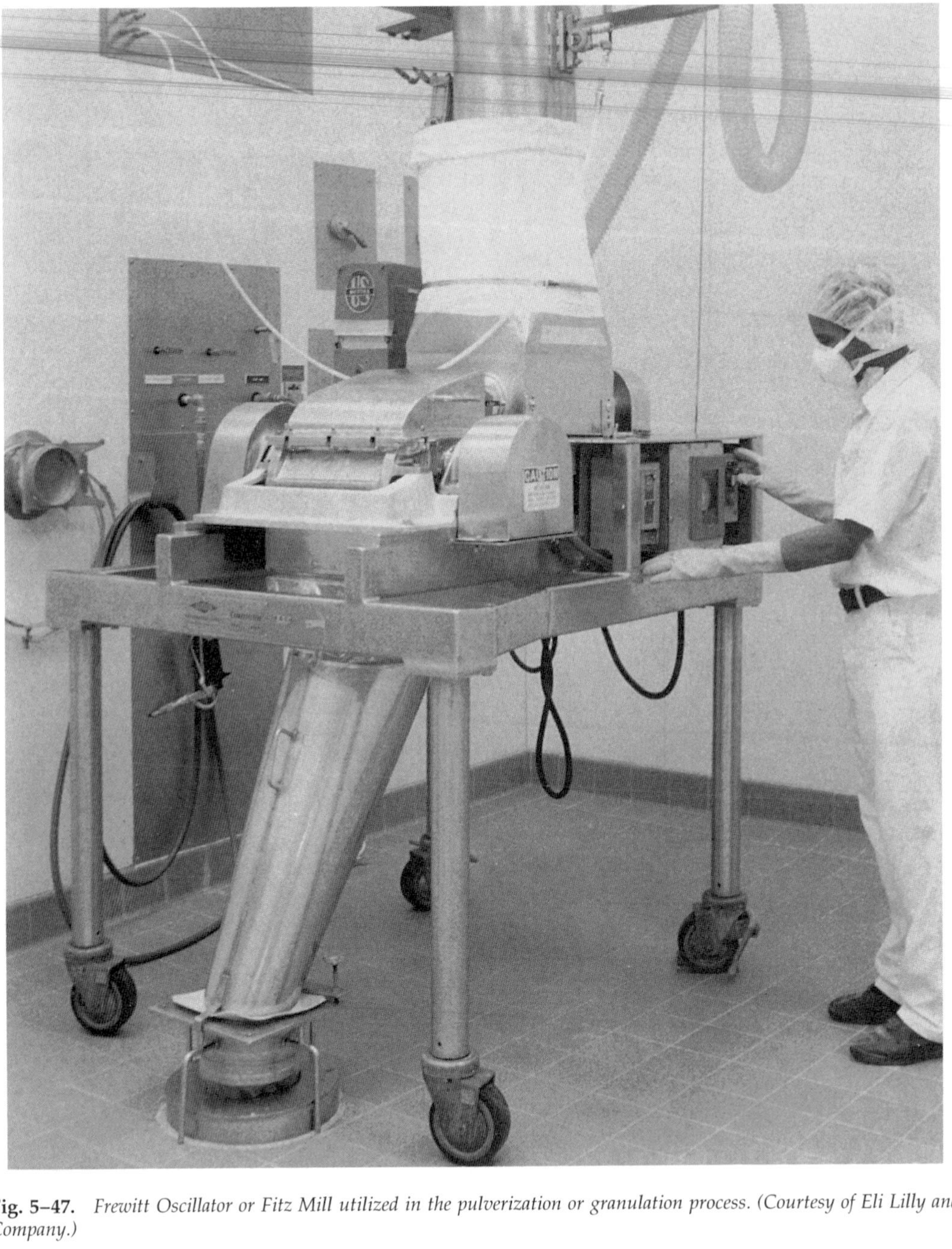

Fig. 5–47. *Frewitt Oscillator or Fitz Mill utilized in the pulverization or granulation process. (Courtesy of Eli Lilly and Company.)*

a tablet deduster. An example of this type of apparatus are shown in Figure 5–49.

Tablet Coating

Tablets are coated for a number of reasons, including the protection of the medicinal agent against destructive exposure to air and/or humidity; to mask the taste of the drug upon swallowing; to provide special characteristics of drug release (e.g., enteric coatings); and to provide aesthetics or distinction to the product.

Some tablets are coated to prevent inadvertent contact with the drug substance and the conse-

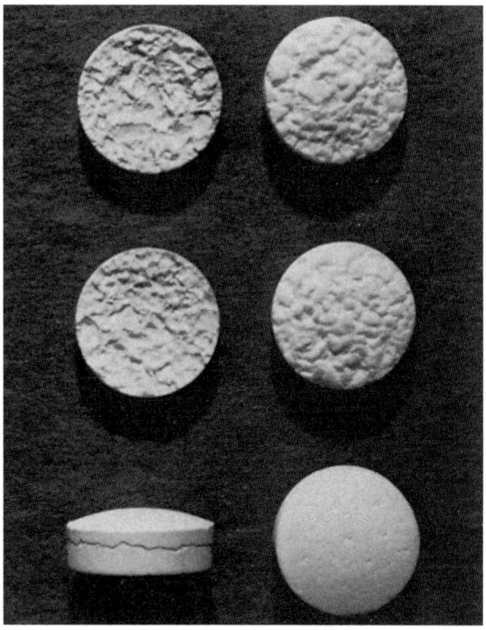

Fig. 5–48. *Tablets which have split on aging, due to conditions of manufacture or storage.*

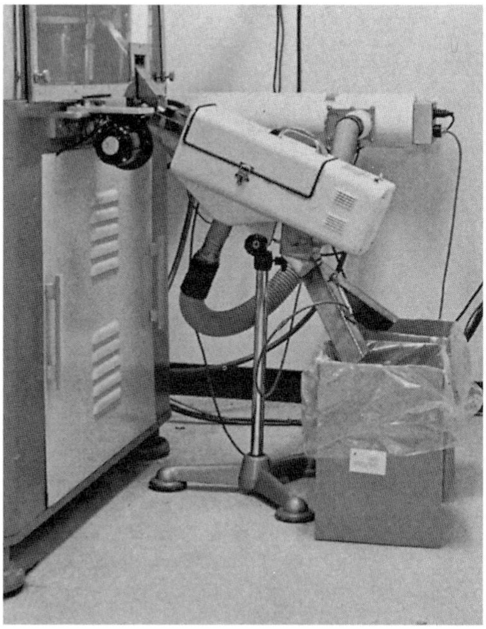

Fig. 5–49. *Model 25 Manesty Tablet Deduster. Tablets leaving tableting machine are dedusted and passed into collection containers. (Courtesy of Eli Lilly and Company.)*

quent effects of drug absorption. Proscar (finasteride, Merck) tablets, for example, are coated for just this reason. The drug is used by men in the treatment of benign prostatic hyperplasia. The labeling instructions warn that women who are pregnant or who could become pregnant should not come into contact with the drug. Drug contact can occur through the handling of broken tablets or through sexual contact, by virtue of traces of drug in semen. If finasteride is absorbed by a woman who is pregnant with a male baby, the drug has the capacity to cause abnormalities in the child's sex organs.

The general methods involved in coating tablets are as follows.

Sugarcoating Tablets

The sugarcoating of tablets may be divided into the following steps: (1) waterproofing and sealing (if needed), (2) subcoating, (3) smoothing and final rounding, (4) finishing and coloring (if desired), and (5) polishing. Generally the entire coating process is conducted in a series of mechanically operated coating pans, which are acorn-shaped vessels of galvanized iron, stainless steel, or copper partially open in the front and with diameters ranging from about 1 to 4 feet and therefore of various capacities (Figs. 5–50 and 5–51). The smaller pans are used for experimental, developmental, and pilot plant operations; the larger pans, for industrial production. The pans are fixed and operate at about a 40° angle, which permits the tablets to remain inside the pan during its revolutions yet also permits the operator to observe and handle the tablets from the open end of the pan. During each of the operations involved in the coating of tablets, the pan is rotated by a motor at moderate speeds, allowing the tablets to tumble and roll about in the pan and make contact with each other and with the coating solutions. As they rotate, the coating solution is gently poured or sprayed onto the tablets in portions, with warm air introduced to hasten the drying of the coat. Tablets may require a number of coats of material, with each coat applied only after the previous coat has dried. Tablets intended to be coated are generally compressed tablets that have been prepared to be highly convex and have as thin an edge as possible to permit the coatings to form rounded rather than angular edges.

WATERPROOFING AND SEALING COATS. For tablets containing components that may absorb moisture or be adversely affected on contact with

Fig. 5–50. *Tablet coating, an older style coating pan, showing the warm air supply and the exhaust. (Courtesy of Wyeth Laboratories.)*

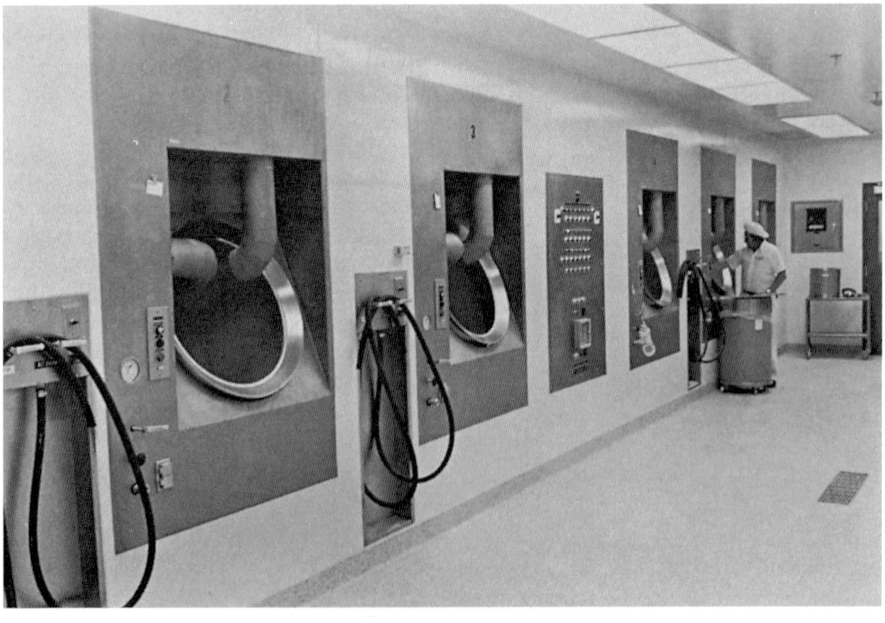

Fig. 5–51. *Modern tablet coating facility. Air and exhaust ducts to assist drying are automatically operated from central board. (Courtesy of Eli Lilly and Company.)*

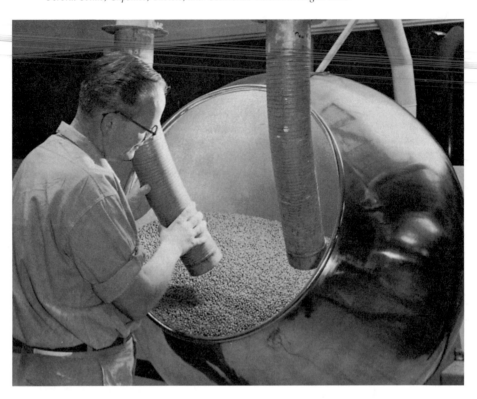

moisture, a waterproofing layer or coating of a material such as shellac is placed on the compressed tablets before the subcoating application. The shellac or other waterproofing agent is applied in solution (usually alcoholic) form and is gently poured on the compressed tablets rotating in the coating pans or is sprayed on as a fine spray. Warm air is blown into the pan during the coating to hasten the drying and to prevent tablets from sticking together. A second coat of the waterproofing substance may be added to the tablets after the first coat has dried to ensure against moisture penetration into the compressed tablets.

SUBCOATING. After the waterproofing or sealing coats (if they are necessary) have been applied, the tablets are given about 3 to 5 subcoats of a sugar-based syrup for the purpose of rounding the tablets and bonding the sugar coating to the compressed tablet. In applying the subcoating, a heavy syrup generally containing gelatin or polyvinylpyrollidone (PVP), or sometimes acacia is added to the tablets as they roll in the coating pan. When the tablets are partially dry they are sprinkled with a dusting powder, which is usually a mixture of powdered sugar and starch but may also contain talc, acacia, or precipitated chalk. Warm air is applied to the rolling tablets, and when they are dry, the subcoating process is repeated and repeated again until the tablets are of the desired shape and size (Fig. 5–52). At this point, the tablets are usually removed from the coating pan, the excess powder is shaken off the tablets by gently jostling them on a cloth screen, and the coating pan is then washed to remove extraneous coating material.

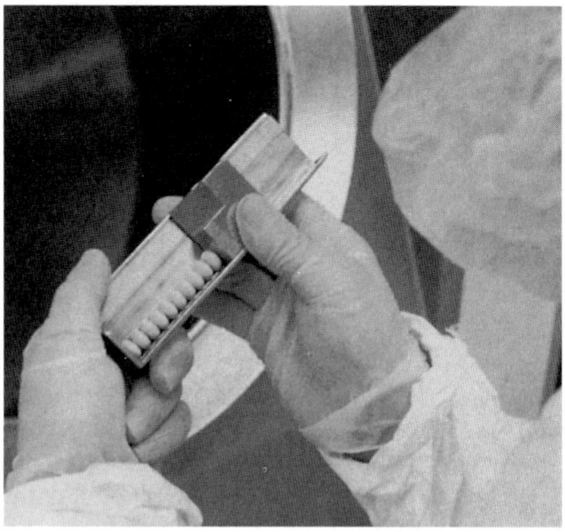

Fig. 5–52. *Tablet gauge used to measure the size of coated tablets. (Courtesy of Eli Lilly and Company.)*

SMOOTHING AND FINAL ROUNDING. After the tablets have been subcoated to the desired shape (roundness), 5 to 10 additional coatings of a very thick syrup are applied to the rolling tablets for the purpose of completing the rounding of the tablets and smoothing the coatings. This syrup may be composed of a sucrose-based simple syrup, or it may have additional components like starch and calcium carbonate. As the syrup is applied, the operator moves his hand through the rolling tablets to distribute the syrup and to prevent the sticking of the tablets to one another. A dusting powder may or may not be used between syrup applications, but warm air is generally applied to hasten the drying time of each coat. If the coating is to be colored, the suitable dye may be added to the syrup during this step of the coating process as well as during the next step.

FINISHING AND COLORING. To attain final smoothness and the appropriate color to the tablets, several coats of a thin syrup containing the desired colorant (if any) are applied. This step is usually performed in a clean pan, free from previous coating materials.

IMPRINTING. Solid dosage forms may be passed through special imprinting machines (Fig. 5–53) to impart identification codes and other distinctive symbols. By FDA regulation, effective in 1995, all solid dosage forms for human consumption, including both prescription-only and over-the-counter drug products, must be imprinted with product-specific identification codes. Some exemptions to this requirement are allowed, namely: solid dosage forms used in most clinical investigations; drugs that are extemporaneously compounded in the course of pharmacy practice; radiopharmaceutical drug products; and products that, because of their size, shape, texture or other physical characteristics, make imprinting technologically infeasible.

Code imprints, in conjunction with a product's size, shape, and color, permit the unique identification of a drug product and its manufacturer or distributor. Code imprints may contain any combination of letters and numbers, or the product's National Drug Code number, and any marks, symbols, logos, or monograms assigned by the drug company to the product. Each product's imprint must be registered with the FDA.

Technically, the imprint may be *debossed, em-*

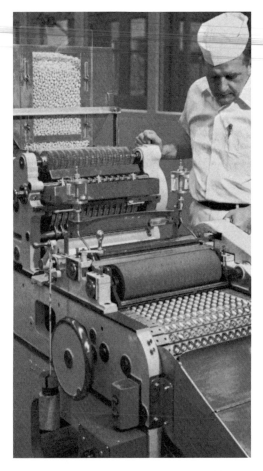

Fig. 5–53. *Branding of coated compression tablets on a Hartnett branding machine. (Courtesy of The Upjohn Company.)*

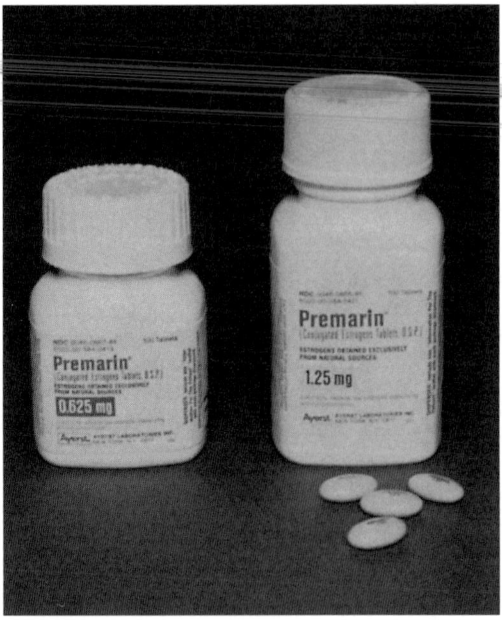

Fig. 5–54. *Example of coated, polished, and monogrammed tablets. (Courtesy of Wyeth-Ayerst Laboratories.)*

bossed, engraved, or printed on the surface with ink. *Debossed* means imprinted with a mark below the dosage form surface; *embossed* means imprinted with a mark raised above the dosage form surface; and *engraved* means imprinted with a code that is cut into the dosage form surface after it has been fabricated.

POLISHING. Coated tablets may be polished in special drum-shaped pans made by stretching a cloth fabric over a metal frame or in ordinary coating pans lined with canvas. The fabric or the canvas may be impregnated with a wax such as carnauba wax with or without the addition of beeswax and the tablets polished as they roll about in the pan. Or, the wax may be dissolved in a nonaqueous solvent such as acetone or petroleum benzin and sprayed on the rolling tablets in small amounts. After each coat has dried, the addition of a small amount of talc to the tumbling tablets contributes to their high luster (Fig. 5–54). Two or three coats of wax may be applied depending upon the desired gloss. Another method of polishing tablets simply involves placing pieces of wax in the polishing pan along with the tablets and permitting the tablets to tumble over the wax until the desired sheen is attained.

Film-Coating Tablets

As one can ascertain from the previous discussion of sugarcoating, the process is not only tedious and time-consuming, requiring the expertise of a highly skilled technician, but it also results in the preparation of coated tablets that may be twice the size and weight of the original uncoated compressed tablets. These factors are important to a manufacturer in his consideration of the expense of both packaging materials and shipping. From a patient's point of view, large tablets are not as convenient to swallow as are small tablets. Also, the coating of tablets by the application of the sugarcoating may vary slightly from batch to batch and within the batch. The film-coating process, which places a thin, skin-tight coating of a plastic-like material over the compressed tablet, was developed to produce coated tablets having essentially the same weight, shape, and size as the originally compressed tablet. The coating is thin enough to reveal any depressed or raised monograms punched into the tablet by the tablet punches. In addition, film-coated tablets are far more resistant to destruction by abrasion than are sugar-coated tablets, and like sugar-coated tablets, the coating may be colored to make the tablets attractive and distinctive.

Film-coating solutions may be nonaqueous or aqueous. The nonaqueous solutions generally contain the following types of materials to provide the desired coating to the tablets:

1. A *film former* capable of producing smooth, thin films reproducible under conventional coating conditions and applicable to a variety of tablet shapes. Example: cellulose acetate phthalate.
2. An *alloying substance* providing water solubility or permeability to the film to ensure penetration by body fluids and therapeutic availability of the drug. Example: polyethylene glycol.
3. A *plasticizer* to produce flexibility and elasticity of the coating and thus provide durability. Example: castor oil.
4. A *surfactant* to enhance spreadability of the film during application. Example: polyoxyethylene sorbitan derivatives.
5. *Opaquants* and *colorants* to make the appearance of the coated tablets handsome and distinctive. Examples: Opaquant, titanium dioxide; colorant, F.D.&C. or D.&C. dyes.
6. *Sweeteners, flavors,* and *aromas* to enhance the acceptability of the tablet to the patient. Examples: sweeteners, saccharin; flavors and aromas, vanillin.
7. A *glossant* to provide luster to the tablets without a separate polishing operation. Example: beeswax.
8. A *volatile solvent* to allow the spread of the other components over the tablets while allowing rapid evaporation to permit an effective yet speedy operation. Example: alcohol-acetone mixture.

Tablets are film coated by the application or spraying of the film-coating solution upon the tablets in ordinary coating pans. The volatility of the solvent enables the film to adhere quickly to the surface of the tablets.

Due to both the expense of the volatile solvents used in the film-coating process and the problem of the release of these potentially toxic agents into the atmosphere, the high cost of solvent recovery systems, and their explosiveness, pharmaceutical manufacturers are favoring the use of aqueous-based film-coating solutions. One of the problems attendant to these, however, is the slow evaporation of the water-base compared to the volatile organic solvent-based film-coating solutions. One commercially available (to the pharmaceutical industry) water-based, colloidal coating dispersion, is called AQUACOAT® (FMC Corporation) and contains a 30% ethyl cellulose pseudolatex. Pseudolatex dispersions have the advantage of high solids content (for greater coating ability) and relatively low viscosity. The low viscosity allows less water to be used in the coating dispersion, resulting in a lesser requirement for water-evaporation and a reduced likelihood of water interference with the tablet formulation. In addition, the low viscosity permits greater coat penetration into the crevices of monogrammed or scored tablets. In using the pseudolatex coating dispersion, a plasticizer is incorporated to assist in the production of a denser, less-permeable film, with higher gloss and greater mechanical strength. Other aqueous systems utilized to film-coat tablets include the use of cellulosic materials as methylcellulose, hydroxypropyl cellulose, and hydroxypropyl methylcellulose.

A typical aqueous film-coating formulation contains the following:[21]

1. *Film-forming polymer* (7–18%). Examples: cellulose ether polymers as hydroxypropyl methylcellulose, hydroxypropyl cellulose, and methylcellulose.
2. *Plasticizer* (0.5–2.0%). Examples: glycerin, propylene glycol, polyethylene glycol, and dibutyl subacetate.
3. *Colorant and opacifier* (2.5–8%). Examples: FD&C or D&C Lakes and iron oxide pigments.
4. *Vehicle* (water, to make 100%).

There are some problems attendant to aqueous film-coating, including: the appearance of small amounts *(picking)* or larger amounts *(peeling)* of film fragments flaking from the tablet surface; roughness of the tablet surface due to failure of spray droplets to coalesce *(orange peel effect);* an uneven distribution of color on the tablet surface *(mottling);* filling-in of the score-line or indented logo on the tablet by the film *(bridging);* and the disfiguration of the core tablet when subjected for too long a period of time to the coating solution (tablet *erosion*). The cause of each of these problems can be determined and rectified through appropriate changes in formulation, equipment, technique or process.[21]

Enteric Coating

The purpose of enteric coating for solid dosage forms has already been discussed. The design of an enteric coating may be based upon the transit time required for the passage of the dosage form from the stomach into the intestines. This may be accomplished through coatings of sufficient thickness to resist dissolution in the stomach. More usually, an enteric coating is based upon the pH of the environment, being designed to resist dissolution in the highly acid environment of the stomach but yielding to the less acid environment of the intestine. Some enteric coatings are designed to dissolve at pH 4.8 and greater.

Enteric coating materials may be applied to either whole compressed tablets or to drug particles or granules used in the subsequent fabrication of tablets or capsules. The coatings may be applied in multiple portions to build a thick coating or they may be applied as a thin film coat. The coating systems may be aqueous-based or organic-solvent–based so long as the coating material resists breakdown in the gastric fluid.

Among the materials used in enteric coatings are shellac, hydroxypropyl methylcellulose phthalate, polyvinyl acetate phthalate, and cellulose acetate phthalate.

Fluid-Bed or Air Suspension Coating

This process, utilizing equipment of the type shown in Figure 5–55, involves the spray coating of pellets, beads, granules, powders, or tablets held in suspension by a column of air. The fluid bed processing equipment used is multifunctional and may be used in preparing tablet granulations as well, as noted earlier in this chapter.

In the Wurster process, named after its developer, the items to be coated are fed into a vertical cylinder and are supported by a column of air that enters from the bottom of the cylinder. Within the air stream, the solids rotate both vertically and horizontally. As the coating solution enters the system from the bottom, it is rapidly placed on the suspended, rotating solids, with rounding coats being applied in less than an hour with the assistance of warm air blasts released in the chamber.

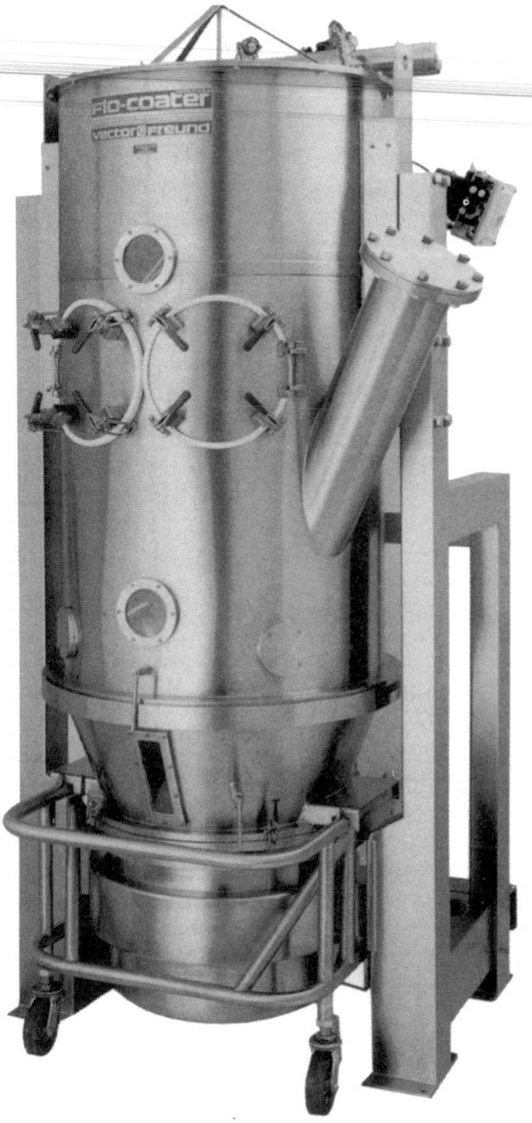

Fig. 5–55. *Vector/Freund Flo-Coater production system. A fluid bed system used in the application of coatings to beads, granules, powders, and tablets. Capacity of models ranges from 5 kg to 700 kg. (Courtesy of Vector Corporation.)*

In another type of fluidized bed system, the coating solution is sprayed downward onto the particles to be coated as they are suspended by air from below. This method is commonly referred to as the *top-spray* method. This method provided greater capacity, up to 1500 kg, than do the other air suspension coating methods.[22] Both the top-spray and bottom-spray methods

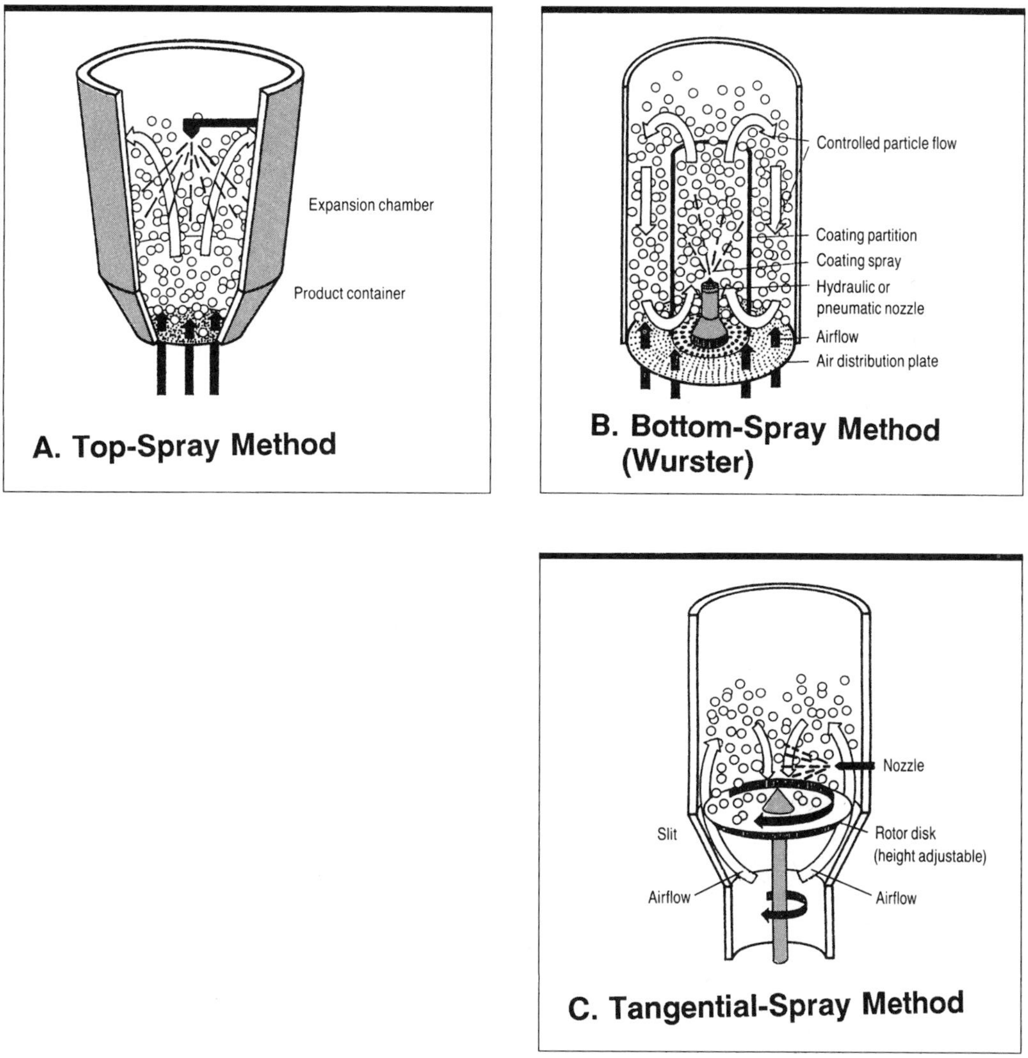

Fig. 5–56. *(A) Top-spray, (B) bottom-spray (Wurster), and (C) tangential-spray methods in the fluid-bed coating of solid particles. (Courtesy of Glatt Air Techniques, Inc.)*

may be employed using a modified apparatus used for fluidized bed granulation. A third method, the *tangential-spray technique*, is used in rotary fluid-bed coaters. The bottom-, top-, and tangential-spray methods are depicted in Figure 5–56.

The three systems are increasingly used for the application of aqueous- or organic-solvent–based polymers as film coatings. The top-spray coating method is particularly recommended for taste masking, enteric release, and barrier films on particles or tablets. The method is most effective when coatings are applied from aqueous solutions, latexes, or hotmelts.[22,23] The bottom-spray coating method is recommended for sustained-release and enteric-release products; and the tangential method for layering coatings, and for sustained-release and enteric-coated products.[23]

Among the variables requiring control in order to produce product of desired and consistent quality are: equipment used and the method of spraying (e.g., top, bottom, tangential), spray-nozzle distance from spraying bed, spray (droplet) size, spray rate, spray pressure, volume of fluidization air, batch size, method(s) and time for drying, air temperature and moisture content in processing compartment.[23]

Compression Coating

In a manner similar to the preparation of multiple compressed tablets having an inner core and an outer shell of drug material, core tablets may be sugarcoated by compression. The coating material in the form of a granulation or a powder is compressed onto a tablet core of drug with a special tablet press. This method eliminates the time-consuming and tedious operation previously described in this section. Compression coating is an anhydrous operation and thus may be safely employed in the coating of tablets having a drug that is sensitive to moisture. The resulting coat is more uniform than the usual sugarcoating applied using pans, and less of a coating is required. Resulting tablets are lighter and smaller and are therefore easier to swallow and less expensive to package and ship.

Irrespective of the method used in coating, all tablets are visually or electronically inspected for physical imperfections (Fig. 5–57).

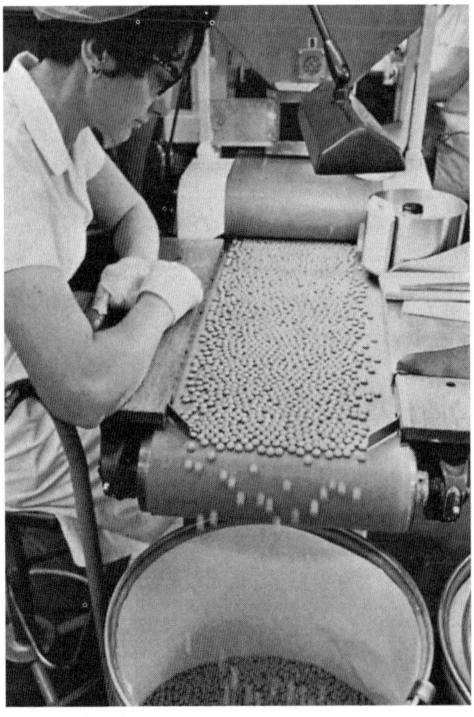

Fig. 5–57. *Checking for physical imperfections in coated tablets. (Courtesy of Smith, Kline & French.)*

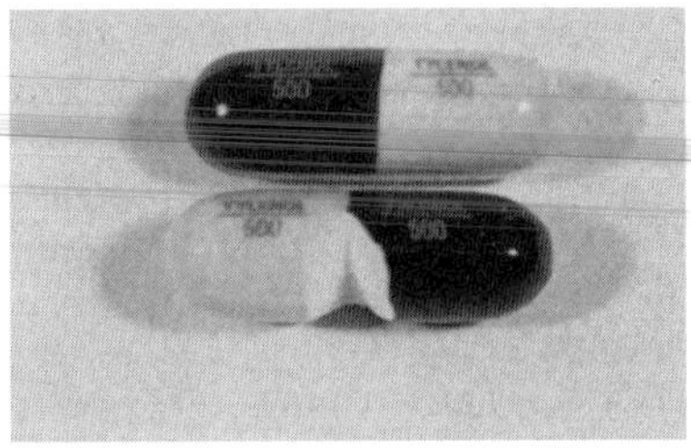

Fig. 5–58. *Cut-away view of "Gelcaps" dosage form. A gelatin-coated capsule-shaped tablet. Dosage form is more easily swallowed than a comparable tablet, smaller than an equivalent capsule, and tamper-evident. (Courtesy of McNeil Consumer Products Co.)*

Gelatin Coated Tablets

A recent innovation in tablet coating is the gelatin-coated tablet. Termed GELCAPS®, the innovator product is a gelatin-coated capsule-shaped tablet (Fig. 5–58). The use of a tablet makes the size of the product about one-third smaller than a capsule filled with an equivalent amount of powder. The gelatin coating facilitates ease of swallowing. Compared to dry-filled, unsealed capsules, GELCAPS are more tamper-resistant and tamper-evident.

Chewable Tablets

Chewable tablets are tablets which are intended to disintegrate smoothly in the mouth at a moderate rate, either with or without actual chewing. Characteristically, chewable tablets have a smooth texture upon disintegration, are pleasant tasting, and leave no bitter or unpleasant aftertaste. Mannitol, a white crystalline hexahydric alcohol, which possesses many of the characteristics desired for the excipient in chewable tablets, is widely employed for this purpose. Mannitol is about 70% as sweet as sucrose with a cool taste and mouth-feel, the latter resulting from its negative heat of solution and a moderate solubility in water. Mannitol's nonhygroscopicity also makes it an ideal excipient for the preparation of chewable tablets containing moisture-sensitive drugs. Chewable tablets are prepared by wet granulation and compression, using minimum degrees of tablet hardness. In many chewable tablet formulations, mannitol may account for 50% or more of the weight of the formulation. Sometimes, other sweetening agents, as sorbitol, lactose, dextrose and glucose, may be substituted for part or all of the mannitol. Lubricants and binders which do not detract from the texture or desired hardness of the tablet are used in formulating chewable tablets. To enhance the appeal of the tablets, colorants and tart or fruity flavorants are commonly employed. Among the types of products prepared into chewable tablets are antacids and vitamins, analgesic and cold tablets intended for children.

The following is a formula for a typical chewable antacid tablet:[24]

	Per Tablet
Aluminum hydroxide	325.0 mg
Mannitol	812.0 mg
Sodium saccharin	0.4 mg
Sorbitol (10% w/v solution)	32.5 mg
Magnesium stearate	35.0 mg
Mint flavor concentrate	4.0 mg

Preparation: Blend the aluminum hydroxide, mannitol, and sodium saccharin. Prepare a wet granulation with the sorbitol solution. Dry at 120°F and screen through a 12-mesh screen. Add the flavor and magnesium stearate, blend, and compress into tablets.

Molded Tablets

The commercial preparation of tablets by molding has been replaced by the tablet compression process.

Official Tablets

Examples of official tablets are presented in Table 5–4.

Rate-Controlled Dosage Forms and Drug Delivery Systems

Some solid dosage forms are designed to release their medication to the body for absorption rapidly and completely, whereas other products are designed to release the drug slowly for more prolonged drug release and sustained drug action. The latter types of dosage forms are commonly referred to as *controlled-release, sustained-release, prolonged-release, timed-release, slow-release, sustained-action, prolonged-action, extended-action,* or *rate-controlled* tablets or capsules.

Although these terms have been frequently used interchangeably, the meaning of "sustained-release" and "controlled-release" are different. Sustained release describes the release of a drug substance from a dosage form or delivery system over an extended period of time. Controlled-release describes a system in which the *rate* of the drug's release is more precisely controlled compared to the sustained release product.

The term "drug delivery systems" refers to the technology utilized to present the drug to the desired body site for drug release and absorption. The modern transdermal patch, discussed in Chapter 10 is an example of a drug delivery system. The first drug delivery system developed was the *syringe,* invented in 1855, used to deliver medication by injection.

The goal of rate-controlled technology is to produce a convenient, generally self-administered dosage form that yields a constant infusion of the drug. The advantages of rate-controlled drug delivery are presented in Table 5–5.

Controlled-release dosage forms that provide sustained drug release require less frequent drug administration than ordinary dosage forms (Fig. 5–59A). This is considered an advantage in assuring patient compliance in the taking of medication. Patients required to take 1 or 2 dosage units a day are less likely to forget a dose than if they were required to take their medication 3 or 4 times a day.[25] Further, controlled-release dosage forms allow whole day coverage and help to reduce the need for the patient to be awakened for a night-time dose. Also, depending upon the medication and the dosage form, the daily cost to the patient may be less with less frequent dosage administration.

Rather than providing *sustained-release,* some solid dosage forms are designed to sequentially release two full doses of a drug. Such dosage forms also enable the patient to be maintained on the drug for longer than usual periods following the administration of a single dosage unit. These types of products are usually termed *repeat-action* tablets or capsules (Fig. 5–59B).

Many of these specialized types of dosage forms are protected by patents and have been given trademark names that help to identify both the manufacturer and the type of pharmaceutical product.

Sustained-Release Forms

Most sustained-release forms are designed so that the administration of a single dosage unit provides the immediate release of an amount of drug that promptly produces the desired therapeutic effect and gradual and continual release of additional amounts of drug to maintain this

Table 5–4. Examples of Some Official Tablets

Official Tablet	*Some Representative Commercial Products*	*Tablet Strengths Usually Available*	*Category and Comments*
Acetaminophen	Tylenol (McNeil)	325 mg	Analgesic and antipyretic
Allopurinol	Zyloprim (Burroughs Wellcome)	100 and 300 mg	Antigout; antiurolithic
Amitriptyline HCl	Elavil HCl (Stuart)	10, 25, 50, 100, and 150 mg	Antidepressant
Bisacodyl	Dulcolax (Ciba)	5 mg	Cathartic; enteric coated tablets
Carbamazepine	Tegretol (Basel)	200 mg	Anticonvulsant
Chlorambucil	Leukeran (Burroughs Wellcome)	2 mg	Antineoplastic
Chlorpheniramine Maleate	Chlor-Trimeton Maleate (Schering-Plough)	4, 8, and 12 mg	Antihistaminic; some tablets (8 and 12 mg) controlled-release
Chlorpropamide	Diabinese (Pfizer)	100 and 250 mg	Antidiabetic
Cimetidine	Tagament (SmithKline Beecham)	200 and 300 mg	Histamine H_2 receptor antagonist
Diazepam	Valium (Roche)	2, 5, and 10 mg	Sedative; skeletal muscle relaxant
Digoxin	Lanoxin (Burroughs Wellcome)	0.125, 0.25, and 0.5 mg	Cardiotonic
Dimenhydrinate	Dramamine (Upjohn)	50 mg	Antinauseant
		25 and 30 mg	Bronchodilator; vasoconstrictor
Furosemide	Lasix (Hoechst-Roussel)	20, 40, and 80 mg	Diuretic; antihypercalemic; antihypertensive
Griseofulvin	Fulvicin U/F (Schering)	250 and 500 mg	Antifungal
Haloperidol	Haldol (McNeil)	0.5, 1, 2, 5, 10 and 20 mg	Tranquilizer
Hydrochlorothiazide	Hydro-Diuril (Merck & Co.)	25, 50, and 100 mg	Diuretic; antihypertensive
Ibuprofen	Motrin (Upjohn)	300, 400, 600, and 800 mg	Analgesic; antipyretic
Levodopa	Larodopa (Roche)	100, 250, and 500 mg	Antidyskinetic
Levothyroxine sodium	Synthroid (Boots)	0.025, 0.05, 0.075, 0.1, 0.125, 0.15, 0.2, and 0.3 mg	Thyroid hormone
Meclizine HCl	Antivert (Roerig)	12.5, 25, and 50 mg	Antivertigo
Meperidine Hydrochloride	Demerol (Sanofi Winthrop)	50 and 100 mg	Narcotic analgesic
Meprobamate	Equanil (Wyeth-Ayerst)	200 and 400 mg	Sedative; hypnotic
Methyldopa	Aldomet (Merck & Co.)	125, 250, and 500 mg	Antihypertensive
Metronidazole	Flagyl (Searle)	250 and 500 mg	Antiamebic; antitrichomonal
Nitroglycerin	Nitrostat (Parke-Davis)	0.150, 0.3, 0.4, and 0.6 mg	Anti-anginal sublingual tablets
Penicillin V Potassium	Pen Vee (Wyeth-Ayerst)	250 and 500 mg	Antibacterial
Prednisone	Deltasone (Upjohn)	1 mg	Adrenocorticoid
Prochlorperazine Maleate	Compazine (SmithKline Beecham)	5, 10, and 25 mg	Antiemetic
Propanolol HCl	Inderal (Wyeth-Ayerst)	10, 20, 40, 60, 80, and 90 mg	Antianginal; antiarrhythmic; antihypertensive
Sulindac	Clinoril (Merck & Co.)	150 and 200 mg	Antirheumatic, antiinflammatory
Terbutaline sulfate	Brethine (Geigy)	2.5 and 5 mg	Antiasthmatic
Tolbutamide	Orinase (Upjohn)	250 and 500 mg	Antidiabetic
Warfarin Sodium	Coumadin (DuPont)	2, 2.5, 7.5, and 10 mg	Anticoagulant

Table 5–5. Advantages of Rate-Controlled Drug-Delivery Systems Over Conventional Dosage Forms

Advantage	*Explanation*
Reduction in drug blood level fluctuations	By controlling the rate of drug release, "peaks and valleys" of drug-blood or serum levels are eliminated.
Reduction in dosing frequency	Rate-controlled products deliver more than a single dose of medication and thus are taken less often than conventional forms.
Enhanced patient convenience and compliance	With less frequency of dose administration, the patient is less apt to neglect taking a dose. There is also greater patient convenience with daytime and nighttime medication, and control of chronic illness.
Reduction in adverse side effects	Because there are seldom drug blood level peaks above the drug's therapeutic range, and into the toxic range, adverse side effects are less frequently encountered.
Reduction in health care costs i.e., economy	Although the initial cost of rate-controlled drug delivery systems is usually greater than conventional dosage forms, the average cost of treatment over an extended time period may be less. With less frequency of dosing, enhanced therapeutic benefit, and reduced side-effects, the time required of health care personnel to dispense, administer and monitor patients is reduced.

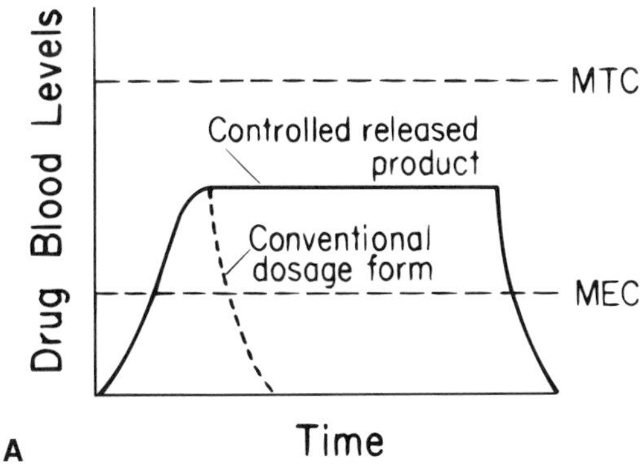

Fig. 5–59A. *Hypothetical drug blood level-time curves for a conventional solid dosage form and a controlled release product.*

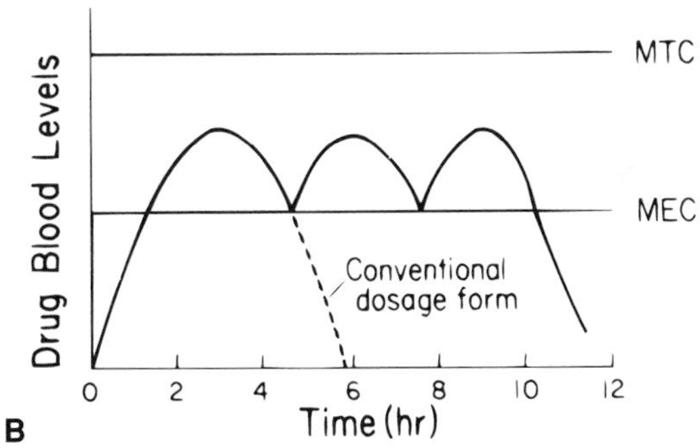

Fig. 5–59B. *Hypothetical drug blood level-time curves for a conventional solid dosage form and a multiple-action product.*

level of effect over an extended period, usually 8 to 12 hours.

In this type of dosage form, the design is based on the particular qualities of each individual drug. What may be an effective type of dosage form design for one drug may be ineffective in promoting the sustained release of another drug because of peculiar physical, chemical, and biological qualities. To maintain the constant level of drug in the system, the drug must be released from the dosage form at a rate that will replace the amount of drug being metabolized and excreted from the body. For each drug, this is a highly individualized quality. In general, the drugs best suited for incorporation into a sustained release product have the following characteristics.

1. *They exhibit neither very slow nor very fast rates of absorption and excretion.* Drugs with slow rates of absorption and excretion are usually inherently long-acting and their preparation into sustained-action type dosage forms is not necessary. Similarly, a drug with a short half life, i.e., $<$2 hours, should not be formulated into a sustained release product because such a delivery system would require unacceptably large release rates and doses.
2. *They are uniformly absorbed from the gastrointestinal tract.* Drugs absorbed poorly or at varying and unpredictable rates are not good candidates for sustained-release products, because their drug release and therefore drug absorption will fluctuate, depending upon the position of the drug in the gastroin-

testinal tract and the dosage form's rate of movement within the tract.

3. *They are administered in relatively small doses.* Drugs with large single doses frequently are not suitable for the preparation of the sustained-action product because the individual dosage unit needed to maintain the extended therapeutic blood level of the drug would have to be too large for the patient to easily swallow.
4. *They possess a good margin of safety.* The most widely used measure of the margin of safety is its therapeutic index, i.e., median toxic dose, TD50/median effective dose, ED50. This index can range from one (where the effective dose produces toxic effects) to several thousand. For very "potent" drugs when therapeutic concentration is narrow, the value of the therapeutic index is very small. The larger the therapeutic index the safer the drug. Thus, those drugs which are potent in very small doses or possess very narrow or small therapeutic indices are poor candidates for formulation into controlled-release formulations because of technologic limitations of precise control over release rates.
5. *They are used in the treatment of chronic rather than acute conditions.* Drugs for acute conditions generally require more physician control of the dosage than that provided by sustained-release products.

The most common mechanisms utilized in rate-controlled pharmaceutical products are: solvent action of biologic fluids on coated drug particles, osmotic systems controlled by the diffusion of biologic fluids through a polymer, erodible systems controlled by the erosion of a polymeric matrix, diffusion systems controlled by the diffusion of the drug through a polymeric membrane or monolithic matrix, and chemical reaction or interaction between the drug substance or its pharmaceutical barrier and site-specific biologic fluids. These mechanisms are utilized in the development of dosage forms and drug delivery systems for oral and other routes of administration.

Examples of the pharmaceutical technology utilized to achieve rate-controlled and sustained release solid dosage forms are described below.

COATED BEADS OR GRANULES OR MICROENCAPSULATED DRUG. In this method a solution of the drug substance in a non-aqueous solvent such as a mixture of acetone and alcohol is coated (by pan or air-suspension coating) onto small inert non-pareil seeds or beads made of a combination of sugar and starch. In instances in which the dose of the drug is large, the starting granules of material may be composed of the drug itself. Then with some of the beads or granules remaining uncoated and intended to provide the immediately released dose of drug when taken, coats of a lipid material like beeswax or a cellulosic material like ethylcellulose are applied to the remainder (about two-thirds to three-fourths) of the granules, with some granules receiving a few coats and others many coats. Then the beads or granules of different thicknesses of coatings are blended in the desired proportions to achieve the proper blend. The coating material may be colored with a dye material so that the beads of different coating thicknesses will be darker in color and distinguishable from those having fewer coats and being lighter in color. When properly blended, the granules may be placed in capsules or tableted. The variation in the thickness of the coats and in the type of material used in the coating is reflected in the rate at which the body fluids are capable of penetrating the coating and in dissolving the drug. Naturally, the thicker the coat, the more resistant to penetration and the more delayed will be the drug release. The presence of drug granules of various coating thicknesses therefore produces the sustained drug release. The time-blood level profile is similar to that obtained with multiple dosing. An example of this type of dosage form is the *Spansule* capsule, shown in Figure 5–60.

Microencapsulation is a process by which solids, liquids, or even gases may be encapsulated into microscopic size particles through the formation of thin coatings of "wall" material around the substance being encapsulated. The process had its early origin in the late 1930s as a "clean" substitute for carbon paper and carbon ribbons as sought by the business machines industry. The ultimate development in the 1950s of reproduction paper and ribbons which contained dyes in tiny gelatin capsules released upon impact by a typewriter key or the pressure of a pen or pencil was the stimulus for the development of a host of microencapsulated materials, including drugs. Gelatin is a common wall-forming material but synthetic polymers as polyvinyl alcohol, ethylcellulose, or polyvinyl chloride have been used. The typical encapsulation process usually begins with the dissolving of the prospective wall material, say gelatin, in water. The material to be encapsulated is added and the two-phase mixture thoroughly stirred. With the material to

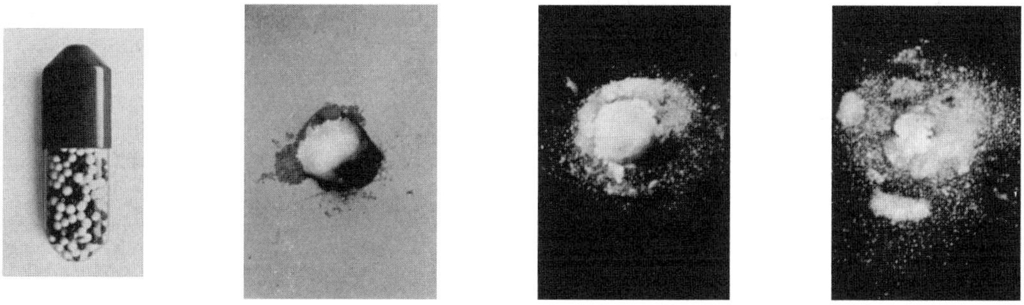

Fig. 5–60. *The* Spansule *capsule showing the hard gelatin capsule containing hundreds of tiny pellets for sustained drug release and the rupturing of one of the pellets as occurs in the gastric fluid. (Courtesy of SmithKline Beecham.)*

be encapsulated broken up to the desired particle size, a solution of a second material is added, usually acacia. This additive material is chosen to have the ability to concentrate the gelatin (polymer) into tiny liquid droplets. These droplets (coacervate) then form a film or coat around the particles of the substance to be encapsulated as a consequence of the extremely low interfacial tension of the residual water or solvent in the wall material so that a continuous, tight, film coating remains on the particle (Fig. 5–61). The final dry microcapsules are free-flowing, discrete particles of coated material. Of the total particle weight, the wall material usually represents between 2 and 20%. By varying the wall thickness of microencapsulated drug particles, their dissolution rates may be altered and sustained release obtained. An example of a drug commercially available in microencapsulated dosage form is potassium chloride as Micro-K (A. H. Robins).

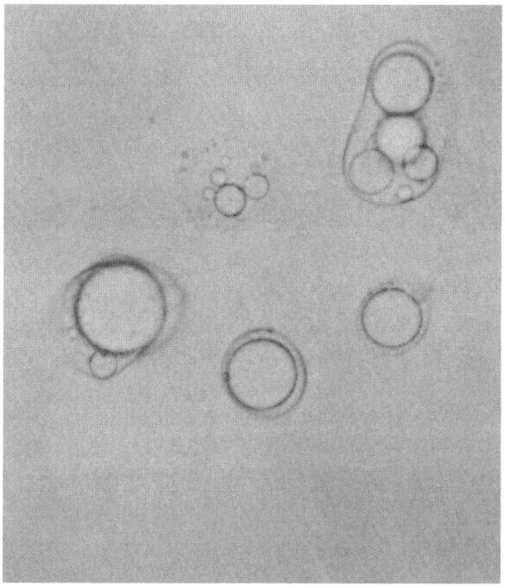

Fig. 5–61. *Microcapsules of mineral oil in a gelatin-acacia coacervate. (Photo courtesy of James C. Price, Ph.D., College of Pharmacy, The University of Georgia.)*

EMBEDDING DRUG IN SLOWLY ERODING MATRIX. By this process, the portion of the drug intended to have sustained action is combined with lipid or cellulosic material processed into granules that can be placed into capsules or tableted. When these granules are combined with granules of drug prepared without the special lipid or cellulosic excipient, the untreated portion provides the immediate drug effect, and the treated portion the prolonged effect. The treated granules slowly erode in the body fluids. The types of materials used in the preparation of the granules may be varied to achieve different rates of erosion. The product SLOW-K (Summit) is a sugar-coated tablet containing 8 mEq of potassium chloride in a wax matrix. The formulation is intended to provide a controlled release of potassium from the matrix to minimize the likelihood of producing high (and irritating) localized concentrations of potassium within the gastrointestinal tract.

Two-layered tablets may be prepared from the granules, with one layer containing the untreated drug for immediate release and the other layer having the drug for sustained release. Three-layered tablets may be similarly prepared, with both outer layers containing the drug for immediate release. Some commercial tablets are prepared with an inner core containing the sustained release portion of drug and an outer shell completely enclosing the core and containing the drug portion for immediate release. Tablets prepared from the type of material described in the next method may be similarly constructed.

EMBEDDING DRUG IN INERT PLASTIC MATRIX. By this method, the drug is granulated with an inert plastic material such as polyethylene, polyvinyl acetate, or polymethacrylate, and the granulation is compressed into tablets. The drug is slowly released from the inert plastic matrix by leaching to the body fluids. The compression of the tablet creates the matrix or plastic form that retains its shape during the leaching of the drug and through its elimination from the alimentary tract. The initially released drug is present on the surfaces of the tablet or is only superficially embedded. The primary example of a dosage form of this type is the *Gradumet* (Abbott).

COMPLEX FORMATION. Certain drug substances when chemically combined with certain other chemical agents form chemical complexes that may be only slowly soluble in body fluids, depending upon the pH of the environment. This slow dissolution rate is effective to provide the sustained action of the drug.

It should be remembered that certain drug substances that are only slowly soluble in body fluids without special complexation or other treatment are inherently long acting.

ION-EXCHANGE RESINS. A solution of the cationic drug is passed through a column containing the ion-exchange resin, to which it complexes by the replacement of hydrogen atoms. The resin-drug complex is then washed and may be tableted, encapsulated, or suspended in an aqueous vehicle. The release of the drug is dependent upon the pH and the electrolyte concentration in the gastrointestinal tract. Generally, release is greater in the acidity of the stomach than the less acidic small intestine. Examples of drug products of this type include *Tussionex* suspension (hydrocodone polistirex) and *Ionamin* capsules (phentermine resin) both by Fisons.

The mechanism of action of drug release from ion exchange resins may be depicted as follows.

In the stomach:

(1) Drug resinate + HCl$\rightleftharpoons$acidic resin + drug hydrochloride
(2) Resin salt + HCl$\rightleftharpoons$resin chloride + acidic drug

In the intestine:

(1) Drug resinate + NaCl$\rightleftharpoons$sodium resinate + drug hydrochloride
(2) Resin salt + NaCl$\rightleftharpoons$resin chloride + sodium salt of drug.

This system incorporates a polymer barrier coating and bead technology in addition to the ion-exchange mechanism. The initial dose comes from an uncoated portion, and the remainder from the coated beads. The coating does not dissolve, and release is controlled over a 12-hour period by ionic exchange. The drug-containing polymer particles are minute, and may be suspended to produce a liquid with controlled-release characteristics [e.g., Tussionex (Fisons)] as well as solid dosage forms.

HYDROCOLLOID SYSTEM. Hydrocolloids can play a significant role in the design of a controlled-release product. An example is the product Valrelease, a 15-mg slow-release dosage form of Valium (diazepam/Roche). Valrelease has been formulated using a unique Hydro-dynamically Balanced drug-delivery System (HBS). This dosage form was designed to achieve, in one administration, plasma concentrations of diazepam equivalent to those obtained with conventional Valium 5 mg tablets taken 3 times daily. The Hydrodynamically Balanced drug-delivery System consists of a matrix so designed that upon contact with gastric fluid, the dosage form demonstrates a bulk density of less than one and, thus, remains buoyant. Capsules and tables prepared to have this characteristic are sometimes referred to as "floating" capsules or tablets. When the Valrelease capsule shell dissolves, the outermost hydrocolloids come in contact with gastric fluid. They swell to form a boundary layer, which prevents immediate penetration of fluid into the formulation. The outer hydrocolloid boundary layer gradually erodes, with the subsequent formation of another "outer" boundary layer. This is a continuous process causing the gelatinous mass to constantly erode, while diazepam is gradually released through each layer as the fluid slowly penetrates the matrix. Valrelease remains in the stomach for a variable period of time, depending on individual physiologic characteristics. However, when Valrelease passes into the intestine, gradual release of the active drug and absorption continue.

OSMOTIC PUMP. The Oros system, developed by Alza, is an *or*al *os*motic pump composed of a core tablet and a semi-permeable coating with a 0.4 mm diameter hole for drug exit. The hole is produced by a laser beam and the product operates on the principle of osmotic pressure (Fig. 5–62A). The semi-permeable membrane permits water to enter from the patient's stomach into the core, dissolving the drug. The pressure that is built up forces or pumps the drug solution out of the delivery orifice (Fig. 5–63).

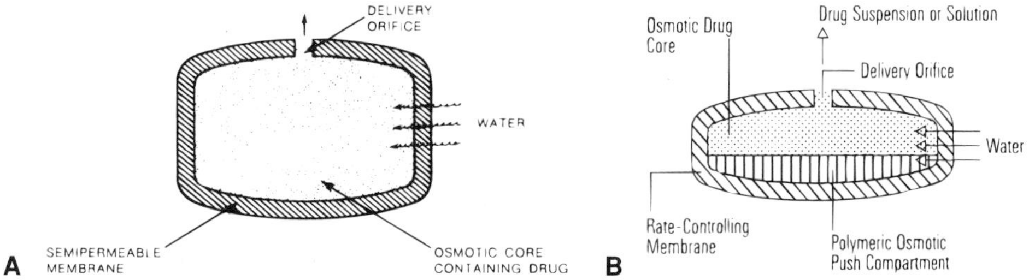

Fig. 5–62. *A, Depiction of the elementary OROS osmotic pump drug delivery system, and B, the OROS Push-Pull Osmotic System. (Courtesy of Alza Corporation.)*

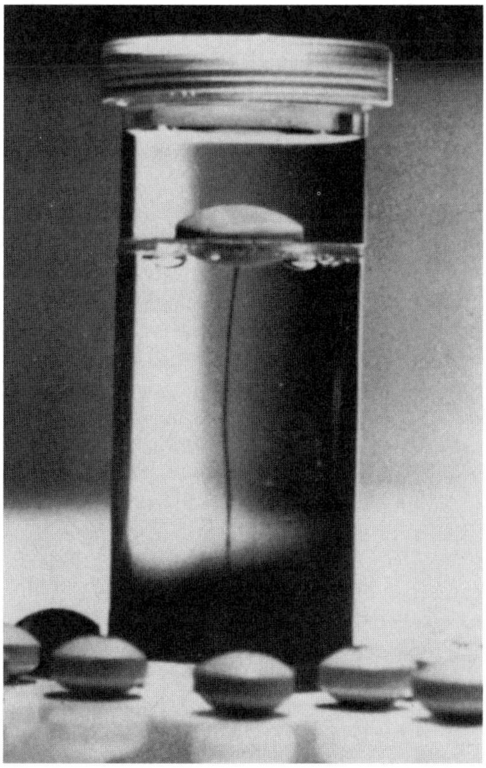

Fig. 5–63. *The OROS (Oral Osmotic) drug delivery system. A tablet core of drug is surrounded by a semipermeable membrane that is pierced by a small laser-drilled hole. After ingestion, water is drawn into the tablet from the digestive tract by osmosis. As water enters the tablet core, the drug gradually goes into solution. The solution is pushed out through the small hole at a controlled rate of about 1 to 2 drops per hour. (Courtesy of ALZA Corporation.)*

The rate of inflow of water and the outflow of drug solution are controlled by the properties of the membrane. Only the drug solution (not the undissolved drug) passes through the hole in the tablet. The rate of drug solution release is approximately one to two drops per hour. The drug-release rate is not affected by the acidity, alkalinity, or movement of the gastrointestinal tract. A currently marketed product of this type is Acutrim (CIBA Consumer).

Oros is a sophisticated oral controlled release drug delivery system in which the release rate may be controlled by changing the *surface area, the thickness* or *the nature* of the membrane and/or by changing the diameter of the drug release orifice.

The *OROS Push-Pull Osmotic System* has two layers (Fig. 5–62B) that are surrounded by a semi-permeable membrane. One layer contains the drug and the other contains a polymeric osmotic agent. When the tablet is swallowed, it draws in a few drops of water every hour across the membrane, slowly dissolving or suspending the drug, and expanding the polymeric osmotic compartment to release the drug through one or more laser-drilled holes at a controlled rate.

Other pharmaceutical companies have developed similar osmotic systems. For example, Elan Pharmaceutical has developed a system called Modas—*Multidirectional Osmotic Drug Absorption System*. Modas is an osmotic device with solubilized drug delivered through a fixed permeable membrane designed to admit moisture and excrete the soluble drug back through the same membrane at constant pressure. The drug comes out of the entire surface area of the tablet at a constant rate.

Repeat Action Forms

Some specialized tablets are prepared so that an initial dose of the drug is released from the tablet shell and a second dose from an inner core of the tablet, which is separated from the outer shell by a slowly permeable barrier coating. Generally the barrier coating is penetrated and drug from the inner core is exposed to the body fluids some 4 to 6 hours after the swallowing of the tablet. Such a tablet permits the release of two doses of drug from a single tablet, eliminating the need for more frequent drug administration. An example of this type of dosage form is *Repetabs* (Schering). As for the sustained-action type of dosage forms, the repeat-action forms are best suited for those drugs having low dosage and employed in chronic conditions and for drugs having regular absorption patterns with fairly rapid rates of absorption and excretion.

Delayed Action Forms

The release of a drug from a dosage form may be intentionally delayed until it reaches the intestinal environment for any of several reasons. Among these may be the fact that the drug is destroyed by the gastric juices, or it may be excessively irritating to the lining of the stomach or a nauseating drug, or it may be better absorbed from the intestines than from the stomach. Capsules and tablets coated so as to remain intact in the stomach but yield their ingredients in the intestines are said to be *enteric coated.* The coating may be composed of a material that is pH dependent and breaks down in the less acidic environment of the intestine, or the coating may erode due to moisture and on a time basis coinciding with the time required for the tablet or capsule to reach the intestines. Other coatings may deteriorate due to the hydrolysis-catalyzing action of certain intestinal enzymes. Among the many agents used to enteric coat tablets and capsules are fats, fatty acids, waxes and mixtures of these, shellac, and cellulose acetate phthalate. An example of a commercially prepared brand of enteric coated tablets is *Enseals* (Lilly). A popular enteric-coated aspirin tablet is Ecotrin (SmithKline Beecham Consumer Brands).

Liposomes

In the early 1960s, research scientists noted that various phospholipids formed multilayered vesicles (sacs) when dispersed in water. These cell-like structures become known as *liposomes.* Like a biologic cell, a liposome is composed of a thin but durable membrane that surrounds an aqueous compartment, protecting it from the outside environment. Both cellular and liposome membranes are capable of regulating the transport of molecules in and out of the enclosed compartment. Thus liposomes may be used to control the passage of drugs, entrapped in the aqueous phase, through the membrane and to the intended body site for absorption or action. In recent years, drug-containing liposome systems have been developed for the delivery of drugs by various routes of administration including inhalation, ocular, injectable, dermal, and oral.

Liposomes may be constructed to have a single aqueous compartment surrounded by a lipid layer *(unilamellar)* or they may consist of concentric lipid and aqueous layers *(multilamellar).* The structure of liposomes permits the incorporation of fat-soluble drugs in the lipid layer and water-soluble drugs in the interior aqueous compartment. Drugs encapsulated in the aqueous phase are released by slowly diffusing through the lipid membrane. Lipid-soluble drugs embedded in the lipid membrane or bound to the membrane surface are slowly released as the membrane is broken down by body fluids. Because lipids from natural sources are used to form the liposome membrane, liposomes are considered biocompatible and biodegradable.

Liposomes are produced by dispersing the lipid (usually phospholipids) phase in the drug solution. Simple mixing to vigorous agitation is applied to the system. Upon dispersion, the lipid molecules align to form the biomolecular membrane. The lipophilic ends of the lipid molecules intercalcate to form the inside of the membrane and the hydrophilic ends line up on the two outer surfaces. The membrane then wraps around, encapsulating the drug solution as the liposome is formed.

Generally, simple hand mixing of the phospholipid and aqueous phase produces a dispersion of multilamellar vesicles of large and widely mixed size. Various homogenizers and pressure flow-through devices have been utilized to achieve a more narrowly defined liposome size distribution. For use as drug carriers, liposomes should be homogeneous and reproducible in batch-to-batch production, stability, and drug release characteristics. Recently, microfluidization techniques have been used to produce liposomes of well-defined size distribution. This process involves the ultra high velocity interaction of two fluid streams in closely defined interaction. The pressures of the system, as high as 8000 psi, result in the jet interaction of the phases and liposome formation rates of as high as 75%, in contrast to other mixing systems which may result in a capture of the aqueous phase between 8 to 25%.

Because of the variation in the method of preparation, the size of liposomes varies from about 0.3 to 10 microns. The size of liposomes influences both their distribution in the body and their deposition. For instance, following injection, large size liposomes can have the tendency to deposit in the lungs whereas smaller particles may concentrate in other body sites, such as the liver. Alterations in the membrane composition, the phospholipid configuration, or in the electrical charge on liposomes can also greatly influence their distribution in the body. Agents such as cholesterol and cetylphosphate have been incorporated into the phospholipid bilayers to alter the liposome's properties, changing not only the diffusion characteristics of the membrane but also the distribution of the liposome within the body following administration.

Several liposome products are under commercial development for inhalation, ocular, dermal and parenteral routes of administration. For example, liposome-based bronchodilators, delivered as nebulized and aerosolized solutions, are being designed to treat bronchospasm. Ocular delivery products containing "bioadhesive" liposomes that adhere to the eye's surface are being developed to provide lubricating eye drops and sustained effects for glaucoma medication. Liposome products for application of therapeutic agents to the skin and scalp to provide extended drug release and perhaps greater percutaneous absorption are being investigated. Liposome-based products are also being developed to target drugs to specific body organs following intravenous administration. The objective is to concentrate the drug's action at the desired body site to maximize therapeutic action and minimize toxicity. Drugs being studied include anticancer agents, antibiotics, and peptide hormones.

Other technologies for rate-controlled targeted delivery include the use of transdermal drug delivery systems, implantable (subcutaneous) drug delivery systems, ocular drug delivery systems, intravenous infusion pumps, and monoclonal antibodies which are utilized as specific carriers for drugs, enzymes, and radiopharmaceuticals in the diagnosis and treatment of disease. These technologies are discussed elsewhere in this text.

Pharmacist Monitoring of Patients Using Controlled-Release Drugs

When a patient is prescribed a controlled-release drug the attainment of the peak and therapeutic concentration of the drug might be somewhat delayed. If an immediate effect is desirable, either an intravenous dose or immediate-release dosage form of the drug would be preferable. Thus, a pharmacist when consulted about a dosing recommendation should keep this in mind as it relates to patient needs.

As mentioned earlier in this chapter variations in the bioavailability from a controlled-release product are possible so the pharmacist must be cognizant of patient complaints of unusual adverse effects or possible ineffectiveness. Therapeutic levels of the certain drugs, e.g., theophylline, must be maintained for the desired therapeutic outcome to occur and once a patient is stabilized on a controlled-release product it should not be substituted. A different product, even with an identical amount of active ingredient, could cause a marked shift in the patient's drug blood/serum level due to different release characteristics of the dosage form. Unless two controlled-release products of the same drug have demonstrated similar bioavailability and therapeutic effect they should not be used interchangeably or substituted for one another.

Packaging and Storing Tablets

Tablets are best stored in tight containers and in places of low humidity protected from extremes in temperature. Products that are especially prone to decomposition by moisture may be copackaged with a desiccant. Drugs that are adversely affected by light are packaged in light-resistant containers. With a few exceptions, solid dosage forms that are properly stored will be stable for several years or more.

In most instances of dispensing, the pharmacist is well advised to use a similar type of container as provided by the manufacturer of the product and the patient advised to maintain the drug in the container dispensed. Proper storage conditions as recommended for the particular drug should be maintained by the pharmacist and patient and expiration dates observed.

The pharmacist should be aware also that the hardness of certain tablets may change upon aging usually resulting in a decrease in the disintegration and dissolution rates of the product.

The increase in tablet hardness can frequently be attributed to the increased adhesion of the binding agent and other formulative components within the tablet. Examples of increased tablet hardening with age have been reported for a number of drugs including aluminum hydroxide, sodium salicylate and phenylbutazone.[26]

Certain tablets containing volatile drugs, as nitroglycerin, may experience the migration of the drug between tablets in the container thereby resulting in a lack of uniformity among the tablets.[27] Further, packing materials, as cotton and rayon, in contact with nitroglycerin tablets may absorb varying amounts of nitroglycerin rendering the tablets sub-potent.[28]

In 1972, the Food and Drug Administration issued a number of regulations covering the packaging, labeling, and dispensing of nitroglycerin products. These regulations include:

1. All nitroglycerin tablets must be packaged in glass containers with tightly-fitting metal screw caps.
2. No more than 100 tablets may be packaged in each container.
3. Nitroglycerin tablets must be dispensed in their original containers and bear the label–"Warning: To prevent loss of potency, keep these tablets in the original container. Close tightly immediately after use."
4. All nitroglyercin tablets should be stored at controlled room temperatures of between 59° and 86°F.

Implementation of these regulations contributed to the maintenance of better content uniformity standards for nitroglycerin tablets than had been previously achieved. However, since nitroglycerin is a volatile liquid at room temperature, some nitroglycerin is lost to the atmosphere when the containers are opened and particularly if they are not tightly closed. In a further effort to reduce the loss of nitroglycerin from tablets and to prevent the migration of the substance from tablet to tablet, pharmaceutical manufacturers of these tablets have recently been developing "stabilized" nitroglycerin tablets. The main method used is to include a small amount of a nonvolatile substance in the formulation which has the effect of reducing the vapor pressure of the nitroglycerin and thus its tendency to escape from the tablet. One such marked product is *Nitrostat* by Parke-Davis which contains polyethylene glycol as the stabilizer.

Other Solid Dosage Forms for Oral Administration

Pills

Pills are small, round, solid dosage forms containing a medicinal agent and intended to be administered orally. Although the manufacture and administration of pills was at one time quite prevalent, today pills have been replaced by compressed tablets and capsules. A procedure for the extemporaneous preparation of pills on a small-scale may be found in the first edition of this text.

Lozenges

Lozenges are disc-shaped, solid dosage forms containing a medicinal agent and generally a flavoring substance and intended to be slowly dissolved in the oral cavity for localized effects. Lozenges are frequently called *troches* and less frequently referred to as *pastilles*. Many of the commercially available lozenges have a hard candy as the base or a base of sugar and an adhesive substance such as mucilage or gum.

Commercially, lozenges may be made by compression, using a tablet machine and large, flat punches. The machine is operated at a high degree of compression to produce lozenges that are harder than ordinary tablets so that they slowly dissolve or disintegrate in the mouth. Medicinal substances that are heat stable may be prepared into a hard, sugar candy lozenge by candy-making machines that process a warm, highly concentrated, flavored syrup as the base and form the lozenges by molding and drying.

Lozenges are gaining renewed acceptance as a means to deliver a multitude of different drugs. As an example, for the treatment of oropharyngeal candidiasis a lozenge dosage form is available with either nystatin or clotrimazole (e.g. Mycelex Troche, Miles) as its active ingredient. The patient allows the lozenge (or troche) to slowly dissolve in the mouth, and the dosage form is much more convenient to the patient when compared to the necessity of swishing an oral suspension in the mouth. Further, these lozenges maintain adequate salivary levels of the antifungal drug for about 3 hours and help to promote effectiveness of therapy. Lozenge dosage forms are also available for self-care drugs, e.g., benzocaine, dextromethorphan, phenylpropanolamine, to treat acute, self-limiting conditions ranging from minor sore throat to cough and congestion. These forms are particularly advantageous for those persons who find it difficult to swallow solid dosage forms and for young children.

Proper Administration of Peroral Dosage Forms

The dosage forms discussed in this chapter are all to be administered by mouth. The easiest way is to place the dosage form upon the tongue and swallow it with a glassful of water. Most patients will understand this method of administration and do so with water. However, some persons do not realize that these dosage forms should be taken with water and may proceed to merely swallow the tablet or the capsule. This can be dangerous because it is possible for the tablet or capsule to lodge within the esophagus. Several documented cases of esophageal ulceration in young women, for example, have occurred with the ingestion of tetracycline and tetracycline derivatives, particularly when taken just before bedtime. Thus, it is important to counsel the patient to take all oral dosage forms with at least some water. This is particularly so with those dosage forms that contain aspirin, ferrous sulfate, any nonsteroidal antiinflammatory drug (NSAID), potassium chloride and any tetracycline drug, to ensure passage of the medicine into the stomach. It is equally important to also instruct patients to take these medications no later than at least 1 hour before retiring for the evening.

Senior citizens are at an increased risk because the process of swallowing medications like those mentioned takes longer, and if they have esophageal strictures, there is the potential for these to lodge in the esophagus. Further, patients who suffer from gastroesophageal reflux disease must also be cautioned to take medicines with water and at least 1 hour before retiring. Otherwise, there is a possibility that some of the medicine may be refluxed back into the esophagus from the stomach once the patient retires for the evening.

As mentioned earlier in this chapter, certain oral dosage forms have protective coatings, e.g., enteric-coated, or may be formulated to provide delayed or continuous release of the active ingredient. The patient must be advised not to chew or crush these tablets as the amount and the rate of release of the drug may be dramatically altered. The patient should also be forewarned that they may notice remnants of these types of dosage forms in the stool. They should be told not to be concerned as the drug portion of the preparation has already been absorbed.

When a tablet can be crushed or a capsule opened to facilitate oral administration the pharmacist must keep in mind that medicines usually have an unpleasant taste. The bitter taste of the drug could be masked partially by recommending to the patient to mix the drug with applesauce, fruit juice, or carbonated beverages. However, the patient must be advised to consume the entire mixture. Otherwise the patient will not receive the total dose.

For those who experience gagging or choking when taking a solid dosage form, there is an innovative product called the Drink-A-Pill Drinking Glass. This contains a specially-designed shelf on which a tablet or capsule is placed after the glass is filled with water. When the patient drinks the content of the glass, the dosage form flows with the water into the mouth and goes right down without the gag reflex. Alternatively, if the patient simply cannot swallow the solid dosage form, the pharmacist can suggest to the prescribing physician a liquid form of the drug. If such a preparation is not available, it may be possible to extemporaneously compound the drug into a liquid vehicle. Several liquid formulations from solid dosage forms are listed in the *Handbook on Extemporaneous Formulations.* If this is not possible, the pharmacist could recommend the use of an available liquid dosage form of a different chemical compound with similar therapeutic effect.

Solid Dosage Forms for Nonoral Route of Administration

There are a few solid dosage forms which are used by routes of administration other than oral. For instance, dosage forms called *pellets* or *inserts* are implanted under the skin by special injectors or by surgical incision for the purpose of providing for the continuous release of medication. Such implants provide the patient with an economical means of obtaining long-lasting effects and obviate the need for frequent injections or oral dosage administration. Hormonal substances are most frequently administered in this manner. For example, the Norplant® system (Wyeth-Ayerst) of levonorgestrel implants provides up to five years of protection from pregnancy after subcutaneous insertion. The implants are closed capsules made of a di-

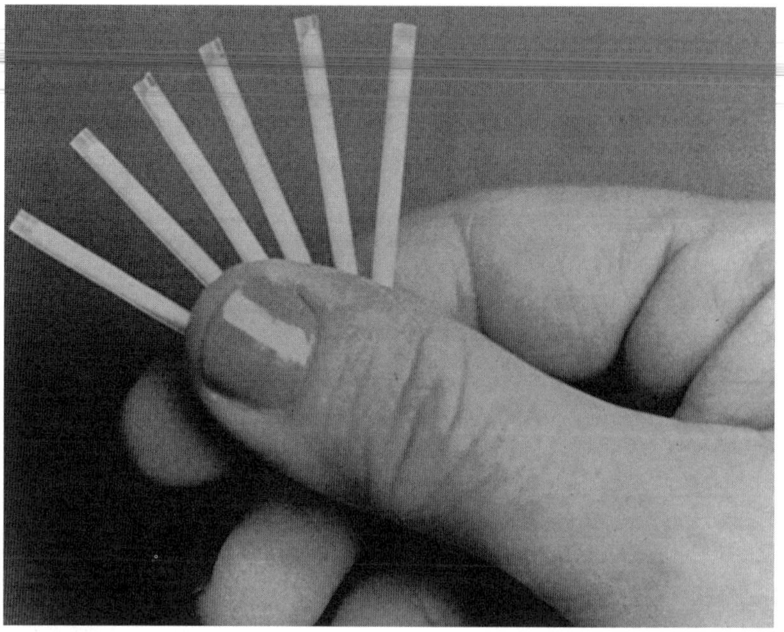

Fig. 5–64. *Norplant® System of levonorgestrel implants for the long-term (up to 5 years) prevention of pregnancy. Six implants are inserted subdermally in the midportion of the inner upper arm about 8 to 10 cm above the elbow crease. The implants are inserted in a fanlike pattern about 15 degrees apart. (Courtesy of Wyeth-Ayerst Laboratories.)*

methylsiloxane/methylvinylsiloxane copolymer containing 36 mg of the synthetic progestin levonorgestrel (Fig. 5–64). Each capsule is 2.4 mm in diameter and 34 mm in length. Six capsules are inserted in a plane beneath the skin of the upper arm by small incision and special injector. Following their term of use, the capsules are removed and may be replaced with fresh capsules.[29]

Other solid dosage forms, *vaginal tablets* or *inserts*, are specially formulated and shaped tablets intended to be placed in the vagina by special applicators, where the medication is released, generally for localized effects. Another example of a solid dosage form intended for use by means other than swallowing is a specially prepared capsule containing a micronized powder [Intal (Fisons)] intended to be released from the capsule and inhaled deep into the lungs through the use of a special inhaler-device (Spinhaler turbo-inhaler). These dosage forms and drug delivery systems will be discussed in subsequent chapters.

References

1. *The United States Pharmacopeia 23/National Formulary 18,* The United States Pharmacopeial Convention, Inc., Rockville, MD, 1995, 1823.
2. Yalkowsky, S.H., and Bolton, S.: Particle Size and Content Uniformity. *Pharm Res., 7*:962–966, 1990.
3. Jager, P.D., DeStefano, G.A., and McNamara, D.P.: Particle-Size Measurement Using Right-Angle Light Scattering. *Pharm. Tech., 17*:102–110, 1993.
4. Carver, L.D.: Particle Size Analysis. *Industrial Research,* 39–43, August 1971.
5. Evans, R.: Determination of Drug Particle Size and Morphology Using Optical Microscopy. *Pharm. Tech., 17*:146–152, 1993.
6. Houghton, M.E., and Amidon, G.E.: Microscopic Characterization of Particle Size and Shape: An Inexpensive and Versatile Method. *Pharm. Res., 9*: 856–863, 1992.
7. Gorman, W.G., and Carroll, F.A.: Aerosol Particle-Size Determination Using Laser Holography. *Pharm. Tech., 17*:34–37, 1993.
8. Milosovich, S.M.: Particle-Size Determination via Cascade Impaction. *Pharm. Tech., 16*:82–86, 1992.
9. Jones, B.E.: Hard Gelatin Capsules and the Pharmaceutical Formulator. *Pharm. Tech., 9*:106–112, 1985.
10. Caldwell, H.C.: Dissolution of Lithium and Magnesium from Lithium Carbonate Capsules Containing Magnesium Stearate. *J. Pharm. Sci., 63*:770–773, 1974.
11. *The United States Pharmacopeia 23/National Formulary 18,* The United States Pharmacopeial Convention, Rockville, MD, 1995, 1838–1839.
12. Capsule Sealing with the Lipcaps™ Sealing Process. Capsugel, Greenwood SC, 1986.
13. Stanley, J.P.: Soft Gelatin Capsules. *The Theory and Practice of Industrial Pharmacy,* 3rd ed., L. Lachman,

H.A. Lieberman, and J.L. Kanig, eds., Lea & Febiger, Philadelphia, 1986, 398–429.
14. *The United States Pharmacopeia 23/National Formulary 18,* The United States Pharmacopeial Convention, Rockville, MD, 1995, 1790.
15. Shangraw, R.F., and Demarest, D.A.: A Survey of Current Industrial Practices in the Formulation and Manufacture of Tablets and Capsules. *Pharm. Tech., 17:*32–44, 1993.
16. Kahn, K.A., and Rhodes, C.T.: Water-Sorption Properties of Tablet Disintegrants. *J. Pharm. Sci., 64:*447, 1975.
17. Lowenthal, W., and Wood, J.H.: Mechanism of Action of Starch as a Tablet Disintegrant VI: Location and Structure of Starch in Tablets. *J. Pharm. Sci., 62:*287, 1973.
18. Rubinstein, M.H.: Lubricant Behaviour of Magnesium Stearate. *Acta Pharmaceutica Suecica 24:*43, 1987.
19. Rubinstein, M.: Tableting Machines—The Need for a Quantum Leap in Design. *Pharm. Tech., 4:* 42–50, 1992.
20. Shangraw, R.R., Wallace, J.W., and Bowers, F.M.: Morphology and Functionality in Tablet Excipients for Direct Compression. *Pharm. Tech., 11:*136, 1987.
21. Mathur, L.K., Forbes, S.J., and Yelvigi, M.: Characterization Techniques for the Aqueous Film Coating Process. *Pharm. Tech., 8:*42, 1984.
22. Jones, D.M.: Factors to Consider in Fluid-Bed Processing. *Pharm. Tech., 9:*50–62, 1985.
23. Mehta, A.M.: Scale-Up Considerations in the Fluid-Bed Process for Controlled-Release Products. *Pharm. Tech., 12:*1988.
24. "Atlas Mannitol, USP Tablet Excipient," ICI Americas Inc., Wilmington, Delaware, 1973.
25. Eisen, S.A., et al.: The Effect of Prescribed Daily Dose Frequency on Patient Medication Compliance. *Arch. Intern. Med., 150:*1881, 1990.
26. Barrett, D., and Fell, J.T.: Effect of Aging on Physical Properties of Phenbutazone Tablets. *J. Pharm. Sci., 64:*335, 1975.
27. Page, D.P., et al.: Stability Study of Nitroglycerin Sublingual Tablets. *J. Pharm. Sci., 64:*140, 1975.
28. Fusari, S.A.: Nitroglycerin Sublingual Tablets I: Stability of Conventional Tablets. *J. Pharm. Sci., 62:* 122, 1973.
29. Norplant® System, Product Information. Wyeth-Ayerst Laboratories, Philadelphia, PA, 1993.

6

Oral Solutions, Syrups, and Elixirs

IN PHYSICOCHEMICAL terms, solutions may be prepared from any combination of solid, liquid, and gas, the three states of matter. For example, a solid solute may be dissolved in either another solid, a liquid, or a gas, and with the same being true for a liquid solute and for a gas, nine types of homogeneous mixtures are possible. In pharmacy, however, interest in solutions is for the most part limited to preparations of a solid, a liquid, and less frequently a gas solute dissolved in a liquid solvent.

In pharmaceutical terms, *solutions* are "liquid preparations that contain one or more chemical substances dissolved in a suitable solvent or mixture of mutually miscible solvents."[1] Because of a particular pharmaceutical solution's use, it may be classified as an *oral solution, otic solution, ophthalmic solution,* or *topical solution.* Still other solutions, because of their composition or use, may be classified as other pharmaceutical dosage forms. For example, aqueous solutions containing a sugar are classified as *syrups;* sweetened hydroalcoholic (combinations of water and ethanol) solutions are termed *elixirs;* solutions of aromatic materials are termed *spirits* if the solvent is alcoholic or *aromatic waters* if the solvent is aqueous. Solutions prepared by extracting active constituents from crude drugs are termed *tinctures* or *fluidextracts,* depending upon their method of preparation and their concentration. *Tinctures* may also be solutions of chemical substances dissolved in alcohol or in a hydroalcoholic solvent. Certain solutions prepared to be sterile and pyrogen-free and intended for parenteral administration are classified as *injections.* Although other examples could be cited, it is apparent that a solution, as a distinct type of pharmaceutical preparation, is much further defined than is the physicochemical definition of the term *solution.*

This chapter deals with the general area of solution preparation and focuses on the oral solution and the two other dosage forms most frequently utilized in the administration of oral medication in solution, the syrup and elixir. Solutions employed topically, by injection, ophthalmically, and by other means are covered in subsequent chapters.

Oral solutions, syrups, and elixirs are prepared and utilized for the specific effects of the medicinal agents present. In these preparations the medicinal agents are intended to provide systemic effects. The fact that they are administered in solution form usually means that their absorption from the gastrointestinal tract into the systemic circulation may be expected to occur more rapidly than from suspension or solid dosage forms of the same medicinal agent.

Solutes other than the medicinal agent are usually present in orally administered solutions. These additional agents usually are included to provide color, flavor, sweetness, or stability to the solution. In formulating or compounding a pharmaceutical solution, the pharmacist must utilize information on the solubility and stability of each of the solutes present with regard to the solvent or solvent system employed. Combinations of medicinal or pharmaceutic agents which will result in chemical or physical interactions affecting the therapeutic quality or pharmaceutic stability of the product must be avoided.

For single-solute solutions and especially for multiple-solute solutions, the pharmacist must be aware of the solubility characteristics of the solutes and the features of the common pharmaceutical solvents. Each chemical agent has its own solubility in a given solvent. For many medicinal agents, their solubilities in the usual solvents are stated in the USP as well as in other reference books.

Solubility

Attractive forces between atoms lead to the formation of molecules and ions. The intermolecular forces, which are developed between like molecules, are responsible for the physical state (i.e., solid, liquid, or gas) of the substance under given conditions, as temperature and pressure. Under ordinary conditions, most organic compounds, and thus most drug substances, form molecular solids.

When molecules interact, attractive forces and repulsive forces are in effect. The attractive forces cause the molecules to cohere, whereas the repulsive forces prevent molecular interpenetration and destruction. When the attractive and repulsive forces are equal, the potential energy between two molecules is minimum and the system is most stable.

Dipolar molecules frequently tend to align themselves with other dipolar molecules such that the negative pole of one molecule points toward the positive pole of the other. Large groups of molecules may be associated through these weak attractions known as *dipole-dipole* or van der Waals forces. In addition to the dipolar interactions, other attractions occur between polar and nonpolar molecules and ions. These include ion-dipole forces and hydrogen bonding. The latter is of particular interest. Because of small size and large electrostatic field, the hydrogen atom can move in close to an electronegative atom, forming an electrostatic type of association referred to as a *hydrogen bond* or *hydrogen bridge.* Hydrogen bonding involves strongly electronegative atoms as oxygen, nitrogen, and fluorine. Such a bond exists in water, represented by the dotted lines:

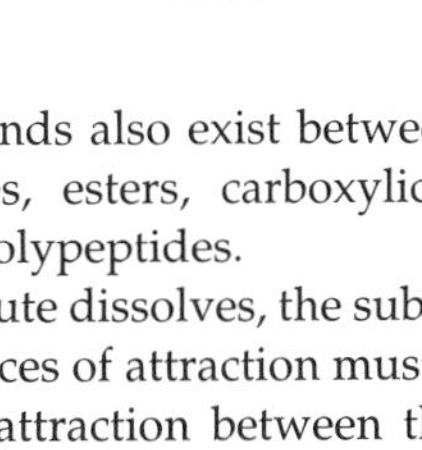

Water

Hydrogen bonds also exist between some alcohol molecules, esters, carboxylic acids, aldehydes, and polypeptides.

When a solute dissolves, the substance's intermolecular forces of attraction must be overcome by forces of attraction between the solute and solvent molecules. This involves breaking the solute-solute forces and the solvent-solvent forces to achieve the solute-solvent attraction.

The *solubility* of an agent in a particular solvent indicates the *maximum* concentration to which a solution may be prepared with that agent and that solvent. When a solvent, at a given temperature, has dissolved all of the solute it can, it is said to be *saturated.* In order to emphasize the possible variation in solubility between two chemical agents and therefore in the amounts of each required to prepare a saturated solution, two official aqueous saturated solutions are cited as examples, Calcium Hydroxide Topical Solution, USP, and Potassium Iodide Oral Solution, USP. The first solution, prepared by agitating an excess amount of calcium hydroxide with purified water, contains only about 140 mg of dissolved solute per 100 mL of solution at 25°C, whereas the latter solution contains about 100 g of solute per 100 mL of solution, over 700 times as much solute as present in the calcium hydroxide topical solution. It is apparent from this comparison that the maximum possible concentration to which a pharmacist may prepare a solution varies greatly and is dependent, in part, on the chemical constitution of the solute. Through selection of a different solubilizing agent or a different chemical salt form of the medicinal agent, alteration of the pH of a solution, or substitution, in part or in whole, of the solvent, a pharmacist can in certain instances dissolve greater quantities of a solute than would otherwise be possible. For example, iodine granules are soluble in water only to the extent of 1 g in about 3000 mL of water. Using only these two agents, the maximum concentration possible would be approximately 0.03% of iodine in aqueous solution. However, through the use of an aqueous solution of potassium or sodium iodide as the solvent, much larger amounts of iodine may be dissolved as the result of the formation of a water-soluble complex with the iodide salt. This reaction is taken advantage of, for example, in Iodine Topical Solution, USP, prepared to contain about 2% of iodine and 2.4% of sodium iodide.

Temperature is an important factor in determining the solubility of a drug and in preparing its solution. Most chemicals absorb heat when they are dissolved and are said to have a *positive heat of solution*, resulting in increased solubility with a rise in temperature. A few chemicals have a *negative heat of solution* and exhibit a decrease in solubility with a rise in temperature. Other factors, in addition to temperature, affect solubility. These include the various chemical and other physical properties of both the solute and the solvent, factors of pressure, the acidity or basicity of the solution, the state of subdivision of the solute, and the physical agitation applied to the solution during the dissolving process. The solubility of a pure chemical substance at a given temperature and pressure is constant; however, its *rate of solution*, that is, the speed at which it dissolves, depends upon the particle size of the substance and the extent of agitation. The finer the powder, the greater the surface area that comes in contact with the solvent, and the more rapid the dissolving process. Also, the greater the agitation, the more unsaturated solvent passes over the drug, and the faster the formation of the solution.

The solubility of a substance in a given solvent may be determined by preparing a saturated solution of it at a specific temperature and determining by chemical analysis the amount of chemical dissolved in a given weight of solution. By simple calculation, the amount of solvent required to dissolve the amount of solute can be determined. The solubility may then be expressed as grams of solute dissolving in milliliters of solvent—for example, "1 g of sodium chloride dissolves in 2.8 mL of water." When the exact solubility has not been determined, general expressions of relative solubility may be used. These terms are defined in the USP as presented in Table 6–1.

A great many of the important organic medicinal agents are either weak acids or weak bases, and their solubility is dependent to a large measure upon the pH of the solvent. These drugs react either with strong acids or strong bases to form water-soluble salts. For instance, the weak bases, including many of the alkaloids (atropine, codeine, and morphine), antihistamines (diphenyhydramine and tripelennamine), local anesthetics (cocaine, procaine, and tetracaine), and other important drugs are not very water-soluble, but they are soluble in dilute solutions of acids. Pharmaceutical manufacturers have prepared many acid salts of these organic bases to enable the preparation of aqueous solutions. It must be recognized, however, that if the pH of the aqueous solutions of these salts is changed by the addition of alkali, the free base may separate from solution unless it has adequate solubility in water. Organic medicinals that are weak acids include the barbiturate drugs (as phenobarbital and pentobarbital) and the sulfonamides (as sulfadiazine and sulfacetamide). These and other weak acids form water-soluble salts in basic solution and may separate from solution by a lowering of the pH. Table 6–2 presents the comparative solubilities of some typical examples of weak acids and weak bases and their salts.

Although there are no exact rules for predicting unerringly the solubility of a chemical agent in a particular liquid, experienced pharmaceutical chemists can estimate the general solubility of a chemical compound based on its molecular structure and functional groups. The information gathered on a great number of individual chemical compounds has led to the characterization of the solubilities of groups of compounds, and though there may be an occasional inaccuracy with respect to an individual member of a group of compounds, the generalizations none-

Table 6–1. Relative Terms of Solubility[2]

Descriptive Term	*Parts of Solvent Required for 1 Part of Solute*
Very soluble	Less than 1
Freely soluble	From 1 to 10
Soluble	From 10 to 30
Sparingly soluble	From 30 to 100
Slightly soluble	From 100 to 1000
Very slightly soluble	From 1000 to 10,000
Practically insoluble, or insoluble	10,000 and over

Table 6–2. Water and Alcohol Solubilities of Some Selected Weak Acids, Weak Bases, and Their Salts

	Number of mL of Solvent Required to Dissolve 1 g of Drug	
Drug	*Water*	*Alcohol*
Atropine	455	2
Atropine sulfate	0.5	5
Codeine	120	2
Codeine sulfate	30	1,280
Codeine phosphate	2.5	325
Morphine	5,000	210
Morphine sulfate	16	565
Phenobarbital	1,000	8
Phenobarbital sodium	1	10
Procaine	200	soluble
Procaine hydrochloride	1	15
Sulfadiazine	13,000	sparingly soluble
Sodium sulfadiazine	2	slightly soluble

theless serve a useful function. As demonstrated by the data in Table 6–2 and other similar data, salts of organic compounds are generally more soluble in water than are the corresponding organic bases. Conversely, the organic bases are generally more soluble in organic solvents, including alcohol, than are the corresponding salt forms. Perhaps the most written guideline for the prediction of solubility is that "like dissolves like," meaning that a solvent having a chemical structure most similar to that of the intended solute will be most likely to dissolve it. Thus, organic compounds are more soluble in organic solvents than in water. Organic compounds may, however, be somewhat water-soluble if they contain polar groups capable of forming hydrogen bonds with water. In fact, the greater the number of polar groups present, the greater will likely be the organic compound's solubility in water. Polar groups include OH, CHO, COH, CHOH, CH_2OH, COOH, NO_2, CO, NH_2 and SO_3H. The introduction of halogen atoms into a molecule tends to decrease water-solubility because of an increase in the molecular weight of the compound without a proportionate increase in polarity. An increase in the molecular weight of an organic compound without a change in polarity generally results in decreased solubility in water. Table 6–3 demonstrates some of these generalities through the use of specific chemical examples.

As with organic compounds, the pharmacist is aware of some general patterns of solubility that apply to inorganic compounds. For instance, most salts of monovalent cations such as sodium, potassium, and ammonium are water soluble, whereas the divalent cations like calcium, magnesium, and barium usually form water-soluble compounds with nitrate, acetate, and chloride anions but not with carbonate, phosphate, or hydroxide anions. To be sure, there are certain combinations of anion and cation which would seem to be quite similar in make-up but which do not have similar solubility characteristics. For instance, magnesium sulfate (Epsom salt) is soluble, but calcium sulfate is only slightly soluble; barium sulfate is very insoluble (1 g dissolves in about 400,000 mL of water) and is used as an opaque media for x-ray observation of the intestinal tract, but barium sulfide and barium sulfite are not as insoluble, and their oral use can result in poisoning; mercurous chloride (HgCl) is insoluble and was formerly used as a cathartic, but mercuric chloride ($HgCl_2$) is soluble in water and is a deadly poison if taken internally. There are many instances in which solubilities of certain drugs and their differentiation from other drugs are critical to the pharmacist in order that he might avoid compounding failures or therapeutic disasters.

For organic as well as for inorganic solutes, the ability of a solvent to dissolve them depends upon its effectiveness in overcoming the electronic forces that hold the atoms of the solute together and the corresponding lack of resolute on the part of the atoms themselves to resist the solvent action. During the dissolution process, the molecules of the solvent and the solute become uniformly mixed and cohesive forces of the atoms are replaced by new forces due to the attraction of the solute and solvent molecules for one another.

The student may find the following general rules of solubility useful.

Table 6–3. Solubilities of Selected Organic Compounds in Water as a Demonstration of Chemical Structure-Solubility Relationship

Compound	*Formula*	*Number of mL of Water Required to Dissolve 1 g of Compound*
Benzene	C_6H_6	1430
Benzoic acid	C_6H_5COOH	275
Benzyl alcohol	$C_6H_5CH_2OH$	25
Phenol	C_6H_5OH	15
Pyrocatechol	$C_6H_4(OH)_2$	2.3
Pyrogallol	$C_6H_3(OH)_3$	1.7
Carbon tetrachloride	CCl_4	2000
Chloroform	$CHCl_3$	200
Methylene chloride	CH_2Cl_2	50

A. For Inorganic Molecules

1. If *both* the cation and anion of an ionic compound are *monovalent*, the solute-solute attractive forces are usually easily overcome, and therefore, these compounds are generally water soluble. (Examples, NaCl, LiBr, KI, NH_4NO_3, $NaNO_2$)
2. If only *one* of the two ions in an ionic compound is *monovalent*, the solute-solute interactions are also usually easily overcome and the compounds are generally water soluble. (Examples: $BaCl_2$, MgI_2, Na_2SO_4, Na_3PO_4)
3. If *both* the cation and anion are *multivalent* the solute-solute interaction may be too great

to be overcome by the solute-solvent interaction and the compound may have poor water solubility. (Examples: $CaSO_4$, $BaSO_4$, $BiPO_4$; Exceptions: $ZnSO_4$, $FeSO_4$)

4. Common salts of alkali metals (Na, K, Li, Cs, Rb) are usually water soluble. (Exception: Li_2CO_3)
5. Ammonium and quaternary ammonium salts are water soluble.
6. Nitrates, nitrites, acetates, chlorates, and lactates are generally water soluble. (Exceptions: silver and mercurous acetate)
7. Sulfates, sulfites, and thiosulfates are generally water soluble. (Exceptions: calcium and barium salts)
8. Chlorides, bromides, and iodides are generally water soluble. (Exceptions: salts of silver and mercurous ions)
9. Acid salts corresponding to an insoluble salt will be more water soluble than the original salt.
10. Hydroxides and oxides of compounds other than alkali metal cations and the ammonium ion are generally water insoluble.
11. Sulfides are water insoluble except for their alkali metal salts.
12. Phosphates, carbonates, silicates, borates, and hypochlorites are water insoluble except for their alkali metal salts and ammonium salts.

B. For Organic Molecules

1. Molecules having one polar functional group are usually soluble to total chain lengths of five carbons.
2. Molecules having branched chains are more soluble than the corresponding straight-chain compound.
3. Water solubility decreases with an increase in molecular weight.
4. Increased structural similarity between solute and solvent is accompanied by increased solubility.

It is the pharmacist's knowledge of the chemical characteristics of drugs that permits the selection of the proper solvent for a particular solute. However, in addition to the factors of solubility, the selection is based on such additional solvent characteristics as clarity, low toxicity, viscosity, compatibility with other formulative ingredients, chemical inertness, palatability, odor, color, and economy. In most instances, and especially for solutions to be taken orally, used ophthalmically, or injected, water is the preferred solvent, because it comes closer to meeting the majority of the above criteria than the other available solvents. In many instances, when water is used as the primary solvent, an auxiliary solvent is also employed to augment the solvent action of water or to contribute to a product's chemical or physical stability. Alcohol, glycerin, and propylene glycol, perhaps the most used auxiliary solvents, have been quite effective in contributing to the desired characteristics of pharmaceutical solutions and in maintaining their stability.

Other solvents, as acetone, ethyl oxide, and isopropyl alcohol, are too toxic to be permitted in pharmaceutical preparations to be taken internally, but they are useful as reagent solvents in organic chemistry and in the preparatory stages of drug development, as in the extraction or removal of active constituents from medicinal plants. For purposes such as this, certain solvents are officially recognized in the compendia. A number of fixed oils, as corn oil, cottonseed oil, peanut oil, and sesame oil, serve useful solvent functions particularly in the preparation of oleaginous injections and are recognized in the official compendia for this purpose.

Some Solvents For Oral Preparations

The following official agents find use as solvents in the preparation of oral solutions, syrups, and elixirs.

Alcohol, USP (Ethyl Alcohol, Ethanol, C_2H_5OH)

Next to water, alcohol is the most useful solvent in pharmacy. It is used as a primary solvent for many organic compounds. Together with water it forms a hydroalcoholic mixture that dissolves both alcohol-soluble and water-soluble substances, a feature especially useful in the extraction of active constituents from crude drugs. By varying the proportion of the two agents, the active constituents may be selectively dissolved and extracted or allowed to remain behind according to their particular solubility characteristics in the menstruum. Alcohol, USP, is 94.9 to 96.0% C_2H_5OH by volume (i.e., v/v) when determined at 15.56°C, the U.S. Government's standard temperature for alcohol determinations. *Dehydrated Alcohol*, USP, contains not less than 99.5% C_2H_5OH by volume and is utilized in instances in which an essentially water-free alcohol is desired.

Alcohol has been well recognized as a solvent and excipient in the formulation of oral pharmaceutical products. Certain drugs are insoluble in water and must be dissolved in an alternate vehicle. Alcohol is often preferred because of its miscibility with water and its ability to dissolve many water-insoluble ingredients, including drug substances, flavorants, and antimicrobial preservatives. Alcohol is frequently used with other solvents, as glycols and glycerin, to reduce the amount of alcohol required. It also is used in liquid products as an antimicrobial preservative alone or as a copreservative with parabens, benzoates, sorbates, and other agents.

However, aside from its pharmaceutic advantages as a solvent and preservative, concern has been expressed over the undesired pharmacologic and potential toxic effects of alcohol when ingested in pharmaceutical products particularly by children. Thus, the FDA has proposed that manufacturers of OTC oral drug products restrict, insofar as possible, the use of alcohol and include appropriate warnings in the labeling. For OTC oral products intended for children under 6 years of age, the recommended alcohol-content limit is 0.5%; for products intended for children 6 to 12 years of age, the recommended limit is 5%; and for products recommended for children over 12 years of age and for adults, the recommended limit is 10%.

Diluted Alcohol, NF

Diluted Alcohol, NF, is prepared by mixing equal volumes of Alcohol, USP, and Purified Water, USP. The final volume of such mixtures is not the sum of the individual volumes of the two components, but due to contraction of the liquids upon mixing, the final volume is generally about 3% less than what would normally be expected. Thus when 50 mL of each component is combined, the resulting product measures approximately 97 mL. It is for this reason that the strength of Diluted Alcohol, NF, is not exactly half that of the more concentrated alcohol, but slightly greater, approximately 49%. Diluted alcohol is a useful hydroalcoholic solvent in various pharmaceutical processes and preparations.

Glycerin, USP (Glycerol), $CH_2OH{\bullet}CHOH{\bullet}CH_2OH$

Glycerin is a clear syrupy liquid with a sweet taste. It is miscible both with water and alcohol. As a solvent, it is comparable with alcohol, but because of its viscosity, solutes are slowly soluble in it unless it is rendered less viscous by heating. Glycerin has preservative qualities and if often used as a stabilizer and as an auxiliary solvent in conjunction with water or alcohol. It is used in many internal preparations.

Propylene Glycol, USP, $Ch_3CH(OH)CH_2OH$

Propylene glycol, a viscous liquid, is miscible with water and alcohol. It is a useful solvent with a wide range of application and is frequently substituted for glycerin in modern pharmaceutical formulations.

Purified Water, USP, H_2O

Naturally occurring water exerts its solvent effect on most substances it contacts and thus is impure and contains varying amounts of dissolved inorganic salts, usually sodium, potassium, calcium, magnesium, and iron, chlorides, sulfates, and bicarbonates, as well as dissolved and undissolved organic matter and microorganisms. Water found in most cities and towns where water is purified for drinking purposes usually contains less than 0.1% of total solids, determined by evaporating a 100 mL sample of water to dryness and weighing the residue (which would weigh less than 100 mg). Drinking water must meet the United States Public Health Service regulations with respect to bacteriological purity. Acceptable drinking water should be clear, colorless, odorless, and neutral or only slightly acid or alkaline, the deviation from neutral being due to the nature of the dissolved solids and gases (carbon dioxide contributing to the acidity and ammonia to the alkalinity of water).

Ordinary drinking water obtained from the tap is not generally acceptable for the manufacture of most aqueous pharmaceutical preparations or for the extemporaneous compounding of prescriptions because of the chemical incompatibilities that may result from the combination of dissolved solids present and the medicinal agents being added. Signs of such incompatibilities are precipitation, discoloration, and occasionally effervescence. Its use is permitted in the washing and in the extraction of crude vegetable drugs, in the preparation of certain products for external use, and in other instances in which the difference between the use of water and purified water is of no consequence. Naturally, when large volumes of water are required to clean pharmaceutical machinery and equipment, tap water may be economically employed so long as a residue of solids is prevented by using purified water as the final rinse or by wiping the water dry with a meticulously clean cloth.

Purified Water, USP is obtained by distillation, ion-exchange treatment, reverse osmosis, or other suitable process. It is prepared from water complying with the federal Environmental Protection Agency with respect to drinking water. Compared to ordinary drinking water, Purified Water, USP is more free of solid impurities. When evaporated to dryness, it must not yield greater than 0.001% of residue (1 mg of total solids per 100 mL of sample evaporated). Thus purified water is 100 times more free of dissolved solids than is water. Purified Water, USP is intended for use in the preparation of aqueous dosage forms, *except* those intended for parenteral administration (injections). For the latter purpose, Water for Injection, USP, Bacteriostatic Water for Injection, USP, or Sterile Water for Injection, USP, are utilized. These are discussed in Chapter 8.

The main methods used in the preparation of purified water are distillation and ion-exchange; these methods are described briefly as follows.

DISTILLATION METHOD. To prepare purified water, there are many commercially available stills in various sizes and styles with various capacities of from about one-half to 100 gallons of distillate per hour. Generally the first portion of aqueous distillate (about the first 10 to 20%) must be discarded, since it contains many foreign volatile substances usually found in urban drinking water, the usual starting material in the preparation of purified water. Also, the last portion of water (about 10% of the original volume of water) remaining in the distillation apparatus must be discarded and not subjected to further distillation because distillation to dryness would undoubtedly result in the decomposition of the remaining solid impurities to volatile substances that would distill and contaminate the previously collected portion of distillate.

ION-EXCHANGE METHOD. On a large or small scale, the ion-exchange method for the preparation of purified water offers a number of advantages over the distillation method. For one thing, the requirement of heat is eliminated and with it costly and troublesome maintenance frequently encountered in the operation of the more complex distillation apparatus. Because of the simpler equipment and the nature of the method, the ion-exchange process permits ease of operation, minimal maintenance, and a more mobile facility. Many pharmacies and small laboratories which purchase large volumes of distilled water from commercial suppliers for use in their work would no doubt benefit financially and in convenience through the installation of an ion-exchange demineralizer in the work area.

The ion-exchange equipment in use today generally involves the passage of water through a column of cation and anion exchangers, consisting of water-insoluble, synthetic, polymerized phenolic, carboxylic, amino, or sulfonated resins of high molecular weight. These resins are mainly of two types: (a) the cation, or acid exchangers, which permit the exchange of the cations in solution (in the tap water) with hydrogen ion from the resin; (b) the anion, or base exchange resins, which permit the removal of anions. These two processes are successively or simultaneously employed to remove both cations and anions from water. The processes are indicated as follows, with M^+ indicating the metal or cation (as Na^+) and the $X-$ indicating the anion (as Cl^-).

(a) Cation Exchange:

$$\text{H-Resin} + M^+ + X^- + H_2O \rightarrow \text{M-Resin} + H^+ + X^- + H_2O$$

(b) Anion Exchange:

$$\text{Resin-NH}_2 + H^+ + X^- + H_2O \rightarrow \text{Resin-NH}_2 \cdot HX + H_2O \text{ (pure)}$$

Water purified in this manner is referred to as *demineralized* or *de-ionized water*, and may be used in any pharmaceutical preparation or prescription calling for distilled water.

REVERSE OSMOSIS. This is one of the processes referred to in the industry as crossflow (or tangential flow) membrane filtration.[3] In this process, a pressurized stream of water is passed *parallel to* the inner side of a filter membrane core. A portion of the feed water, or influent, permeates the membrane as filtrate, while the balance of the water sweeps tangentially along the membrane to exit the system without being filtered. The filtered portion is called the *permeate* because it has permeated the membrane. The water that has passed through the system is referred to as the *concentrate,* because it contains the concentrated contaminants rejected by the membrane. Whereas, in *osmosis,* the flow through a semi-permeable membrane is from a less concentrated solution to a more concentrated solution, the flow in this crossflow system is from a more concentrated to a less concentrated solution—thus the term *reverse osmosis.* Depending upon their pore size, crossflow filter membranes are capable of removing particles defined in the range of *microfiltration* (0.1 to 2 microns, e.g., bacteria); *ultrafiltration* (0.01 to 0.1 microns, e.g., virus); *nanofiltration* (0.001 to 0.01 microns, e.g., organic compounds in the molecular weight range of 300 to 1000); and *reverse osmosis* (particles smaller than 0.001 microns). Reverse osmosis removes virtually all virus, bacteria, pyrogens, organic molecules, and 90–99% of all ions.[3]

Preparation of Solutions

Most pharmaceutical solutions are unsaturated with solute. Thus the amounts of solute to be dissolved are usually well below the capacity of the volume of solvent employed. The strengths of pharmaceutical preparations are usually expressed in terms of *% strength,* although for very dilute preparations, expressions of *ratio strength* may be used. These expressions and examples are shown in Table 6–4.

The term %, when used without qualification (as with w/v, v/v, or w/w) means % weight-in-volume for solutions or suspensions of solids in liquids; % weight-in-volume for solutions of gases in liquids; % volume-in-volume for solutions of liquids in liquids; and weight-in-weight for mixtures of solids and semisolids.

Some chemical agents that may be soluble in a given solvent are only slowly soluble and require an extended time for dissolving. To hasten the dissolution process, a pharmacist may employ one or several techniques. He may apply heat, reduce the particle size of the solute, utilize a solubilizing agent, or subject the ingredients to rigorous agitation during the preparation of the solution. Normally, most chemical agents are more soluble in solvents at elevated temperatures than at room temperature or below because an endothermic reaction between the solute and the solvent utilizes the energy of the heat to enhance the dissolution process. However, elevated temperatures cannot be maintained for pharmaceuticals, and the net effect of heat is simply an increase in the *rate* of solution rather than an increase in solubility. An increased rate is satisfactory to the pharmacist, because most of his solutions are unsaturated anyhow and do not require the presence of solute above the normal capacity of the solvent at room temperature. Pharmacists are generally reluctant to employ heat to facilitate solution, and when they do, they are careful not to exceed the minimally-required temperature, for many medicinal agents are destroyed at elevated temperatures, and the advantage of rapid solution may be completely offset by drug deterioration. If volatile solutes are to be dissolved or if the solvent is volatile (as alcohol), the heat would encourage the loss of these

Table 6–4. Common Methods of Expressing the Strengths of Pharmaceutical Preparations

Expression	*Abbreviated Expression*	*Meaning and Example*
Percent weight-in-volume	% w/v	number of grams of a constituent in 100 mL of preparation (e.g., 1% w/v = 1 g of constituent in 100 mL of preparation).
Percent volume-in-volume	% v/v	number of mL of a constituent in 100 mL of preparation (e.g., 1% v/v = 1 mL of constituent in 100 mL of preparation).
Percent weight-in-weight	% w/w	number of grams of a constituent in 100 g of preparation (e.g., 1% w/w = 1 g of constituent in 100 g of preparation).
Ratio strength, weight-in-volume	—:— w/v	number of grams of constituent in stated number of mL of preparation (e.g., 1:1000 w/v = 1 g of constituent in 1000 mL of preparation).
Ratio strength, volume-in-volume	—:— v/v	number of mL of constituent in stated number of mL of preparation (e.g., 1:1000 v/v = 1 mL of constituent in 1000 mL of preparation).
Ratio strength, weight-in-weight	—:— w/w	number of grams of constituent in stated number of grams of preparation (e.g., 1:1000 w/w = 1 g of constituent in 1000 g of preparation).

agents to the atmosphere and must therefore be avoided. Pharmacists are aware that certain chemical agents, particularly calcium salts, undergo exothermic reactions as they dissolve and give off heat. For such materials the use of heat would actually discourage the formation of a solution. The best pharmaceutical example of this type of chemical is calcium hydroxide, which is used in the preparation of Calcium Hydroxide Topical Solution, USP. This solute is soluble in water to the extent of 140 mg per 100 mL of solution at 25°C (about 77°F) and 170 mg per 100 mL of solution at 15°C (about 59°F). Obviously the temperature at which the solution is prepared or stored can affect the concentration of the resultant solution.

In addition to, or instead of, raising the temperature of the solvent to increase the rate of solution, a pharmacist may choose to decrease the particle size of the solute. This may be accomplished by the *comminution* (grinding a solid to a fine state of subdivision) of the solute with a mortar and pestle on a small scale or industrial micronizer on a large scale. The reduced particle size causes an increase in the surface area of the substance exposed to the solvent. If the powder is placed in a suitable vessel (as a beaker, graduate cylinder, or bottle) with a portion of the solvent and is stirred or shaken, as suited to the container, the rate of solution may be increased due to the continued circulation of fresh solvent to the drug's surface and the constant removal of newly-formed solution from the drug's surface.

Most solutions prepared for oral administration are prepared by simple solution of the solutes in the solvent or solvent mixture. On an industrial scale, solutions are prepared in large mixing vessels with ports for mechanical stirrers to effect solution (Fig. 6–1). When heat is desired, thermostatically controlled mixing tanks may be utilized.

Oral Solutions and Preparations for Oral Solution

Solutions intended for oral administration usually contain flavorants and colorants to make the medication more attractive and palatable for the patient. When needed, they may also contain stabilizers to maintain the chemical and physical

Fig. 6–1. *Large scale pharmaceutical mixing vessels. (Courtesy of Schering Laboratories.)*

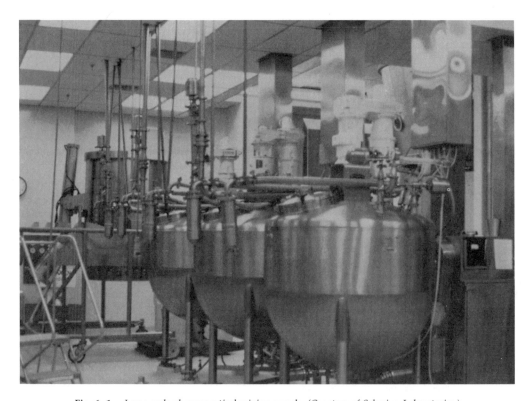

stability of the medicinal agents and preservatives to prevent the growth of microorganisms in the solution. The formulation pharmacist must be wary of chemical interactions which may occur between the various components of a solution which may result in an alteration in the preparation's stability and/or potency. For instance, it has been demonstrated that esters of p-hydroxybenzoic acid (methyl-, ethyl-, propyl-, and butylparabens), frequently used preservatives in oral preparations, have a tendency to partition into certain flavoring oils.[4] This partitioning effect could reduce the effective concentration of the preservatives in the aqueous medium of a pharmaceutical product below the level needed for preservative action.

Liquid pharmaceuticals for oral administration are usually formulated such that the patient receives the usual dose of the medication in a conveniently administered volume, as 5 mL (one teaspoonful), 10 mL or 15 mL (one tablespoonful). A few solutions have unusually large doses, as Magnesium Citrate Oral Solution, USP with a usual adult dose of 200 mL. On the other hand many solutions used in pediatric patients are given by drop, utilizing a calibrated dropper usually furnished by the manufacturer in the product package.

Dry Mixtures for Solution

A number of medicinal agents, particularly certain antibiotics, have insufficient stability in aqueous solution to meet extended shelf-life periods. Thus, commercial manufacturers of these products provide them to the pharmacist in dry powder or granule form for reconstitution with a prescribed amount of purified water immediately before dispensing to the patient. The dry powder mixture contains all of the formulative components including drug, flavorant, colorant, buffers, and others, except for the solvent. Once reconstituted by the pharmacist the resultant solutions remain stable when stored in the refrigerator for the labeled periods, usually from 7 to 14 days depending upon the preparation. This is generally a sufficient period of time for the patient to complete the volume of medication usually prescribed. However, if medication remains after the patient completes his course of therapy, he should be instructed to discard the remaining portion which would be unfit for use at a later date.

Examples of dry powder mixtures intended for reconstitution to oral solutions are the following:

Cloxacillin Sodium for Oral Solution, USP (Biocraft); an antiinfective antibiotic
Nafcillin Sodium for Oral Solution, USP [Unipen (Wyeth-Ayerst)]; a bactericidal semisynthetic penicillin
Oxacillin Sodium for Oral Solution, USP [Prostaphlin (Apothecon)]; an antiinfective antibiotic
Penicillin V Potassium for Oral Solution, USP [Pen-Vee K (Wyeth-Ayerst)]; an antiinfective antibiotic
Potassium Chloride for Oral Solution, USP [K-LOR (Abbott)]; a potassium supplement

Oral Solutions

In the practice of pharmacy, the pharmacist may be called upon to dispense a commercially prepared oral solution; dilute the concentration of a solution, as in the preparation of a pediatric form of an adult product; prepare a solution through the reconstitution of a dry powder mixture; or extemporaneously compound an oral solution from bulk components.

In each instance, the pharmacist should be sufficiently knowledgeable of the dispensed product to expertly advise the patient of the proper use, dosage, method of administration, and storage of the product. Knowledge of the solubility and stability characteristics of the medicinal agents and the solvents employed in the commercial products is useful to the pharmacist in informing the patient of the advisability of mixing the solution with juice, milk, or other beverages upon administration. Information regarding the solvents used in each commercial product appears on the product label and in the accompanying package insert. Table 6–5 presents examples of some oral solutions. Some solutions of special pharmaceutical interest are also described in this text.

Oral Rehydration Solutions

Rapid fluid loss associated with diarrhea can lead to dehydration and ultimately death in some patients, particularly infants. It has been estimated that over five million children under 4 years of age die due to diarrheal illnesses each year worldwide.[5] Diarrhea is characterized by an increased frequency of loose, watery stools, and because there is an intensive fluid loss, dehy-

Table 6–5. Examples of Oral Solutions by Category

Oral Solution	*Some Representative Commercial Products*	*Concentration of Commercial Product*	*Comments*
Anticonvulsants			
Trimethadione Oral Solution	Tridone Oral Solution (Abbott)	200 mg trimethadione/5 mL	A sweetened and flavored aqueous solution used in the treatment of petit mal seizures.
Antidepressants			
Nortriptyline HCl Oral Solution	Pamelor Oral Solution (Sandoz)	10 mg nortriptyline/5 mL	Tricyclic antidepressant
Fluoxetine HCl	Prozac Liquid (Dista)	20 mg fluoxetine/5 mL	Used in the treatment of depression and for obsessive-compulsive disorder
Antihistamine/Decongestant			
Pseudoephedrine HCl and Chlorpheniramine Maleate Liquid	Dorcol Children's Liquid Cold Formula (Sandoz)	15 mg of pseudoephedrine HCl and 1 mg of chlorpheniramine maleate per 5 mL	This solution is used in children for the temporary relief of nasal congestion, running nose and sneezing due to the common cold, hay fever and other upper respiratory allergies.
Antiperistaltic			
Diphenoxylate HCl and Atropine Sulfate Oral Solution	Lomotil Liquid (Searle)	2.5 mg of diphenoxylate HCl and 0.025 mg of atropine sulfate/5 mL	This preparation is indicated in the management of diarrhea. Diphenoxylate is related structurally and pharmacologically to the narcotic meperidine. Atropine sulfate is added to the solution in subtherapeutic amounts to discourage (by virtue of side effects) deliberate overdosage.
Loperamide HCl Oral Solution	Imodium A-D Liquid (McNeil)	1 mg of loperamide HCl per 5 mL	This preparation is indicated for the treatment of diarrhea for both adults and children 6 years of age and older. Loperamide is structurally related to haloperidol.
Antipsychotics			
Haloperidol Oral Solution	Haldol Concentrate (McNeil)	2 mg haloperidol/mL	These solutions are used primarily in severe neuropsychiatric conditions when oral medication is preferred and other oral dosage forms (as tablets and capsules) are considered impractical. The concentrated solutions are employed by adding the desired amount of the concentrate by calibrated dropper to soup or a beverage as tomato or fruit juices, milk, coffee, tea, or carbonated beverages.
Perphenazine Oral Solution	Trilafon Concentrate (Schering)	16 mg perphenazine/5 mL	
Thiordazine HCl Oral Solution	Mellaril Concentrate (Sandoz)	30 and 100 mg thioridazine HCl/mL	
Thiothixene HCl Oral Solution	Navane Concentrate (Roerig)	equivalent of 5 mg thiothixene/mL	
Bronchodilator			
Theophylline Oral Solution	Theophylline Oral Solution (Roxane)	80 mg of theophylline per 15 mL	This alcohol-free solution is used for the treatment of bronchial asthma and reversible bronchospasm associated with chronic bronchitis and emphysema.
Cathartics			
Magnesium Citrate Oral Solution, USP	—	amount of magnesium citrate equivalent to between 1.55 g and 1.9 g/100 mL of magnesium oxide	Discussed in text
Sodium Phosphate Oral Solution	Phospho-Soda (Fleet)	18 g sodium phosphate and 48 g sodium biphosphate/100 mL	Works as laxative within 1 hour when taken before meals or overnight when taken at bedtime. Usual dose is 10 to 20 mL of solution, best taken diluted with one-half glass of water and followed with a full glass of water.
Corticosteroid			
Prednisolone Sodium Phosphate Oral Liquid	Pediapred Oral Liquid (Fisons)	5 mg prednisolone (as sodium phosphate) per 5 mL	Synthetic adrenocortical steroid with predominantly glucocorticoid properties indicated in the treatment of endocrine, rheumatic, collagen, allergic, and other disorders.
Dental Caries Protectant			
Sodium Fluoride Oral Solution	Pediaflor Drops (Ross)	0.5 mg/mL	Prophylaxis of dental caries; intended for use when community water supplies are inadequately fluoridated.
Diuretic			
Furosemide Oral Solution	Lasix Oral Solution (Hoeschst-Roussel)	10 mg of furosemide per mL	This preparation is indicated to treat edema and hypertension in adults and in children.

Table 6–5. Continued

Oral Solution	Some Representative Commercial Products	Concentration of Commercial Product	Comments
Electrolyte Replenisher			
Potassium Chloride Oral Solution	Klorvess 10% Liquid (Sandoz)	20 mEq of KCl/15 mL in a flavored aqueous vehicle	Used in conditions of hypopotassemia (low level of potassium in the blood). Condition may be prompted by severe or chronic diarrhea, a low level of potassium intake in the diet, increased renal excretion of potassium, and other causes. The solution is diluted with water or fruit juice before taking.
Fecal Softener			
Docusate Sodium Solution	Colace Liquid (Apothecon)	10 mg docusate sodium/mL	Usually 50 to 200 mg of the drug is measured by calibrated dropper and mixed with milk, fruit juice, or other liquid (to mask the taste) before administration. The drug softens the fecal mass by lowering the surface tension, thus permitting normal bowel habits, particularly in geriatric, pediatric, cardiac, obstetric, and surgical patients. Dosage is taken for several days or until bowel movements are normal.
Hematinic			
Ferrous Sulfate Oral Solution	Fer-In-Sol Drops (Mead Johnson Nutritional)	75 mg ferrous sulfate/0.6 mL	Used for prevention and treatment of iron deficiency anemias. Usual prophylactic dose of 0.3 or 0.6 mL measured by calibrated dropper and mixed with water, fruit juice, or vegetable juice before administration. Dosage form intended primarily for infants and children.
Histamine H_2 Antagonist			
Cimetidine HCl Liquid	Tagamet HCl Liquid (SKB)	300 mg of cimetidine HCl per 5 mL	This preparation is indicated to treat peptic ulcer disease and pathological hypersecretory conditions, e.g., Zollinger-Ellison syndrome.
Narcotic Agonist Analgesic			
Methadone HCl Oral Solution	Methadone HCL (Roxane)	1 or 2 mg/mL	For relief of severe pain; detoxification and maintenance treatment of narcotic addiction.
Psychotherapeutic Agent			
Ergoloid Mesylate Oral Solution	Hydergine Liquid (Sandoz)	1 mg/mL	Utilized in symptomatic treatment of idiopathic decline in mental capacity.
Vitamin D Source			
Ergocalciferol Solution	Calciferol Drops (Kremers-Urban)	8,000 units/mL	A solution of water-insoluble ergocalciferol (vitamin D_2) in propylene glycol. The usual prophylactic dose of ergocalciferol is about 400 units and the therapeutic dose may be as high as 200,000 to 500,000 units daily in treating rickets.

dration can be an outcome. During diarrhea, the small intestine secretes far above the normal amount of fluid and electrolytes, and this simply exceeds the ability of the large intestine to reabsorb it. This fluid loss occurs mostly from the body's extracellular fluid compartment and can lead to a progressive loss of blood volume culminating in hypovolemic shock.

Diarrhea is a normal physiologic body response to rid itself of a noxious or toxic substance, e.g., *Rotavirus, Escherichia coli.* Thus, the treatment approach is to allow the diarrhea to proceed and not to terminate it too quickly, but promptly replace the fluid and electrolytes that are lost to prevent dehydration. The loss of fluid during diarrhea is accompanied by a depletion of sodium, potassium and bicarbonate ions, which if severe can result, as mentioned, in hypovolemic shock, as well as acidosis, hyperpnea and vomiting. If continuous, bouts of vomiting and diarrhea can cause malnutrition as well. Consequently, the goal is to replace lost fecal water with an oral rehydration solution and utilize nutritional foods such as soybean formula and bran.

Oral rehydration solutions are usually effective in treatment of patients with mild volume depletion of 5 to 10% of body weight. These are available over-the-counter, are relatively inexpensive and their use has diminished the incidence of complications associated with parenterally-administered electrolyte solutions. Therapy with these solutions is based on the observation that glucose is actively absorbed from the small intestine, even during bouts of diarrhea. This active transport of glucose is advantageous because it is coupled with sodium absorption. Almost like in domino fashion, sodium absorption promotes anion absorption which in turn promotes water absorption to short circuit dehydration. To produce maximal absorption of sodium and water studies have demonstrated that the optimal concentrations of glucose and sodium in an isotonic solution are 110 mM (2%) glucose and 60 mEq/L of sodium ion, respectively. Bicarbonate and/or citrate ions are also included in these solutions to help correct the subsequent metabolic acidosis which is caused by diarrhea and dehydration.

A typical oral rehydration solution contains 45 mEq Na^+, 20 mEq K^+, 35 mEq Cl^-, 30 mEq citrate, and 25 g of dextrose per liter. These formulations are available in liquid or powder/packet form for reconstitution. It is important that the user add the specific amount of water needed to prepare the powder forms. Further, these products should not be mixed with or given with other electrolyte-containing liquids, such as milk or fruit juices. Otherwise, there is no method to calculate how much electrolyte the patient actually received. Commercially available, ready-to-use oral electrolyte solutions to prevent dehydration or achieve rehydration include Resol Solution (Wyeth-Ayerst), Pedialyte Solution (Ross), and Rehydrate Solution (Ross). These products also contain dextrose or glucose. Ricelyte Oral Solution (Mead Johnson) contains electrolytes in a syrup of rice solids. The rice-based formula produces a lower osmotic effect than the dextrose- or glucose-based formulas and is thought to be more effective in reducing stool output and shortening the duration of diarrhea. The pharmacist must discourage the production of homemade versions of electrolyte solutions. The success of the commercial solutions is based on the accuracy of the formulation. If prepared incorrectly, homemade preparations could cause hypernatremia or cause the diarrhea to worsen.

Oral Colonic Lavage Solution

Traditionally, the preparation of the bowel for procedures such as a colonoscopy have consisted of the administration of clear liquid diets for 24 to 48 hours preceding the procedure, the administration of oral laxatives, e.g., magnesium citrate or bisacodyl, the night before, and cleansing enemas administered 2 to 4 hours prior to procedure commencement. Typically, to circumvent the cost of having to hospitalize the patient the night prior to the procedure, patients were allowed to perform this regimen at home. However, while the results have been generally satisfactory, that is, the bowel is cleared for the procedure, poor patient compliance with and acceptance of this regimen can cause problems during the procedure. Further, additive effects of malnutrition and poor oral intake prior to the procedure can cause more patient problems.

Consequently, an alternative method to prepare the gastrointestinal tract has been devised. This procedure requires less time and dietary restriction and obviates the need for cleansing enemas. This method involves the oral administration of a balanced solution of electrolytes with polyethylene glycol (PEG-3350). Prior to its dispensing to the patient, the pharmacist reconstitutes this powder with water creating an iso-osmotic solution having a mildly salty taste. The polyethylene glycol acts as an osmotic agent within the gastrointestinal tract and the balanced electrolyte concentration results in virtually no net absorption or secretion of ions. Thus, a large volume of this solution can be administered without a significant change in water or electrolyte balance.

The formulation of this oral colonic lavage solution is as follows:

Polyethylene Glycol 3350	236.00 g
Sodium Sulfate	22.74 g
Sodium Bicarbonate	6.74 g
Sodium Chloride	5.86 g
Potassium Chloride	2.97 g

In 4800 mL disposable container

The recommended adult dosage of this product is 4 L of solution prior to the gastrointestinal procedure. The patient is instructed to drink 240 mL of solution every 10 minutes until about 4 L are consumed. The patient is advised to drink each portion quickly rather than sipping it continuously. Usually, the first bowel movement will occur within 1 hour. Several regimens are utilized, and one method is to schedule patients for a midmorning procedure, allowing the patient 3 hours for drinking and a 1-hour waiting period to complete bowel evacuation.

To date this approach to bowel evacuation has been associated with a low incidence of side effects, primarily nausea, transient abdominal fullness, bloating, and occasionally, cramps and vomiting. Ideally, the patient should not have taken any food 3 to 4 hours before beginning the administration of the solution. In no case should solid foods be taken by the patient for at least 2 hours before the solution is administered. No foods, except clear liquids, are permitted after this product is administered and prior to the examination. The product must be stored in the refrigerator after reconstitution, and this aids somewhat in decreasing the salty taste of the product.

Magnesium Citrate Oral Solution

Magnesium citrate oral solution is a colorless to slightly yellow, clear, effervescent liquid having a sweet, acidulous taste and a lemon flavor. It is commonly referred to as "Citrate" or as "Citrate of Magnesia." It is required to contain an amount of magnesium citrate equivalent to between 1.55 and 1.9 g of magnesium oxide in each 100 mL.

The solution is prepared by reacting official magnesium carbonate with an excess of citric acid (equation 1), flavoring and sweetening the solution with lemon oil and syrup, filtering with talc, and then carbonating it by the addition of either potassium or sodium bicarbonate (equation 2). The solution may be further carbonated by the use of carbon dioxide under pressure.

$$(MgCO_3)_4 \cdot Mg(OH)_2 + 5H_3C_6H_5O_7 \rightarrow 5MgHC_6H_5O_7 + 4CO_2 + 6H_2O \quad (1)$$

$$3KHCO_3 + H_3C_6H_5O_7 \rightarrow K_3C_6H_5O_7 + 3CO_2 + 3H_2O \quad (2)$$

The solution provides an excellent medium for the growth of molds, and any mold spores present during the manufacture of the solution must be killed if the preparation is to remain stable. For this reason, during the preparation of the solution the liquid is heated to boiling (prior to carbonation), boiled water is employed to bring the solution to its proper volume, and boiling water is used to rinse the final container. The final solution may be sterilized.

Magnesium citrate solution has always been troublesome, since it has a tendency to deposit a crystalline solid upon standing. Apparently this is due to the formation of some almost insoluble, normal magnesium citrate (rather than the exclusively dibasic form as in equation 1). The cause of the problem has largely been attributed to the indefinite composition of the official magnesium carbonate, which by definition is "a basic hydrated magnesium carbonate or a normal hydrated magnesium carbonate" (see equation 1). It contains the equivalent of 40 to 43.5% of magnesium oxide. Apparently solutions prepared from magnesium carbonates with differing equivalents of magnesium oxide vary in stability, with the most stable ones being prepared from samples of magnesium carbonate having the lower equivalent of magnesium oxide. The formula for the preparation of 350 mL of magnesium citrate solution calls for the use of 15 g of official magnesium carbonate, which corresponds to approximately 6.0 to 6.47 g of magnesium oxide.

In carbonating the solution, the bicarbonate may be added in tablet form rather than as a powder in order to delay the effervescence resulting from its contact with the citric acid. If the powder were used, the reaction would be immediate and violent, and it would be virtually impossible to close the bottle in time to prevent the loss of carbon dioxide or solution. The solution may be further carbonated by the use of CO_2 under pressure. Most of the magnesium citrate solutions prepared commercially today are packaged in the same type of bottles as "soft drink" carbonated beverages. The solution is generally packaged in bottles of 300 mL. Since the solution is carbonated, it loses some of its character if allowed to stand for a period of time after the container has been opened. Magnesium citrate solution is generally stored in a cold place, preferably in a refrigerator, keeping the bottle on its side so the cork or rubber liners of the caps are kept moist and swollen, thereby maintaining the airtight seal between the cap and the bottle.

The solution is employed as a saline cathartic, with the citric acid, lemon oil, syrup, carbonation, and the low temperature of the refrigerated solution all contributing to the patient's acceptance of the large volume of medication. For many patients it represents a pleasant way of taking an otherwise bitter saline cathartic.

Sodium Citrate and Citric Acid Oral Solution

This official solution contains 100 mg of sodium citrate and 67 mg of citric acid in each mL of aqueous solution. The solution is administered orally in doses of 10 to 30 mL as frequently as four times daily as a systemic alkalinizer. Systemic alkalinization is useful in patients having conditions in which long term maintenance of an alkaline urine is desirable, such as patients with uric acid and cystine calculi of the urinary tract. The solution is also a useful adjuvant when administered with uricosuric agents in gout therapy since urates tend to crystallize out of an acid urine.

Syrups

Syrups are concentrated, aqueous preparations of a sugar or sugar-substitute with or without added flavoring agents and medicinal substances. Syrups containing flavoring agents but not medicinal substances are called *nonmedicated* or *flavored vehicles* (syrups). Some official, previously official and examples of commercially available nonmedicated syrups are presented in Table 6–6. These syrups are intended to serve as pleasant-tasting vehicles for medicinal substances to be added in the extemporaneous compounding of prescriptions or in the preparation of a standard formula for a *medicated syrup,* which is a syrup containing a therapeutic agent. Due to the inability of some children and elderly people to swallow solid dosage forms, it is not unusual today for a pharmacist to be asked to prepare an oral liquid dosage form of a medication available in the pharmacy only as tablets or capsules. In doing so, considerations of drug solubility, stability, and bioavailability must be considered case by case.[6,7] The liquid dosage form selected for compounding may be a solution or a suspension, depending upon the chemical and physical characteristics of the particular drug and its solid dosage form. Vehicles are commercially available for this purpose.[7]

Medicated syrups are commercially prepared from the starting materials; that is, by combining each of the individual components of the syrup, as sucrose, purified water, flavoring agents, coloring agents, the therapeutic agent, and other necessary and desirable ingredients. Naturally, medicated syrups are employed in therapeutics for the value of the medicinal agent present in the syrup.

Syrups provide a pleasant means of administering a liquid form of a disagreeable tasting drug. They are particularly effective in the administration of drugs to youngsters, since their pleasant taste usually dissipates any reluctance on the part of the child to take the medicine. The fact that syrups contain little or no alcohol adds to their favor among parents.

Any water-soluble drug that is stable in aqueous solution may be added to a flavored syrup. However care must be exercised to insure the compatibility between the medicinal drug substance and the other formulative components of the syrup. Also, certain flavored syrups have an

Table 6–6. Examples of Nonmedicated Syrups (Vehicles)

Nonmedicated Syrup	*Comments*
Cherry Syrup	A sucrose-based syrup containing about 47% by volume of cherry juice. The syrup's tart and fruit flavor is attractive to most patients and the acidic pH of the syrup makes it useful as a vehicle for drugs requiring an acid medium.
Cocoa Syrup	This syrup is a suspension of cocoa powder in an aqueous vehicle sweetened and thickened with sucrose, liquid glucose, and glycerin, and flavored with vanillin and sodium chloride. The syrup is particularly effective in administering bitter tasting drugs to children.
Orange Syrup	This sucrose-based syrup utilizes sweet orange peel tincture, and citric acid as the source of flavor and tartness. The syrup resembles orange juice in taste and is a good vehicle for drugs stable in an acidic medium.
Ora-Sweet and Ora-Sweet SF (Paddock Laboratories)	Commercially available vehicles for the extemporaneous compounding of syrups. Both vehicles have a pH between 4 and 4.5 and are alcohol free. Ora-Sweet SF syrup is sugar free.
Raspberry Syrup	A sucrose-based syrup containing about 48% by volume of raspberry juice. It is a pleasantly flavored vehicle used to disguise the salty or sour taste of saline medicaments.
Syrup	This is an 85% solution of sucrose in purified water. This "simple syrup" may be used as the basis for the preparation of flavored or medicated syrups.

acidic medium, whereas others may be neutral or slightly basic and the proper selection must be made to insure the stability of any added medicinal agent. Perhaps the most frequently found types of medications administered as medicated syrups are antitussive agents and antihistamines. This is not to imply that other types of drugs are not formulated into syrups; indeed, a wide variety of medicinal substances can be found in syrup form and among the many commercial products. Examples of medicated syrups are presented in Table 6–7.

Components of Syrups

Most syrups contain the following components in addition to the purified water and any medicinal agents present: (1) the sugar, usually sucrose, or sugar-substitutes used to provide sweetness and viscosity, (2) antimicrobial preservatives, (3) flavorants, and (4) colorants. Also, many syrups, especially those prepared commercially, contain special solvents, solubilizing agents, thickeners, or stabilizers.

Sucrose and Non-Sucrose Based Syrups

Sucrose is the sugar most frequently employed in syrups, although in special circumstances it may be replaced in whole or in part by other sugars, as dextrose, or non-sugars as sorbitol, glycerin and propylene glycol. In some instances, all glycogenetic substances (materials converted to glucose in the body), including those agents mentioned above, are replaced by nonglycogenetic substances such as methylcellulose or hydroxyethylcellulose. These two materials are not hydrolyzed and absorbed into the blood stream, and their use results in an excellent syrup-like vehicle for medications intended for use by diabetic patients and others whose diets must be controlled and restricted to nonglycogenetic substances. The viscosity generally resulting from the use of these cellulose derivatives is much like that of a sucrose syrup. The addition of one or more artificial sweeteners usually produces an excellent facsimile of a true syrup.

The characteristic "body" that the sucrose and the alternative agents seek to impart to the syrup is essentially the result of attaining the proper viscosity. This quality, together with the sweetness and the flavorants generally added, results in a type of pharmaceutical preparation that is quite effective in masking the taste of added medicinal agents. When the syrup is swallowed, only a portion of dissolved drug actually makes contact with the taste buds, the remainder of the drug being carried past them and down the throat in the containment of the viscous syrup. This type of physical concealment of the taste is not possible for a solution of a drug in an unthickened, mobile, aqueous preparation. In the case of antitussive syrups, the thick sweet syrup has a soothing effect on the irritated tissues of the throat as it passes over them.

Most syrups contain a high proportion of sucrose, usually 60 to 80%, not only because of the desirable sweetness and viscosity of such solutions but also because of their inherent stability in contrast to the unstable character of dilute sucrose solutions. The aqueous sugar medium of dilute sucrose solutions is an efficient nutrient medium for the growth of microorganisms, particularly yeasts and molds. On the other hand, concentrated sugar solutions are quite resistant to microbial growth, due to the unavailability of the water required for the growth of microorganisms. This aspect of syrups is best demonstrated by the simplest of all syrups, Syrup NF, which has the synonym of "simple syrup" and is prepared by dissolving 85 g of sucrose in enough purified water to make 100 mL of syrup. The resulting preparation requires no additional preservation; in fact, preservatives may not be added to this official syrup. When properly prepared and maintained, the syrup is inherently stable and resistant to the growth of microorganisms. An examination of this syrup reveals its concentrated nature and the relative absence of available water for microbial growth. Syrup has a specific gravity of about 1.313, which means that each 100 mL of syrup weighs 131.3 g. Because 85 g of sucrose are present, the difference between 85 g and 131.3 g or 46.3 g, represents the weight of the purified water present. Thus, 46.3 g, or mL, of purified water are used to dissolve the 85 g of sucrose. The solubility of sucrose in water is 1 g in 0.5 mL of water; therefore, to dissolve 85 g of sucrose, about 42.5 mL of water would be required. Thus, only a very slight excess of water (about 3.8 mL per 100 mL of syrup) is employed in the preparation of syrup. Although not enough to be particularly amenable to the growth of microorganisms, the slight excess of water permits the syrup to remain physically stable under conditions of varying temperatures. If the syrup were completely saturated with sucrose, under cool storage conditions some sucrose might crystallize from solution

Table 6–7. Examples of Medicated Syrups by Category

Syrup	*Some Representative Commercial Products*	*Concentration of Commercial Product**	*Comments*
Analgesic			
Meperidine HCl Syrup	Demerol Syrup (Sanofi Winthrop)	50 mg meperidine HCl/5 mL	Narcotic analgesic indicated for relief of moderate to severe pain and as an adjunct to general anethesia.
Anticholinergics			
Dicyclomine HCl Syrup	Bentyl Syrup (Marion Merrell Dow)	10 mg dicyclomine HCl/5 mL	Used as adjunctive therapy in treatment of peptic ulcer.
Oxybutynin Chloride Syrup	Ditropan Syrup (Marion Merrell Dow)	5 mg of oxybutynin chloride per 5 mL	Used for the relief of symptoms associated with voiding in patients with uninhibited neurogenic and reflex neurogenic bladder.
Antiemetics			
Chlorpromazine HCl Syrup	Thorazine Syrup (SmithKline Beecham)	10 mg chlorpromazine HCl/5 mL	Used to control nausea and vomiting.
Dimenhydrinate Syrup	D-M-H Syrup (Alra)	15 mg dimenhydrinate/5 mL	Used to control nausea, vomiting, and motion sickness.
Prochlorperazine Edisylate Syrup	Compazine Syrup (SmithKline Beecham)	5 mg prochlorperazine edisylate/5 mL	Used to control nausea and vomiting.
Promethazine HCl Syrup	Phenergan Syrup (Wyeth-Ayerst)	6.25 mg, 12.5 mg, and 25 mg promethazine HCl/5 mL	Used to control nausea, vomiting, motion sickness, and allergic reactions.
Anticonvulsant			
Sodium Valproate Syrup	Depakene Syrup (Abbott)	250 mg of valproic acid (as sodium salt) per 5 mL	Used as the sole or adjunctive therapy in simple (petit mal) and complex absence seizure disorders.
Antihistamines			
Chlorpheniramine Maleate Syrup	Chlor-Trimeton Allergy Syrup (Schering-Plough)	2 mg chlorpheniramine maleate/5 mL	
Cyproheptadine HCl Syrup	Periactin Syrup (Merck & Co.)	2 mg cyproheptadine HCl/5 mL	
Hydroxyzine HCl Syrup	Atarax Syrup (Roerig)	10 mg hydroxyzine HCl/5 mL	All of the antihistamines listed are used for prevention and treatment of allergic reactions.
Triprolidine HCl Syrup	Actidil Syrup (Burroughs Wellcome)	1.25 mg triprolidine HCl/5 mL	
Antipruritics			
Trimeprazine Tartrate Syrup	Temaril Syrup (Allergan Herbert)	2.5 mg trimeprazine tartrate/5 mL	Used for relief of itching in urticaria.
Antipsychotic			
Lithium Citrate Syrup	Cibalith-S (CIBA)	8 mEq lithium/5 mL	Used in the management of psychotic disorders.
Antitussives			
Dextromethorphan Syrup	Delsym (Fisons)	30 mg dextromethrophan/5 mL	For relief of cough.
Diphenhydramine Syrup	Benylin Cough Syrup (Parke-Davis Consumer)	12.5 mg of diphenhydramine HCl per 5 mL	Used for the control of coughs due to colds or allergy.
Antiviral			
Amantadine HCl Syrup	Symmetrel Syrup (DuPont)	50 mg amantadine HCl/5 mL	Prevention of respiratory infections caused by A_2 (Asian) viral strains. Treatment of idiopathic Parkinson's disease.
Bronchodilators			
Albuterol Sulfate Syrup	Proventil Syrup (Schering)	2 mg of albuterol sulfate per 5 mL	
	Ventolin Syrup (Allen & Hanburys)		Used for the relief of bronchospasm in patients with obstructive airway disease, and for the prevention of exercise induced bronchospasm.
Metaproterenol Sulfate Syrup	Alupent Syrup (Boehringer Ingelheim)	10 mg of metaproterenol sulfate per 5 mL	
Cathartic			
Lactulose Syrup	Chronulac Syrup (Marion Merrell Dow)	10 g of lactulose per 15 mL	Dose is 15 to 30 mL daily as a laxative.
Cholinergic			
Pyridostigmine Bromide Syrup	Mestinon Syrup (ICN Pharmaceuticals)	60 mg pyridostigmine bromide/5 mL	Used in treatment of myasthenia gravis.
Decongestant			
Pseudoephedrine Hydrochloride Syrup	Children's Sudafed Liquid (Burroughs Wellcome)	30 mg of pseudoephedrine hydrochloride per 5 mL	Used for the temporary relief of nasal congestion due to the common cold, hay fever or other upper respiratory allergies, and nasal congestion associated with sinusitis.

Table 6–7. Continued

Syrup	Some Representative Commercial Products	Concentration of Commercial Product*	Comments
Emetic			
Ipecac Syrup	Ipecac Syrup (Roxane)	21 mg ether-soluble alkaloids of ipecac/15 mL	Used to induce vomiting in poisoning. The dose of 15 mL may be repeated in 20 minutes if vomiting does not occur. If after the second dose, vomiting does not occur, the stomach should be emptied by gastric lavage.
Expectorant			
Guaifenesin Syrup	Guaifenesin Syrup (Roxane)	100 mg guaifenesin/5 mL	For symptomatic relief of respiratory conditions associated with cough and bronchial congestion.
Fecal Softener			
Docusate Sodium Syrup	Colace Syrup (Apothecon)	20 mg docusate sodium/5 mL	Stool softener by surface-action.
Gastrointestinal Stimulant			
Metoclopramide HCl Monohydrate Syrup	Reglan Syrup (Robins)	5 mg of metoclopramide HCl per 5 mL	Used to provide relief of symptoms associated with diabetic gastroparesis (gastric stasis) and gastroesophageal reflux.
Hemostatic			
Aminocaproic Acid Syrup	Amicar Syrup (Lederle)	1.25 g aminocaproic acid/5 mL	Used in treatment of excessive bleeding resulting from systemic hyperfibrinolysis and urinary fibrinolysis.
Hypnotic/Sedative			
Chloral Hydrate Syrup	Chloral Hydrate Syrup (Roxane)	500 mg chloral hydrate/10 mL	Sedative in doses of 250 mg and hypnotic to induce sleep at doses of 500 mg. Alcoholic beverages should be avoided when taking this syrup. The syrup is usually diluted with water or other beverage before taking.

* The amount per stated volume of syrup constitutes a usual single dose of the medication unless otherwise stated.

and, by acting as nuclei, initiate a type of chain reaction that would result in the separation of an amount of sucrose disproportionate to its solubility at the storage temperature. The syrup would then be very much unsaturated and probably suitable for microbial growth. As formulated, the official syrup is both stable and resistant to crystallization as well as to microbial growth. However, many of the other official syrups and a host of commercial syrups are not intended to be as nearly saturated as Syrup, NF, and therefore must employ added preservative agents to prevent microbial growth and to ensure their stability during their period of use and storage.

As noted earlier, sucrose-based syrup may be substituted in whole or in part by other agents in the preparation of medicated syrups. A solution of a polyol, as sorbitol, or a mixture of polyols, as sorbitol and glycerin, are commonly used. Sorbitol Solution, USP, which contains 64% by weight of the polyhydric alcohol sorbitol is employed as shown in the following example formulations for medicated syrups:[8]

Antihistamine Syrup

Chlorpheniramine Maleate	0.4 g
Glycerin	25.0 mL
Syrup	83.0 mL
Sorbitol Solution	282.0 mL
Sodium Benzoate	1.0 g
Alcohol	60.0 mL
Color and flavor	q.s.
Purified Water, to make	1000.0 mL

Ferrous Sulfate Syrup

Ferrous Sulfate	135.0 g
Citric Acid	12.0 g
Sorbitol Solution	350.0 mL
Glycerin	50.0 mL
Sodium Benzoate	1.0 g
Flavor	q.s.
Purified Water, to make	1000.0 mL

Acetaminophen Syrup

Acetaminophen	24.0 g
Benzoic Acid	1.0 g
Disodium Calcium EDTA	1.0 g
Propylene Glycol	150.0 mL
Alcohol	150.0 mL
Saccharin Sodium	1.8 g
Purified Water	200.0 mL
Flavor	q.s.
Sorbitol Solution, to make	1000.0 mL

Cough-Cold Syrup

Dextromethorphan Hydrobromide	2.0 g
Guaifenesin	10.0 g
Chlorpheniramine Maleate	0.2 g
Phenylephrine Hydrochloride	1.0 g

Sodium Benzoate	1.0 g
Saccharin Sodium	1.9 g
Citric Acid	1.0 g
Sodium Chloride	5.2 g
Alcohol	50.0 mL
Sorbitol Solution	324.0 mL
Syrup	132.0 mL
Liquid Glucose	44.0 mL
Glycerin	50.0 mL
Color	q.s.
Flavor	q.s.
Purified Water, to make	1000.0 mL

All materials used in the extemporaneous compounding and manufacturing of pharmaceuticals should be of USP/NF quality and obtained from FDA-approved sources.

Antimicrobial Preservative

The amount of a preservative required to protect a syrup against microbial growth varies with the proportion of water available for growth, the nature and inherent preservative activity of some formulative materials (as many flavoring oils that are inherently sterile and possess antimicrobial activity), and the capability of the preservative itself. Among the preservatives commonly used in the preservation of syrups with the usually effective concentrations are benzoic acid (0.1 to 0.2%), sodium benzoate (0.1 to 0.2%), and various combinations of methyl-, propyl-, and butylparabens (totaling about 0.1%). Frequently alcohol is used in the preparation of syrups to assist in the dissolving of alcohol-soluble ingredients, but normally it is not present in the final product in amounts that would be considered to be adequate for preservation (15 to 20%). *See accompanying Physical Pharmacy Capsule.*

Flavorant

Most syrups are flavored with synthetic flavorants or with naturally occurring materials as volatile oils (e.g. orange oil), vanillin, and others, to render the syrup pleasant tasting. Because syrups are aqueous preparations, these flavorants must possess sufficient water-solubility. However, sometimes a small amount of alcohol is added to a syrup to ensure the continued solution of a poorly (water) soluble flavorant.

Colorant

To enhance the appeal of the syrup, a coloring agent is generally used which correlates with the flavorant employed (i.e. green with mint, brown with chocolate, etc.). The colorant used is generally water soluble, nonreactive with the other syrup components, and color-stable at the pH range and under the intensity of light that the syrup is likely to encounter during its shelf-life.

Preparation of Syrups

Syrups are most frequently prepared by one of four general methods, depending upon the physical and chemical characteristics of the ingredients. Broadly stated, these methods are (1) solution of the ingredients with the aid of heat, (2) solution of the ingredients by agitation without the use of heat, or the simple admixture of liquid components, (3) addition of sucrose to a prepared medicated liquid or to a flavored liquid, and (4) by percolation of either the source of the medicating substance or of the sucrose. In certain instances a syrup may be successfully prepared by more than one of the above methods, and the selection may simply be a matter of preference on the part of the pharmacist.

For many of the official syrups there is no officially designated method for preparation. This is due to the fact that most official syrups are available on a commercial basis and are not prepared extemporaneously by the pharmacist.

Solution with the Aid of Heat

Syrups are prepared by this method when it is desired to prepare the syrup as quickly as possible and when the syrup's components are not damaged or volatilized by heat. In this method the sugar is generally added to the purified water, and heat is applied until solution is effected. Then, other required heat-stable components are added to the hot syrup, the mixture is allowed to cool, and its volume is adjusted to the proper level by the addition of purified water. In instances in which heat-labile agents or volatile substances, as volatile flavoring oils and alcohol, are to be added, they are generally added to the syrup after the solution of the sugar is effected by heat, and the solution is rapidly cooled to room temperature.

The use of heat facilitates the rapid solution of the sugar as well as certain other components of syrups; however, caution must be exercised against becoming impatient and using excessive heat. Sucrose, a disaccharide, may be hydrolyzed into monosaccharides, dextrose (glucose), and fructose (levulose). This hydrolytic reaction is referred to as *inversion,* and the combination of the

Preservation of Syrups

Syrups can be preserved by (1) storage at low temperature, (2) adding preservatives such as glycerin, benzoic acid, sodium benzoate, methyl paraben or alcohol in the formulation, or (3) by the maintenance of a high concentration of sucrose as a part of the formulation. High sucrose concentrations will usually protect an oral liquid dosage form from growth of most microorganisms. A problem arises, however, when pharmacists must add other ingredients to syrups that can result in a decrease in the sucrose concentration. This may cause a loss of the preservative effectiveness of the sucrose. This can be overcome, however, by calculating the quantity of a preservative (such as alcohol) to add to the formula to maintain the preservative effectiveness of the final product.

EXAMPLE

Rx	Active drug	5 mL volume occupied
	Other drug solids	3 mL volume occupied
	Glycerin	15 mL
	Sucrose	25 g
	Ethanol 95%	q.s.
	Purified Water q.s.	100 mL

How much alcohol would be required to preserve this prescription? We will use the "free water" method to calculate the quantity of alcohol required.

Simple syrup contains 85 g of sucrose per 100 mL of solution, which weighs 131.3 g (Sp. Gr. = 1.313). It takes 46.3 mL of water to prepare the solution (131.3 − 85 = 46.3) and the sucrose occupies a volume of (100 − 46.3 = 53.7) 53.7 mL.

1. Since this solution is preserved, 85 g of sucrose preserves 46.3 mL of water and 1 g of sucrose preserves 0.54 mL of water. With 25 g of sucrose present, the amount of water preserved is:

$$25 \times 0.54 = 13.5 \text{ mL}$$

2. Since 85 g of sucrose occupies a volume of 53.7 mL, 1 g of sucrose will occupy a volume of 0.63 mL. The volume occupied by the sucrose in this prescription is:

$$25 \times 0.63 = 15.75 \text{ mL}$$

3. The active drug and other solids occupy 8 mL (5 + 3) volume.
4. Each mL of glycerin can preserve an equivalent quantity of volume (2 × 15 = 30), so 30 mL would be preserved.
5. The volume taken care of so far is 13.5 + 15.75 + 8 + 30 = 67.25 mL. The quantity of "free water" remaining is:

$$100 - 67.25 = 32.75 \text{ mL}$$

6. Since it requires about 18% alcohol to preserve the water,

$$0.18 \times 32.75 = 5.9 \text{ mL}$$

of alcohol (100%) would be required.
7. If 95% ethanol is used, then 5.9/0.95 = 6.21 mL would be required.

To prepare the prescription, about 6.21 mL of 95% ethanol can be added, with sufficient purified water to make 100 mL of the final solution.

two monosaccharide products is *invert sugar.* When heat is applied in the preparation of a sucrose syrup, some inversion of the sucrose is almost certain. The speed of inversion is greatly increased by the presence of acids, the hydrogen ion acting as a catalyst to the reaction. Should inversion occur, the sweetness of the syrup is altered, because invert sugar is sweeter than sucrose; and the normally colorless syrup darkens due to the effect of heat on the levulose portion of the invert sugar. When the syrup is greatly overheated, it becomes amber colored due to the caramelization of the sucrose. Syrups so decomposed are more susceptible to fermentation and to microbial growth than the stable, nondecomposed syrups. Because of the prospect of decomposition by heat, syrups cannot be sterilized by autoclaving. The use of boiled purified water in the preparation of a syrup can enhance its permanency, and the addition of preservative agents, when permitted, can protect it during its shelf life. Storage in tight containers is a requirement for all syrups.

Solution by Agitation without the Aid of Heat

To avoid heat-induced inversion of sucrose, a syrup may be prepared without heat by agitation. On a small scale, sucrose and other formulative agents may be dissolved in purified water by placing the ingredients in a vessel of greater capacity than the volume of syrup to be prepared, thus permitting the thorough agitation of the mixture. This process is more time-consuming than that utilizing heat to facilitate the solution of sucrose, but the product has maximum stability. Huge glass-lined or stainless steel tanks affixed with mechanical stirrers or agitators are employed in the large-scale preparation of syrups.

Sometimes simple syrup or some other nonmedicated syrup, rather than sucrose, is employed as the sweetening agent and vehicle. In instances such as this, other liquids that are soluble in the syrup or miscible with it may be added and thoroughly mixed to form a uniform product. When solid agents are to be added to a syrup, it is best to dissolve them in a minimal amount of purified water and then incorporate the resulting solution into the syrup. When solid substances are added directly to a syrup, they generally dissolve slowly because the viscous nature of the syrup does not permit the solid substance to distribute readily throughout the syrup to the available solvent and also because a limited amount of available water is present in concentrated syrups.

Addition of Sucrose to a Medicated Liquid or to a Flavored Liquid

Occasionally a medicated liquid, as a tincture or fluidextract, is employed as the source of medication in the preparation of a syrup. Many such tinctures and fluidextracts contain alcohol-soluble constituents and are prepared with alcoholic or hydroalcoholic vehicles. If the alcohol-soluble components are desired medicinal agents to be present in the corresponding syrup, some means of rendering them water-soluble is generally employed. However, if the alcohol-soluble components are undesirable or unnecessary components of the corresponding syrup, they are generally removed by mixing the tincture or fluidextract with water, allowing the mixture to stand until separation of the water-insoluble agents is complete, and filtering them from the mixture. The filtrate then represents the medicated liquid to which the sucrose is added in the preparation of the syrup. In other instances when the tincture or fluidextract is miscible with aqueous preparations, it may be added directly to simple syrup or to a flavored syrup to medicate it.

Percolation

In the percolation method,* either sucrose may be percolated to prepare the syrup, or the source of the medicinal component may be percolated to form an extractive to which sucrose or syrup may be added. This latter method really involves two separate procedures: first the preparation of the extractive of the drug and then the preparation of the syrup.

An example of a syrup prepared by percolation is ipecac syrup. Ipecac syrup is prepared by adding glycerin and syrup to an extractive of powdered ipecac obtained by percolation. The drug ipecac consists of the dried rhizome and roots of *Cephaëlis ipecacuanha* and contains the medicinally active alkaloids, emetine, cephaeline, and psychotrine. These alkaloids are extracted from the powdered ipecac by percolation with a hydroalcoholic solvent.

The syrup is categorized as an emetic with a usual dose of 15 mL. This amount of syrup is commonly used in the management of poisoning in children when the evacuation of the stomach contents is desirable. About 80% of children given this dose will vomit within a half hour. For a household emetic in event of poisoning, 1-oz. bottles of the syrup may be sold without the requirement of a prescription. Ipecac syrup also has some application as a nauseant expectorant, in doses smaller than the emetic dose.

Recent evidence indicates that many bulimics—most commonly young women in their late teens to early 30s—use syrup of ipecac to bring on attacks of vomiting in an attempt to lose

* The process of percolation is discussed in Chapter 14.

more weight.[9] Pharmacists must be aware of this misuse of syrup of ipecac and warn these individuals because one of the active ingredients besides ipecac in the syrup is emetine. With continual use of the syrup, emetine builds up toxic levels within body tissues and in 3 to 4 months can do irreversible damage to heart muscles resulting in symptoms mimicking a heart attack. Shortness of breath is the most common symptom in patients who misuse syrup of ipecac, but some persons may describe low blood pressure-related symptoms and irregularities of heart beat.

Elixirs

Elixirs are clear, sweetened, hydroalcoholic solutions intended for oral use, and are usually flavored to enhance their palatability. *Nonmedicated* elixirs are employed as vehicles and *medicated* elixirs for the therapeutic effect of the medicinal substances they contain. Compared to syrups, elixirs are usually less sweet and less viscous because they contain a lower proportion of sugar and consequently less effective than syrups in masking the taste of medicinal substances. However, because of their hydroalcoholic character, elixirs are better able than aqueous syrups to maintain both water-soluble and alcohol-soluble components in solution. Also because of their stable characteristics and the ease which which they are prepared (by simple solution), from a manufacturing standpoint, elixirs are preferred over syrups.

The proportion of alcohol present in elixirs varies widely since the individual components of the elixirs have different water and alcohol solubility characteristics. Each elixir requires a specific blend of alcohol and water to maintain all of the components in solution. Naturally, for those elixirs containing agents which have poor water-solubility the proportion of alcohol required is greater than for elixirs prepared from components having good water solubility. In addition to alcohol and water, other solvents, as glycerin and propylene glycol, are frequently employed in elixirs as adjunct solvents.

Although many elixirs are sweetened with sucrose or with a sucrose-syrup, some utilize sorbitol, glycerin and/or artificial sweeteners. Elixirs having a high alcoholic content usually utilize an artificial sweetener as saccharin, which is required only in small amounts, rather than sucrose which is only slightly soluble in alcohol and requires greater quantities for equivalent sweetness.

All elixirs contain flavoring materials to increase their palatability and most elixirs have coloring agents to enhance their appearance. Elixirs containing over 10 to 12% of alcohol are usually self-preserving and do not require the addition of an antimicrobial agent for their preservation.

Although the USP monographs for medicated elixirs provide standards, they do not generally provide official formulas. Formulations are left up to the individual manufacturers. Example formulations for some medicated elixirs are as follows:[8]

Phenobarbital Elixir

Phenobarbital	4.00 g
Orange Oil	0.25 mL
Propylene Glycol	100.00 mL
Alcohol	200.00 mL
Sorbitol Solution	600.00 mL
Color	q.s.
Purified Water, to make	1000.00 mL

Theophylline Elixir

Theophylline	5.3 g
Citric Acid	10.0 g
Liquid Glucose	44.0 g
Syrup	132.0 mL
Glycerin	50.0 mL
Sorbitol Solution	324.0 mL
Alcohol	200.00 mL
Saccharin Sodium	5.0 g
Lemon Oil	0.5 g
FDC Yellow No. 5	0.1 g
Purified Water, to make	1000.0 mL

Medicated elixirs are formulated such that a patient receives the usual adult dose of the drug in convenient measure of elixir. For most elixirs, one or two teaspoonfuls (5 or 10 mL) provide the usual adult dose of the drug. One advantage of elixirs over their counterpart drugs in solid dosage forms is the flexibility and ease of dosage administration to patients who have difficulty swallowing solid forms.

A disadvantage of elixirs for children and for adults who choose to avoid alcohol is their alcoholic content. The reader may wish to refer to the discussion of alcohol as a solvent earlier in this chapter for FDA-recommended limits on alcohol content for OTC oral products.

Because of their usual content of volatile oils and alcohol, elixirs should be stored in tight, light-resistant containers and protected from excessive heat.

Preparation of Elixirs

Elixirs are usually prepared by simple solution with agitation and/or by the admixture of two or more liquid ingredients. Alcohol-soluble and water-soluble components are generally dissolved separately in alcohol and in purified water, respectively. Then the aqueous solution is added to the alcoholic solution, rather than the reverse, in order to maintain the highest possible alcoholic strength at all times so that minimal separation of the alcohol-soluble components occurs. When the two solutions are completely mixed the mixture is made to volume with the specified solvent or vehicle. Frequently the final mixture will not be clear, but cloudy, due principally to the separation of some of the flavoring oils by the reduced alcoholic concentration. If this occurs, the elixir is usually permitted to stand for a prescribed number of hours, to ensure the saturation of the hydroalcoholic solvent and to permit the oil globules to coalesce so that they may be more easily removed by filtration. Talc, a frequent filter aid in the preparation of elixirs, has the ability to absorb the excessive amounts of oils and therefore assist in their removal from the solution. The presence of glycerin, syrup, sorbitol, and propylene glycol in elixirs generally contributes to the solvent effect of the hydroalcoholic vehicle, assists in the dissolution of the solute, and enhances the stability of the preparation. However, the presence of these materials adds to the viscosity of the elixir and shows the rate of their filtration.

Nonmedicated Elixirs

Nonmedicated elixirs may be useful to the pharmacist in the extemporaneous filling of prescriptions involving: (1) the addition of a therapeutic agent to a pleasant tasting vehicle, and (2) the dilution of an existing medicated elixir. In selecting a liquid vehicle for a drug substance, the pharmacist should be concerned with the solubility and stability of the drug substance in water and alcohol. If a hydroalcoholic vehicle is selected, the proportion of alcohol present should be only slightly above that amount which is needed to effect and maintain the drug's solution. When a pharmacist is called upon to dilute an existing medicated elixir, the nonmedicated elixir he selects as the diluent should have the approximate alcoholic concentration as the elixir being diluted. Also, the flavor and color characteristics of the diluent should not be in conflict with the medicated elixir and all components should be chemically and physically compatible.

In years past, when pharmacists were called upon more frequently than today to compound prescriptions, the three most commonly used nonmedicated elixirs were: Aromatic Elixir, Compound Benzaldehyde Elixir, and Iso-Alcoholic Elixir.

Medicated Elixirs

As noted previously, medicated elixirs are employed for the therapeutic benefit of the medicinal agent present. In most instances, the official and commercial elixirs contain a single therapeutic agent. The main advantage of having only a single therapeutic agent present is that the dosage taken of that single drug may be increased or decreased by simply taking more or less of the elixir, whereas when two or more therapeutic agents are present in the same preparation, it is impossible to increase or decrease the amount taken of one without an automatic and corresponding adjustment in the dose taken of the other; a change which may not be desired. Thus, for patients required to take more than a single medication, many physicians prefer them to take separate preparations of each drug so that if an adjustment in the dosage of one is desired, it may be accomplished without the concomitant adjustment of the other.

Table 6–8 presents some examples of medicated elixirs. Some of these are briefly discussed below.

Antihistamine Elixirs

As indicated in Table 6–8, antihistamines are useful primarily in the symptomatic relief of certain allergic disorders. In their action, they suppress symptoms caused by histamine, one of the chemical agents released during the antigen-antibody reaction of the allergic response. Although only minor differences exist in the properties of most antihistamines, one or another may be preferred by a prescriber through his experience in managing a specific type of allergic reaction. A prescriber's preference may also be based on the incidence of adverse effects which may be expected to occur. The incidence and severity

Table 6–8. Examples of Medicated Elixirs by Category

Elixir	*Some Representative Commercial Products*	*Usual Adult Dose of Drug/Volume of Commercial Elixir*	*Comments*
Adrenocortical Steroid			
Dexamethasone Elixir	Decadron Elixir (Merck & Co.)	500 μg/5 mL	Dexamethasone is a synthetic analogue of hydrocortisone that is considered to be about 30 times more potent than the latter drug. The commercial dexamethasone elixir is packaged with a calibrated dropper for the accurate measurement of small doses and is intended primarily for children, but also has utility for adults who may have trouble swallowing tablets. The elixir is used for many indications, including the treatment of rheumatoid arthritis, skin diseases, allergies and inflammatory conditions. The commercial product contains 5% alcohol.
Analgesic/Antipyretic			
Acetaminophen Elixir	Children's Tylenol Elixir (McNeil)	160 mg/5 mL	Use for reduction of pain and lowering of fever particularly in patients sensitive to or unable to take aspirin. Elixir especially useful for pediatric patients, and is alcohol-free.
Anticholinergic/Antispasmodic			
Hyoscyamine Sulfate Elixir	Levsin Elixir (Schwarz)	0.125 mg hyoscyamine sulfate/5 mL	Used to control gastric secretion, visceral spasm, hypermotility, and abdominal cramps. The commercial product contains 20% alcohol.
Antihistamine			
Diphenhydramine HCl Elixir	Benadryl Elixir (Parke-Davis)	12.5 mg/5 mL	Antihistamine elixirs are employed for a variety of allergic reactions including: perennial and seasonal allergic rhinitis, vasomotor rhinitis, allergic skin manifestations of urticaria, reactions to insect bites, and others. The commercial product contains 5.6% alcohol.
Antipsychotic			
Fluphenazine HCl Elixir	Prolixin Elixir (Apothecon)	2.5 mg/5 mL	Used in the management of psychotic disorders. The commercial product contains 14% alcohol.
Cardiotonic			
Digoxin Elixir	Lanoxin Pediatric Elixir (Burroughs Wellcome)	50 μg/mL	Among other effects, digoxin increases the force of myocardial contraction. Used in congestive heart failure, atrial fibrillation and other cardiac conditions. See text for additional discussion. The commercial product contains 10% alcohol.
Expectorants			
Terpin Hydrate Elixir	Terpin Hydrate Elixir (Rugby)	170 mg/10 mL	Terpin hydrate has expectorant action. The addition of codeine and dextromethorphan provides antitussive action as well. These elixirs contain between 39% and 44% alcohol.
Terpin Hydrate and Codeine Elixir	Terpin Hydrate and Codeine Elixir (Rugby)	170 mg terpin hydrate and 20 mg codeine/10 mL	
Terpin Hydrate and Dextromethorphan HBr Elixir	Terpin Hydrate and Dextromethorphan Elixir (Rugby)	170 mg terpin hydrate and 20 mg dextromethorphan HBr/10 mL	
Mucolytic Expectorant			
Iodinated Glycerol Elixir	Organidin Elixir (Wallace)	30 mg organically bound iodine/5 mL	Used in respiratory conditions as asthma and bronchitis. It increases the output of thin respiratory tract fluid and helps to liquify mucus in the respiratory tree. The commercial product contains 21.75% alcohol.
Sedative/Hypnotics			
Butabarbital Sodium Elixir	Butisol Sodium Elixir (Wallace)	30 mg/5 mL	The barbiturate elixirs are utilized in low dosage as sedatives and in higher dosage as hypnotics. The butabarbital sodium elixir contains 7% alcohol and the phenobarbital elixir contains 14% alcohol. See text for additional discussion.
Phenobarbital Elixir	Phenobarbital Elixir (Lilly)	20 mg/5 mL	
Smooth Muscle Relaxant			
Theophylline Sodium Glycinate Elixir	Asbron G Elixir (Sandoz)	300 mg/15 mL	Used in bronchial asthma and other conditions requiring smooth muscle relaxation; product literature states that the buffering action of the glycine and the drug's solubility reduce the chance of theophylline precipitation in the stomach, resulting in the product's greater gastric tolerance than aminophylline.

of these effects do vary somewhat with the drug and the dose of each drug. The most common untoward effect is sedation, and patients taking antihistamines should be warned against engaging in activities requiring mental alertness, as driving an automobile or tractor or operating machinery. Other common adverse effects include dryness of the nose, throat, and mouth, dizziness and disturbed concentration. Included among the most sedating antihistamines are diphenhydramine, doxylamine, and methapyrilene. In fact, diphenhydramine is used as a sleep aid in numerous over-the-counter products for its ability to cause drowsiness.

Most antihistaminic agents are basic amines. By forming salts through interaction with acid, the compounds are rendered water soluble. These salt forms are generally used in elixirs and thus the elixirs of the antihistamines are not required to contain a large proportion of alcohol. Because the acid salts of the antihistamines are used, the pH of these elixirs is on the acid side and must remain so if the drugs are to remain freely soluble in water. A pharmacist should keep this in mind when utilizing one of these elixirs in the compounding of a prescription involving adding or mixing other components.

Barbiturate Sedative/Hypnotic Elixirs

The barbiturates are sedative/hypnotic agents which are used to produce various degrees of central nervous system depression. As the dose of these drugs is increased, the effects go from sedation to hypnosis to respiratory depression, the latter being the cause of death in fatal barbiturate overdosage.

Barbiturates are administered in small doses in the daytime hours as sedatives to reduce restlessness and emotional tension. The appropriate dose for this purpose is that amount which alleviates anxiety or tension but does not produce drowsiness or lethargy. Greater doses of the barbiturates may be given before bedtime as hypnotics to relieve insomnia.

Barbiturates have been classified according to the duration of their (hypnotic) effects; that is, *long-acting, intermediate-acting, short-acting*, or *ultrashort-acting* agents. The long-acting barbiturates including phenobarbital are considered most useful in maintaining daytime sedation and in treating some convulsive states and least useful in acting as hypnotics. The intermediate-acting barbiturates include amobarbital and are used primarily for short-term daytime sedation and are effective in treating insomnia. The barbiturates classified as short-acting include pentobarbital and secobarbital and are used similarly to the intermediate-acting barbiturates. The ultrashort-acting barbiturates, as thiopental, are given intravenously to induce anesthesia.

The most common untoward effect noticed in patients taking barbiturates is drowsiness and lethargy. Large doses may produce residual sedation resembling the hangover following alcohol intoxication. Prolonged use of barbiturates may lead to psychic or physical dependence. This dependence, in susceptible individuals, leads to compulsive abuse of the drug with severe withdrawal symptoms following abstinence. In heavy chronic users, abrupt withdrawal may lead to convulsions, delirium, and occasionally to coma and death.

Some pharmaceutic aspects of Phenobarbital Elixir are presented below.

Phenobarbital Elixir

Phenobarbital elixir is formulated to contain 0.4% of phenobarbital, which provides about 20 mg of drug per teaspoonful (5 mL) of elixir. The elixir is commonly flavored with orange oil, colored red with an FDA-approved colorant, and sweetened with syrup. The official elixir contains about 14% of alcohol, which is used to dissolve the phenobarbital. However, this amount represents almost the very minimum required to keep the phenobarbital in solution. Thus glycerin is often added to enhance the solubility of phenobarbital.

Phenobarbital is a long-acting barbiturate with a duration of action of about 4 to 6 hours and a usual adult dose as a sedative of about 30 mg and a hypnotic dose of about 100 mg. The strength of the elixir permits the convenient adjustment of dosage to achieve the proper degree of sedation in the treatment of infants, children, and certain adult patients.

The elixir is commercially available from a variety of manufacturers under its nonproprietary name.

Digoxin Elixir

No official method of preparation is indicated for Digoxin Elixir USP; however, it is required to contain 4.50 mg to 5.25 mg of digoxin per 100 mL of elixir or about 0.25 mg per 5 mL teaspoonful. The usual oral adult dose of digoxin as a cardiotonic agent is about 1.5 mg on initial therapy and about 0.5 mg for maintenance therapy.

Digoxin is a cardiotonic glycoside obtained from the leaves of *Digitalis lanata.* It is a white crystalline powder that is insoluble in water, but soluble in dilute alcohol solutions. The official elixir contains about 10% of alcohol. Digoxin is a poisonous drug, and its dose must be carefully determined and administered to each individual patient. Adults generally take digoxin tablets rather than the elixir, which must be measured by the highly variable household teaspoon. The elixir is generally employed in pediatric practice, and the commercial product available for this purpose is packaged with a calibrated dropper to facilitate accurate dosage measurements.

Digoxin is one of many drugs which is available to the prescriber in more than a single type of dosage form. The prescriber frequently has the choice of selecting a solid dosage form, as a tablet or capsule, or a liquid form of the medication for his patient. The advantages of each have been noted previously but it is important here to point out again that drugs administered in different dosage forms may exhibit different bioavailability characteristics with varying patterns of drug release and rates and extents of drug absorption. Such differences have been noted for digoxin, between tablets from different manufacturers, as well as between tablets and oral liquid dosage forms. Figure 6–2 shows the differences noted in one study of the serum digoxin levels following administration of 0.5 mg of digoxin by oral tablet and oral solution having an elixir-like vehicle. It can be readily seen that the serum digoxin levels following administration of the oral solution were considerably greater than from the oral tablet.

A patient taking a drug known to exhibit bioavailability problems, and whose therapeutic dosage regimen has been successfully established with a particular drug product, should not be changed to another product.

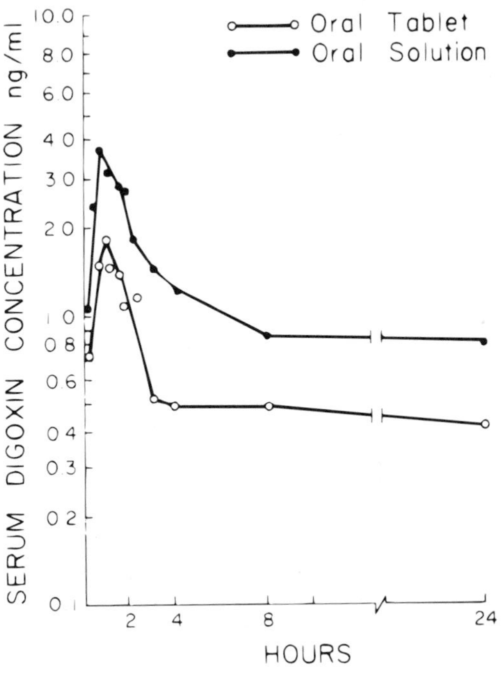

Fig. 6–2. *Serum digoxin concentrations following administration of 0.5 mg of digoxin by oral tablet and elixir-like oral solution. (Adapted from D. H. Huffman and D. L. Azarnoff: Absorption of Orally Given Digoxin Preparations. J.A.M.A., 222:957, 1972.)*

Proper Administration and Use of Liquid Peroral Dosage Forms

The dosage forms discussed in this chapter are all to be administered by mouth. Conveniently, these can be measured in a spoon, i.e., teaspoon, tablespoon, depending upon the desired dosage and swallowed. Perferably, however, these medicines should be measured out in calibrated devices for administration. These devices assure the patient that the correct dose will be received because teaspoons, for example, can vary dramatically in the volume they deliver. Even though these are liquids, it is recommended that the patient follow the administration of the liquid dosage form with a glassful of water.

The pharmacist must be careful in the selection of liquid products given the patient's history and other concurrent medicines. For example, some syrups contain sucrose or another sugar as an ingredient, and the pharmacist must recall that such syrups would not be optimal for use in an oral prescription intended for a diabetic patient. Similarly, a product that is formulated as an elixir would not be advantageous to use in a patient who receives concurrent medicines that possess an antabuse-like activity, i.e., the patient may get violently ill from the concurrent ingestion of alcohol. Metronidazole and chlorpropramide are two drugs that have been implicated to cause this reaction when mixed with alcohol. Further, if the patient is receiving another drug that causes drowsiness the pharmacist must make a decision to intervene and contact the prescribing physician to determine whether the prescribed elixir could be harmful to the patient.

References

1. *United States Pharmacopeia 23/National Formulary 18,* United States Pharmacopeial Convention, Inc., Rockville, MD, 1995, 1947.
2. *United States Pharmacopeia 23/National Formulary 18,* United States Pharmacopeial Convention, Inc., Rockville, MD, 1995, 10.
3. *Pure Water Handbook,* Osmonics, Inc., Minnetonka, MN, 1991.
4. Chemburkar, P.B., and Joslin, R.S.: Effect of Flavoring Oils on Preservative Concentrations in Oral Liquid Dosage Forms. *J. Pharm. Sci., 64:*414–441, 1975.
5. Gossel, T.A.: Oral Rehydration Solutions. *US Pharmacist, 12:*90–98, 1987.
6. *Handbook on Extemporaneous Formulations.* American Society of Hospital Pharmacists, Bethesda, MD, 1987.
7. Pesko, L.J.: Compounding: Oral Liquids. *Amer. Druggist, 208:*49, 1993.
8. *Oral Liquid Pharmaceuticals.* ICI Americas, Inc., Wilmington, DE, 1975.
9. Murphy, D.: Ipecac Misuse by Bulimics: APhA Launches Educational Campaign. *Amer. Pharm. NS25:*264–265, 1985.

7

Oral Suspensions, Emulsions, Magmas, and Gels

This Chapter includes the main types of liquid preparations containing undissolved drug distributed throughout a vehicle and intended for oral administration. In these preparations, the substance distributed is referred to as the *dispersed phase* and the vehicle is termed the *dispersing phase* or *dispersion medium*. Together, they produce a *dispersed system*.

The particles of the dispersed phase are usually solid materials which are insoluble in the dispersion medium. In the case of emulsions, the dispersed phase is a liquid substance which is neither soluble nor miscible with the liquid of the dispersing phase. The emulsification process results in the dispersion of liquid drug as fine droplets throughout the dispersing phase.

The particles of the dispersed phase vary widely in size, from large particles visible to the naked eye down to particles of colloidal dimension, falling between 1.0 nm and 0.5 μm in size. Dispersions containing coarse particles, usually 10–50 μm in size, are referred to as *coarse dispersions* and include the *suspensions* and *emulsions*. Dispersions containing particles of smaller size are termed *fine dispersions* (0.5–10 μm), and, if the particles are in the colloidal range, *colloidal dispersions*. *Magmas* and *gels* represent such fine dispersions.

Largely because of their greater size, dispersed particles in a coarse dispersion have a greater tendency to separate from the dispersion medium than do the particles of a fine dispersion. Most solids in dispersion tend to settle to the bottom of the container because of their greater density than the dispersion medium, whereas most emulsified liquids for oral use are oils and generally have a lesser density than the aqueous medium in which they are dispersed and tend to rise toward the top of the preparation. Complete and uniform redistribution of the dispersed phase is essential to the accurate administration of uniform doses. For a properly prepared dispersion, this should be accomplished by the moderate agitation of the container.

While the focus of this chapter is on dispersions of drugs administered orally, the same basic pharmaceutical characteristics apply to those dispersion systems administered by other routes and discussed later in this text. Included among these are lotions for topical application to the skin, ophthalmic suspensions, and sterile suspensions for injection.

Oral Suspensions

Suspensions may be defined as preparations containing finely divided drug particles (referred to as the *suspensoid*) distributed somewhat uniformly throughout a vehicle in which the drug exhibits a minimum degree of solubility. Some suspensions are available in ready-to-use form—that is, already distributed through a liquid vehicle with or without stabilizers and other pharmaceutical additives (Fig. 7–1). Other preparations are available as dry powders intended for suspensions in liquid vehicles. This type of product generally is a powder mixture containing the drug and suitable suspending and dispersing agents, which upon dilution and agitation with a specified quantity of vehicle (generally purified water) results in the formation of a suspension suitable for administration. Figure 7–2 demonstrates the preparation of this type of product. Drugs that are unstable if maintained for extended periods of time in the presence of an aqueous vehicle (for example, many antibiotic drugs) are most frequently supplied as dry powder mixtures for reconstitution at the time of dispensing. This type of preparation is designated in the USP by a title of the form "... for Oral Suspension." Prepared suspensions not requiring reconstitution at the time of dispensing are simply designated as "... Oral Suspension."

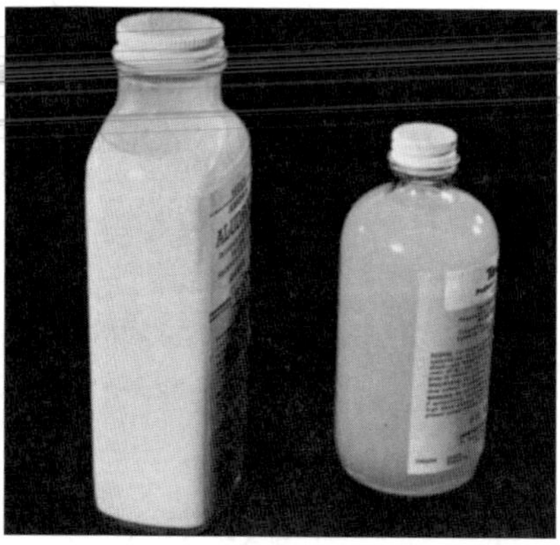

Fig. 7–1. *Examples of some commercial oral suspensions.*

Reasons for Oral Suspension

The reasons for preparing the oral suspension are several. For one thing, certain drugs are chemically unstable when in solution but stable when suspended. In instances such as this, the oral suspension insures chemical stability while permitting liquid therapy. For many patients, the liquid form is preferred over the solid form of the same drug because of the ease of swallowing liquids and the flexibility in the administration of a range of doses. This is particularly advantageous for infants, children and the elderly. The disadvantage of the disagreeable taste of certain drugs when given in solution form is overcome when the drug is administered as undissolved particles of a suspension. In fact, chemical forms of certain poor-tasting drugs have been specifically developed for their insolubility in a desired vehicle for the sole purpose of preparing a palatable liquid dosage form. For example, the water-insoluble ester form of chloramphenicol, chloramphenicol palmitate, was developed to prepare a palatable liquid dosage form of the chloramphenicol, the result being the development of Chloramphenicol Palmitate Oral Suspension, USP. By the creation of insoluble forms of drugs for use in suspensions, the difficult taste-masking problems of developmental pharmacists are greatly reduced, and the selection of the flavorants to be used in a given suspension may be based on taste preference rather than on a particular flavorant's ability to act as a masking agent for an unpleasant tasting drug. For the most part, oral suspensions are aqueous preparations with the vehicle flavored and sweetened to suit the anticipated taste preferences of the intended patient.

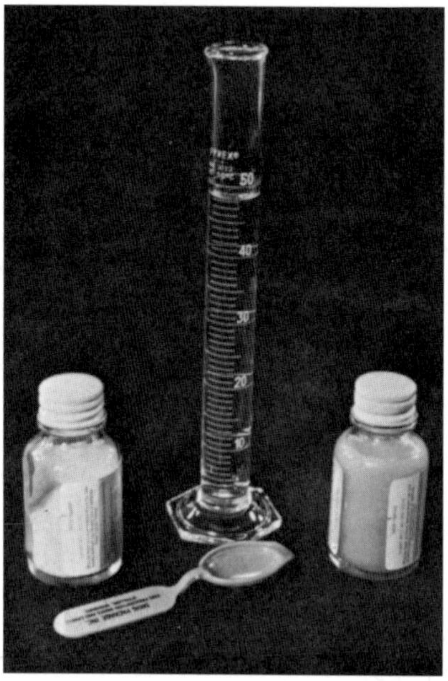

Fig. 7–2. *Commercial antibiotic preparation for oral suspension following reconstitution with purified water. On the left is the dry powder mixture, and on the right the suspension after reconstitution with the specified amount of purified water.*

Features Desired in a Pharmaceutical Suspension

There are many considerations in the development and preparation of a pharmaceutically elegant suspension. In addition to therapeutic efficacy, chemical stability of the components of the formulation, permanency of the preparation, and esthetic appeal of the preparation—desirable qualities in all pharmaceutical preparations—a few other features apply more specifically to the pharmaceutical suspension:

1. A properly prepared pharmaceutical suspension should settle slowly and should be readily redispersed upon the gentle shaking of the container.
2. The characteristics of the suspension should be such that the particle size of the suspensoid remains fairly constant throughout long periods of undisturbed standing.
3. The suspension should pour readily and evenly from its container.

These main features of a suspension, which depend upon the nature of the dispersed phase, the dispersion medium, and pharmaceutical adjuncts, will be discussed briefly.

Sedimentation Rate of the Particles of a Suspension

The various factors involved in the rate of velocity of settling of the particles of a suspension are embodied in the equation of Stokes' law, which is presented in the accompanying Physical Pharmacy Capsule.

Stokes' equation was derived for an ideal situation in which uniform, perfectly spherical particles in a very dilute suspension settle without effecting turbulence in their downward course, without collision of the particles of the suspensoid, and without chemical or physical attraction or affinity for the dispersion medium. Obviously, Stokes' equation does not apply precisely to the usual pharmaceutical suspension in which the suspensoid is irregularly shaped, of various particle diameters, and not spherical, in which the fall of the particles *does* result in both turbulence and collision, and also in which there may be a reasonable amount of affinity of the particles for the suspension medium. However, the basic concepts of the equation do give a valid indication of the factors that are important to the suspension of the particles and a clue to the possible adjustments that can be made to a formulation to decrease the rate of particle sedimentation.

From the equation it is apparent that the velocity of fall of a suspended particle is greater for larger particles than it is for smaller particles, all other factors remaining constant. By reducing the particle size of the dispersed phase, one can expect a slower *rate* of descent of the particles. Also, the greater the density of the particles, the greater the rate of descent, provided the density of the vehicle is not altered. Because aqueous vehicles are generally used in pharmaceutical oral suspensions, the density of the particles is generally greater than that of the vehicle, a desirable feature, for if the particles were less dense than the vehicle, they would tend to float, and floating particles would be quite difficult to distribute uniformly in the vehicle. The rate of sedimentation may be appreciably reduced by increasing the viscosity of the dispersion medium, and within limits of practicality this may be done. However, a product having too high a viscosity is not generally desirable, because it pours with difficulty and it is equally difficult to redisperse the suspensoid. Therefore, if the viscosity of a suspension is increased, it is done so only to a modest extent to avoid these difficulties.

The viscosity characteristics of a suspension may be altered not only by the vehicle used, but also by the solids content. As the proportion of solid particles is increased in a suspension, so is the viscosity. The viscosity of a pharmaceutical preparation may be determined through the use of a Brookfield Viscometer, which measures viscosity by the force required to rotate a spindle in the fluid being tested (Fig. 7–3).

For the most part, the physical stability of a pharmaceutical suspension appears to be most appropriately adjusted by an alteration in the dispersed phase rather than through great changes in the dispersion medium. In most instances, the dispersion medium is supportive to the adjusted dispersed phase. These adjustments mainly are concerned with particle size, uniformity of particle size, and separation of the particles so that they are not likely to become greatly larger or to form a solid cake on standing.

Physical Features of the Dispersed Phase of a Suspension

Probably the most important single consideration in a discussion of suspensions is the size of the drug particles. In most good pharmaceutical suspensions, the particle diameter is between 1 and 50 μm.

Particle size reduction is generally accomplished by dry-milling prior to the incorporation of the dispersed phase into the dispersion medium. One of the most rapid, convenient, and inexpensive methods of producing fine drug powders of about 10 to 50 μm size is *micropulverization*. Micropulverizers are high-speed, attrition or impact mills which are efficient in reducing powders to the size acceptable for most oral and topical suspensions. For still finer particles, under 10 μm, the process of *fluid energy* grinding, sometimes referred to as *jet-milling* or *micronizing*, is quite effective. By this process, the shearing action of high velocity compressed air streams on the particles in a confined space produces the desired ultrafine or micronized particles. The particles to be micronized are swept into violent turbulence by the sonic and supersonic velocity of the air streams. The particles are accelerated into high velocities and collide with one another, resulting in fragmentation and a decrease in the size of the particles. This

Sedimentation Rate & Stokes' Equation

Stokes' Equation:

$$\frac{dx}{dt} = \frac{d^2(\rho_i - \rho_e)g}{18\eta}$$

where dx/dt is the rate of settling,
d^2 is the diameter of the particles,
ρ_i is the density of the particle,
ρ_e is the density of the medium,
g is the gravitational constant, and
η is the viscosity of the medium.

A number of factors can be adjusted to enhance the physical stability of a suspension, including the diameter of the particles and the density and viscosity of the medium. The effect of changing these is illustrated in the following example.

EXAMPLE 1

A powder has a density of 1.3 g/cc and is available as a powder with an average particle diameter of 2.5 microns (assuming the particles to be spheres). According to Stoke's Equation, this powder will settle in water (viscosity of 1 cps assumed) at a rate of:

$$\frac{(2.5 \times 10^{-4})^2(1.3 - 1.0)(980)}{18 \times 0.01} = 1.02 \times 10^{-4} \text{ cm/sec}$$

If the particle size of the powder is reduced to 0.25 μ and water is still used as the dispersion medium, the powder will now settle at a rate of:

$$\frac{(2.5 \times 10^{-5})^2(1.3 - 1.0)(980)}{18 \times 0.01} = 1.02 \times 10^{-6} \text{ cm/sec}$$

As is evident, a decrease in particle size by a factor of 10 results in a reduction in the rate of settling by a factor of 100. This enhanced effect is a result of the "d" factor in Stokes Equation being squared.

Now, if a different dispersion medium, such as glycerin, is used in place of water, a further decrease in settling will result. Glycerin has a density of 1.25 g/cc and a viscosity of 400 cps. The larger particle size powder (2.5 μ) will settle at a rate of:

$$\frac{(2.5 \times 10^{-4})^2(1.3 - 1.25)(980)}{18.4} = 4.25 \times 10^{-8} \text{ cm/sec}$$

The smaller particle size (0.25 μ) powder will now settle at a rate of:

$$\frac{(2.5 \times 10^{-5})^2(1.3 - 1.25)(980)}{18 \times 4} = 4.25 \times 10^{-10} \text{ cm/sec}$$

A summary of these results is shown in the following table:

Condition	*Rate of Settling (cm/sec)*
2.5 μ powder in water	1.02×10^{-4}
0.25 μ powder in water	1.02×10^{-6}
2.5 μ powder in glycerin	4.25×10^{-8}
0.25 μ powder in glycerin	4.25×10^{-10}

As is evident from this table, a change in dispersion medium results in the greatest change in the rate of settling of particles. Particle size reduction also can contribute significantly to suspension stability. These factors are important in the formulation of physically stable suspensions.

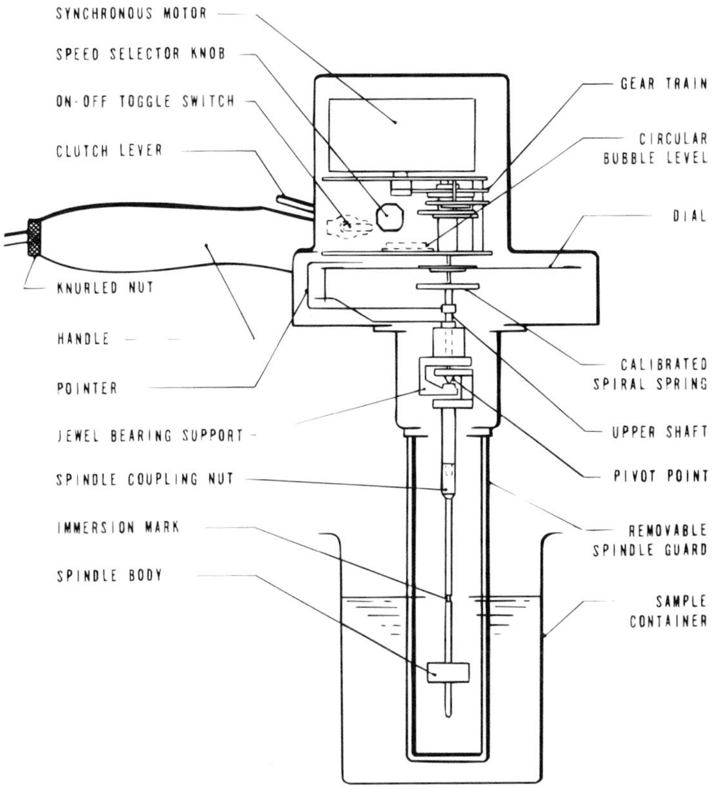

Fig. 7–3. *Schematic drawing of the Brookfield Viscometer. (Courtesy of Brookfield Engineering Laboratories.)*

method may be employed in instances in which the particles are intended for parenteral or ophthalmic suspensions. Particles of extremely small dimensions may also be produced by *spray-drying* techniques. A spray dryer is a cone-shaped piece of apparatus into which a solution of a drug is sprayed and rapidly dried by a current of warmed, dry air circulating in the cone. The resulting dry powder is then collected. It is not possible for a community pharmacist to achieve the same degree of particle-size reduction with such simple comminuting equipment as the mortar and pestle. However, many micronized drugs are commercially available and when needed may be purchased by the pharmacist in bulk quantities.

As shown by Stokes' equation, the reduction in the particle size of a suspensoid is beneficial to the stability of the suspension in that the rate of sedimentation of the solid particles is reduced as the particles are decreased in size. The reduction in particle size produces slow, more uniform rates of settling. However, one should avoid reducing the particle size to too great a degree of fineness, since fine particles have a tendency to form a compact cake upon settling to the bottom of the container. The result may be that the cake resists breakup upon shaking, and forms rigid aggregates of particles which are of larger dimension and less suspendable than the original suspensoid. The particle shape of the suspensoid can also affect caking and product stability. It has been shown that symmetrical barrel-shaped particles of calcium carbonate produced more stable suspensions than did asymmetrical needle-shaped particles of the same agent. The needle-shaped particles formed a tenacious sediment-cake on standing which could not be redistributed whereas the barrel-shaped particles did not cake on standing.[1]

To avoid the formation of a cake, measures must be take to prevent the agglomeration of the particles into larger crystals or into masses. One common method of preventing the rigid cohesion of small articles of a suspension is through the intentional formation of a less rigid or loose aggregation of the particles held together by comparatively weak particle-to-particle bonding forces. Such an aggregation of particles is termed a *floc* or a *floccule*, with flocculated particles forming a type of lattice structure that resists complete settling (although flocs settle more rapidly than fine, individual particles) and thus are less prone to compaction than unflocculated particles. The flocs settle to form a higher sediment volume than unflocculated particles, the loose structure of which permits the aggregates to break up easily and distribute readily with a small amount of agitation.

There are several methods of preparing flocculated suspensions, the choice depending on the type of drug involved and the type of product desired. For instance, in the preparation of an oral suspension of a drug, clays such as diluted bentonite magma are commonly employed as the flocculating agent. The structure of the bentonite magma and of other clays used for this purpose also assists the suspension by helping to support the floc once formed. When clays are unsuitable as agents, as in a parenteral suspension, frequently a floc of the dispersed phase can be produced by an alteration in the pH of the preparation (generally to the region of minimum drug solubility). Electrolytes can also act as flocculating agents, apparently by reducing the electrical barrier between the particles of the suspensoid and forming a bridge so as to link them together. The carefully determined concentration of nonionic and ionic surface-active agents (surfactants) can also induce the flocculation of particles in suspension and increase the sedimentation volume.

Dispersion Medium

Oftentimes, as with highly flocculated suspensions, the particles of a suspension settle too rapidly to be consistent with what might be termed a pharmaceutically elegant preparation. The rapid settling hinders the accurate measurement of dosage and from an esthetic point of view produces too unsightly a supernatant layer. In many of the commercial suspensions, suspending agents are added to the dispersion medium to lend it a structure to assist in the suspension of the dispersed phase. Carboxymethylcellulose, methylcellulose, microcrystalline cellulose, polyvinyl pyrrolidone, xanthan gum, and bentonite are a few of the agents employed to thicken the dispersion medium and help suspend the suspensoid. When polymeric substances and hydrophilic colloids are used as suspending agents, appropriate tests must be performed to show that the agent does not interfere with the availability for therapeutic effects of the suspension's medicinal substance. These materials have been found to bind certain medicinal agents, rendering them unavailable or more slowly available for their therapeutic function. Also, the amount of the suspending agent must not be such to render the suspension too viscous to agitate (to distribute the *suspensoid*) or to pour. The study of the flow characteristics is termed *rheology*. *A summary of the concepts of rheology is found in the accompanying Physical Pharmacy Capsule.*

Support of the suspensoid by the dispersion medium may depend upon several factors: the density of the suspensoid, whether it is flocculated, and the amount of material requiring support.

The solid content of a suspension intended for oral administration may vary considerably, depending on the dose of the drug to be administered, the volume of product desired to be administered, and also on the ability of the dispersion medium to support the concentration of drug while maintaining desirable features of viscosity and flow. The usual adult oral suspension is frequently designed to supply the dose of the particular drug in a convenient measure of 5 mL or one teaspoonful. Pediatric suspensions are formulated to deliver the appropriate dose of drug by administering a dose-calibrated number of drops. Figure 7–4 shows commonly packaged oral suspensions administered as pediatric drops. Some are accompanied by a calibrated dropper, whereas other packages have the drop capability built into the container. On administration the drops may be placed directly into the infant's mouth or mixed with a small

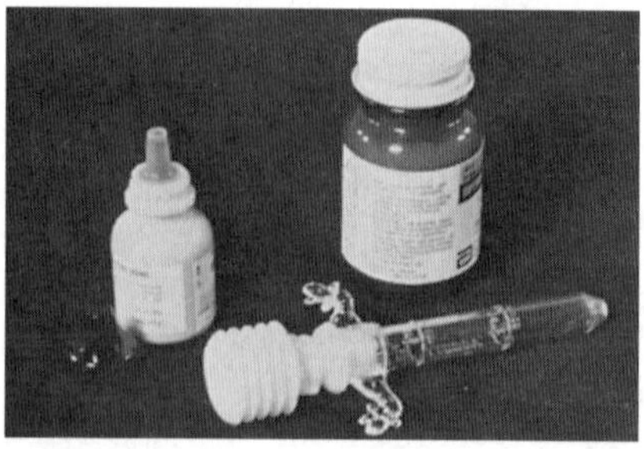

Fig. 7–4. *Examples of oral pediatric suspensions showing package designs of a built-in dropper device and a calibrated dropper accompanying the medication container.*

Rheology

Rheology is the study of flow and involves the viscosity characteristics of powders, fluids, and semisolids. Materials are divided into two general categories depending upon their flow characteristics: Newtonian and non-Newtonian. Newtonian flow is characterized by a constant viscosity, regardless of the shear rates applied. Non-Newtonian flow is characterized by a change in viscosity characteristics with increasing shear rates. Non-Newtonian flow includes plastic, pseudoplastic and dilatant flow.

Newton's Law of Flow relates parallel layers of liquid, with the bottom layer fixed, when a force is placed on the top layer and the top plane moves at constant velocity and each lower layer moves with a velocity directly proportional to its distance from the stationary bottom layer. The velocity gradient, or rate of shear (dv/dr), is the difference of velocity dv between two planes of liquid separated by the distance dr. The force (F′/A) applied to the top layer that is required to result in flow (rate of shear, G) is called the shearing stress (F). The relationship can be expressed.

$$\frac{F'}{A} = \eta \frac{dv}{dr}$$

where η is the viscosity coefficient, or viscosity. This relationship is often written

$$\eta = \frac{F}{G}$$

where F = F′/A and G = dv/dr. The higher the viscosity of a liquid, the greater the shearing stress required to produce a certain rate of shear. A plot of F vs G yields a rheogram. A Newtonian fluid will plot as a straight line with the slope of the line being η. The unit of viscosity is the *poise,* which is the shearing force required to produce a velocity of 1 cm/sec between two parallel planes of liquid, each 1 cm^2 in area and separated by a distance of 1 cm. The most convenient unit to use is the centipoise, or cp (equivalent to 0.01 poise).

These basic concepts can be illustrated in the following two graphs.

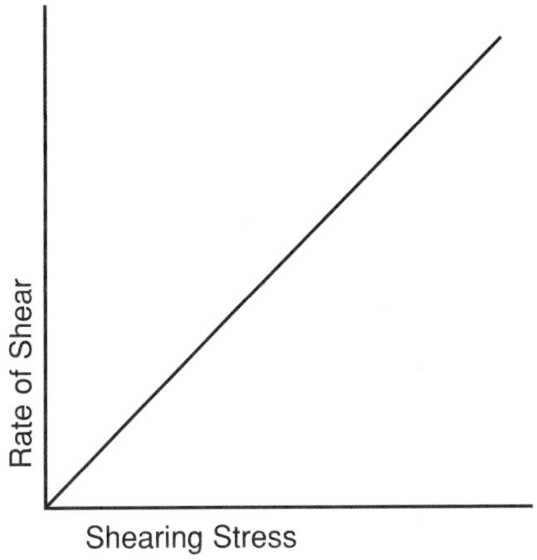

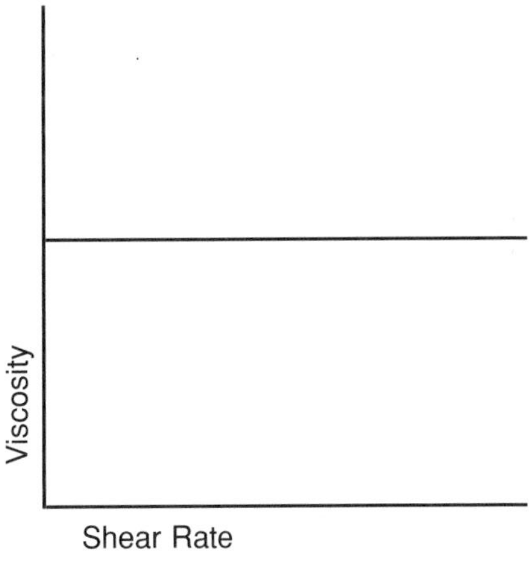

EXAMPLE 1

What is the shear rate when an oil is rubbed into the skin with a relative rate of motion between the fingers and the skin of about 10 cm/sec and the film thickness is about 0.02 cm?

$$G = \frac{10 \text{ cm/sec}}{0.02} = 500 \text{ sec}^{-1}$$

The viscosity of Newtonian materials can be easily determined using a capillary viscometer, such as the Ostwald Pipet, and the following relationship:

$$\eta' = ktd$$

Rheology (Continued)

where η' = viscosity,
k = a coefficient, including such factors as the radius and length of the capillary, volume of the liquid flowing, pressure head, etc,
t = time, and
d = density of the material.

The official compendia, the USP–NF, utilize Kinematic Viscosity, which is the absolute viscosity divided by the density of the liquid, as follows:

$$\text{Kinematic Viscosity} = \eta'/\rho$$

The relative viscosity of a liquid can be obtained by utilizing a capillary viscometer and comparing data with a second liquid of known viscosity, provided the densities of the two liquids are known, as follows:

$$\eta'/\eta'_o = (\rho t)/(\rho_o t_o)$$

EXAMPLE 2

At 25°C, water has a density of 1.0 g/cc and a viscosity of 0.895 cps. The time of flow of water in a capillary viscometer is 15 sec. A 50% aqueous solution of glycerin has a flow time of 750 sec. The density of the glycerin solution is 1.216 g/cc. What is the viscosity of the glycerin solution?

$$\eta' = \frac{(0.895)(750)(1.216)}{(1)(15)} = 54.4 \text{ cps}$$

EXAMPLE 3

The time of flow between marks on an Ostwald viscometer using water ($\rho = 1$) was 120 sec at 20°C. The time for a liquid ($\rho = 1.05$) to flow through the same viscometer was 230 sec. What is the absolute and relative viscosity of the liquid?

$$\eta = (0.01)\frac{(1.05)(230)}{(1.0)(120)}$$

$$\eta = 0.020 \text{ poise} = 2.0 \text{ centipoise}$$

Viscosity is related to temperature according to:

$$\eta' = Ae^{Ev/RT}$$

where A = a constant depending on the molecular weight and molar volume of the material,
Ev = the activation energy required to initiate flow between molecules,
R = the gas constant, and
T = the absolute temperature.

Viscosity is additive in ideal solutions, as follows:

$$\frac{1}{\eta} = \frac{1}{\eta}V_1 + \frac{1}{\eta}V_2$$

where η = the viscosity of the solutions, and
V_1 and V_2 = the volume fractions of the pure liquids.

EXAMPLE 4

What is the viscosity of the liquid resulting from mixing 300 mL of liquid A ($\eta = 1.0$ cp) and 200 mL of liquid B ($\eta = 3.4$ cp)?

$$\frac{1}{\eta} = \frac{1(0.6)}{1.0} + \frac{1}{3.4}(0.4)$$

$$\eta = 1.4 \text{ cps}$$

Non-Newtonian substances are those that fail to follow Newton's Equation of Flow. Example materials include colloidal solutions, emulsions, liquid suspensions, and ointments. There are three general types of non-Newtonian materials: plastic, pseudoplastic, and dilatant.

Rheology (Continued)

Substances that exhibit plastic flow are called *Bingham bodies. Plastic flow* does not begin until a shearing stress, corresponding to a certain yield value, is exceeded. The flow curve intersects the shearing stress axis and does not pass through the origin. The materials are "elastic" below the yield value.

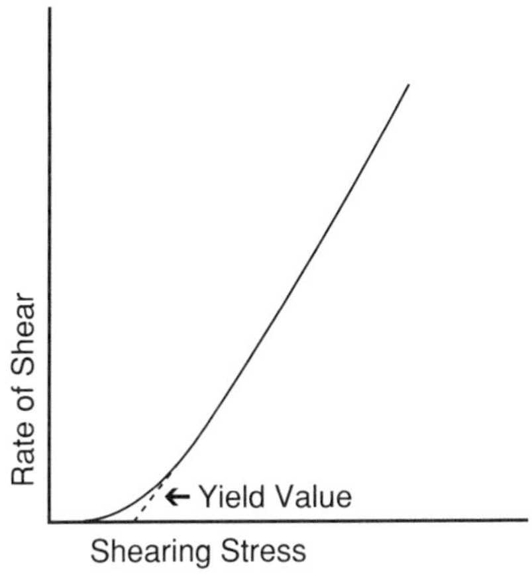

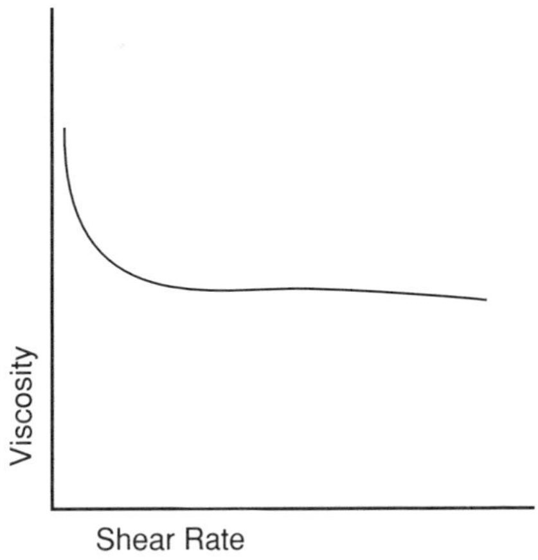

Pseudoplastic substances begin flow when a shearing stress is applied; therefore, they exhibit no yield value. With increasing shearing stress, the rate of shear increases; consequently, these materials are also called "shear-thinning" systems. It is postulated that this occurs as the molecules, primarily polymers, align themselves along the long axis and slip or slide past each other.

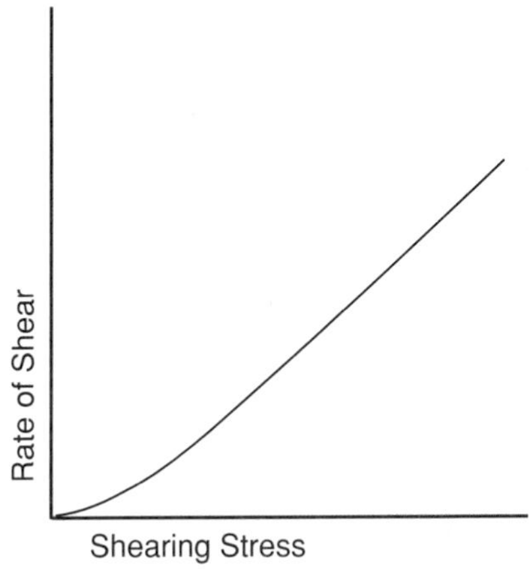

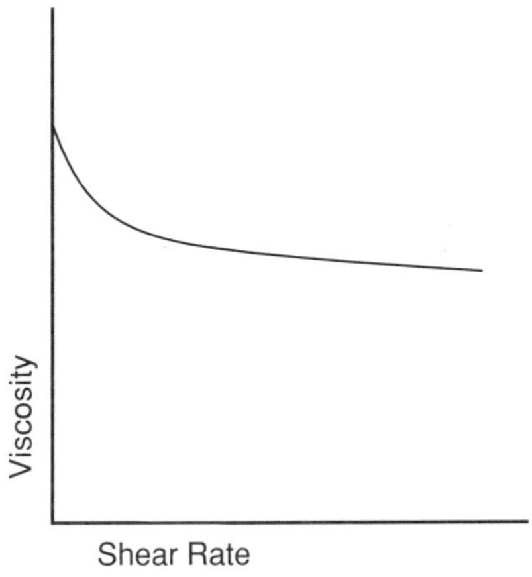

Dilatant materials are those that increase in volume when sheared, and the viscosity increases with increasing shear rate. These are also called "shear thickening" systems. Dilatant systems are usually characterized by having a high percentage of solids in the formulation.

Rheology (Continued)

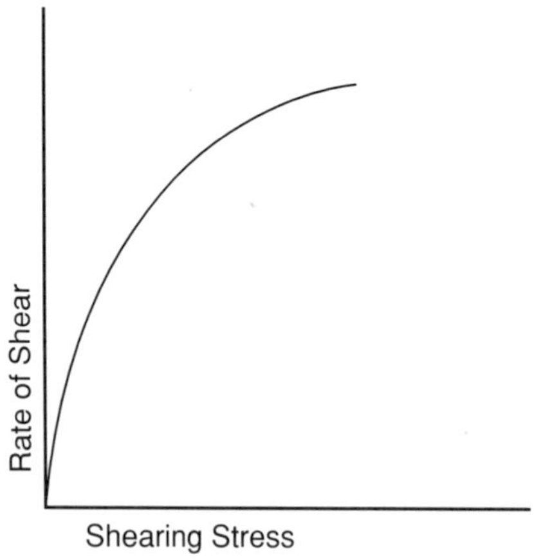

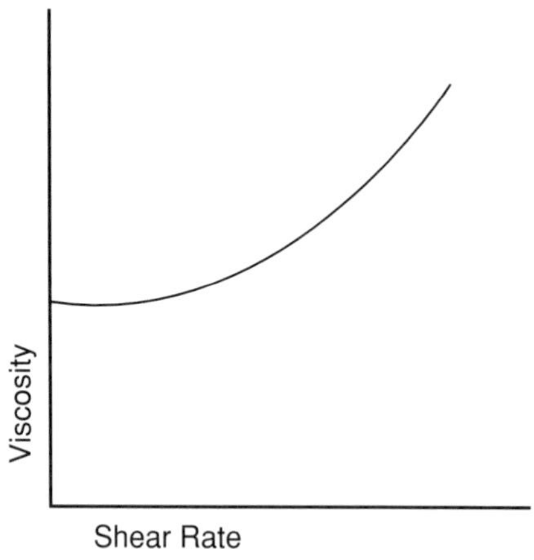

The viscosity of non-Newtonian materials is determined using a viscometer capable of producing differing shear rates, measuring the shear stress, and plotting the results. Other types of flow not detailed here include *thixotropic, antithixotropic,* and *rheopexic.* Thixotropic flow is used in some pharmaceutical formulations to advantage. It is a reversible gel-sol transformation. Upon setting, a network gel is formed that provides a rigid matrix that will stabilize suspensions and gels. When stressed (by shaking), the matrix relaxes and forms a sol, with the characteristics of a liquid dosage form for ease of use. All these unique flow types can be characterized by studying their respective rheograms.

portion of food. Because many of the suspensions of antibiotic drugs intended for pediatric use are prepared in a highly flavored, sweetened, colored base, they are frequently referred to by their manufacturers and also popularly as ''syrups,'' even though in fact they are suspensions.

The Preparation of the Suspension

In the preparation of a suspension, the pharmacist must be acquainted with the characteristics of both the intended dispersed phase and the dispersion medium. In some instances the dispersed phase has an affinity for the vehicle to be employed and is readily ''wetted'' by it upon its addition. Other drugs are not penetrated easily by the vehicle and have a tendency to clump together or to float on top of the vehicle. In the latter case, the powder must first be wetted by a so-called ''wetting agent'' to make the powder more penetrable by the dispersion medium. Alcohol, glycerin, and other hygroscopic liquids are employed as wetting agents when an aqueous vehicle is to be used as the dispersion phase. They function by displacing the air in the crevices of the particles, dispersing the particles, and subsequently allowing the penetration of dispersion medium into the powder. In the large-scale preparation of suspensions the wetting agents are mixed with the particles by an apparatus such as a colloid mill; on a small scale in the pharmacy, they are mixed with a mortar and pestle. Once the powder is wetted, the dispersion medium (to which have been added all of the formulation's soluble components such as colorants, flavorants, and preservatives) is added in portions to the powder, and the mixture is thoroughly blended before subsequent additions of vehicle. A portion of the vehicle is used to wash the mixing equipment free of suspensoid, and this portion is used to bring the suspension to final volume and insure that the suspension contains the desired concentration of solid matter. The final product is then passed through a colloid mill or other blender or mixing device to insure uniformity.

Whenever appropriate, suitable preservatives should be included in the formulation of suspensions to preserve against bacterial and mold contamination.

An example formula for an oral suspension follows.[2] In the example, the suspensoid is the antacid aluminum hydroxide, the preservatives are methylparaben and propylparaben, with syrup and sorbitol solution providing the viscosity as well as the sweetness.

Aluminum Hydroxide Compressed Gel	326.8 g
Sorbitol Solution	282.0 mL
Syrup	93.0 mL
Glycerin	25.0 mL
Methylparaben	0.9 g
Propylparaben	0.3 g
Flavor	q.s.
Purified Water, to make	1000.0 mL

In preparing a formula such as this, the parabens are dissolved in a heated mixture of the sorbitol solution, glycerin, syrup, and a portion of the water. The mixture is then cooled and the aluminum hydroxide added with stirring. The flavor is added and sufficient purified water to volume. The suspension is then homogenized, using a hand homogenizer, homomixer, or colloid mill. An example of a high-speed, industrial-size mixer used to prepare dispersions of various types including suspensions and emulsions is shown in Fig. 7–5.

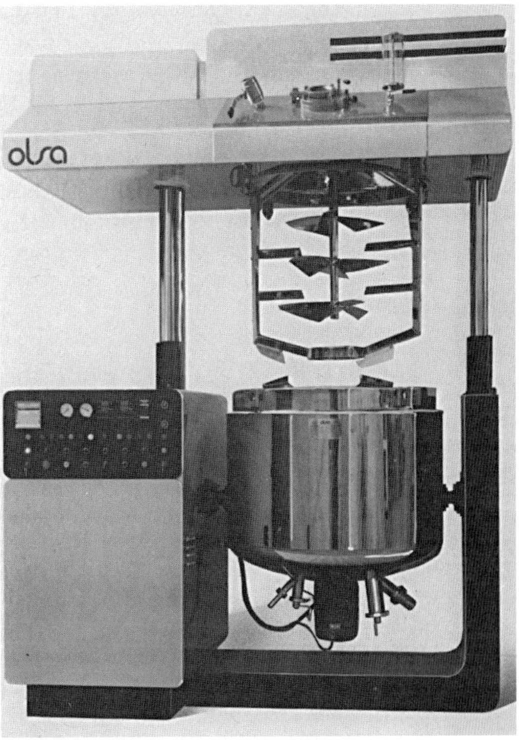

Fig. 7–5. *An example of an industrial mixer for the manufacture of disperse systems including suspensions and emulsions. (Courtesy of Key International, Inc.)*

Sustained-Release Suspensions

The formulation of liquid oral suspensions having sustained-release capabilities has resulted in only limited success due to the difficulty in maintaining the stability of sustained-release particles when present in liquid dispersal systems.[3] Product development research has centered around the same types of technologies used in preparing sustained-release tablets and capsules (i.e., coated beads, drug impregnated wax matrix, microencapsulation, ion-exchange resins, etc.). The use of a combination of ion-exchange resin complex and particle coating *has* resulted in product success via the so-called Pennkinetic system. By this technique, ionic drugs are complexed with ion-exchange resins and the drug-resin complex particles coated with ethyl cellulose.[3] In liquid formulations (suspensions) of the coated particles, the drug remains adsorbed onto the resin, but is slowly released by the ion-exchange process when taken into the gastrointestinal tract. An example of this product type is hydrocodone polistirex [Tussionex Pennkinetic Extended-Release Suspension (Fisons)].

Extemporaneous Compounding of Suspensions

Unfortunately, not all medicines are available in a convenient, easy to take liquid dosage form. Consequently, patients who are not able to swallow solid medicines, e.g., infants, the elderly, may present a special need. Thus, the pharmacist may have to use a solid dosage form, e.g., tablet, capsule, of the drug and extemporaneously compound a liquid product. A difficulty that confronts the pharmacist is a lack of ready information of stability of a drug when it is incorporated into a liquid vehicle. It is known that drugs in liquid form have faster decomposition rates than when in solid form, and some are affected by the pH of the medium. Leucovorin calcium when compounded from crushed tablets or the injectable form is most stable in milk or antacid and is unstable in acidic solutions.

To overcome this information gap, the pharmacist can attempt to contact the pharmaceutical manufacturer of the solid dosage form to attain stability information. A number of extemporaneous formulations have appeared in the professional literature (e.g., for prednisone oral suspension[4] and ketoconazole suspension[5]) and some manufacturers may provide within the package insert a formula for the preparation of an oral liquid form, e.g., Rifadin [Marion Merrell Dow]. Further, the Committee on Extemporaneous Formulations, an American Society of Hospital Pharmacy special interest group, has compiled and published a listing of extemporaneous formulations in a text titled, *Handbook of Extemporaneous Formulations.* It is a compilation of formulations based upon documented stability data and unpublished data compiled by pharmaceutical manufacturers and practitioners.

Typically, when formulating an extemporaneous suspension, the contents of a capsule are emptied into a mortar or the tablets of the drug crushed in a mortar with a pestle. The selected vehicle is then slowly added to and mixed with the powder to create a paste and then diluted to the desired volume. The selected vehicle can be commercially available for this purpose, e.g., Roxane's Diluent (Flavored) for Oral Use (Roxane) or Suspendol-S (Paddock).

The extent of the formulation depends upon the patient for whom the product is intended. For example, a liquid suspension for a neonate does not necessitate the inclusion of preservatives, colorings, flavorings and alcohol because of the potential for each of these to cause either acute or long-term adverse effects. Because this liquid product will probably be administered through a tube feeding threaded through the mouth into the stomach, and because taste sensation is usually underdeveloped in the neonate a flavoring agent is not required.

In the neonate, alcohol can alter liver function, cause gastric irritation and effect neurologic depression. So unless it is absolutely necessary it should be omitted from an extemporaneous formulation. Pharmacists must be cautious because some vehicles such as Aromatic Elixir, NF contain a significant amount of alcohol, i.e., 21 to 23%, and would not be preferable for use in this patient type. The same problem would hold for liquid formulations for the elderly or any patient who may be receiving another medication that depresses the central nervous system.

Preservatives have been implicated for deleterious adverse effects in preterm infants. Benzyl alcohol should be omitted from neonate formulations because this agent can cause a gasping syndrome characterized by a deterioration of multiple organ systems and eventually death. Propylene glycol has also been implicated to cause problems, i.e., seizures, stupor, in some preterm infants. Thus, formulations for neonates should be purposely kept simple, and not compounded to supply more than just a few days of medicine.

To minimize stability problems of the extemporaneously prepared product, it should be placed in air-tight, light-resistant containers by the pharmacist and subsequently stored in the refrigerator by the patient. Because it is a suspension, the patient should be instructed to shake it well prior to use and on a daily basis watch for any color change or consistency change that might indicate a stability problem with the formulation.

Packaging and Storage of Suspensions

All suspensions should be packaged in wide mouth containers having adequate airspace above the liquid to permit adequate shaking and ease of pouring (Fig. 7–6).

Most suspensions should be stored in tight containers protected from freezing, excessive heat, and light. It is important that suspensions be shaken before each use to ensure a uniform distribution of solid in the vehicle and thereby uniform and proper dosage.

Examples of Oral Suspensions

Examples of official and commercial oral suspensions are presented in Table 7–1. Antacid and antibacterial suspensions are briefly discussed below as examples of this dosage form.

Antacid Oral Suspensions

Antacids are intended to counteract the effects of gastric hyperacidity and as such are employed by persons, as peptic ulcer patients, who must reduce the level of acidity in the stomach. They are also widely employed and sold over-the-

Fig. 7–6. *Liquid filling. The 1000-gallon portable storage tank holding the bulk product is shown in the background. The fluid preparation is pumped from the bottom of the tank through sanitary piping to the large stainless steel hopper located in the foreground. Immediately below the hopper are eight piston-type filling cylinders. Extending from the filling heads are eight filling tubes, each with a bottle-centering bell. On the left, bottles are shown being conveyed after cleaning. As they pass through an indexing worm, the bottles are then spaced accurately for transfer by a pusher bar to the filling position. After filling, incoming bottles push those filled onto the conveyor to the bottle-capping operation. (Courtesy of The Upjohn Company.)*

counter to patients suffering from conditions popularly referred to as "acid indigestion," "heartburn," and "sour stomach." Many patients belch or otherwise reflux acid from the stomach to the esophagus and take antacids to counter the acid brought to the esophagus and throat.

Most antacid preparations are composed of water-insoluble materials that act within the confines of the gastrointestinal tract to counteract the acid and/or soothe the irritated or inflamed linings of the gastrointestinal tract. There are a few water-soluble agents employed, as sodium bicarbonate, but for the most part, water-insoluble salts of aluminum, calcium, and magnesium are employed, as aluminum hydroxide, aluminum phosphate, dihydroxyaluminum aminoacetate, calcium carbonate, calcium phosphate, magaldrate, magnesium carbonate, magnesium oxide and magnesium hydroxide. The ability of each of these to neutralize gastric acid varies with the chemical agent. For instance, sodium bicarbonate, calcium carbonate, and magnesium hydroxide neutralize acid effectively, whereas magnesium trisilicate and aluminum hydroxide do so less effectively and much more slowly. In selecting an antacid, it is also important to consider the possible adverse effects of each agent in

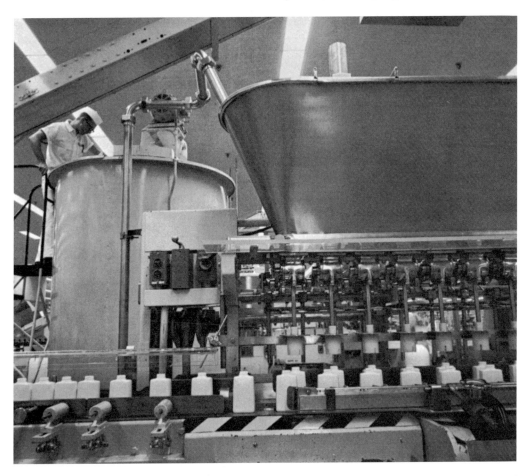

Table 7–1. Examples of Oral Suspensions by Category

Oral Suspension	*Some Representative Commercial Products*	*Concentration of Respective Drug in Commercial Oral Suspension*	*Comments*
Analgesic			
Propoxyphene Napsylate Oral Suspension	Darvon-N Suspension (Lilly)	50 mg/5 mL	Propoxyphene napsylate is a water-insoluble agent that differs from propoxyphene HCl (Darvon) in solubility (the HCl salt is water-soluble) and allows more stable liquid dosage forms and tablet formulations. The drug is employed as an analgesic in the relief of mild to moderate pain. It is related structurally to the narcotic methadone.
Antacids			
Alumina, Magnesia, and Simethicone Oral Suspension	Mylanta Liquid (Johnson & Johnson Merck)	Aluminum hydroxide, 200 mg; magnesium hydroxide, 200 mg; and simethicone, 20 mg/5 mL	These preparations are used to counteract gastric hyperacidity and to relieve distress in the upper gastrointestinal tract. See text for additional discussion.
Alumina Magnesia and Calcium Carbonate Oral Suspension	Camalox Suspension (Rorer)	225 mg of aluminum hydroxide, 200 mg of magnesium hydroxide, and 250 mg of calcium carbonate/5 mL	
Magaldrate Oral Suspension	Riopan Oral Suspension (Whitehall)	540 mg of hydroxymagnesium aluminate, a chemical entity of aluminum and magnesium hydroxides	
Magnesia and Alumina Oral Suspension	Maalox Suspension (Rhône-Poulenc Rorer)	225 mg of aluminum hydroxide and 200 mg of magnesium hydroxide/5 mL	
Aluminum Hydroxide and Magnesium Carbonate Oral Suspension	Gaviscon Liquid Antacid (Marion Merrell Dow)	Aluminum hydroxide, 95 mg, magnesium carbonate, 412 mg/15 mL, and sodium alginate	
Anthelmintics			
Pyrantel Pamoate Oral Suspension	Antiminth Oral Suspension (Pfizer)	250 mg/5 mL	These anthelmintics are employed to rid the body of worm infections. See text for additional discussion.
Thiabenzadole Oral Suspension	Mintezol Oral Suspension (Merck Sharp & Dohme)	500 mg/5 mL	
Antibacterials (Antibiotics)			
Chloramphenicol Palmitate Oral Suspension	Chloromycetin Palmitate Oral Suspension (Parke-Davis)	150 mg/5 mL	A broad-spectrum antibiotic reserved for serious infections by susceptible organisms when less potentially hazardous agents are ineffective or contraindicated. The tasteless palmitate ester of chloramphenicol is hydrolyzed in the gut to chloramphenicol before absorption.
Erythromycin Estolate Oral Suspension	Ibosone Oral Suspension (Dista)	125 and 500 mg/5 mL	Broad-spectrum macrolide antibiotic having bacteriostatic and bacteriocidal activity.
Tetracycline HCl Oral Suspension	Tetracycline HCl Syrup (Rugby)	125 mg/5 mL	Tetracycline antibiotics act by inhibiting microorganisms' protein synthesis. They are effective against a wide range of gram-positive and gram-negative microorganisms.

Table 7–1. Continued

Oral Suspension	*Some Representative Commercial Products*	*Concentration of Respective Drug in Commercial Oral Suspension*	*Comments*
Antibacterials (Non-antibiotic Anti-infectives)			
Methenamine Mandelate Oral Suspension	Mandelamine Suspension and Mandelamine Suspension Forte (Parke-Davis)	250 and 500 mg (Forte)/5 mL	Methenamine mandelate oral suspension is prepared with an oleaginous vehicle. Methenamine mandelate is a chemical combination of approximately equal parts of methenamine and mandelic acid which is effective in destroying most of the pathogens commonly found to infect the urinary tract. An acid urine is essential for the activity of the drug, with maximum efficacy occurring at pH 5.5. The methenamine component of the drug in an acid urine is hydrolyzed to ammonia and the bactericidal agent, formaldehyde. The mandelic acid component meantime exerts its antibacterial action and contributes to the acidification of the urine. The usual dose of the drug is 1 g, up to four times a day. The suspension form of the drug is especially useful in treating pediatric patients as well as those adults who cannot or will not swallow a tablet (also official and commercially available).
Sulfamethoxazole and Trimethoprim Suspension	Bactrim Suspension (Roche) Septra Suspension (Burroughs-Wellcome)	40 mg of trimethoprim and 200 mg of sulfamethoxazole per 5 mL	This suspension is used to treat acute middle ear infection (otitis media) in children and urinary tract infections due to susceptible microorganisms.
Sulfamethoxazole Oral Suspension	Gantanol Suspension (Roche)	500 mg/5 mL	These sulfa-drug suspensions are bacteriostatic agents particularly useful in the treatment of urinary tract infections. Sulfonamides competitively inhibit bacterial synthesis of folic acid and para-aminobenzoic acid.
Sulfisoxazole Acetyl Oral Suspension	Gantrisin Syrup and Gantrisin Pediatric Suspension (Roche)	500 mg/5 mL	
Anticonvulsants			
Primidone Oral Suspension	Mysoline Suspension (Wyeth-Ayerst)	250 mg/5 mL	This drug is useful in the management of grand mal epilepsy and psychomotor attacks.
Antidiarrheal			
Bismuth Subsalicylate Suspension	Pepto-Bismol Liquid (Procter & Gamble)	262 mg/5 mL	For indigestion without causing constipation, nausea, and control of diarrhea. An unlabeled use has been for the prevention and treatment of traveler's (enterotoxigenic *Escherichia coli*) diarrhea, but in neither case is it the first line of therapy.
Antiflatulent			
Simethicone Oral Suspension	Mylicon Drops (Johnson & Johnson Merck)	40 mg/0.6 mL	Used for the symptomatic treatment of gastrointestinal distress due to entrapment of gas. The drug acts by reducing the surface tension of gas bubbles, enabling them to coalesce and to be released through belching or passing flatus.
Antifungals			
Nystatin Oral Suspension	Nystatin Oral Suspension (Roxane)	100,000 units/mL	Mycostatin is an antibiotic with antifungal activity. The suspension is held in the mouth as long as possible before swallowing in the treatment of infections of the oral cavity caused by *Candida* (Monilia) *albicans* and other Candida species.
Griseofulvin Oral Suspension	Grifulvin V Oral Suspension (Ortho)	125 mg/mL	Microsize griseofulvin acts systemically as an antifungal (fungistatic).
Antihypertensive			
Methyldopa Oral Solution	Aldomet Oral Suspension (Merck & Co.)	250 mg/5 mL	Antihypertensive agent useful in lowering high blood pressure.
Antipsychotics, Sedatives, Antiemetics			
Chlorprothixene Oral Suspension, USP	Taractan Concentrate (Roche)	100 mg/5 mL	Used in the control of moderate to severe agitation, anxiety, and tension, when such symptoms are manifestations of schizophrenia.

Table 7–1. Continued

Oral Suspension	*Some Representative Commercial Products*	*Concentration of Respective Drug in Commercial Oral Suspension*	*Comments*
Hydroxyzine Pamoate Oral Suspension	Vistaril Oral Suspension (Pfizer)	25 mg/5 mL	Used in the management of anxiety, tension, and psychomotor agitation.
Thioridazine Oral Suspension	Mellaril-S Oral Suspension (Sandoz)	25 mg/5 mL	For the management of manifestations of psychotic disorders and short-term treatments of moderate to marked depression with variable degrees of anxiety in adults.
Diuretic			
Chlorothiazide Oral Suspension	Diuril Oral Suspension (Merck & Co.)	250 mg/5 mL	Acts as a diuretic by interfering with the renal tubular mechanism of electrolyte reabsorption (increases excretion of sodium and chloride).
Nonsteroidal Anti-inflammatory			
Indomethacin Oral Suspension	Indocin Oral Suspension (Merck & Co.)	25 mg/5 mL	For the active treatment of moderate to severe rheumatoid arthritis (including acute flares of chronic illness), moderate to severe osteoarthritis, acute painful shoulder (bursitis or tendinitis), and acute gouty arthritis.

relation to the individual patient being treated. Each agent has its own peculiar potential for adverse effects. For instance, sodium bicarbonate possesses the capability for sodium overload and systemic alkalosis which is of potential hazard to patients on sodium-restricted diets. Magnesium preparations may lead to diarrhea and are dangerous to patients with diminished renal function due to the patients' inability to excrete all of the magnesium which may be absorbed (the gastric acid converts insoluble magnesium hydroxide to magnesium chloride which is water-soluble and is partially absorbed). Calcium carbonate carries the potential for inducing hypercalcemia and stimulation of gastric secretion and acid production, the latter effect known as "acid rebound." Excessive use of aluminum hydroxide may lead to constipation and phosphate depletion with consequent muscle weakness, bone resorption, and hypercalciuria.

The use to which an antacid is to be put is a major consideration in its selection. For instance, in the occasional treatment of heartburn, or other infrequent episodes of gastric distress, a single dose of sodium bicarbonate or a magnesium hydroxide preparation may be desired, but for the treatment of acute peptic ulcer or duodenal ulcer in which the therapeutic regimen includes the frequent administration of antacids, sodium bicarbonate would provide too great an amount of sodium and the magnesium hydroxide would induce diarrhea. Thus, in the treatment of ulcerative conditions, a combination of magnesium hydroxide and aluminum hydroxide is frequently used because the latter agent possesses some constipating effects which counter the diarrhea effects of the magnesium hydroxide.

In instances in which frequent dosage administration is required, and in cases in which gastroesophageal reflux is being treated, liquid antacids generally are preferred over tablet forms. For one thing, the liquid suspensions assert more immediate action—they do not require the time needed for tablets to disintegrate. It is important that an antacid preparation have a reasonably fast onset of action because its presence in the stomach may not last long due to gastric emptying into the intestines. It has been shown by endoscopic studies that on a fasting stomach very little antacid remains in the stomach 1 hour following administration. It is for this reason that the FDA has set the requirement that antacid tablets that are not intended to be chewed upon administration must disintegrate within 10 minutes in simulated gastric conditions. Frequent food snacks generally prolong the time an antacid remains in the stomach and can prolong its action.

Because many antacid materials, especially aluminum and calcium-containing products, interfere with the absorption of other drugs, especially the tetracycline group of antibiotics, pharmacists must caution their patients against taking such drugs concomitantly.

In addition to the suspension forms of antacids, a number of liquid antacid preparations of the magma and gel type are official and commercially available and will be mentioned later in this chapter. All of these liquid forms are usually pleasantly flavored (generally with peppermint) to enhance their palatability and patient appeal. Because liquid antacid preparations characteristically contain a large amount of solid material, they must be shaken vigorously to redistribute the antacid prior to administration. Also, a large dose of antacids is frequently required. Thus, many patients would prefer to swallow one or two tablespoonfuls of a liquid antacid preparation than to swallow whole or chew the corresponding number of tablets (commonly 3 to 6) for the equivalent dose of drug.

Antibacterial Oral Suspensions

The antibacterial oral suspensions include preparations of antibiotic substances (e.g., chloramphenicol palmitate, erythromycin derivatives, and tetracycline and its derivatives), sulfonamides (e.g., sulfamethoxazole, sulfisoxazole acetyl), other chemotherapeutic agents (e.g., methenamine mandelate and nitrofurantoin), or combinations of these (e.g., sulfamethoxazole-trimethoprim).

Many antibiotic materials are unstable when maintained in solution for an appreciable length of time and therefore, from a stability standpoint, insoluble forms of the drug substances in aqueous suspension or as dry powders for reconstitution (discussed next) are attractive to pharmaceutical manufacturers. The antibiotic oral suspensions, including those prepared by reconstitution, provide a convenient way to administer dosages to infants and children as well as to adult patients who may prefer liquid preparations to solid dosage forms. Many of the oral suspensions that are intended primarily for infants are packaged with a calibrated dropper to assist in the delivery of the prescribed dose. Examples of some commercial pediatric antibiotic oral suspensions are pictured in Figure 7–4, and examples of calibrated droppers in Figure 7–7.

The dispersing phase of antibiotic suspensions is aqueous, and usually colored, sweetened and flavored to render the liquid more appealing and palatable. As noted previously, the palmitate form of chloramphenicol was selected from the suspension dosage form not only because of its water-insolubility, but also because of its quality of being flavorless, thereby eliminating the formulating problem of trying to mask the otherwise bitter taste of the chloramphenicol base.

Dry Powders for Oral Suspension

A number of official and commercial preparations consist of dry powder mixtures or granules, which are intended to be suspended in water or some other vehicle prior to oral administration. As indicated previously, these official preparations have "for Oral Suspension" in their official title to distinguish them from already prepared suspensions.

The majority of drugs prepared as a dry mix for oral suspension are antibiotics. The dry products are prepared commercially to contain the antibiotic drug, colorants (FD&C dyes), flavorants, sweeteners (as sucrose or sodium saccharin), stabilizing agents (as citric acid, sodium citrate), suspending agents (as guar gum, xanthan gum, methylcellulose), and preserving agents (as methylparaben, sodium benzoate) that may be needed to enhance the stability of either the dry powder or granule mixture or the ultimate liquid suspension. When called upon to "reconstitute" and dispense one of these products, the pharmacist loosens the powder at the bottom of the container by lightly tapping it against a hard surface, and then adds the label-designated amount of purified water, usually in portions, and shakes until all of the dry powder

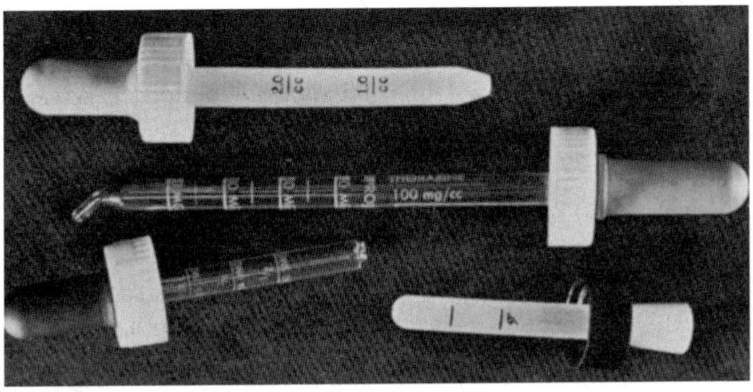

Fig. 7–7. *Examples of calibrated droppers utilized in the administration of pediatric medications.*

has been suspended (Fig. 7–2). It is important for the pharmacist to add precisely the prescribed amount of purified water to the dry mixture if the proper drug concentration per dosage unit is to be achieved. Also, the use of purified water rather than tap water is needed to avoid the addition of possible offending impurities which could adversely affect the stability of the resulting preparation. Generally, manufacturers provide the dry powder or granule mixture in a slightly oversized container to permit the adequate shaking of the contents after the entire amount of purified water has been added. Pharmacists must realize that an oversized bottle is provided with each of these products and they must carefully measure out the required amount of purified water. They should not "eyeball" the amount of water to be added or mistakenly fill up the bottle with purified water. Among the official antibiotic drugs for oral suspension are the following:

Amoxicillin for Oral Suspension, USP
 [Amoxil for Oral Suspension (SmithKline Beecham)]
Ampicillin for Oral Suspension, USP
 [Omnipen for Oral Suspension (Wyeth-Ayerst)]
Bacampicillin for Oral Suspension, USP
 [Spectrobid for Oral Suspension (Roerig)]
Cefaclor for Oral Suspension, USP
 [Ceclor for Oral Suspension (Lilly)]
Cefixime for Oral Suspension, USP
 [Suprax Powder for Oral Suspension (Lederle)]
Cephadrine for Oral Suspension, USP
Cephalexin for Oral Suspension, USP
 [Keflex for Oral Suspension (Dista)]
Dicloxacillin Sodium for Oral Suspension, USP
 [Pathocil for Oral Suspension (Wyeth-Ayerst)]
Doxycycline for Oral Suspension, USP
 [Vibramycin Monohydrate for Oral Suspension (Pfizer)]
Erythromycin Ethylsuccinate for Oral Suspension, USP
 [E.E.S. Granules for Oral Suspension (Abbott)]
Penicillin V for Oral Suspension, USP

There are also several official combinations of antibiotics for oral suspension combined with other drugs. For example, the combination of erythromycin ethyl succinate and acetylsulfisoxazole granules for oral suspension is indicated for the treatment of acute middle ear infection caused by susceptible strains of *Hemophilus influenzae*. Probenecid is combined with ampicillin for reconstitution and ultimate use for the treatment of uncomplicated infections (urethral, endocervical or rectal) caused by *Neisseria gonorrhoeae* in adults.

Among the official drugs other than antibiotics prepared as dry powder mixtures for reconstitution to oral suspension are the following: cholestyramine [Questran (Bristol)], a drug used in the management of high cholesterol levels; and barium sulfate [Barosperse (Mallinckrodt)], used orally or rectally as a radiopaque contrast medium to visualize the gastrointestinal tract as an aid to diagnosis. Barium sulfate was introduced into medicine about 1910 as a contrast medium in the roentgen-ray examination of the gastrointestinal tract. It is practically insoluble in water and thus its administration, even in the large doses required, is safe because it is not absorbed from the gastrointestinal tract. The pharmacist must be careful not to confuse "barium sulfate," with other forms of barium as the *sulfide* and *sulfite* which are soluble salts and *are* poisonous. Barium sulfate is a fine, non-gritty, white, odorless and tasteless powder. When prepared into a suspension and administered orally, it is used to diagnose conditions of the hypopharynx, esophagus, stomach, small intestine and colon. The barium sulfate renders the gastrointestinal tract opaque to the x ray so that it may be photographed, revealing any abnormality in the anatomic features of the tract. When administered rectally, the barium sulfate allows visualization of the features of the rectum and colon.

Commercially, barium sulfate for diagnostic use is available as a bulk powder containing the required suspending agents for effective reconstitution to an oral suspension or enema prior to administration. Enema units, which contain prepared suspension in a ready-to-use and disposable bag, are also available.

Emulsions

An emulsion is a dispersion in which the dispersed phase is composed of small globules of a liquid distributed throughout a vehicle in which it is immiscible (Fig. 7–8). In emulsion terminology, the dispersed phase is referred to as the *internal phase*, and the dispersion medium as the *external* or *continuous phase*. Emulsions having an oleaginous internal phase and an aqueous

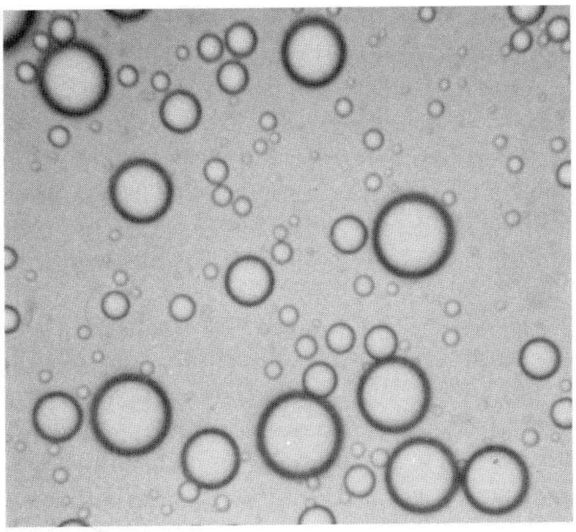

Fig. 7–8. *Mineral oil in water emulsion. The largest oil globule in the photograph measures approximately 0.04 mm. (Courtesy of James C. Price, Ph.D., College of Pharmacy, The University of Georgia.)*

external phase are referred to as *oil-in-water* emulsions, and are commonly designated as "o/w" emulsions. Conversely, emulsions having an aqueous internal phase and an oleaginous external phase are termed *water-in-oil* emulsions and are referred to as "w/o" emulsions. Because the external phase of an emulsion is continuous, an oil-in-water emulsion may be diluted or extended with water or an aqueous preparation, and a water-in-oil emulsion with an oleaginous or oil-miscible liquid. Generally, to prepare a stable emulsion, a third phase is necessary, that being an *emulsifying agent.* Depending upon their constituents, the viscosity of emulsions can vary greatly, and pharmaceutical emulsions may be prepared as liquids or semisolids. Based on the constituents and the intended application, liquid emulsions may be employed orally, topically, or parenterally; semisolid emulsions, topically. Many pharmaceutical preparations that may actually be emulsions may not be classified as such because they fit some other pharmaceutical category more appropriately. For instance, certain lotions, liniments, creams, ointments, and commercial vitamin drops may be emulsions but may be referred to in the terms indicated and will be discussed in this book under these various designations.

Purpose of Emulsions and of Emulsification

Pharmaceutically, the process of emulsification enables the pharmacist to prepare relatively stable and homogeneous mixtures of two immiscible liquids. It permits the administration of a liquid drug in the form of minute globules rather than in bulk. For orally administered emulsions, the oil-in-water type of emulsion permits the palatable administration of an otherwise distasteful oil by dispersing it in a sweetened, flavored aqueous vehicle in which it may be carried past the taste buds and into the stomach. The reduced particle size of the oil globules may render the oil more digestible and more readily absorbed, or if that is not the intent, more effective in its task, as for example the increased efficacy of mineral oil as a cathartic when in the emulsified form.

Emulsions to be applied externally to the skin may be prepared as o/w or w/o emulsions, depending upon such factors as the nature of the therapeutic agents to be incorporated into the emulsions, the desirability for an emollient or tissue softening effect of the preparation, and the condition of the skin surface. Medicinal agents that are irritating to the skin generally are less irritating if present in the internal phase of an emulsified topical preparation than in the external phase from which direct contact with the skin is more prevalent. Naturally, the miscibility or the solubility in oil and in water of a medicinal agent to be used in an emulsified preparation would dictate to a great extent the vehicle in which it must be present, and its nature would in turn suggest the phase of the emulsion that the resulting solution should become. On the unbroken skin, a water-in-oil emulsion can usually be applied more evenly because the skin is covered with a thin film of sebum, and this surface is more readily wetted by oil than by water. A water-in-oil emulsion is also more softening to the skin, because it resists drying out and is resistant to removal by contact with water. On the other hand, if it is desirable to have a preparation that is more easily removed from the skin with water, an oil-in-water emulsion would be preferred. As for absorption, absorption through the skin (percutaneous absorption) may be enhanced by the diminished particle size of the internal phase. Other aspects of topical preparations are discussed in Chapter 10.

Theories of Emulsification

Many theories have been advanced in an attempt to explain how emulsifying agents act in promoting emulsification and in maintaining the stability of the resulting emulsion. Although certain of these theories apply rather specifically to certain types of emulsifying agents and to certain conditions (as the pH of the phases of the system and the nature and relative proportions of the internal and external phases), they may be viewed in a general way to describe the manner in which emulsions may be produced and stabilized. Among the most prevalent theories are the *surface-tension theory*, the *oriented-wedge theory*, and the *plastic* or *interfacial film theory*.

All liquids have a tendency to assume a shape having the least amount of surface area exposed. For a drop of a liquid, that shape is spherical. In a spherical drop of liquid there are internal forces that tend to promote the association of the molecules of the substance to resist the distortion of the drop into a less spherical form. If two or more drops of the same liquid come into contact with one another, the tendency is for them to join or to *coalesce*, making one larger drop having a lesser surface area than the total surface area of the individual drops. This tendency of liquids may be measured quantitatively, and when the surrounding of the liquid is air, it is referred to as the liquid's *surface tension*. *When the liquid is in contact with a second liquid in which it is insoluble and immiscible, the force causing each liquid to resist breaking up into smaller particles is called interfacial tension*. Substances that can promote the lowering of this resistance to breakup can encourage a liquid to be reduced to smaller drops or particles. These tension-lowering substances are referred to as *surface-active* (surfactants) or *wetting agents*. According to the *surface-tension theory* of emulsification, the use of these substances as emulsifiers and stabilizers results in the lowering of the interfacial tension of the two immiscible liquids, reducing the repellent force between the liquids and diminishing each liquid's attraction for its own molecules. Thus the surface-active agents facilitate the breaking up of large globules into smaller ones, which then have a lesser than usual tendency to reunite or coalesce.

The *oriented-wedge* theory assumes monomolecular layers of emulsifying agent curved around a droplet of the internal phase of the emulsion. The theory is based on the presumption that certain emulsifying agents orient themselves about and within a liquid in a manner reflective of their solubility in that particular liquid. In a system containing two immiscible liquids, presumably the emulsifying agent would be preferentially soluble in one of the phases and would be embedded more deeply and tenaciously in that phase than the other. Since many molecules of substances upon which this theory is based (for example, soaps) have a hydrophilic or water-loving portion and a hydrophobic or water-hating portion (but usually lipophilic or oil-loving), the molecules will position or orient themselves into each phase. Depending upon the shape and size of the molecules, their solubility characteristics, and thus their orientation, the wedge-shape arrangement envisioned for the molecules will cause the surrounding of either oil globules or water globules. Generally an emulsifying agent having a greater hydrophilic character than hydrophobic character will promote an oil-in-water emulsion, and a water-in-oil emulsion results through the use of an emulsifying agent that is more hydrophobic than hydrophilic. Putting it another way, the phase in which the emulsifying agent is more soluble will generally become the continuous or external phase of the emulsion. Although this theory may not represent a totally accurate depiction of the molecular arrangement of the emulsifier molecules, the concept that water-soluble emulsifiers generally do form oil-in-water emulsions is important and is generally found in practice.

The *plastic-* or *interfacial-film theory* places the emulsifying agent at the interface between the oil and water, surrounding the droplets of the internal phase as a thin layer of film adsorbed on the surface of the drops. The film prevents the contact and coalescing of the dispersed phase; the tougher and more pliable the film, the greater the stability of the emulsion. Naturally, enough of the film-forming material must be available to coat the entire surface of each drop of internal phase. Here again, the formation of an oil-in-water or a water-in-oil emulsion is dependent upon the degree of solubility of the agent in the two phases, with water-soluble agents encouraging oil-in-water emulsions and oil-soluble emulsifiers the reverse.

In actuality, it is unlikely that a single theory of emulsification may be used to explain the means by which the many and varied emulsifiers promote emulsion formation and stability. It is more than likely that even within a given emulsion system, more than one of the aforementioned theories of emulsification is applicable and plays a part. For instance, lowering of the interfacial tension is important in the initial formation of an emulsion, but the formation of a protective wedge of molecules or film of emulsifier is important for continued emulsion stability. No doubt certain emulsifiers are capable of both tasks.

Preparation of Emulsions

Emulsifying Agents

The initial step in preparation of an emulsion is the selection of the emulsifier. To be useful in a pharmaceutical preparation, the emulsifying agent must possess certain qualities. For one thing, it must be compatible with the other formulative ingredients and must not interfere with the stability or efficacy of the therapeutic agent. It should be stable and not deteriorate in the preparation. The emulsifier should be nontoxic with respect to its intended use and the amount to be consumed by the patient. Also, it should possess little odor, taste, or color. Of prime importance is the capability of the emulsifying agent to promote emulsification and to maintain the stability of the emulsion for the intended shelf life of the product.

Various types of materials have been used in pharmacy as emulsifying agents, with hundreds, if not thousands, of individual agents tested for their emulsification capabilities. Although no attempt will be made here to try to discuss the merits of each of these agents in pharmaceutical emulsion, it would be well to point out the types of materials that are commonly used and their general application. Among the emulsifiers and stabilizers for pharmaceutical systems are the following:

1. Carbohydrate materials such as the naturally occurring agents acacia, tragacanth, agar, chondrus, and pectin. These materials form hydrophilic colloids when added to water and generally produce o/w emulsions. Acacia is perhaps the most frequently used emulsifier in the preparation of extemporaneous emulsions by the community pharmacist. Tragacanth and agar are commonly employed as thickening agents in acacia-emulsified products. Microcrystalline cellulose is employed in a number of commercially prepared suspensions and emulsions as a viscosity regulator to retard particle settling and provide dispersion stability.
2. Protein substances such as gelatin, egg yolk, and casein. These substances produce o/w emulsions. The disadvantage of gelatin as an emulsifier is that the emulsions prepared from it frequently are too fluid and become more fluid upon standing.
3. High molecular weight alcohols such as stearyl alcohol, cetyl alcohol, and glyceryl monostearate. These are employed primarily as thickening agents and stabilizers for o/w emulsions of certain lotions and ointments used externally. Cholesterol and cholesterol derivatives may also be employed in externally used emulsions and promote w/o emulsions.
4. Wetting agents, which may be anionic, cationic, or nonionic. These agents contain both hydrophilic and lipophilic groups, with the lipophilic protein of the molecule generally accounting for the surface-activity of the molecule. In anionic agents, this lipophilic portion is negatively charged, but in the cationic agent it is positively charged. Owing to their opposing ionic charges, anionic and cationic agents tend to neutralize each other if present in the same system and are thus considered incompatible with one another. Nonionic emulsifiers show no inclination to ionize. Depending upon their individual nature, certain of the members of these groups form o/w emulsions and others w/o emulsions. Anionic emulsifiers include various monovalent, polyvalent, and organic soaps such as triethanolamine oleate and sulfonates such as sodium lauryl sulfate. Benzalkonium chloride, known primarily for its bactericidal properties, may be employed as a cationic-type of emulsifier. Agents of the nonionic type include the sorbitan esters and the polyoxyethylene derivatives, some of which appear in Table 7–2.

   The ionic nature of a surfactant is of prime consideration in the selection of a surfactant to utilize in forming an emulsion. Nonionic surfactants are effective over pH range 3 to 10; cationic surfactants are effective over pH range 3 to 7; and, anionic surfactants require a pH of greater than 8.[6]
5. Finely divided solids such as colloidal clays including bentonite, magnesium hydroxide, and aluminum hydroxide. These generally form o/w emulsions when the insoluble material is added to the aqueous phase if there is a greater volume of the aqueous phase than of the oleaginous phase. However, if the powdered solid is added to the oil and the oleaginous phase volume predominates, a substance like bentonite is capable of forming w/o emulsion.

The relative volume of internal and external phases of an emulsion is important, regardless of the type of emulsifier used. As the internal concentration of an emulsion is increased, there is an increase in the viscosity of the emulsion to a certain point, after which the viscosity decreases sharply. At this point the emulsion has undergone *inversion;* that is, it has changed from an o/w emulsion to a w/o, or vice versa. In practice, emulsions may be prepared without inversion with as much as about 75% of the volume of the product being internal phase.

The HLB System

Generally, each emulsifying agent has a hydrophilic portion and a lipophilic portion with one or the other being more or less predominant and influencing in the manner already described the type of emulsion. A method has been devised[7] whereby emulsifying or surface-active agents may be categorized on the basis of their chemical make-up as to their hydrophile-lipophile balance or "HLB." By this method, each agent is assigned an HLB value or number which is indicative of the substance's polarity. Although the numbers have been assigned up to about 40, the usual range is between 1 and 20. Materials that are highly polar or hydrophilic have been assigned higher numbers than materials that are less polar and more lipophilic. Generally, those surface-active agents having an assigned HLB value of from 3 to 6 are greatly lipophilic and produce water-in-oil emulsions, and those agents have HLB values of from about 8 to 18 produce oil-in-water emulsions. Examples of some assigned HLB values for some selected surfactants are shown in Table 7–2. The type of activity to be expected from surfactants of assigned HLB numbers is presented in Table 7–3.

In the HLB system, in addition to assigning values to the emulsifying agents, values are also assigned to oils and oil-like substances. In using the HLB concept in the preparation of an emulsion, one selects emulsifying agents having the same or nearly the same HLB value as the oleaginous phase of the intended emulsion. For example, mineral oil has an assigned HLB value of 4 if a w/o emulsion is desired and a value of 10.5 if an o/w emulsion is to be prepared. To prepare a stable emulsion, the emulsifying agent selected should have an HLB value similar to the one for mineral oil, depending on the type of emulsion desired. When needed, two or more emulsifiers may be combined to achieve the proper HLB value.

The accompanying Physical Pharmacy Capsules summarize the activities of surfactants and the calculations involved in determining the quantity of surfactant required to prepare a stable emulsion.

Table 7–2. Examples of HLB Values for Selected Emulsifiers

Agent	*HLB*
Ethylene glycol distearate	1.5
Sorbitan tristearate (Span 65*)	2.1
Propylene glycol monostearate	3.4
Triton X-15†	3.6
Sorbitan monooleate (Span 80*)	4.3
Sorbitan monostearate (Span 60*)	4.7
Diethylene glycol monolaurate	6.1
Sorbitan monopalmitate (Span 40*)	6.7
Sucrose dioleate	7.1
Acacia	8.0
Amercol L-101‡	8.0
Polyoxyethylene lauryl ether (Brij 30*)	9.7
Gelatin	9.8
Triton X-45†	10.4
Methylcellulose	10.5
Polyoxyethylene monostearate (Myrj 45*)	11.1
Triethanolamine oleate	12.0
Tragacanth	13.2
Triton X-100†	13.5
Polyoxyethylene sorbitan monostearate (Tween 60*)	14.9
Polyoxyethylene sorbitan monooleate (Tween 80*)	15.0
Polyoxyethylene sorbitan monolaurate (Tween 20*)	16.7
Pluronic F 68§	17.0
Sodium oleate	18.0
Potassium oleate	20.0
Sodium lauryl sulfate	40.0

* ICI Americas, Inc., Wilmington, DE
† Rohm and Haas, Philadelphia, PA
‡ Amerchol Corporation, Edison, NJ
§ BASF-Wyandotte Chemical Corporation, Parsippany, NJ

Table 7–3. Activity and HLB Value of Surfactants

Activity	*Assigned HLB*
Antifoaming	1 to 3
Emulsifiers (w/o)	3 to 6
Wetting agents	7 to 9
Emulsifiers (o/w)	8 to 18
Solubilizers	15 to 20
Detergents	13 to 15

Blending of Surfactants

Wetting agents are surfactants with HLB values of **7 to 9.** Wetting agents aid in attaining intimate contact between solid particles and liquids.

Emulsifying agents are surfactants with HLB values of **3 to 6.** Emulsifying agents reduce interfacial tension between oil and water, resulting in minimizing surface energy through the formation of globules.

Detergents are surfactants with HLB values of **13 to 16.** Detergents will reduce the surface tension and aid in wetting the surface and the dirt. The soil will be emulsified, and foaming generally occurs and a washing away of the dirt.

Solubilizing agents have HLB values of **16 to 18.**

HLB values are additive, and often surfactants are blended. For example if 20 mL of an HLB of 9.0 are required, then two surfactants (with HLB values of 8.0 and 12.0) can be blended in a 3:1 ratio. The following quantities of each will be required:

$$\tfrac{3}{4} \times 8.0 = 6.0$$
$$\tfrac{1}{4} \times 12.0 = 3.0$$
$$\text{Total HLB} = 9.0$$

Methods of Emulsion Preparation

Emulsions may be prepared by several methods, depending upon the nature of the emulsion components and the equipment available for use. On a small scale, as in the laboratory or pharmacy, emulsions may be prepared using a dry Wedgewood or porcelain mortar and pestle, a mechanical blender or mixer such as a Waring blender or a milk-shake mixer, a hand homogenizer (Fig. 7–9), or sometimes a simple prescription bottle. On a large scale, large volume mixing tanks (Fig. 7–5) may be used to form the emulsion through the action of a highspeed impeller. As desired, the product may be rendered finer by passage through a colloid mill, in which the particles are sheared between the small gap separating a high speed rotor and the stator, or by passage through a large homogenizer, in which the liquid is forced under great pressure through a small valve opening. Industrial homogenizers have the capacity to handle as much as 100,000 liters of product per hour (Fig. 7–10).

In the small-scale extemporaneous preparation of emulsions, three methods may be used. They are the *continental* or *dry gum method*, the *English* or *wet gum method*, and the *bottle* or the *Forbes bottle method*. In the first method, the emulsifying agent (usually acacia) is mixed with the oil before the addition of water. In the second method, the emulsifying agent is added to the water (in which it is soluble) to form a mucilage, and then the oil is slowly incorporated to form the emulsion. The bottle method is reserved for volatile oils or less viscous oils and is a variation of the dry gum method.

CONTINENTAL OR DRY GUM METHOD. The method is also referred to as the "4:2:1" method

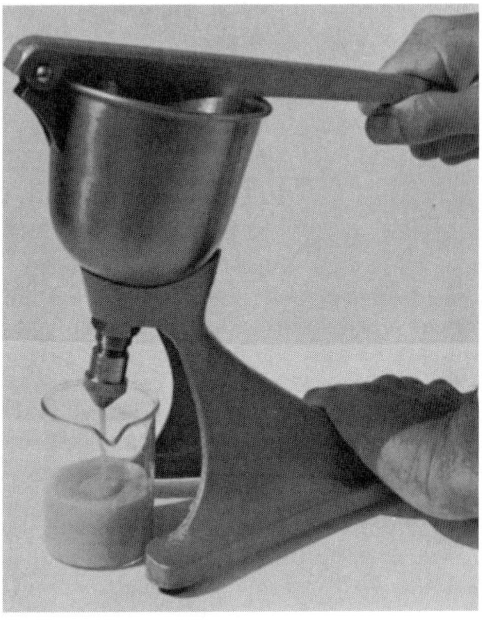

Fig. 7–9. *The laboratory preparation of an emulsion, using a hand homogenizer.*

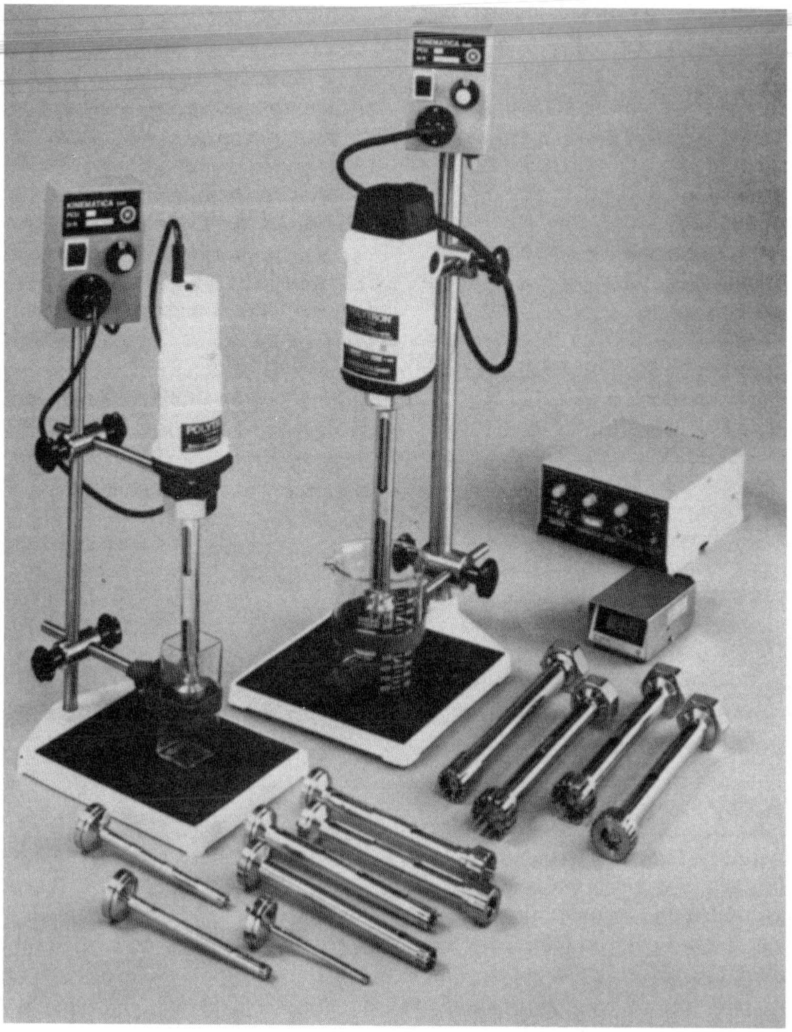

Fig. 7–10. *Brinkmann Homogenizer Models PT 10/35 and PT 45/80 with accessories. The equipment is used for the homogenization, dispersion and emulsification of solids or liquids. Volumes can be processed ranging from 0.5 mL to 25 liters. (Courtesy of Brinkmann Instruments Co., Division of Sybron Corporation.)*

because for every 4 parts (volumes) of oil, 2 parts of water and 1 part of gum are added in preparing the initial or *primary emulsion*. For instance, if 40 mL of oil are to be emulsified, 20 mL of water and 10 g of gum would be employed, with any additional water or other formulation ingredients being added afterward to the primary emulsion. In this method the acacia or other o/w emulsifier is triturated with the oil in a perfectly dry Wedgewood or procelain mortar until thoroughly mixed. A mortar with a rough rather than smooth inner surface must be used to ensure proper grinding action and the reduction of the globule size during the preparation of the emulsion. A glass mortar has too smooth a surface to produce the proper size reduction of the internal phase. After the oil and gum have been mixed, the two parts of water are then added all at once, and the mixture is triturated immediately, rapidly, and continuously until the primary emulsion that forms is creamy white and produces a crackling sound to the movement of the pestle. Generally, about 3 minutes of mixing are required to produce such a primary emulsion. Other liquid formulative ingredients that are soluble in or miscible with the external phase may then be added to the primary emulsion with mixing. Solid substances such as preservatives, stabilizers, colorants, and any flavoring material are usually dissolved in a suitable volume of water (assuming water is the external phase) and added as a solution to the primary emulsion. Any substances that might interfere with the stability of the emulsion or the emulsifying agent are added as near last as is practically possible. For instance, since alcohol has a precipitating action on gums such as acacia, alcohol or any solution containing alcohol should not be added directly to the primary emulsion, since the total alcoholic concentration of the mixture would be greater at that point than it would be after other diluents had been previously added. When all necessary agents have been added, the emulsion is transferred to a graduate and made to volume with water previously swirled about in the mortar to remove the last portion of emulsion.

Provided the dispersion of the acacia in the oil is adequate, the dry gum method can almost be guaranteed to produce an acceptable emulsion. Sometimes, however, the amount of acacia needs to be adjusted upward to ensure an emulsion can be produced. For example, volatile oils, liquid petrolatum (mineral oil) and linseed oil usually require a "3:2:1 or 2:2:1" ratio for adequate preparation.

Rather than use a mortar and pestle, the pharmacist can generally prepare an excellent emulsion using the dry gum method and an electric mixer or blender.

ENGLISH OR WET GUM METHOD. By this method, the same proportions of oil, water, and gum are used as in the continental or dry gum method, but the order of mixing is different, and the proportion of ingredients may be varied during the preparation of the primary emulsion as is deemed necessary by the operator. Generally a mucilage of the gum is prepared by triturating granular acacia with twice its weight of water in a mortar. The oil is then added slowly in portions, and the mixture is triturated to emulsify the oil. Should the mixture become too thick during the process, additional water may be blended into the mixture before another successive portion of oil is added. After all of the oil has been added, the mixture is thoroughly mixed for several minutes to insure uniformity. Then, as with the continental or dry gum method, the other formulative materials are added, and the emulsion is transferred to a graduate and made to volume with water.

BOTTLE OR FORBES BOTTLE METHOD. For the extemporaneous preparation of emulsions from volatile oils or oleaginous substances of low viscosities, the bottle method is useful. In this method, powdered acacia is placed in a dry bottle, two parts of oil are then added, and the mixture is thoroughly shaken in the capped container. A volume of water approximately equal to the oil is then added in portions, the mixture being thoroughly shaken after each addition. When all of the water has been added, the primary emulsion thus formed may be diluted to the proper volume with water or an aqueous solution of other formulative agents.

This method is not suited for viscous oils, because they cannot be thoroughly agitated in the bottle when mixed with the emulsifying agent. In instances in which the intended dispersed phase is a mixture of part fixed oil and part volatile oil, the dry gum method is generally employed for emulsification.

AUXILIARY METHODS. An emulsion prepared by either the wet gum or the dry gum methods can generally be increased in quality by passing it through a hand homogenizer. In this apparatus, the pumping action of the handle forces the emulsion through a very small orifice which reduces the globules of the internal phase to about 5 μm and sometimes less. The hand homogenizer is less efficient in reducing the particle size of very thick emulsions, and it should not be employed for emulsions containing a high proportion of solid matter because of possible damage to the valve.

IN SITU SOAP METHOD. The two types of soaps developed by this method are calcium soaps and soft soaps. Calcium soaps are water-in-oil emulsions which contain certain vegetable oils, e.g., oleic acid, in combination with lime water (syn: Calcium Hydroxide Solution USP), and are prepared simply by mixing equal volumes of the oil and lime water. The emulsifying agent in this instance is the calcium salt of the free fatty acid which is formed from the combination of the two entities. In the case of olive oil, the free fatty acid is oleic acid, and the resultant emulsifying agent formed is calcium oleate. A difficulty which sometimes arises when preparing this self-emulsifying product is that the amount of free fatty acids in the oil may be insufficient on a 1:1 basis with calcium hydroxide and typically to make up for this deficiency a little excess of the oil is needed to ensure a nice, homogeneous emulsion results. Otherwise, tiny droplets of water form

Surface Area of Globules

The following is an example calculation for determining the quantity of surfactant required to prepare a stable oil-in-water emulsion.

A surface-active agent will spread itself as a single layer when applied to the surface of still water. The dimensions of a molecule can be determined by their surface orientation. For example, if a micropipet is used to deliver 3 μL of a surfactant onto the clean, quiet surface of water, the area over which it spreads, determined experimentally using a film balance, is 12,000 cm^2. The actual thickness of the film can be calculated by dividing the volume of surfactant applied by the surface area, as follows:

$$\frac{0.003\ \text{cm}^3}{12{,}000\ \text{cm}^2} = 2.5 \times 10^{-7}\ \text{cm}$$

The surfactant has a density of 0.910 g/cc and a molecular weight of 325 g/mole. To calculate the cross-sectional area occupied by each molecule, one can divide the area of the monomolecular film by the number of molecules present in the 3 μL of surfactant comprising the film, as follows:

1. The weight of the surfactant can be obtained by multiplying the volume by the density (0.003 mL $\times$ 0.910 g/cc = 0.00273 g).
2. To calculate the number of moles present, divide the weight of the surfactant by its molecular weight (0.00273 g/325 g/mole = 8.4×10^{-6} moles).
3. The number of molecules present is the number of moles times Avogadro's Number ($8.4 \times 10^{-6} \times 6.02 \times 10^{23} = 5.0568 \times 10^{18}$ molecules).
4. The cross-sectional area can now be calculated by dividing the surface area by the number of molecules (12,000 cm^2/$5.0568 \times 10^{18} = 2.373 \times 10^{-15}$ cm^2 = 23.73×10^{-16}, or approximately 24 square angstroms.

The quantity of surfactant required to emulsify selected quantity of oil for the preparation of an oil in water emulsion can be calculated as follows.

EXAMPLE

To emulsify 50 mL of oil to an average globular diameter of 1 micron, the volume of each globule is:

$$V_i = \frac{4}{3}\pi r^3 = \frac{4}{3}\pi(0.5 \times 10^{-4})^3 = 0.524 \times 10^{-12}\ \text{ml}$$

To calculate the number of globules present per mL, divide 1 mL by the volume of each globule:

$$\frac{1\ \text{mL}}{0.524 \times 10^{-12}\ \text{mL/globule}} = 1.91 \times 10^{12}\ \text{globules per mL}$$

The surface area (S) of each individual globule will be:

$$S = 4\pi r^2 = 4\pi(0.5 \times 10^{-4})^2 = 3.14 \times 10^{-8}\ \text{cm}^2$$

and the surface area of all the globules in 1 mL of oil is:

$$(1.91 \times 10^{12}) \times (3.14 \times 10^{-8}) = 6 \times 10^4\ \text{cm}^2$$

The number of surfactant molecules that will be adsorbed at the interface of the oil globules, and the dispersion medium from 1 cc of oil, is equal to the total surface area divided by the cross-sectional area of the surfactant:

$$\frac{6 \times 10^4\ \text{cm}^2}{2.373 \times 10^{-15}\ \text{cm}^2/\text{molecule}} = 2.528 \times 10^{19}\ \text{molecules}$$

Surface Area of Globules (Continued)

To calculate the number of moles of surfactant that will be required to emulsify 1 mL of oil is equal to the number of molecules adsorbed at the interface divided by Avogadro's number:

$$\frac{2.528 \times 10^{19} \text{ molecules}}{6.02 \times 10^{23} \text{ molecules/mole}} = 4.199 \times 10^{-5} \text{ moles}$$

and the quantity required for 50 mL will be:

$$50 \text{ mL} \times 4.199 \times 10^{-5} \text{ moles/mL} = 2.095 \times 10^{-3} \text{ moles}$$

$$2.095 \times 10^{-3} \text{ moles} \times 325 \text{ g/mole} = 0.681 \text{ g, or } 681 \text{ mg}$$

Therefore, 681 mg of surfactant will be required to emulsify 50 mL of the oil.

on the surface of the preparation. Because the oil phase is the external phase, this formulation is ideal where occlusion and skin softening are desired, e.g., itchy, dry skin or sunburned skin. A typical example of this emulsion is calamine liniment:

Calamine	
Zinc Oxide aa	80.0 g
Olive Oil	
Calcium Hydroxide Sol'n aa qs ad	1000.0 mL

Microemulsions

Microemulsions are thermodynamically stable, optically transparent, isotropic mixtures of a biphasic oil-water system stabilized with surfactants. The diameter of droplets in a *micro*-emulsion may be in the range of 100 Å (10 millimicrons) to 1000 Å whereas in a *micro*emulsion the droplets may be 5000 Å in diameter.[6] Both o/w and w/o microemulsions may be formed spontaneously by agitating the oil and water phases with carefully selected surfactants. The type of emulsion produced depends upon the properties of the oil and surfactants utilized.

Hydrophilic surfactants may be used to produce "transparent" o/w emulsions of many oils, including flavor oils and vitamin oils such as A, D, and E. Surfactants in the HLB range of 15 to 18 have been used most extensively in the preparation of such emulsions. These emulsions are dispersions of oil, not true solutions; however, because of the appearance of the product, the surfactant is commonly said to "solubilize" the oil. Surfactants commonly used in the preparation of such oral liquid formulations are polysorbate 60 and polysorbate 80.

Amount the advantages cited for the use of microemulsions in drug delivery are: more rapid and efficient oral absorption of drugs than through solid dosage forms; enhanced transdermal drug delivery through increased drug diffusion into the skin; and the unique potential application of microemulsions in the development of artificial red blood cells and in the targeting of cytotoxic drugs to cancer cells.[6]

Stability of Emulsions

Generally speaking, an emulsion is considered to be physically unstable if: (a) the internal or dispersed phase upon standing tends to form aggregates of globules, (b) large globules or aggregates of globules rise to the top or fall to the bottom of the emulsion to form a concentrated layer of the internal phase, and (c) if all or part of the liquid of the internal phase becomes "unemulsified" and forms a distinct layer on the top or bottom of the emulsion as a result of the coalescing of the globules of the internal phase. In addition, an emulsion may be adversely affected by microbial contamination and growth and by other chemical and physical alterations.

AGGREGATION AND COALESCENCE. Aggregates of globules of the internal phase have a greater tendency than do individual particles to rise to the top of the emulsion or fall to the bottom. Such a preparation of the globules is termed the "creaming" of the emulsion, and provided coalescence is absent, it is a reversible process. The term is taken from the dairy industry and is analogous to the creaming or the rising to the top of cream in milk that is allowed to stand. The creamed portion of an emulsion may be redistributed rather homogeneously upon shaking, but if the aggregates are difficult to disassemble or if insufficient shaking is employed before each dose, improper dosage of the internal phase substance may result. Further, the creaming of pharmaceutical emulsion is not esthetically acceptable to the pharmacist nor appealing to the consumer. More importantly, it increases the risk of the coalescing of the globules.

According to the Stokes' equation (p. 256), the rate of separation of the dispersed phase of an emulsion may be related to such factors as the particle size of the dispersed phase, the difference in the density between the phases, and the viscosity of the external phase. It is important to recall that the rate of separation is increased by increased particle size of the internal phase, a larger density difference between the two phases, and a decreased viscosity of the external phase. Therefore, to increase the stability of an emulsion, the globule or particle size should be reduced as fine as is practically possible, the density difference between the internal and external phases should be minimal, and the viscosity of the external phase should be reasonably high. Thickeners such as tragacanth and microcrystalline cellulose are frequently added to emulsions to increase the viscosity of the external phase. Upward creaming takes place in unstable emulsions of the o/w or w/o type in which the internal phase has a lesser density than the external phase. Downward creaming takes place in unstable emulsions in which the opposite is true.

Of greater destruction to an emulsion than creaming is the coalescence of the globules of the internal phase and the separation of that phase into a layer. The separation of the internal phase from the emulsion is called the "breaking" of the emulsion, and the emulsions is described as being "cracked" or "broken." This is irreversible, because the protective sheath about the globules of the internal phase no longer exists. Attempts to reestablish the emulsion by agitation of the two separate layers are generally unsuccessful. Additional emulsifying agent and reprocessing through appropriate machinery are usually necessary to reproduce an emulsion.

Generally, care must be taken to protect emulsions against the extremes of cold and heat. Freezing and thawing result in the coarsening of an emulsion and sometimes in its breaking. Excessive heat has the same effect. Because emulsion products may be transported to and used in various geographic locations having varying climates and conditions of extremely high and low temperature, pharmaceutical manufacturers must have predetermined knowledge of their emulsion stability before they may be shipped. For most emulsions, the industry performs tests of evaluation under experimental conditions of 5° C, 40° C, and 50° C to determine the product's stability. Stability at both 5° C and 40° C for 3 months is considered the minimal stability that an emulsion should possess. Shorter exposure periods at 50° C may be used as an alternate test.

Because other environmental conditions such as the presence of light, air, and contaminating microorganisms can adversely affect the stability of an emulsion, appropriate formulative and packaging steps are usually taken to minimize such possible hazards to product stability. For light-sensitive emulsions, light-resistant containers are used. For emulsions susceptible to oxidative decomposition, antioxidants may be included in the formulation and adequate label warning provided to ensure that the container is tightly closed to air after each use. Many molds, yeasts, and bacteria can bring about the decomposition of the emulsifying agent of an emulsion, thereby causing the disruption of the system. In cases in which the emulsifier is not affected by the microbes, the product can be rendered unsightly by their presence and growth and will of course not be efficacious from a pharmaceutical or therapeutic standpoint. Fungistatic preservatives are generally included in the aqueous phase of an o/w emulsion, since fungi (molds and yeasts) are more likely to contaminate emulsions than are bacteria. Combinations of methylparaben and propylparaben are frequently employed to serve this function. Alcohol in the amount of 12 to 15% based on the external phase volume is frequently added to orally used o/w emulsions for preservation.

Examples of Oral Emulsions

Mineral Oil Emulsion

This emulsion, also referred to as liquid petrolatum emulsion, is an oil-in-water emulsion prepared from the following formula:

Mineral Oil	500 mL
Acacia (finely powdered)	125 g
Syrup	100 mL
Vanillin	40 mg
Alcohol	60 mL
Purified Water, a sufficient quantity, to make	1000 mL

The emulsion is prepared by the dry gum method (4:2:1), mixing the oil with the acacia and adding 250 mL of purified water all at once to effect the primary emulsion. To this is slowly added with trituration the remainder of the ingredients, with the vanillin dissolved in the alcohol. A substitute flavorant for the vanillin, a substitute preservative for the alcohol, and a substitute emulsifying agent for the acacia and an alternative method of emulsification may be used as desired.

The emulsion is employed as a lubricating cathartic with an usual dose of 30 mL. The usual dose of the plain (unemulsified) mineral oil for the same purpose is 15 mL. The emulsion is much more palatable than is the unemulsified oil. Both are best taken at bedtime. There are a number of commercial preparations of emulsified oil, with many containing additional cathartic agents as phenolphthalein, milk of magnesia, agar, and others.

Castor Oil Emulsion

This emulsion is utilized as a laxative, for isolated bouts of constipation, and in preparation of the colon for x-ray and endoscopic examination. The castor oil present in the emulsion works directly on the small intestine to promote bowel movement. This, and other laxatives, should not be used regularly or excessively as they can lead to dependence for bowel movement. Castor oil may cause excessive loss of water and body electrolytes if used excessively which can have a debilitating effect. Laxatives should not be used when nausea, vomiting, or abdominal pain is present since these symptoms may indicate appendicitis, and use of a laxative in this instance could promote rupturing of the appendix.

The amount of castor oil in commercial castor oil emulsions varies from about 35 to 67%. The amount of oil present influences the dose of the emulsion required. Generally, for an emulsion containing about two-thirds oil, the adult dose would be 45 mL, about 3 tablespoonfuls. For children 2 to 6 years of age, 15 mL is usually sufficient and for children less than 2 years of age, 5 mL may be given. Castor oil is best taken on an empty stomach, followed with one full glass of water.

Simethicone Emulsion

Simethicone emulsion is a water-dispersible form of simethicone used as a defoaming agent for the relief of painful symptoms of excess gas in the gastrointestinal tract. Simethicone emulsion works in the stomach and intestines by changing the surface tension of gas bubbles enabling them to coalesce; thus, freeing the gas for easier elimination. The emulsion, in drop form, is useful for the relief of gas in infants due to colic, air swallowing, or lactose intolerance. The commercial product [Mylicon Drops (Johnson & Johnson Merck)] contains 40 mg of simethicone per 0.6 mL. Simethicone is also present in a number of antacid formulations [e.g., Mylanta (Johnson & Johnson Merck)] as a therapeutic adjunct to relieve the discomfort of gas.

Gels and Magmas

Gels are defined as semisolid systems consisting of dispersions made up of either small inorganic particles or large organic molecules enclosing and interpenetrated by a liquid. Gels in which the macromolecules are distributed throughout the liquid in such a manner that no apparent boundaries exist between them and the liquid are called *single-phase gels.* In instances in which the gel mass consists of floccules of small distinct particles, the gel is classified as a two-phase system and frequently called a *magma* or a *milk.* Gels and magmas are considered colloidal dispersions since they each contain particles of colloidal dimension.

Colloidal Dispersions

Many of the various types of colloidal dispersions have been given appropriate names. For instance, *sol* is a general term to designate a dispersion of a solid substance in either a liquid, a solid, or a gaseous dispersion medium. However, more often than not it is used to describe the solid-liquid dispersion system. To be more descriptive, a prefix such as *hydro-* for water *(hydrosol)* or *alco-* for alcohol *(alcosol)* may be employed to indicate the dispersion medium. The term *aerosol* has similarly been developed to indicate a dispersion of a solid or a liquid in a gaseous phase.

Although there is no precise point at which the size of a particle in a dispersion can be considered to be "colloidal," there is a generally accepted size range. A substance is said to be colloidal when its particles fall between 1 nm and 0.5 μm. Colloidal particles are usually larger than atoms, ions, or molecules and generally consist of aggregates of many molecules, although in certain proteins and organic polymers single, large molecules may be of colloidal dimension and form colloidal dispersions. One difference between colloidal dispersions and true solutions is the larger particle size of the disperse phase of the former type of preparation. Another difference is the optical properties of the two systems. True solutions do not scatter light and therefore appear clear, but colloidal dispersions contain opaque particles that do scatter light and thus appear turbid. This turbidity is easily seen, even with dilute preparations, when the dispersion is observed at right angles to a beam of light passed through the dispersion (Tyndall effect). Although reference is made here to dilute colloidal dispersions, most pharmaceutical preparations contain high concentrations of particles within the colloidal size range, and in these instances there is no difficulty in observing turbidity. In fact, certain preparations may be quite opaque, depending upon the concentration of the disperse phase. Also, the particle size of the disperse phase in some pharmaceutical preparations may not be uniform, and a preparation may contain particles within and outside of the colloidal range, giving the preparation more of an opaque appearance than if all particles were uniformly colloidal.

Particle size is not the only important criterion for establishing the colloidal state. The nature of the dispersing phase with respect to the disperse phase is also of great importance. The attraction or lack of attraction between the disperse phase and the dispersion medium affects the ease of preparation of a colloidal dispersion as well as the character of the dispersion. Certain terminology has been developed to characterize the various degrees of attraction between the phases of a colloidal dispersion. If the disperse phase interacts appreciably with the dispersion medium, it is referred to as being *lyophilic,* meaning "solvent-loving." If the degree of attraction is small, the colloid is termed *lyophobic,* or "solvent-hating." These terms are more suitably used when reference is made to the specific dispersion medium, for a single substance may be lyophobic with respect to one dispersion medium and lyophilic with respect to another. For instance, starch is lyophilic in water but lyophobic in alcohol. Terms such as *hydrophilic* and *hydrophobic,* which are more descriptive of the nature of the colloidal property, have therefore been developed to refer to the attraction or lack of attraction of the substance specifically to water. Generally speaking, because of the attraction to the solvent of lyophilic substances in contrast to the lack of attraction of lyophobic substances, lyophilic colloidal systems are usually easier to prepare and have the greater stability. A third type of colloidal sol, termed as *association* or *amphiphilic colloid,* is formed by the grouping or association of molecules that exhibit both lyophilic and lyophobic properties.

Lyophilic colloids are generally large organic molecules capable of being solvated or associated with the molecules of the dispersing phase. These substances disperse readily upon addition to the dispersion medium to form colloidal dispersions. As more molecules of the substance are added to the sol, the viscosity is characteristically increased and when the concentration of molecules is sufficiently high, the liquid sol may become a semisolid or solid dispersion, termed a *gel.* Gels owe their rigidity to an intertwining network of the disperse phase which entraps and holds the dispersion medium. A change in the temperature can cause certain gels to resume the sol or liquid state. Also, some gels may become fluid after agitation only to resume their solid or semisolid state after remaining undisturbed for a period of time, a phenomenon known as *thixotrophy.*

Lyophobic colloids are generally composed of inorganic particles. When these are added to the dispersing phase, there is little if any interaction between the two phases. Unlike lyophilic colloids, lyophobic materials do not spontaneously disperse but must be encouraged to do so by special, individualized procedures. Their addition to the dispersion medium does not greatly affect the viscosity of the vehicle. Amphiphilic colloids form dispersions in both aqueous and nonaqueous media. Depending upon their individual character and the nature of the dispersion medium, they may or may not become greatly solvated. However, they generally cause an increase in the viscosity of the dispersion medium with an increase in concentration.

For the most part, the colloidal sols and gels used in pharmacy are aqueous preparations. The various preparations composed of colloidal dispersions are prepared, not according to any general method but according to the means best suited to the individual preparation. Some substances such as acacia are termed *natural colloids* because they are self-dispersing upon addition to the dispersing medium. Other materials that require special means for prompt dispersion are termed *artificial colloids.* They may require fine pulverization of coarse particles to colloidal size by a colloid mill or a micropulverizer, or colloidal size particles may be formed by chemical reaction under highly controlled conditions.

Preparation of Magmas and Gels

Many magmas and gels are prepared by freshly precipitating the disperse phase in order to achieve a fine degree of subdivision of the particles and a gelatinous character to those particles. The desired gelatinous precipitate results when solutions of inorganic agents react to form an insoluble chemical having a high attraction for water. As the microcrystalline particles of the precipitate develop, they strongly attract water to yield gelatinous particles, which combine to form the desired gelantinous precipitate. Other magmas and gels may be prepared by the direct hydration in water of the inorganic chemical, the hydrated form constituting the disperse phase of the dispersion. In addition to the water vehicle, other agents as propylene glycol, propylgallate and hydroxypropylcellulose may be used to enhance gel formation.

Because of the high degree of attraction between the disperse phase and the aqueous medium in both magmas and gels, these preparations remain fairly uniform on standing with little settling of the disperse phase. However, on long standing a supernatant layer of the dispersion medium develops, but the uniformity of the preparation is easily reestablished by moderate shaking. To ensure uniform dosage, magmas and gels should be shaken before use, and a statement to that effect must be included on the label of such preparations. The medicinal magmas and gels are used orally for the value of the disperse phase.

Examples of Magmas and Gels

One official magma, Bentonite Magma, NF, is used as a suspending agent and finds application in the extemporaneous compounding of prescriptions calling for the suspension of medicinal agents. Sodium Fluoride and Phosphoric Acid Gel, USP, is applied topically to the teeth as a dental care prophylactic. Other official gels applied topically include Fluocinonide Gel, USP, an antiinflammatory corticosteroid, and Tretinoin Gel, USP, an irritant which stimulates epidermal cell turnover and causes peeling and is effective in the treatment of acne. Other official magmas and gels are employed as antacids, namely: Aluminum Phosphate Gel, USP, Aluminum Hydroxide Gel, USP; Dihydroxyaluminum Aminoacetate Magma, USP, and Milk of Magnesia (Magnesia Magma), USP. Some of these preparations are discussed briefly below.

Bentonite Magma, NF

Bentonite magma is a preparation of 5% bentonite, a native, colloidal hydrated aluminum silicate, in purified water. It may be prepared mechanically in a blender with the bentonite added directly to the purified water while the machine is running, or it may be prepared by sprinkling the bentonite, in portions, upon hot purified water, allowing each portion to become thoroughly wetted without stirring before another portion is added. By the latter method, the mixture must be allowed to stand for 24 hours before it may be stirred. The standing period ensures the complete hydration and swelling of the bentonite. Bentonite, which is insoluble in water, swells to approximately twelve times its volume upon addition to water. The NF monograph for bentonite contains a test for "swelling power," in which 2 g of a bentonite sample is added in portions to 100 mL of water contained in a 100-mL glass-stoppered cylinder. At the end of a 2-hour period, the mass at the bottom of the cylinder is required to occupy an apparent volume of not less than 24 mL. Other required tests are for gel formation, fineness of powder, and pH, the latter being between 9.5 and 10.5. After bentonite magma has been allowed to stand undisturbed for some period of time, it sets to a gel. Upon agitation the sol form returns. The process may be repeated indefinitely. As mentioned earlier, this phenomenon is termed *thixotropy*, and bentonite magma is termed a *thixotropic gel*. The thixotropy occurs only when the bentonite concentration is somewhat above 4%.

Bentonite magma is employed as a suspending agent. Its alkaline pH must be considered, because this might be undesirable for certain drugs. Further, because the suspending capacity of the magma is drastically reduced if the pH is lowered to about pH7, another suspending agent should be selected for drugs requiring a less alkaline medium rather than make bentonite magma more acidic.

Aluminum Hydroxide Gel, USP

Aluminum Hydroxide Gel, USP, is an aqueous suspension of a gelatinous precipitate composed of insoluble aluminum hydroxide and the hydrated aluminum oxide, equivalent to about 4% of aluminum oxide. The disperse phase of the gel is generally prepared by chemical reaction, using various reactants. Usually the aluminum source of the reaction is aluminum chloride or aluminum alum, which yields the insoluble aluminum oxide and aluminum hydroxide precipitate. To the gel, the USP permits the addition of peppermint oil, glycerin, sorbitol, sucrose, saccharin, or other flavorants and sweeteners as well as suitable antimicrobial agents.

This antacid preparation is a white, viscous suspension. It is effective in neutralizing a portion of the gastric hydrochloric acid and by virtue of its gelatinous, viscous, and insoluble character, coats the inflamed and perhaps ulcerated gastric surface and is useful in the treatment of hyperacidity and peptic ulcers. The main disadvantage to its use is its constipating effects. The usual dose is 10 mL, four or more times a day. Ten mL of the analogous commercial product (Amphojel, Wyeth-Ayerst) has the capacity to neutralize about 13 mEq of acid. The preparation should be stored in tight containers, and freezing should be avoided.

Because it possesses a trivalent cation, aluminum hydroxide has the capability to interfere with the bioavailability of tetracycline by chelating with the antibiotic in the gastrointestinal tract. Thus, when these two medicines are indicated for patient use, the doses of each should be staggered to ensure the patient receives the benefit of both drugs. Aluminum hydroxide gel has also been implicated at decreasing the bioavailability of other drugs as well by adsorption onto the gel. This is usually illustrated by a decrease in the area under the concentration time curve (AUC) for the concomitantly administered drug. Suffice to say that the clinical significance of the interaction might not be that great, but observation of the patient to insure the proper therapeutic outcome from the other drug is important. Thus, for example, if aluminum hydroxide gel is suspected of causing incomplete absorption of the second drug, then an upward alteration in the dose of the drug might be necessary provided the aluminum hydroxide gel administration remains the same.

Milk of Magnesia, USP

Milk of Magnesia, USP, is a preparation containing between 7 and 8.5% of magnesium hydroxide. Although there is no method of preparation indicated in the USP for this preparation, it may be prepared by a reaction between sodium hydroxide and magnesium sulfate (1), diluted solutions being used to ensure a fine, flocculent, gelatinous precipitate of magnesium hydroxide. The precipitate so produced is washed with purified water to remove the sodium sulfate prior to its incorporation with additional purified water to prepare the required volume of product. Commercially, the product is more economically produced by the direct hydration of magnesium oxide (2).

(1) $2NaOH + MgSO_4 \rightarrow Mg(OH)_2 + Na_2SO_4$

(2) $MgO + H_2O \rightarrow Mg(OH)_2$

Irrespective of its method of preparation, milk of magnesia is a white, opaque, viscous preparation from which varying proportions of water separate on standing. For this reason it should be shaken before use. The preparation has a pH of about 10, which may bring about a reaction between the magma and the glass container imparting a bitter taste to the preparation. To minimize such an occurrence, 0.1% citric acid may be added to the preparation. Also, flavoring oils at a concentration not exceeding 0.05% may be added to enhance the palatability of the preparation.

Milk of Magnesia possesses reasonable acid-neutralizing ability and a dose of 5 mL will neutralize about 10 mEq of stomach acid. However, to neutralize more acid a higher dose, e.g., 15 mL is usually necessary, and this may predispose the patient to the development diarrhea, a common side effect of this drug. Thus, to circumvent the problem of diarrhea from magnesium hydroxide and the constipating effects of aluminum hydroxide, frequently these two drugs are combined in an antacid preparation. The combination results in a more palatable product with optimum buffering of stomach contents between a pH of 4 to 5, and less of a chance for either diarrhea or constipation to occur. When a laxative effect is desired a bedtime dose of 30 to 60 mL of milk of magnesia will suffice very nicely by the next morning.

The preparation is best stored in tight containers preferably at a temperature above freezing and below 35°C. Freezing results in a coarsening of the disperse phase, and temperatures above 35°C decrease the gel structure.

Proper Administration and Use of Peroral Disperse Systems

The variety of dosage forms discussed in this chapter are for oral consumption, and like those liquid dosage forms from the previous chapter, these can be measured in a spoon, i.e., teaspoon, tablespoon, depending upon the desired dosage. With these dosage forms it is very important that the patient understand how much of the product to use. For example, differences in dosage can occur between product category, e.g., OTC antidiarrheal suspensions [tablespoonfuls] *vs* OTC antacid suspensions [teaspoonfuls]. Differences in dosage can also occur within a category, most notably antacid suspensions. Some are recommended in teaspoon doses because of higher concentration whereas others are suggested in tablespoon quantities. It is important, therefore, that the pharmacist ensure that the patient knows how much to use, and then use a calibrated device to make sure the right amount is taken.

Reconstituted products, as mentioned earlier in the chapter frequently are suspensions. Several potential problems can emerge if the pharmacist is not careful to counsel the patient about them. Usually the patient or the guardian of the patient receives the product in an oversized bottle that allows for the proper shaking of the product prior to its use. To allay fears that all of the medicine may not be in the bottle, the pharmacist must make the patient or the guardian aware of this, and indicate this feature enhances the shakability before its administration. Further, some patients do not make the connection that the medicine should be administered by mouth. Oral antibiotic suspensions intended to treat a middle ear infection have been mistakenly administered directly into the ear by some patients or guardians. Thus, the pharmacist should review with the patient the proper administration. Lastly, because these are reconstituted with purified water stability problems with the drug usually dictate it be stored in the refrigerator until it is consumed. The patient has to be informed of this. Tiny labels on the container directing one to store the product in the refrigerator are sometimes overlooked by the consumer. Alternatively, not all suspensions need to be stored in the refrigerator but because or prior experience with other liquid suspensions that necessitated refrigeration a patient or guardian may assume this is necessary.

Certain suspensions by virtue of their active ingredients, e.g., aluminum hydroxide gel, cholestyramine, kaolin, have the ability to interfere with the absorption of other drugs that might be concurrently administered. For example, cholestyramine has been shown to interfere with and decrease the bioavailability of such drugs as warfarin, digitoxin and thyroid hormones. The pharmacist should be aware of this and make recommendations to help avoid this drug interaction whenever possible. The typical suggestion would be to stagger the administration of the liquid cholestyramine away from other drug administration by several hours, and in the case of warfarin, giving warfarin at least 6 hours after the cholestyramine reportedly avoids the impaired warfarin bioavailability.[8] However, warfarin is a drug that undergoes enterohepatic recycling in the body, and if cholestyramine were present in the intestine because of earlier administration it could bind it and decrease warfarin's subsequent reabsorption. In this instance, concomitant use of one of the two drugs should be discontinued by the physician. However, if concurrent use is necessary, the pharmacist should monitor the patient more frequently for the possibility of an altered anticoagulant response. This is important because if adjustments in warfarin dosage were made on the basis of cholestyramine interference and then the cholestyramine was discontinued, the warfarin dosage also would have to be decreased accordingly, i.e., based on the patient's prothrombin time.

References

1. Heyd, A., and Dhabhar, D.: Particle Shape Effect on Caking of Coarse Granulated Antacid Suspensions. *Drug & Cosmetic Industry, 125:*42, 1979.
2. *Oral Liquid Pharmaceuticals:* Wilmington, DE, ICI Americas Inc., 1975.
3. Chang, R.K.: Formulation Approaches for Sustained-Release Oral Suspensions. *Pharm. Tech. 16:* 134–136, 1992.
4. Allen, L.V.: Prednisone Oral Suspension, *U.S. Pharmacist, 14:*84, 1989.
5. Allen, L.V.: Ketoconazole Oral Suspension. *US Pharmacist, 18:*98, 1993.
6. Bhargava, H.N., Narurkar, A., and Lieb, L.M.: Using Microemulsions for Drug Delivery. *Pharm. Tech., 11:* 46, 1987.
7. Griffin, W.C.: *J. Soc. Cosmetics Chemists, 1:*311, 1949; *ibid, 5:*1, 1954.
8. Hansten, P.D., and Horn, J.R.: *Drug Interactions.* 6th Ed., Philadelphia, Lea & Febiger, 1989, p. 80.

8

Parenteral Medications and Sterile Fluids

Considered in this chapter are important pharmaceutical dosage forms that have the common characteristic of being prepared to be sterile; that is, free from contaminating microorganisms. Among these sterile dosage forms are the various small- and large-volume injectable preparations, irrigation fluids intended to bathe body wounds or surgical openings, dialysis solutions, biological preparations as vaccines, toxoids, antitoxins, and blood replenishment products. Sterility in these preparations is of utmost importance because they are placed in direct contact with the internal body fluids or tissues where infection can easily arise. Ophthalmic preparations which are also prepared to be sterile will be discussed separately in Chapter 11.

Injections

Injections are sterile, pyrogen-free preparations intended to be administered parenterally. The term *parenteral* refers to the injectable routes of administration. The term has its derivation from the Greek words *para* and *enteron*, meaning outside of the intestine, and denotes routes of administration other than the oral route. *Pyrogens* are fever-producing organic substances arising from microbial contamination and are responsible for many of the febrile reactions which occur in patients following intravenous injection. Pyrogens and the determination of their presence in parenteral preparations will be discussed later in this chapter. In general, the parenteral routes of administration are undertaken when rapid drug action is desired, as in emergency situations, when the patient is uncooperative, unconscious, or unable to accept or tolerate medication by the oral route, or when the drug itself is ineffective by other routes. With the exception of insulin injections, which are commonly *self*-administered by diabetic patients, most injections are administered by the physician, his assistant, or nurse in the course of medical treatment. Thus injections are employed mostly in the hospital, extended care facility, and clinic and less frequently in the home. An exception would be in *home health care* programs in which health professionals pay scheduled visits to patients in their homes, providing needed treatment, including intravenous medications. These programs enable patients who do not require or are unable to pay for more expensive hospitalization to remain in the familiar surroundings of their homes while receiving appropriate medical care. The pharmacist supplies injectable preparations to the physician and nurse, as required for their use in the institutional setting, clinic, office, or home health care program.

Perhaps the earliest injectable drug to receive official recognition was the hypodermic morphine solution which appeared first in the 1874 addendum to the 1867 British Pharmacopeia, and later, in 1888 in the first edition of the National Formulary of the United States. Today, there are literally hundreds of drugs and drug products available for parenteral administration.

Interesting historical accounts of the origin and development of injection therapy may be found in the references cited.

Parenteral Routes of Administration

Drugs may be injected into almost any organ or area of the body, including the joints *(intra-articular)*, a joint-fluid area *(intrasynovial)*, the spinal column *(intraspinal)*, into spinal fluid *(intrathecal)*, arteries *(intra-arterial)*, and in an emergency, even into the heart *(intracardiac)*. However, most commonly injections are performed into a vein *(intravenous, I.V.)*, into a muscle *(intramuscular, I.M.)*, into the skin *(Intradermal, I.D., intracutaneous)*, or under the skin *(subcutaneous, S.C., Sub-Q, S.Q., hypodermic, "Hypo.")* (Fig. 8–1).

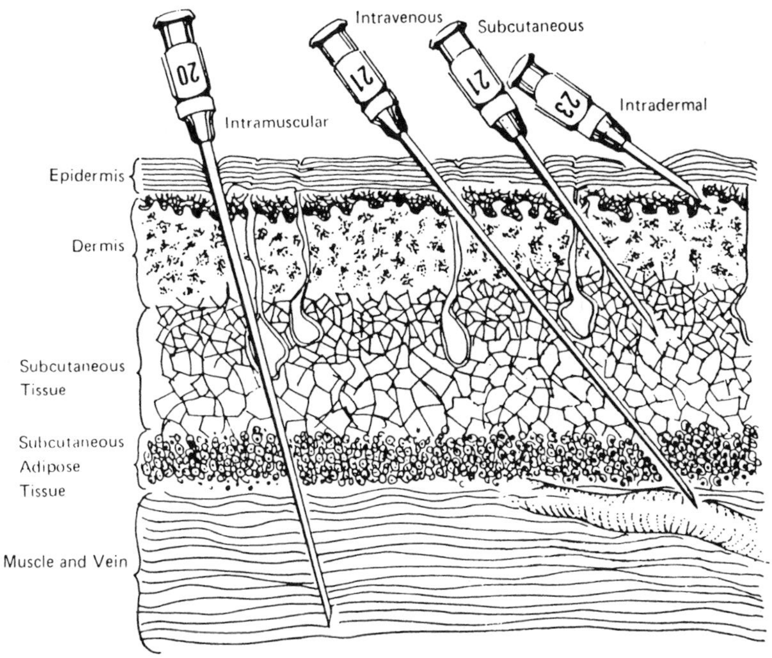

Fig. 8–1. *Routes of parenteral administration. Numbers on needles indicate size or gauge of needle based on outside diameter of needle shaft. (Turco, S. and King, R.E., Sterile Dosage Forms: Their Preparation and Clinical Applications. 3rd Ed., Courtesy of Lea & Febiger, 1987.)*

Intravenous Route

The intravenous injection of drugs had its scientific origin in 1656 in the experiments of Sir Christopher Wren, architect of St. Paul's Cathedral and amateur physiologist. Using a bladder and quill for a syringe and needle, he injected wine, ale, opium, and other substances into the veins of dogs and studied their effects. Intravenous medication was first given to man by Johann Daniel Major of Kiel in 1662, but was abandoned for a period because of the occurrence of thrombosis and embolism in the patients so treated. The invention of the hypodermic syringe toward the middle of the 19th century created a new interest in intravenous techniques and toward the turn of the century, intravenous administration of solutions of sodium chloride and glucose became popular. Today, the intravenous administration of drugs is a routine occurrence in the hospital, although there are still recognized dangers associated with the practice. Thrombus and embolus formation may be induced by intravenous needles and catheters, and the possibility of particulate matter in parenteral solutions poses concern for those involved in the development, administration, and use of intravenous solutions.

Intravenously administered drugs provide rapid action compared to other routes of administration and because drug absorption is not a factor, optimum blood levels may be achieved with the accuracy and immediacy not possible by other routes. In emergency situations, the intravenous administration of a drug may be a lifesaving procedure because of the placement of the drug directly into the circulation and the prompt action which ensues. On the negative side, once a drug is administered intravenously, it cannot be retrieved. In the case of an adverse reaction to the drug, for instance, the drug cannot be easily removed from the circulation as it could, for example, by the induction of vomiting following the oral administration of the same drug.

Although most superficial veins are suitable for venipuncture, the veins of the antecubital area (situated in front of the elbow) are usually selected for direct intravenous injection. The veins in this location are large, superficial and easy to see and enter. Most clinicians insert the needle with the bevel facing upward, at the most acute angle possible with the vein, to ensure that the direction of flow of the injectable is that of the flow of the blood. Strict aseptic precautions must be taken at all times to avoid risk of infection. Not only are the injectable solutions sterile, the syringes and needles employed must also be sterilized and the point of entrance must be disinfected to reduce the chance of carrying bacteria from the skin into the blood via the needle. Prior to injection, administration personnel must withdraw the plunger of the syringe or squeeze a special bulb found on most I.V. sets to ensure that the needle has been properly located. In both instances, a "flashback" of blood into the administration set or the syringe indicates proper placement of the needle within the vein.

Both small and large volumes of drug solutions may be administered intravenously. The use of 1000-mL containers of solutions for intravenous infusion is commonplace in the hospital. These solutions containing such agents as nutrients, blood extenders, electrolytes, amino acids, and other therapeutic agents are generally administered through an indwelling needle or catheter by continuous drip. The drip or flow rates may be adjusted by the clinician according to the needs of the patient. Generally, flow rates of 2 to 3 mL per minute are employed. For intravenous infusion, the needle or catheter is generally placed in the prominent veins of the forearm or leg and taped firmly to the patient so that it will not slip from place during infusion. The main hazard of intravenous infusion is the possibility of thrombus formation induced by the touching of the wall of the vein by the catheter or needle. Thrombi are more likely to occur when the infusion solution is of an irritating nature to the biologic tissues. A *thrombus* is a blood clot formed within the blood vessel (or heart) due usually to a slowing of the circulation or to an alteration of the blood or vessel wall. Once such a clot circulates, it becomes an *embolus*, carried by the blood stream until it lodges in a blood vessel, obstructing it, and resulting in a blockage or occlusion referred to as an *embolism*. Such an obstruction may be a critical hazard to the patient, depending upon the site and severity of the obstruction.

Intravenously administered drugs ordinarily must be in aqueous solution; they must mix with the circulating blood and not precipitate from solution. Such an event could lead to pulmonary microcapillary occlusion and the subsequent blockage of blood passage. An intravenously delivered fat emulsion (Intralipid, 10%, Clintec) has gained acceptance for use as a source of calories and essential fatty acids for patients requiring parenteral nutrition for extended periods of time (usually for more than 5 days). The product contains up to 20% soybean oil emulsified with egg yolk phospholipids, in a vehicle of glycerin in water for injection. The emulsion is administered via a peripheral vein or by central venous infusion.

Naturally, the intravenous route is utilized in the administration of blood transfusions and it also serves as the point of exit in the removal of blood from patients for diagnostic work and for obtaining blood from donors.

In the late 1980s, automated intravenous delivery systems became commercially available for intermittent, self-administration of analgesics. Patient-controlled analgesia (PCA) has been used to control the pain associated with postoperative pain from a variety of surgical procedures, labor, sickle cell crisis, and chronic pain associated with cancer. For patients with chronic malignant pain, PCA allows a greater degree of ambulation and independence.[1]

The typical PCA device includes a syringe or chamber that contains the analgesic drug and a programmable electomechanical unit. The unit, which might be compact enough to be worn on a belt or carried in a pocket (e.g., WalkMed™ PCA–Medex, Inc.), controls the delivery of drug by advancing a piston when the patient presses a button. The drug can be loaded into the device by a health care professional or dispensed from preloaded cartridges available through the manufacturer. The devices take advantage of intravenous bolus injections to produce rapid analgesia, along with slower infusion to produce steady-state opiate concentrations for sustained pain control.

The advantage of the PCA is its ability to provide constant and uniform analgesia. The typical intramuscular injection of an opiod into a depot muscular site may result in variable absorption, leading to unpredictable blood concentrations. Further, these injections are usually given when needed and are often inadequate to treat the pain. The PCA can prevent pharmacokinetic and pharmacodynamic differences between patients from interfering with the effectiveness of analgesia. Because opiod kinetics differ greatly between patients, the rates of infusion must be tailored.[2]

PCA devices can be used for intravenous, subcutaneous, or epidural administration. Gener-

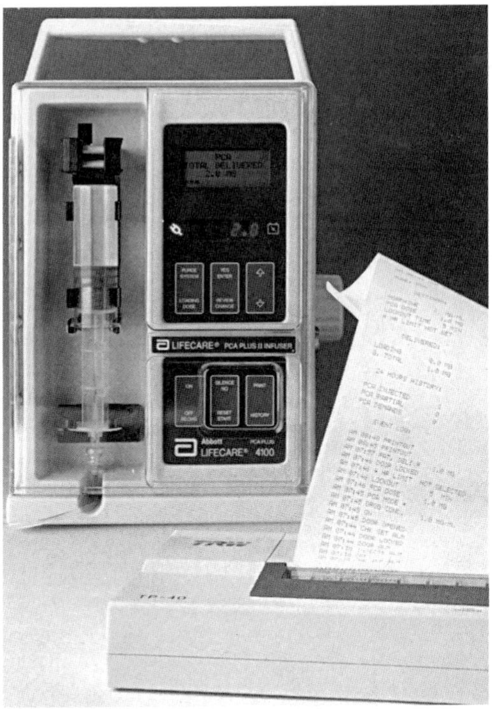

Fig. 8–2. *PCA Plus II (LifeCare 4100)-Patient-controlled analgesic infuser. (Courtesy of Abbott Hospital Products Division.)*

ally, these devices are either *demand dosing* (i.e., a fixed dose of drug is injected intermittently) or *constant-rate infusion plus demand dosing*.[2] Regardless of type utilized, the physician or nurse establishes the loading dose, the rate of background infusion, dose per demand, lockout interval (i.e., minimum time between demand doses), and maximum dosage over a specified time interval. Fig. 8–2 demonstrates the PCA Plus II (Lifecare 4100) infuser. With this device the patient pushes a button on a pendant to deliver a prescribed quantity of the analgesic.

Intramuscular Route

Intramuscular injections of drugs provide drug effects that are less rapid, but generally of greater duration than those obtained from intravenous administration.[3] Aqueous or oleaginous solutions or suspensions of drug substances may be administered intramuscularly. Depending upon the type of preparation employed, the absorption rates may vary widely. Generally it would be expected that drugs in solution would be more rapidly absorbed than those in suspension and that drugs in aqueous preparations would be more rapidly absorbed than when in oleaginous preparations. The physical type of preparation employed is based on the properties of the drug itself and on the therapeutic goals desired.

Intramuscular injections are performed deep into the skeletal muscles. The point of injection should be as far as possible from major nerves and blood vessels. Injuries to patients from intramuscular injection usually are related to the point at which the needle entered and where the medication was deposited. Such injuries include paralysis resulting from neural damage, abscesses, cysts, embolism, hematoma, sloughing of the skin, and scar formation.

In adults, the upper outer quadrant of the gluteus maximus is the most frequently used site for intramuscular injection. In infants, the gluteal area is small and composed primarily of fat, not muscle. What muscle there is is poorly developed. An injection in this area might be presented dangerously close to the sciatic nerve, especially if the child is resisting the injection and squirming or fighting. Thus, in infants and young children, the deltoid muscles of the upper arm or the midlateral muscles of the thigh are preferred. An injection given in the upper or lower portion of the deltoid would be well away from the radial nerve. The deltoid may also be used in adults, but the pain is more noticeable here than in the gluteal area. If a series of injections are to be given, the injection site is usually varied. To be certain that a blood vessel has not been entered, the clinician may aspirate slightly on the syringe following insertion of the needle to observe if blood enters the syringe. Usually, the volume of medication which may be conveniently administered by the intramuscular route is limited; generally a maximum of 5 mL is administered intramuscularly in the gluteal region and 2 mL in the deltoid of the arm.

The Z-Track Injection technique is useful for intramuscular injections of medications that stain upper tissue, e.g., iron dextran injection, or those that irritate tissue, e.g., Valium, by sealing these medications in the lower muscle. Because of its staining qualities, iron dextran injection, for example, must be injected only into the muscle mass of the upper outer quadrant of the buttock. The skin is displaced laterally prior to injection, then the needle is inserted and syringe aspirated, and the injection performed slowly and smoothly. The needle is then withdrawn and the skin released. This creates a "Z" pattern that blocks infiltration of medication into the subcutaneous tissue. The injection is 2 to 3 inches deep, and a 19- to 20-gauge needle is utilized. To further prevent any staining of upper tissue, usually one needle is used to withdraw the iron dextran from its ampul, and then replaced with another for the purposes of the injection.

Subcutaneous Route

The subcutaneous route may be utilized for the injection of small amounts of medication. The injection of a drug beneath the surface of the skin is usually made in the loose interstitial tissues of the outer surface of the upper arm, the anterior surface of the thigh, and the lower portion of the abdomen. The site of injection is usually rotated when injections are frequently given, e.g., daily insulin injections. Prior to injection, the skin at the injection site should be thoroughly cleansed. The maximum amount of medication that can be comfortably injected subcutaneously is about 1.3 mL and amounts greater than 2 mL will most likely cause painful pressure. Syringes with up to 3 mL capacities and utilizing needles with 24 to 26 gauges are used for subcutaneous injections. These needles will have cannula lengths that vary between ⅜ inch to 1 inch. Most typically, subcutaneous insulin needles are between 25 to 28 gauge with needle length between ⅜ to ⅝ inch. Upon insertion, if blood appears in the syringe a new site should be selected.

Drugs which are irritating or those which are present in thick suspension form may produce induration, sloughing, or abscess formation and may be painful to the patient. Such preparations should be considered not suitable for subcutaneous injection.

Intradermal Route

A number of substances may be effectively injected into the corium, the more vascular layer of the skin just beneath the epidermis. These substances include various agents for diagnostic determinations, desensitization, or immunization. The usual site for intradermal injection is the anterior surface of the forearm. A short (⅜ in.) and narrow gauge (23- to 26-gauge) needle is usually employed. The needle is inserted horizontally into the skin with the bevel facing upward. The injection is made when the bevel just disappears into the corium. Usually only about 0.1 mL volumes may be administered in this manner.

Official Types of Injections

According to the USP, injections are separated into five distinct types, generally defined as follows:

1. Medicaments or solutions, or emulsions suitable for injection, bearing titles of the form, "________ *Injection.*" (Ex: Insulin Injection, USP)
2. Dry solids or liquid concentrates containing no buffers, diluents, or other added substances, and which, upon the addition of suitable solvents, yield solutions conforming in all aspects to the requirements for injections, and which are distinguished by titles of the form, *"Sterile ________"* (Ex: Sterile Ampicillin Sodium, USP)
3. Preparations the same as those described in (2) except that they contain one or more buffers, diluents, or other added substances, and which are distinguished by titles of the form, "________ *for Injection*" (Ex: Methicillin Sodium for Injection, USP)
4. Solids which are suspended in a suitable fluid medium and which are not to be injected intravenously or into the spinal canal, distinguished by titles of the form, *"Sterile ________ Suspension."* (Ex: Sterile Dexamethasone Acetate Suspension, USP)
5. Dry solids, which, upon the addition of suitable vehicles, yield preparations conforming in all respects to the requirements for Sterile Suspensions, and which are distinguished by titles of the form, *"Sterile ________ for Suspension."* (Ex: Sterile Ampicillin for Suspension, USP)

The form in which a given drug is prepared for parenteral use by the manufacturer depends upon the nature of the drug itself, with respect to its physical and chemical characteristics, and also upon certain therapeutic considerations. Generally, if a drug is unstable in solution, it may be prepared as a dry powder intended for reconstitution with the proper solvent at the time of its administration, or it may be prepared as a suspension of the drug particles in a vehicle in which the drug is insoluble. If the drug is unstable in the presence of water, that solvent may be replaced in part or totally by a solvent in which the drug is insoluble. If the drug is insoluble in water, an injection may be prepared as an aqueous suspension or as a solution of the drug in a suitable nonaqueous solvent, such as a vegetable oil. If an aqueous solution is desired, a water-soluble salt form of the insoluble drug is frequently prepared to satisfy the required solubility characteristics. Aqueous or blood-miscible solutions may be injected directly into the blood stream. Blood-immiscible liquids, e.g., oleaginous injections and suspensions, can interrupt the normal flow of blood within the circulatory system, and their use is generally restricted to other than intravenous administration. The onset and duration of action of a drug may be somewhat controlled by the chemical form of the drug used, the physical state of the injection (solution or suspension), and the vehicle employed. Drugs that are very soluble in body fluids generally have the most rapid absorption and onset of action. Thus, drugs in aqueous solution have a more rapid onset of action than do drugs in oleaginous solution. Drugs in aqueous suspension are also more rapid acting than drugs in oleaginous suspension due to the greater miscibility of the aqueous preparation with the body fluids after injection and the subsequent more rapid contact of the drug particles with the body fluids. Oftentimes more prolonged drug action is desired to reduce the necessity of frequently repeated injections. These long-acting types of injections are commonly referred to as repository or "depot" types of preparations.

The solutions and suspensions of drugs intended for injection are prepared in the same general manner as was discussed previously in this text for oral solutions (Chapter 6) and oral suspensions (Chapter 7), with the following differences:

1. Solvents or vehicles used must meet special purity and other standards assuring their safety by injection.
2. The use of added substances, as buffers, stabilizers, and antimicrobial preservatives, fall under specific guidelines of use and are restricted in certain parenteral products. The use of coloring agents is strictly prohibited.
3. Parenteral products are always sterilized and meet sterility standards and must be pyrogen-free.
4. Parenteral solutions must meet compendial standards for particulate matter.
5. Parenteral products must be prepared in environmentally controlled areas, under strict sanitation standards, and by personnel specially trained and clothed to maintain the sanitation standards.
6. Parenteral products are packaged in special hermetic containers of specific and high quality. Special quality control procedures are utilized to ensure their hermetic seal and sterile condition.
7. Each container of an injection is filled to a volume in slight excess of the labeled "size" or volume to be withdrawn. This overfill permits the ease of withdrawal and administration of the labeled volumes.
8. There are restrictions over the volume of injection permitted in multiple-dose containers and also a limitation over the types of containers (single-dose or multiple-dose) which may be used for certain injections.
9. Specific labeling regulations apply to injections.
10. Sterile powders intended for solution or suspension immediately prior to injection are frequently packaged as *lyophilized* or freeze-dried powders to permit ease of solution or suspension upon the addition of the solvent or vehicle.

Solvents and Vehicles for Injections

The most frequently used solvent in the large-scale manufacturer of injections is *Water for Injection, USP.* This water is purified by distillation or by reverse osmosis and meets the same standards for the presence of total solids as does *Purified Water, USP,* not more than 1 mg per 100 mL Water for Injection, USP and may not contain added substances. Although water for injection is not required to be sterile, it must be pyrogen-free. The water is intended to be used in the manufacture of injectable products which are to be sterilized after their preparation. Water for injection should be stored in tight containers at temperatures below or above the range in which microbial growth occurs. Water for injection is intended to be used within 24 hours following its collection. Naturally, the water should be collected in sterile and pyrogen-free containers. The containers are usually glass or glass-lined.

Sterile Water for Injection, USP is water for injection which has been sterilized and packaged in single-dose containers of not greater than 1-liter size. As water for injection, it must be pyrogen-free and may not contain an antimicrobial agent or other added substance. This water may contain a slightly greater amount of total solids than water for injection due to the leaching of solids from the glass-lined tanks during the sterilization process. This water is intended to be used as a solvent, vehicle or diluent for already-sterilized and packaged injectable medications. The one-liter bottles cannot be administered intravenously because they have no tonicity. Thus, they are used for reconstitution of multiple antibiotics. In use, the water is aseptically added to the vial of medication to prepare the desired injection. For instance, a suitable injection may be prepared from the dry powder, Sterile Ampicillin Sodium, USP, by the aseptic addition of sterile water for injection.

Bacteriostatic Water for Injection, USP is sterile water for injection containing one or more suitable antimicrobial agents. It is packaged in prefilled syringes or in vials containing not more than 30 mL of the water. The container label must state the name and proportion of the antimicrobial agent(s) present. The water is employed as a sterile vehicle in the preparation of small volumes of injectable preparations. The presence of the bacteriostatic agent gives the flexibility for multiple-dose vials. If the first person to withdraw medication inadvertently contaminates the vial contents, the preservative will destroy the microorganism. Because of the presence of antimicrobial agents the water must only be used in parenterals that are administered in small volumes. Its use in parenterals administered in large volume is restricted due to the excessive and perhaps toxic amounts of the antimicrobial agents which would be injected along with the medication. Generally, if volumes of greater than 5 mL of solvent are required, sterile water for injection rather than bacteriostatic water for injection is preferred. In using bacteriostatic water for injection, due regard must also be given to the chemical compatibility of the bacteriostatic agent(s) present with the particular medicinal agent being dissolved or suspended.

Sodium Chloride Injection, USP is a sterile isotonic solution of sodium chloride in Water for Injection. It contains no antimicrobial agents. The sodium and chloride ion contents of the injection are approximately 154 mEq of each per liter. The solution may be used as a sterile vehicle in preparing solutions or suspensions of drugs for parenteral administration.

Bacteriostatic Sodium Chloride Injection, USP is a sterile isotonic solution of sodium chloride in Water for Injection. It contains one or more suitable antimicrobial agents which must be specified on the labeling. Sodium chloride is present at 0.9% concentration to render the solution isotonic. For the reasons noted previously for bacteriostatic water for injection, this solution may not be packaged in containers greater than 30 mL in size. When this solution is used as a vehicle, care must be exercised to assure the compatibility of the added medicinal agent with the preservative(s) present as well as with the sodium chloride. Further, USP labeling requirements demand that the label state, "Not for Use in Newborns." This new labeling statement was the result of problems encountered with neonates and the toxicity of the bacteriostat, i.e., benzyl alcohol. This toxicity may result from the high cumulative amounts (mg/kg) of benzyl alcohol and the limited detoxification capacity of the neonate liver. This solution has not been reported to cause problems in older infants, children, or adults.

Ringer's Injection, USP is a sterile solution of sodium chloride, potassium chloride, and calcium chloride in water for injection. The three agents are present in concentrations similar to that found in physiologic fluids. The solution is employed as a vehicle for other drugs, or alone as an electrolyte replenisher and fluid extender. *Lactated Ringer's Injection, USP* has different quantities of the same three salts in Ringer's Injection and contains sodium lactate. This injection is a fluid and electrolyte replenisher and a systemic alkalizer.

Nonaqueous Vehicles

Although an aqueous vehicle is generally preferred for an injection, its use may be precluded in a formulation due to the limited water solubility of a medicinal substance or its susceptibility to hydrolysis. When such physical or chemical factors limit the use of a wholly aqueous vehicle, the pharmaceutical formulator must turn to one or more nonaqueous vehicles.

The selected vehicle must be nonirritating, nontoxic in the amounts administered, and nonsensitizing. Like water, it must not exert a pharmacologic activity of its own, nor may it adversely affect the activity of the medicinal agent. In addition, the physical and chemical properties of the solvent or vehicle must be considered, evaluated, and determined to be suitable for the task at hand before it may be employed. Among the many considerations are the solvent's physical and chemical stability at various pH levels, its viscosity, which must be such as to allow ease of injection (syringeability), its fluidity, which must be maintained over a fairly wide temperature range, its boiling point, which should be sufficiently high to permit heat sterilization, its miscibility with body fluids, its low vapor pressure to avoid problems during heat sterilization, and its constant purity or ease of purification and standardization. There is no single solvent that is free of limitations, and thus the cross-consideration and the assessment of each solvent's advantages and disadvantages help the formulator determine the most appropriate solvent for use in a given preparation. Among the nonaqueous solvents presently employed in parenteral products are fixed vegetable oils, glycerin, polyethylene glycols, propylene glycol, alcohol, and a number of lesser used agents as ethyl oleate, isopropyl myristate, and dimethylacetamide. These and other nonaqueous vehicles may be used provided they are safe in the amounts administered and do not interfere with the therapeutic efficacy of the preparation or with its response to prescribed assays and tests.

The USP specifies restrictions on the fixed vegetable oils which may be employed in parenteral products. For one thing, they must remain clear when cooled to 10°C to ensure the stability and clarity of the injectable product upon storage under refrigeration. The oils must not contain mineral oil or paraffin, as these materials are not absorbed by body tissues. The fluidity of a vegetable oil generally depends upon the proportion of unsaturated fatty acids, such as oleic acid, to saturated acids, such as stearic acid. Oils to be employed in injections must meet officially stated requirements of iodine number and saponification number.

Although the toxicities of vegetable oils are generally considered to be relatively low, some patients exhibit allergic reactions to specific oils. Thus, when vegetable oils are employed in parenteral products, the label must state the specific oil present. The most commonly used fixed oils in injections are corn oil, cottonseed oil, peanut oil, and sesame oil. Castor oil and olive oil have been used on occasion.

By the selective employment of solvent or vehicle, a pharmacist can prepare injectable preparations as solutions or suspensions of a medicinal substance in either an aqueous or nonaqueous vehicle. For the most part, oleaginous injections are administered intramuscularly. They must not be administered intravenously as the oil globules will occlude the pulmonary microcirculation. Some examples of official injections employing oil as the vehicle are presented in Table 8–1.

Added Substances

The USP permits the addition of suitable substances to the official preparations intended for injection for the purpose of increasing their stability or usefulness, provided the substances are not interdicted in the individual monographs and are harmless in the amounts administered and do not interfere with the therapeutic efficacy of the preparation or with specified assays and tests. Many of these added substances are antibacterial preservatives, buffers, solubilizers, antioxidants, and other pharmaceutical adjuncts. Agents employed solely for their coloring effect are strictly prohibited in parenteral products.

The USP requires that one or more suitable substances be added to parenteral products that are packaged in multiple-dose containers, to prevent the growth of microorganisms regardless of the method of sterilization employed, unless

Table 8–1. Examples of Some Injections in Oil

Injection	*Oil*	*Category*
Dimercaprol Injection	Peanut	Antidote to arsenic, gold and mercury poisoning
Estradiol Cypionate Injection	Cottonseed	Estrogen
Estradiol Valerate Injection	Sesame or Castor	Estrogen
Fluphenazine Decanoate Injection	Sesame	Antipsychotic
Fluphenazine Enanthate Injection	Sesame	Antipsychotic
Hydroxyprogesterone Caproate Injection	Sesame or Castor	Progestin
Progesterone in Oil Injection	Sesame	Progestin
Testosterone Cypionate Injection	Cottonseed	Androgen
Testosterone Cypionate plus Estradiol Cypionate Injection	Cottonseed	Androgen plus Estrogen
Testosterone Enanthate Injection	Sesame	Androgen

otherwise directed in the individual monograph or unless the injection's active ingredients are themselves bacteriostatic. Such substances are used in concentrations that prevent the growth of or kill microorganisms in the preparations. Because many of the usual preservative agents are toxic when given in excessive amounts or irritating when parenterally administered, special care must be exercised in the selection of the appropriate preservative agents. For the following preservatives, the indicated maximum limits prevail for use in a parenteral product unless otherwise directed: for agents containing mercury and the cationic, surface-active compounds, 0.01%; for agents like chlorobutanol, cresol, and phenol, 0.5%; for sulfur dioxide as an antioxidant, or for an equivalent amount of the sulfite, bisulfite, or metabisulfite of potassium or sodium, 0.2%.

In addition to the stabilizing effect of the additives, the air within an injectable product is frequently replaced with an inert gas, such as nitrogen, to enhance the stability of the product by preventing chemical reaction between the oxygen in the air and the drug.

Methods of Sterilization

The term *sterilization,* as applied to pharmaceutical preparations, means the complete destruction of all living organisms and their spores or their complete removal from the preparation. Five general methods are used for the sterilization of pharmaceutical products:

1. Steam sterilization
2. Dry-heat sterilization
3. Sterilization by filtration
4. Gas sterilization
5. Sterilization by ionizing radiation

The method used in attaining sterility in a pharmaceutical preparation is determined largely by the nature of the preparation and its ingredients. However, regardless of the method used, the resulting product must pass a test for sterility as proof of the effectiveness of the method and the performance of the equipment and the personnel.

Steam Sterilization

Steam sterilization is conducted in an autoclave and employs steam under pressure. It is recognized as the method of choice in most cases where the product is capable of withstanding such treatment (Fig. 8–3).

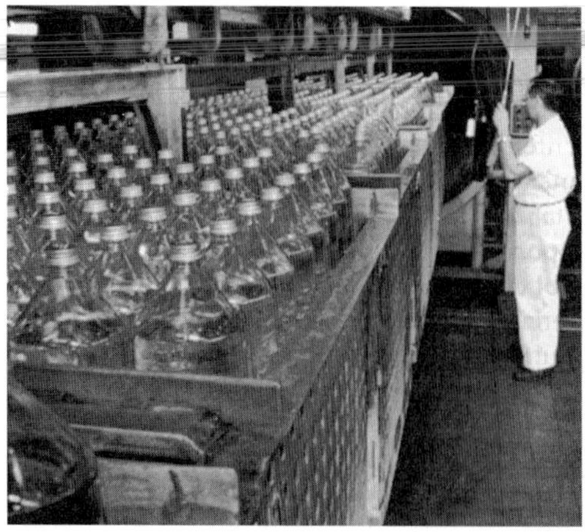

Fig. 8–3. *Autoclaving of intravenous electrolyte solutions. (Courtesy of Abbott Laboratories.)*

Most pharmaceutical products are adversely affected by heat and cannot be heated safely to the temperature required for dry-heat sterilization (about 170°C). When moisture is present, bacteria are coagulated and destroyed at a considerably lower temperature than when a moisture is absent. In fact, bacterial cells with a large percentage of water are generally killed rather easily. Spores, which contain a relatively low percentage of water, are comparatively difficult to destroy. The mechanism of microbial destruction in moist heat is thought to be by denaturation and coagulation of some of the organism's essential protein. It is the presence of the hot moisture within the microbial cell that permits destruction at relatively low temperature. Death by dry heat is thought to be by the dehydration of the microbial cell followed by a slow burning or oxidative process. Because it is not possible to raise the temperature of steam above 100°C under atmospheric conditions, pressure is employed to achieve higher temperatures. It should be recognized that the temperature, not the pressure, is destructive to the microorganisms and that the application of pressure is solely for the purpose of increasing the temperature of the system. Time is another important factor in the destruction of microorganisms by heat. Most modern autoclaves have gauges to indicate to the operator the internal conditions of temperature and pressure and a timing device to permit the desired exposure time for the load. The usual steam pressures, the temperatures obtainable under these pressures, and the approximate length of time required for sterilization after the system reaches the indicated temperatures are as follows:

10 pounds pressure (115.5°C), for 30 minutes
15 pounds pressure (121.5°C), for 20 minutes
20 pounds pressure (126.5°C), for 15 minutes.

As can be seen, the greater the pressure applied, the higher the temperature obtainable and the less the time required for sterilization.

The temperature at which most autoclaves are routinely operated is usually 121°C, as measured at the steam discharge line running from the autoclave. It should be understood that the temperature attained in the chamber of the autoclave must also be reached by the interior of the load being sterilized, and this temperature must be maintained for an adequate time. The penetration time of the moist heat into the load may vary with the nature of the load, and the exposure time must be adjusted to account for this latent period. For example, a solution packaged in a thin-walled 50-mL ampul may reach a temperature of 121°C in from 6 to 8 minutes after that temperature is registered in the steam discharge line, whereas 20 minutes or longer may be required to reach that temperature within a solution packaged in a completely filled thick-walled 1000-mL glass bottle. An estimate of these latent periods must be added to the total time in order to ensure adequate exposure times. Because this sterilization process depends upon the presence of moisture and an elevated temperature, air is removed from the chamber as the sterilization process is begun, because a combination of air and steam yields a lower temperature than does steam alone under the same condition of pressure. For instance, at 15 pounds pressure the temperature of saturated steam is 121.5°C, but a mixture of equal parts of air and steam will reach only about 112°C.

In general, this method of sterilization is applicable to pharmaceutical preparations and materials that can withstand the required temperatures and are penetrated by, but not adversely affected by, moisture. In sterilizing aqueous solutions by this method, the moisture is already present, and all that is required is the elevation of the temperature of the solution for the prescribed period of time. Thus solutions packaged in sealed containers, as ampuls, are readily sterilized by this method. The method is also applicable to bulk solutions, glassware, surgical dressings, and instruments. It is not useful in the sterilization of oils, fats, oleaginous preparations, and other preparations not penetrated by the moisture or the sterilization of exposed powders that may be damaged by the condensed moisture.

Dry-Heat Sterilization

Dry-heat sterilization is usually carried out in sterilizing ovens specifically designed for this purpose. The ovens may be heated either by gas or electricity and are generally thermostatically controlled.

Because dry heat is less effective in killing microorganisms than is moist heat, higher temperatures and longer periods of exposure are required. These must be determined individually for each product with consideration to the size and type of product and the container and its heat distribution characteristics. In general, individual units to be sterilized should be as small as possible, and the sterilizer should be loaded in such a manner as to permit free circulation of heated air throughout the chamber. Dry-heat sterilization is usually conducted at temperatures of 160° to 170°C for periods of not less than 2 hours. Higher temperatures permit shorter exposure times for a given article; conversely, lower temperatures require longer exposure times. For example, if a particular chemical agent melts or decomposes at 170°C, but is unaffected at 140°C, the lower temperature would be employed in its sterilization, and the exposure time would be increased over that required to sterilize another chemical that may be safely heated to 170°C.

Dry-heat sterilization is generally employed for substances that are not effectively sterilized by moist heat. Such substances include fixed oils, glycerin, various petroleum products such as petrolatum, liquid petrolatum (mineral oil), and paraffin and various heat-stable powders such as zinc oxide. Dry-heat sterilization is also an effective method for the sterilization of glassware and surgical instruments. Dry-heat sterilization is the method of choice when dry apparatus or dry containers are required, as in the handling of packaging of dry chemicals or nonaqueous solutions.

Sterilization by Filtration

Sterilization by filtration, which depends upon the physical removal of microorganisms by ad-

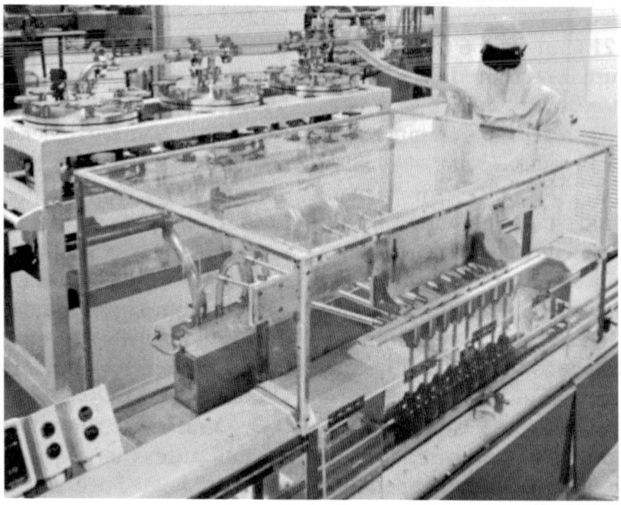

Fig. 8–4. *Sterilization by filtration. An eight-head bottle-filling machine using three large sterilizing filters for sterile filling of bottles in large scale pharmaceutical production. (Courtesy of Millipore Corporation.)*

sorption on the filter medium or by a sieving mechanism, is used for the sterilization of heat-sensitive solutions. Medicinal preparations sterilized by this method are required to undergo severe validation and monitoring since the effectiveness of the filtered product can be greatly influenced by the microbial load in the solution being filtered (Fig. 8–4).

Commercially available filters are produced with a variety of pore-size specifications. It would be well to mention briefly one type of these modern filters, the Millipore filters (Fig. 8–5). Millipore filters are thin plastic membranes

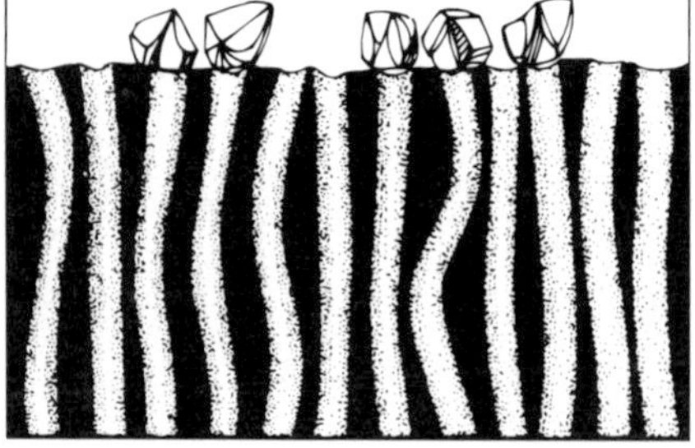

Fig. 8–5. *Membrane filters act as microporous screens that retain all particles and microorganisms larger than the rated pore size on their surface. (Courtesy of Millipore Corporation.)*

of cellulosic esters with millions of pores per square inch of filter surface. The pores are made to be extremely uniform in size and occupy approximately 80% of the filter membrane's volume, the remaining 20% being the solid filter material. This high degree of porosity permits flow rates much in excess of other filters having the same particle-retention capability. Millipore filters are made from a variety of polymers to provide membrane characteristics required for the filtration of almost any liquid or gas system. Also, the filters are made of various pore sizes to meet the selective filtration requirements of the operator. They are available in pore sizes from 14 to 0.025 μm. For comparative purposes, the period that ended the last sentence is approximately 500 μm in size. The size of the smallest particle visible to the naked eye is about 40 μm, a red blood cell is about 6.5 μm, the smallest bacteria, about 0.2 μm, and a polio virus, about 0.025 μm.

Although the pore size of a bacterial filter is of prime importance in the removal of microorganisms from a liquid, there are other factors such as the electrical charge on the filter and that of the microorganism, the pH of the solution, the temperature, and the pressure or vacuum applied to the system.

The major advantages of bacterial filtration include its speed in the filtration of small quantities of solution, its ability to sterilize effectively ther-

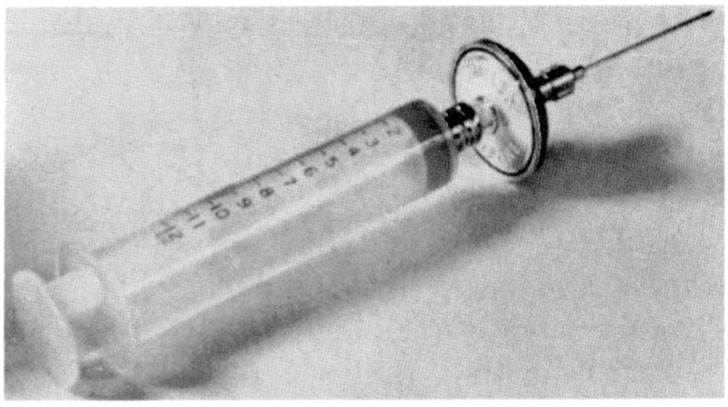

Fig. 8–6. *Luer-Lock syringe adapted with a MILLEX Filter Unit and hypodermic needle. (Courtesy of Millipore Corporation.)*

molabile materials, the relatively inexpensive equipment required, and the complete removal of living and dead microorganisms as well as other particulate matter from the solution. One serious disadvantage to the use of bacterial filters is the possibility of a flaw in the construction of the filter and thus some uncertainty of sterility, a circumstance not true of methods involving dry- or moist-heat sterilization in which the procedures are just about guaranteed to give effective sterilization. Also, filtration of large volumes of liquids would require more time, particularly if the liquid were viscous, than would, say, steam sterilization. In essence, the bacterial filters are useful when heat cannot be used and also for small volumes of liquids.

Bacterial filters may be used conveniently and economically in the community pharmacy to filter extemporaneously prepared solutions (as ophthalmic solutions) that are required to be sterile (Figs. 8–6 and 8–7). Further, membrane filters are the only method of bacterial sterilization used widely by hospital pharmacists.

To date, there has been limited information about drug adsorption to membrane filters. Several recent studies, however, have demonstrated that membrane filters have the capacity to remove drug from solution. For example, 0.22 micron filters reduce the in vitro antimicrobial activity of amphotericin B (a colloidal suspension), while filtration of the amphotericin B through 0.85 and 0.45 micron filters did not. Butler et al. demonstrated that the potency of drugs administered intravenously and in small doses could be significantly reduced during in-line filtration with a filter containing a cellulose ester membrane.[4] The pharmaceutical literature indicates that drugs administered in low doses might present the problem of the drug's bonding to the filter. Many filters in clinical use are nitrate or acetate esters of cellulose. These compounds are polar and have residual hydroxyl groups that might become involved with drug adsorption interactions. Hydrophobic interactions between hydrocarbon portions of drug molecules being filtered and linear cellulose molecules of filters are also thought to be involved in drug adsorption.

In general, current information suggests that little or no adsorption takes place with membrane filters. However, it is recommended that minute dosages of drugs (i.e., <5 mg) should not be filtered until sufficient data are available to demonstrate insignificant adsorption. With respect to amphotericin B, it is perhaps better to avoid any type of clinical filter until further research is performed on this phenomenon.

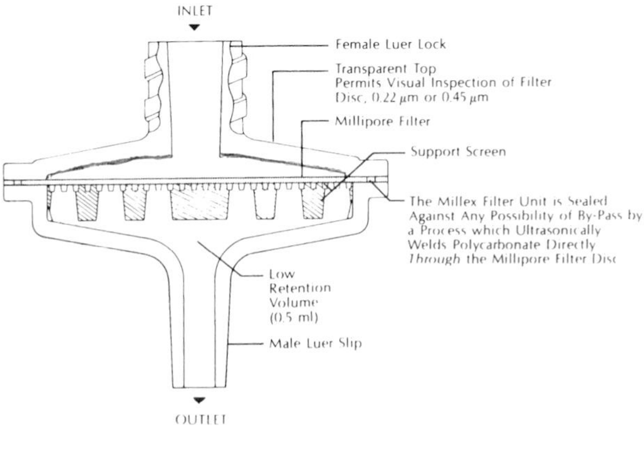

Fig. 8–7. *Cutaway showing composition of the MILLEX filter unit. (Courtesy of Millipore Corporation.)*

Gas Sterilization

Some heat-sensitive and moisture-sensitive materials can be sterilized much better by exposure to ethylene oxide or propylene oxide gas than by other means. These gases are highly flammable when mixed with air but can be employed safely when properly diluted with an inert gas such as carbon dioxide or a suitable fluorinated hydrocarbon. Such mixtures are commercially available.

Sterilization by this process requires specialized equipment resembling autoclaves, and many combination steam autoclaves-ethylene oxide sterilizers are commercially available. Greater precautions are required for this method of sterilization than for some of the others, because the variables—for instance, time, temperature, gas concentration, and humidity—are not as firmly quantitated as those of dry-heat and steam sterilization. In general, sterilization with gas is enhanced, and the exposure time required is reduced, by increasing the relative humidity of the system (to about 60%) and by increasing the exposure temperature (to between 50 and 60°C). If the material being sterilized cannot tolerate either the moisture or the elevated temperature, exposure time will have to be increased. Generally, sterilization with ethylene oxide gas requires from 4 to 16 hours of exposure. Ethylene oxide is thought to function as a sterilizing agent by its interference with the metabolism of the bacterial cell.

The great penetrating qualities of ethylene oxide gas make it a useful sterilizing agent in certain special applications, as in the sterilization of medical and surgical supplies and appliances such as catheters, needles, and plastic disposable syringes in their final plastic packaging just prior to shipment. The gas is also used to sterilize certain heat-labile enzyme preparations, certain antibiotics, and other drugs, with tests being performed to assure of the absence of chemical reaction or other deleterious effects on the drug substance.

Sterilization by Ionizing Radiation

Techniques are available for the sterilization of some types of pharmaceuticals by gamma rays and by cathode rays, but the application of such techniques is limited because of the highly specialized equipment required and the effects of irradiation on products and their containers.

The exact mechanism by which irradiation sterilizes a drug or preparation is still subject to investigation. One of the proposed theories involves an alteration of the chemicals within or supporting the microorganism to form deleterious new chemicals capable of destroying the cell. Another theory proposes that vital structures of the cell, such as the chromosomal nucleoprotein, are disoriented or destroyed. It is probably a combination of irradiation effects that causes the cellular destruction, which is complete and irreversible.

Validation of Sterility

Regardless of the method of sterilization employed, pharmaceutical preparations required to be sterile must undergo sterility tests to confirm the absence of microorganisms. The USP contains monographs and standards for biologic indicators of a sterilization process. A *biologic indicator* is a characterized preparation of specific microorganisms resistant to a particular sterilization process. They may be utilized to monitor a sterilization cycle and/or to periodically revalidate the process. Biologic indicators are generally of two main forms. In one, spores are added to a carrier, as a strip of filter paper, packaged to maintain physical integrity while allowing the sterilization effect. In the other, the spores are added to representative units of the product being sterilized, with sterilization assessed based on these samples. In steam sterilization, spores of suitable strains of *Bacillus stearothermophilus* are commonly employed because of their resistance to this mode of sterilization. In dry-heat, or ethylene oxide sterilization, spores of a subspecies of *Bacillus subtilis* are commonly used. In sterilization by ionizing radiation, spores of suitable strains of *Bacillus pumilus* have been utilized.

The effectiveness of thermal sterilization procedures has been quantified through the determination and calculation of *F value* to express the time of thermal death. *Thermal death time* is defined as the time required to kill a particular organism under specified conditions. The F_0, at a particular temperature *other than 121 °C,* is the time, in minutes, required to provide the lethality equivalent to that provided at 121° for a stated time.

Although heat distribution in an autoclave chamber is usually rapid with 121°C obtained nearly instantaneously throughout the autoclave, the product being sterilized may not achieve identical conditions due to a variety of factors of heat transfer, including the thermal conductivity of the packaging components, the viscosity and density of the product, container proximity, passage of steam around containers and other variables. F values may be computed from biologic data derived from the rate of destruction of known numbers of microorganisms, as shown in the following equation:*

$$F_0 = D_{121}(\text{Log } A - \text{Log } B)$$

where

D_{121} = the time required for a one-log reduction in the microbial population exposed to a temperature of 121°C
A = The initial microbial population
B = the number of microorganisms that survive after a defined heating time.

Pyrogens and Pyrogen Testing

As indicated earlier, *pyrogens* are fever-producing organic substances arising from microbial contamination and responsible for many of the febrile reactions which occur in patients following injection. The causative material is thought to be a lipopolysaccharide from the outer cell wall of the bacteria and endotoxins. Because the material is thermostable, it may remain in water even after sterilization by autoclaving or by bacterial filtration.

Manufacturers of water for injection may employ any suitable method for the removal of pyrogens from their product. Because pyrogens are organic substances, one of the more common means of facilitating their removal is by oxidizing them to easily eliminated gases or to nonvolatile solids, both of which are easily separated from water by fractional distillation. Potassium permanganate is usually employed as the oxidizing agent, with its efficiency being increased by the addition of a small amount of barium hydroxide serving to impart alkalinity to the solution and to make nonvolatile barium salts of any acidic compounds that may be present. These two reagents are added to water that has previously been distilled several times, and the distillation process is repeated with the chemical-free distillate being collected under strict aseptic conditions. When properly conducted, this method results in a highly purified, sterile, and pyrogen-free water. However, in each instance the official pyrogen test must be performed for assurance of the absence of these fever-producing materials.

PYROGEN TEST. The USP Pyrogen Test utilizes healthy rabbits that have been properly maintained in terms of environment and diet prior to performance of the test. Normal, or "control" temperatures are taken for each animal to be used in the test. These temperatures are used as the base for the determination of any temperature increase resulting from the injection of a test solution. In a given test, rabbits are used whose temperatures do not differ by more than one degree from each other and whose body temperatures are considered to be unelevated. A synopsis of the procedure of the test is as follows.

> Render the syringes, needles, and glassware free from pyrogens by heating at 250°C for not less than 30 minutes or by other suitable method. Warm the product to be tested to 37°C ± 2°C.
> Inject into an ear vein of each of three rabbits 10 mL of the product per kg of body weight, completing each injection within 10 minutes after the start of administration. Record the temperature at 30-minute intervals between 1 and 3 hours subsequent to the injection.
> If no rabbit shows an individual rise in temperature of 0.5° or more above its respective control temperature, the product meets the requirements for the absence of pyrogens. If any rabbit shows an individual temperature rise of 0.5° or more, continue the test using five other rabbits. If not more than three of the eight rabbits show individual rises in temperature of 0.5° or more and if the sum of the eight individual maximum temperature rises does not exceed 3.3°, the material under examination meets the requirements for the absence of pyrogens.

In recent years, it has been shown that an extract from the blood cells of the horseshoe crab *(Limulus polyphemus)* contains an enzyme and protein system that coagulates in the presence of low levels of lipopolysaccharides. This discovery has led to the development of the *Limulus* amebocyte lysate (LAL) test for the presence of bacterial endotoxins. The USP Bacterial Endotoxins Test utilizes LAL and is considered generally more sensitive to endotoxin than the rabbit test. The FDA has endorsed the test as a replacement for the rabbit test.

The Industrial Preparation of Parenteral Products

Once the formulation for a particular parenteral product is determined, including the selection of the proper solvents or vehicles and additives, the production pharmacist must follow rigid aseptic procedures in preparing the injecta-

* Akers, M.J., Attia, I.A., and Avis, K.E.: Understanding and Utilizing F_0 Values. *Pharm. Tech., 11*:44–48, 1987.

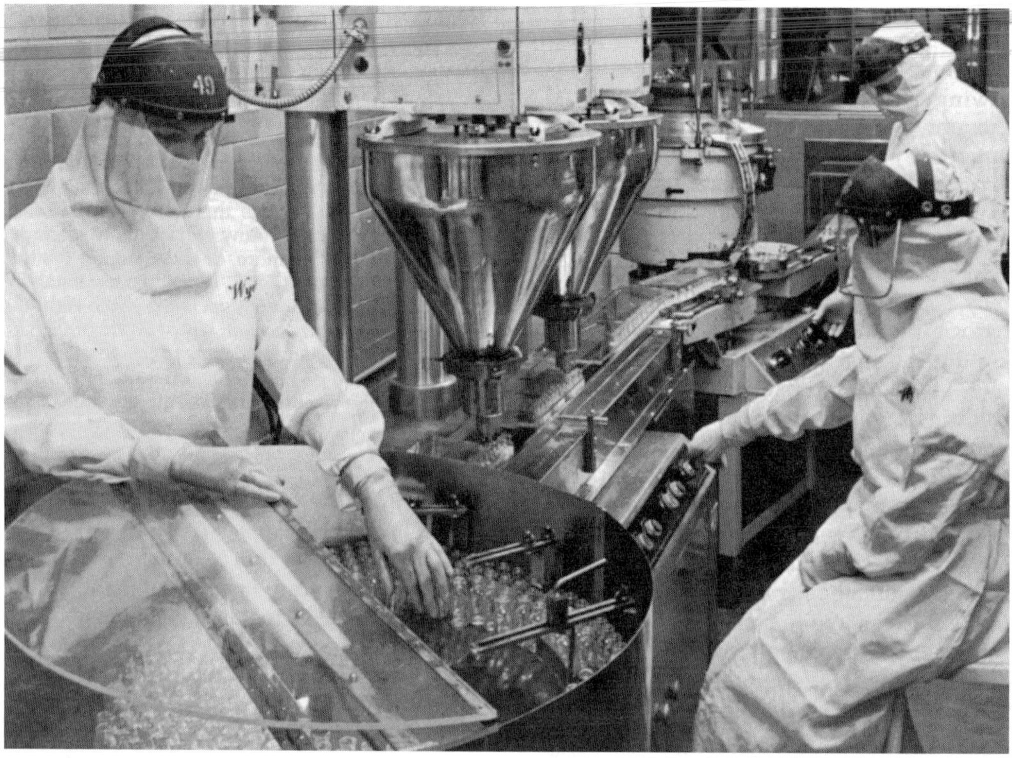

Fig. 8–8. *Sterile filling of vials. (Courtesy of Wyeth Laboratories.)*

ble products. In most manufacturing plants the area in which parenteral products are made is maintained bacteria-free through the use of ultraviolet lights, a filtered air supply, sterile manufacturing equipment, such as flasks, connecting tubes, and filters, and sterilized work clothing worn by the personnel in the area (Fig. 8–8).

In the preparation of parenteral solutions, the required ingredients are dissolved according to good pharmaceutical practice either in water for injection, in one of the alternate solvents, or in a combination of solvents. The solutions are then usually filtered until sparkling clear through a membrane-type filter. After filtration, the solution is transferred as rapidly as possible and with the least possible exposure into the final containers. The product is then sterilized, preferably by autoclaving, and samples of the finished product are tested for sterility and pyrogens. In instances in which sterilization by autoclaving is impractical due to the nature of the ingredients, the individual components of the preparation that are heat or moisture labile may be sterilized by other appropriate means and added aseptically to the sterilized solvent or to a sterile solution of all of the other components sterilizable by autoclaving.

Suspensions of drugs intended for parenteral use may be prepared by reducing the drug to a very fine powder with a ball mill, micronizer, colloid mill, or other appropriate equipment and then suspending the material in a liquid in which it is insoluble. It is frequently necessary to sterilize separately the individual components of a suspension before combining them, as frequently the integrity of a suspension is destroyed by autoclaving. Autoclaving of a parenteral suspension may alter the viscosity of the product, thereby affecting the suspending ability of the vehicle, or change the particle size of the suspended particles, thereby altering both the pharmaceutic and the therapeutic characteristics of the preparation. If a suspension remains unaltered by autoclaving, this method is generally employed to sterilize the final product. Because parenterally administered emulsions, which are dispersions or suspensions of a liquid throughout another liquid, are generally destroyed by

Colligative Properties of Drugs

Drug molecules have properties that are often divided into additive, constitutive, or colligative.

Additive properties depend upon the total contribution of the atoms in the molecule, or upon the sum of the properties of the constituents of the solution. An example is molecular weight.

Constitutive properties depend upon the arrangement and, to a lesser extent, the number and kind of atoms in a molecule. Examples of this are the refraction of light, electrical properties, and surface and interfacial properties.

Colligative properties depend primarily upon the number of particles in solution. Example properties include changes in vapor pressure, boiling point, freezing point and osmotic pressure. These values should be approximately equal for equimolal concentrations of drugs.

LOWERING OF VAPOR PRESSURE

A vapor, when in equilibrium with its pure liquid at a constant temperature, will exert a certain pressure known as the *vapor pressure.* When a solute is added to the pure liquid, it will alter the tendency of the molecules to escape the original liquid. In an ideal solution, or one that is very dilute, the partial vapor pressure of one component (p_1) is proportional to the mole fraction of molecules (N_1) of that component in the mixture:

$$p_1 = N_1 p_1^\circ$$

where p_1° is the vapor pressure of the pure component.

EXAMPLE 1

What is the partial vapor pressure of a solution containing 50 g dextrose in 1000 mL of water (the vapor pressure of water is given as 23.76 mm Hg).

1. (50 g dextrose)/(MW of 180) = 0.28 moles of dextrose
2. (1000 g water)/MW of 18) = 55.56 moles of water
3. 0.28 + 55.56 = 55.84 total moles
4. (55.56)/(55.84) = 0.995 mole fraction of water
5. p_1 = (0.995)(23.76 mm Hg) = 23.64 mm Hg

The vapor pressure of the solution is 23.64 mm Hg. The decrease in vapor pressure by the addition of the 50 g dextrose is 23.76 − 23.64 = 0.12 mm Hg.

INCREASE IN BOILING POINT

The *boiling point* of a liquid is that temperature when the vapor pressure of the liquid comes into equilibrium with the atmospheric pressure. The vapor pressure is reduced when a nonvolatile solute is added to a solvent, so the solution must be heated to a higher temperature to reestablish the equilibrium—hence, an increase in the boiling point. This is described in the following equation:

$$\Delta T_b = k_b m$$

where ΔT_b is the change in boiling point,
k_b is the molal elevation constant of water, and
m is the molality of the solute.

EXAMPLE 2

What is the boiling point elevation of a solution containing 50 g dextrose in 1000 mL of water (the molal elevation constant of water is 0.51).

1. (50 g dextrose)/(MW of 180) = 0.28 moles of dextrose in 1000 mL of water or 0.28 molal solution.
2. ΔT_b = (0.51) (0.28) = 0.143°C.

Colligative Properties of Drugs (Continued)

DECREASE IN FREEZING POINT

The *freezing point* of a pure liquid is the temperature at which the solid and liquid phases are in equilibrium at 1 atmosphere pressure. The freezing point of a solution is that temperature at which the solid phase of pure solvent and the liquid phase of solution are in equilibrium at 1 atmosphere pressure. When a solute is added to a solvent, the decrease in freezing point is proportional to the concentration of the solute. The relationship is described by the following equation:

$$\Delta T_f = k_f m$$

where ΔT_f is the change in freezing point,
k_f is the molal freezing point depression constant of water, and
m is the molality of the solute.

EXAMPLE 3

What is the decrease in freezing point of a solution containing 50 g dextrose in 1000 mL of water (the molal elevation constant of water is −1.86°C).

1. (50 g dextrose)/(MW of 180) = 0.28 moles of dextrose in 1000 mL of water or 0.28 molal solution.
2. $\Delta T_f = (-1.86)\ (0.28) = -0.52°C$.

OSMOTIC PRESSURE

The pressure that must be applied to a more concentrated solution just to prevent the flow of pure solvent into the solution separated by a semipermeable membrane is called the *osmotic pressure.* This relationship can be expressed as follows:

$$PV = nRT$$

where P is the pressure (atm)
V is the volume (L)
n is number of moles of solute
R is the gas constant (0.082 L-atm/mole deg), and
T is the absolute temperature in °C.

EXAMPLE 4

What is the osmotic pressure of 50 g dextrose in 1000 mL of water at room temperature (25°C)?

1. (50 g dextrose)/(MW of 180) = 0.28 moles of dextrose
2. 273°C + 25°C = 298°C
3. Volume will be ≈1 L
4. $P = [(0.28)(0.082)(298)]/(1) = 6.84$ atm

Deviations from reality in the above ideal examples of colligative properties are explained by the use of the Van't Hoff term, i. This "i" term considers that electrolytes exert more pressure than nonelectrolytes and is related to the number of ionic species present. These deviations may be caused by ionic interaction, degree of dissociation of weak electrolytes, or associations of nonelectrolytes.

autoclaving, an alternate method of sterilization must be employed for this type of injectable.

Some injections are packaged as dry solids rather than in conjunction with a solvent or vehicle due to the instability of the therapeutic agent in the presence of the liquid component. These dry powdered drugs are packaged as the sterilized powder in the final containers to be reconstituted with the proper liquid prior to use, generally to form a solution or less frequently a suspension. The method of sterilization of the powder may be dry heat or another method that is appropriate for the particular drug involved. Examples of sterile drugs prepared and packaged *without* the presence of pharmaceutical additives as buffers, preservatives, stabilizers, tonicity agents, and other substances include:

Sterile Ampicillin Sodium
Sterile Ceftizoxime Sodium
Sterile Ceftazidime Sodium
Sterile Cefuroxime Sodium
Sterile Kanamycin Sulfate
Sterile Nafcillin Sodium
Sterile Penicillin G Benzathine
Sterile Streptomycin Sulfate
Sterile Tobramycin Sulfate

Antibiotics are prepared industrially in large fermentation tanks (Fig. 8–9).

Those sterile drugs formulated *with* pharmaceutical additives and intended to be reconstituted prior to injection include the following:

Cephradine for Injection
Cyclophosphamide for Injection
Dactinomycin for Injection
Erythromycin Lactobionate for Injection
Hyaluronidase for Injection
Hydrocortisone Sodium Succinate for Injection
Mitomycin for Injection
Nafcillin Sodium for Injection
Oxytetracycline Hydrochloride for Injection
Penicillin G Potassium for Injection
Vinblastine Sulfate for Injection

In certain instances, a liquid is packaged along with the dry powder for use at the time of reconstitution (Fig. 8–10). This liquid is sterile and may contain some of the desired pharmaceutical additives as the buffering agents. More frequently, the solvent or vehicle is not provided along with the dry product, but the labeling on the injection generally lists suitable solvents. Sodium chloride injection or sterile water for injection are perhaps the most frequently employed solvents used to reconstitute dry-packaged injections. The dry powders are packaged in containers large enough to permit proper shaking with the liquid component when the latter is aseptically injected through the container's rubber closure during its reconstitution. To facilitate the

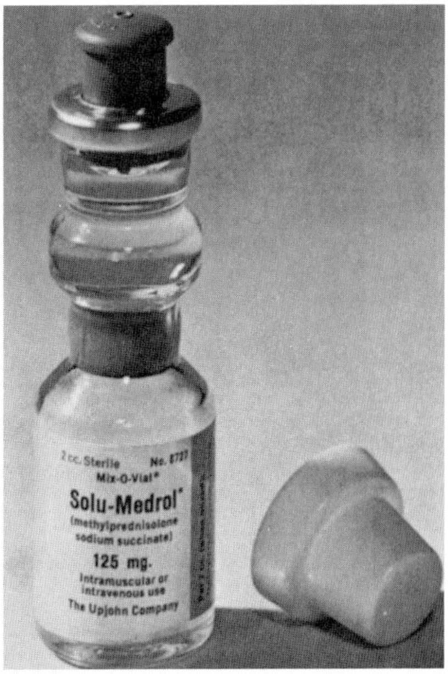

Fig. 8–10. *The Mix-O-Vial shown above is a combination vial containing dry ingredients in the bottom compartment and a liquid diluent in the top compartment, separated by a specially formulated center seal. The bottom compartment can either be liquid filled, frozen and dried to make a lyophilized product, or it may be powder filled. The top diluent contains a preservative and may or may not contain one or more active ingredients.*

To use the vial, the dust cover is removed (as shown above), pressure is applied with the thumb to the top plunger which dislodges the center seal and the vial is shaken until the solution is effected. The top of the plunger is then swabbed with a disinfectant; the syringe needle inserted through the target circle on the plunger and the contents of the vial withdrawn into the syringe.

The Mix-O-Vial offers stability of product (until it is activated), convenience, fast operation and safety as regards the right drug with the proper diluent in the correct proportions. (Courtesy of The Upjohn Company.)

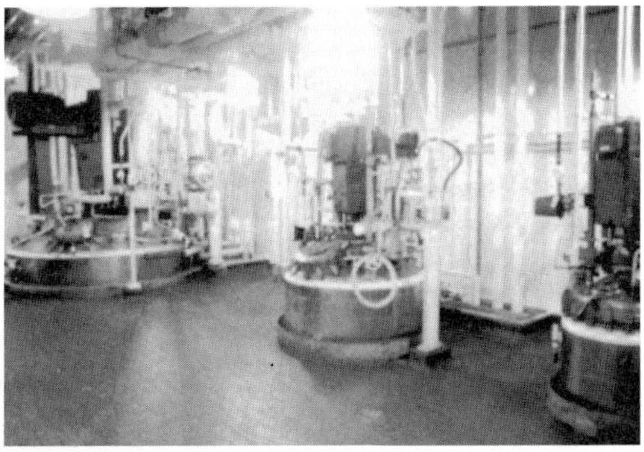

Fig. 8–9. *Fermentation tank in the preparation of antibiotics. (Courtesy of Schering-Plough.)*

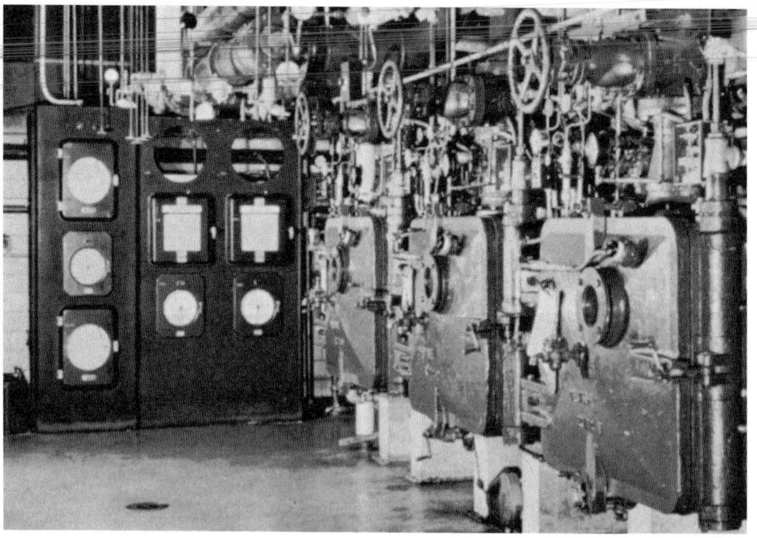

Fig. 8–11. *Antibiotic lyophilizers. (Courtesy of Abbott Laboratories.)*

dissolving process, the dry powder is prevented from caking upon standing by the appropriate means including its preparation by lyophilization (Fig. 8–11). Powders so treated form a honeycomb, lattice structure that is rapidly penetrated by the liquid, and solution is rapidly effected because of the large surface area of powder exposed.

Several manufacturers now ship to the hospital pharmacy reconstituted intravenous antibiotic solutions, e.g., cefazolin sodium, in the frozen state. When thawed these nonpyrogenic solutions are stable for a finite amount of time, e.g., reconstituted cefazolin is stable for 24 hours at room temperature and for 96 hours refrigerated (5°C). The product is packaged in a small plastic bag for piggy-back use in intravenous administration to the patient.

Packaging, Labeling, and Storage of Injections

Containers for injections, including the closures, must not interact physically or chemically with the preparation so as to alter its strength or efficacy (Fig. 8–12). If the container is made of glass, it must be clear and colorless or of a light amber color to permit the inspection of its contents. The type of glass suitable and preferred for each parenteral preparation is usually stated in the individual monograph. Injections are placed either in single-dose containers or in multiple-dose containers (Figs. 8–13 through 8–15). By definition:

Single-dose Container—A single-dose container is a hermetic container holding a quantity of sterile drug intended for parenteral administration as a single dose, and which when opened cannot be re-sealed with assurance that sterility has been maintained.

Multiple-dose Container—A multiple-dose container is a hermetic container that permits withdrawal of successive portions of the contents without changing the strength, quality, or purity of the remaining portion.

Single-dose containers may be ampuls or single-dose vials. Ampuls (Fig. 8–16) are sealed by fusion of the glass container under aseptic conditions (Figs. 8–17 and 8–18). The glass container is made so as to have a neck portion that may be easily separated from the body of the container without fragmentation of the glass. After opening, the contents of the ampul may be drawn into a syringe with a hypodermic needle. Once opened, the ampul cannot be resealed, and any unused portion may not be retained and used at a later time, since the contents would have questionable sterility. Some injectable products are packaged in pre-filled syringes, with or without special administration devices (Figs. 8–13,

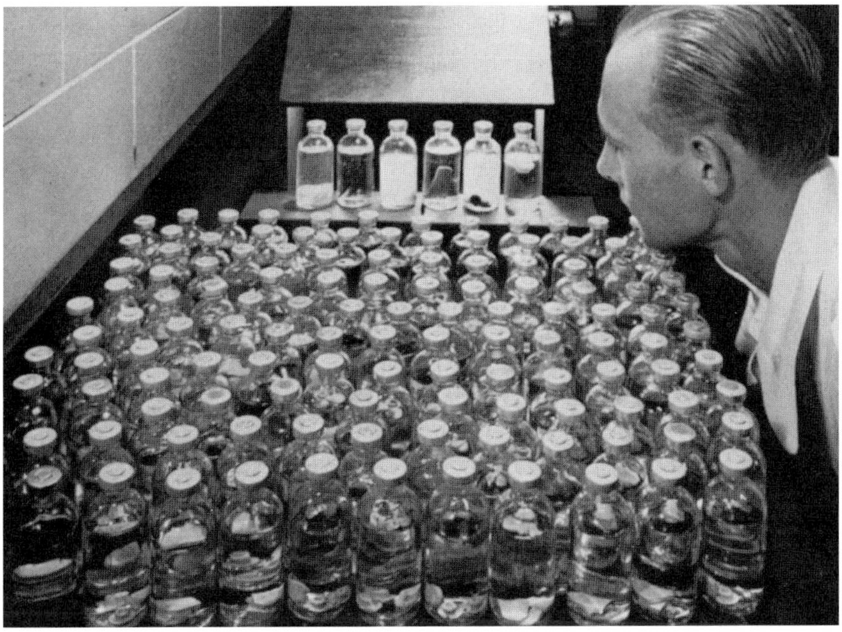

Fig. 8–12. *Testing compatibility of rubber closures with the solution with which they are in contact. (Courtesy of Abbott Laboratories.)*

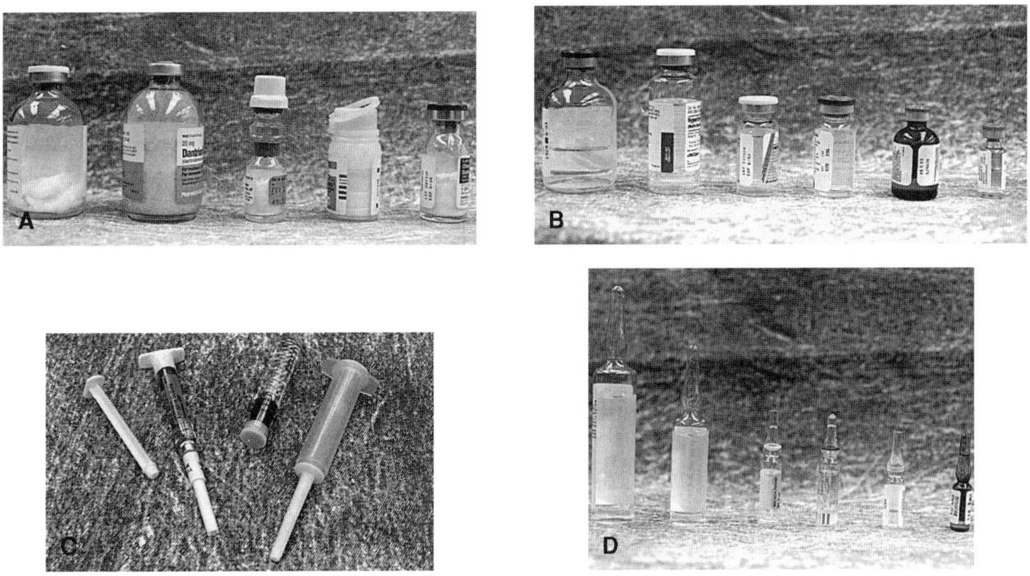

Fig. 8–13. *Examples of packaging of injectable products. A. Multiple-dose vials of suspensions and dry powders. B. Vials for solutions, including one with light-protective glass. C. Unit dose, disposable syringes. D. Various sizes of ampuls. (Courtesy of William B. French, PhD.)*

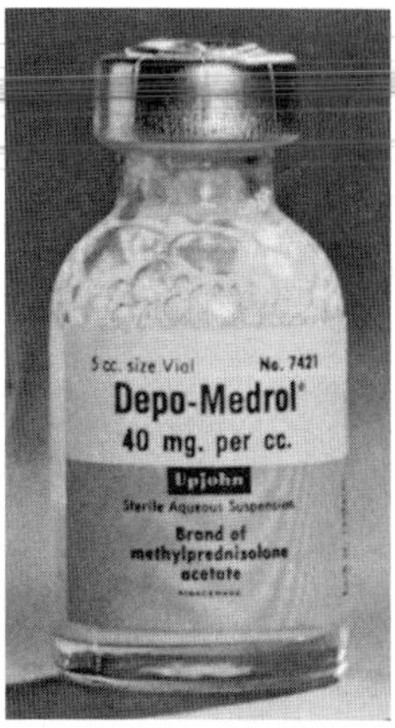

Fig. 8–14. *A typical vial used for sterile injectable products. It is made from Type I (borosilicate) glass. The rubber closure has been specially selected as regards compatibility with the product, desirable physical characteristics, etc. The overseal holds the closure in place and provides a means for ready access to the contents of the vial. (Courtesy of the Upjohn Company.)*

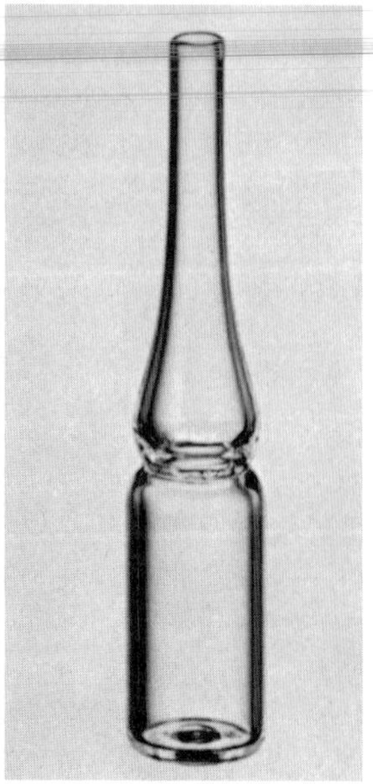

Fig. 8–16. *Ampul, before filling and sealing. (Courtesy of Owens Illinois.)*

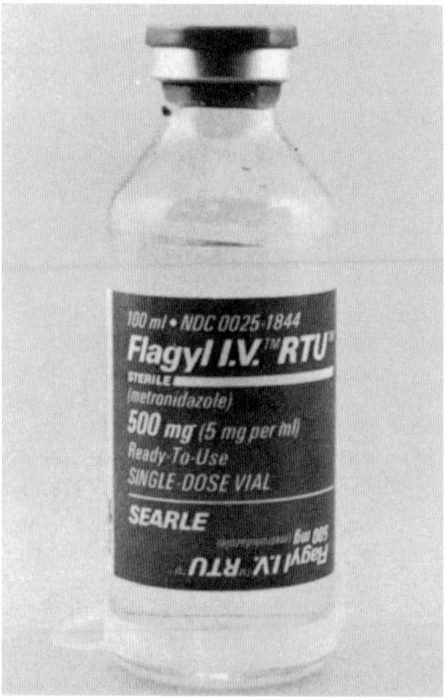

Fig. 8–15. *Example of a 100 mL single-dose vial for intravenous infusion in ready-to-use (RTU) form. (Courtesy of Searle Pharmaceuticals, Inc.)*

8–19, 8–20, 8–21). The types of glass for parenteral product containers have already been pointed out in Chapter 4, and the student should recall that Types I, II, and III are suitable for parenteral products, with Type I being the most resistant to chemical deterioration. The type of glass to be used as the container for a particular injection is indicated in the individual monograph for that preparation.

One of the prime requisites of solutions for parenteral administration is clarity. They should be sparkling clear and free of all particulate matter, that is, all of the mobile, undissolved substances which are unintentionally present. Included are such contaminants as dust, cloth fibers, glass fragments, material leached from the glass or plastic containers or seals, and any other material which may find its way into the product during its manufacture or administration, or develop during storage.

To prevent the entrance of unwanted particles into parenteral products, a number of precautions must be taken during the manufacture, storage, and use of the products. During manufacture, for instance, the parenteral solution is usually final filtered before being placed into the parenteral containers. The containers are carefully selected to be chemically resistant to the solution being added and of the highest available

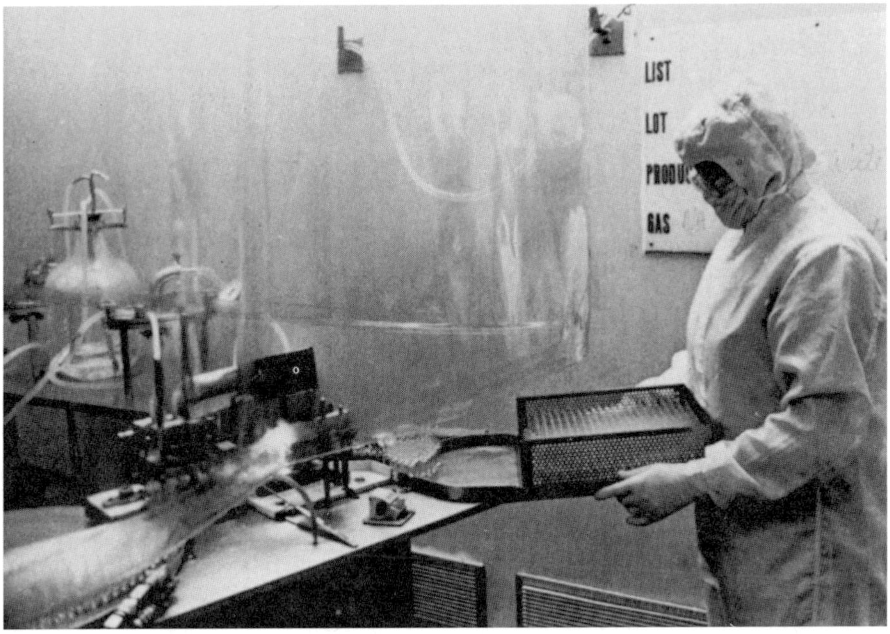

Fig. 8–17. *Ampul filling. (Courtesy of Abbott Laboratories.)*

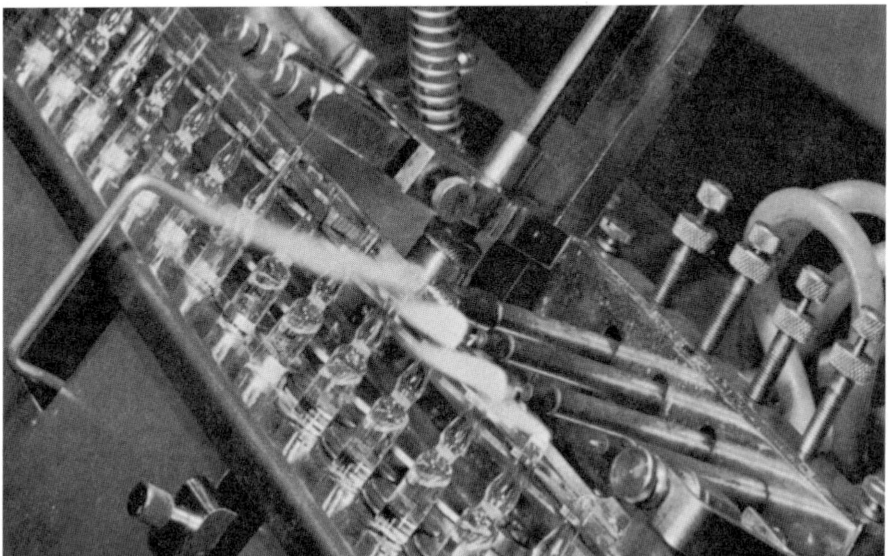

Fig. 8–18. *Ampul sealing. (Courtesy of Abbott Laboratories.)*

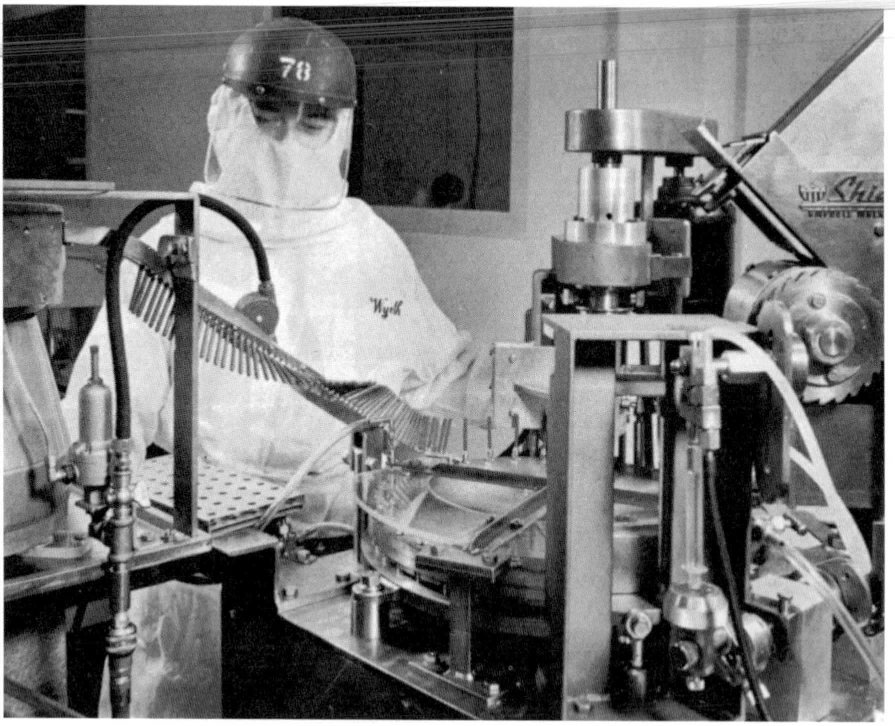

Fig. 8–19. *Operation of a TUBEX filling machine. (Courtesy of Wyeth Laboratories.)*

quality to minimize the chances of container components being leached into the solution. It has been recognized for some time, that some of the particulate matter found in parenteral products is generated from leached material from the glass or plastic containers. Once the container is selected for use, it must be carefully cleaned to be free of all extraneous matter (Fig. 8–22). During container-filling, extreme care must be exercised to prevent the entrance of air-borne dust, lint or other contaminants into the container. The provision of filtered and directed air flow in production areas is useful in reducing the likelihood of contamination. Laminar flow hoods have been developed which allow for the draft-free flow of clean, filtered air over the work area. These

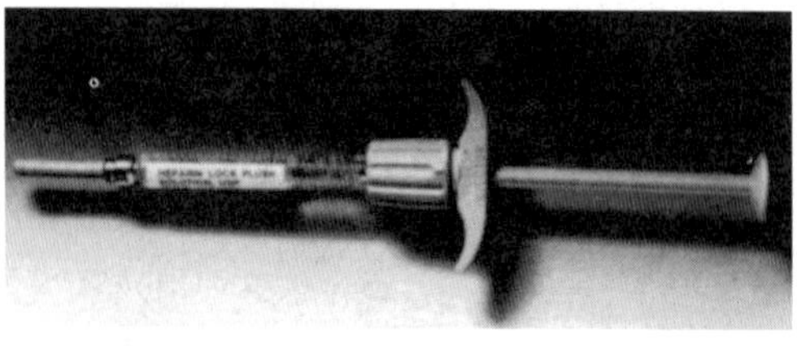

Fig. 8–20. *The Tubex Injector. The ribbed collar and plunger rod securely hold a glass sterile cartridge-needle unit. Each pre-filled unit contains a dose of medication with an attached sterile needle. After administration, the cartridge-needle unit is discarded; the Injector is reusable. (Courtesy of Wyeth-Ayerst Laboratories.)*

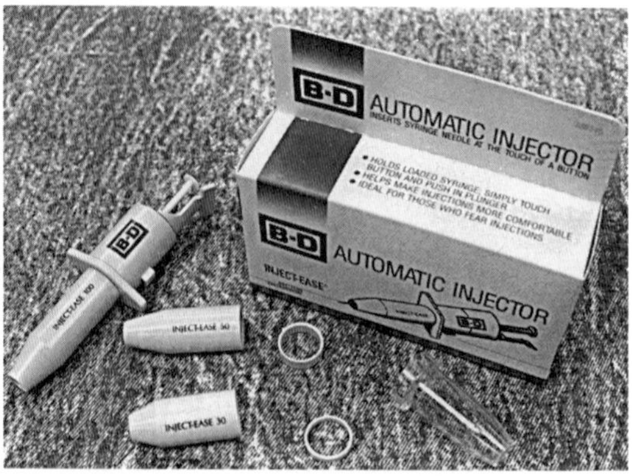

Fig. 8–21. *Inject-Ease automatically inserts the needle of an insulin syringe into the skin when activated. (Courtesy of William B. French, PhD.)*

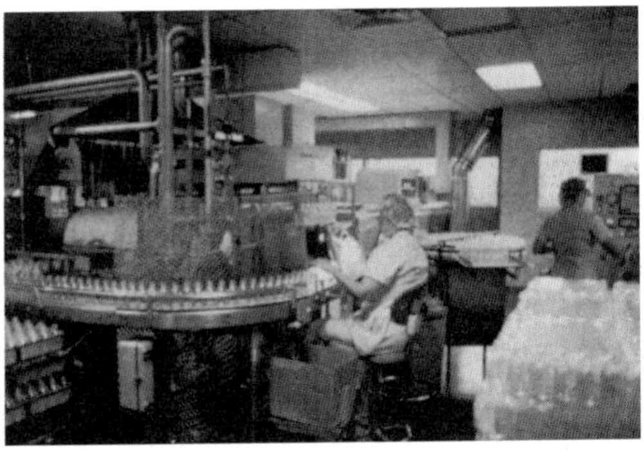

Fig. 8–22. *Production line in the preparation of vials for sterilization and filling. (Courtesy of Schering-Plough.)*

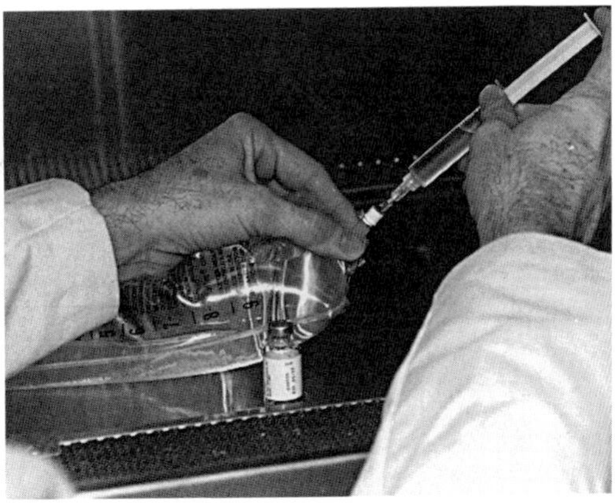

Fig. 8–24. *Pharmacist preparing a parenteral admixture in a laminar flow hood. (Courtesy of William B. French, PhD.)*

hoods are commonly found in the hospital setting for both the manufacture and the incorporation of additives into parenteral and ophthalmic products (Fig. 8–23). The personnel involved in the manufacture of parenterals must be made acutely aware of the importance of cleanliness and aseptic techniques. They are provided uniforms made of monofilament fabrics that do not shed lint. They wear face hoods, caps, gloves, and disposable shoe covers to prevent contamination (Fig. 8–24).

After the containers are filled and hermetically sealed, they are visually (Fig. 8–25) or automatically (Fig. 8–26) inspected for particulate matter. Usually an inspector passes the filled container

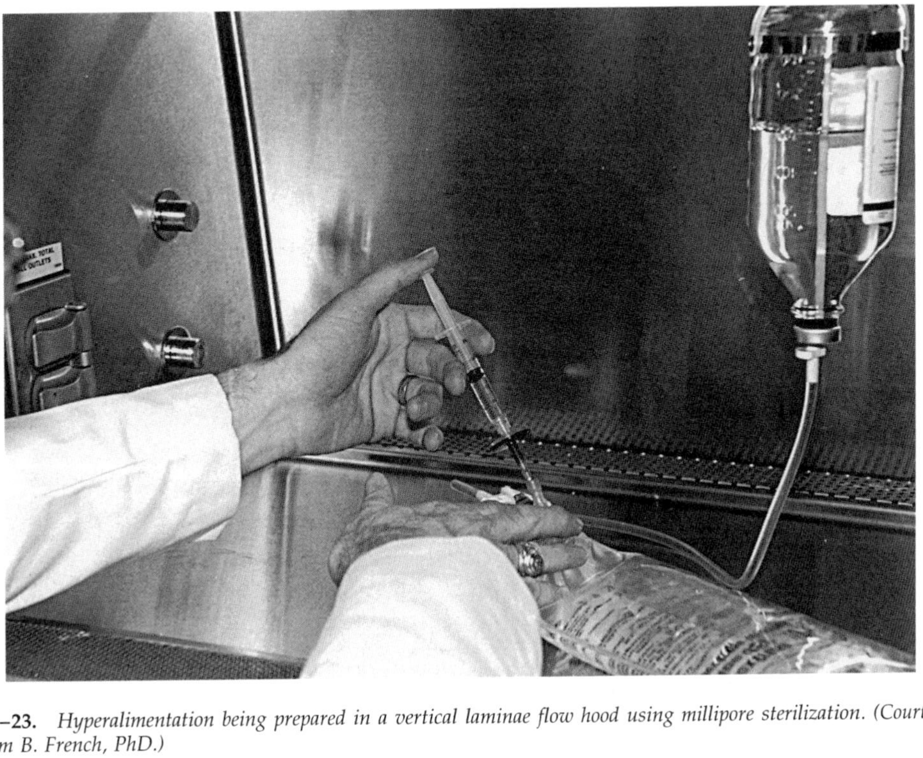

Fig. 8–23. *Hyperalimentation being prepared in a vertical laminae flow hood using millipore sterilization. (Courtesy of William B. French, PhD.)*

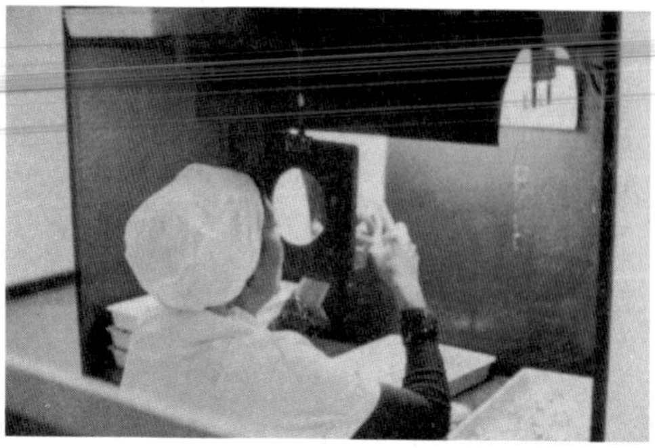

Fig. 8–25. *Industrial inspection of parenteral fluid for particulate matter. (Courtesy of Schering-Plough.)*

past a light source with a black background to observe for mobile particles. Particles of approximately 50 μm in size may be detected in this manner. Reflective particles, such as fragments of glass, may be visualized in smaller size, about 25 μm in size. Other methods are used to detect particulate matter smaller than that which may be detected by the unaided eye including microscopic examinations as well as the use of sophisticated equipment as the Coulter Counter which electronically counts particles present in a sample presented to it. Once past the inspection following production the product may be labeled. Prior to its use, however, the pharmacist should inspect each parenteral solution dispensed for evidence of particulate matter.

Although the total significance of injecting or infusing parenteral solutions containing particulate matter into a patient has not been ascertained, it is apparent that particulate matter has the potential of inducing thrombi and vessel blockage and depending upon the chemical composition of the particles the additional potential for introducing into the patient chemical agents which are undesired and possibly toxic.

In formulating a single-dose parenteral product, the pharmacist must consider not only the physicochemical aspects of the drug, but also the intended therapeutic use of the product itself. Some single-dose preparations are prepared to be administered rapidly in small volumes, but other preparations are allowed to drip slowly into the circulatory system over a period of hours. Most small-volume parenterals are formulated so that a convenient amount of solution, say 0.5 to 2 mL, contains the usual dose of the drug although larger volumes of more diluted solutions are frequently administered intrave-

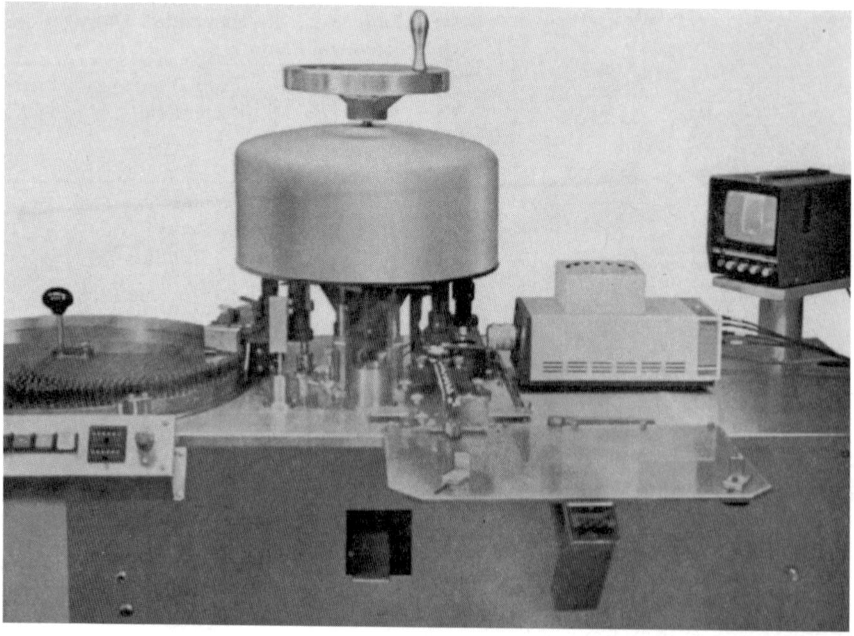

Fig. 8–26. *The AUTOSKAN industrial automatic inspection machine which detects the presence of particulate matter in injectables with a television camera and electronics, and automatically rejects them from the production line. (Courtesy of Lakso Company, Inc.)*

nously and intramuscularly. Generally, several strengths of injections of a given drug are marketed to permit a wider dosage selection by the physician without being wasteful of the drug as would be the case if he administered only part of a given single-dose parenteral solution. The large-volume, single-dose preparations generally are those solutions used to expand the blood volume or to replenish nutrients or electrolytes and are given by slow intravenous drip. However, in no instance may a single-dose parenteral container permit the withdrawal and administration of greater than 1000 mL. In addition, preparations intended for intraspinal, intracisternal, or peridural administration must be packaged only in single-dose containers as a precaution against contamination.

Frequently in the hospital, a physician may order an additional agent to be placed in a large-volume parenteral solution for infusion. In these instances, the person filling such an order must be certain that aseptic conditions are employed and that the additive is compatible with the contents of the original large volume parenteral solution.[5] Care must also be exercised not to introduce particulate matter into the solution. Many pharmaceutical companies have developed special devices for the aseptic transfer of pharmaceutical additives to large volume parenterals. An ordinary sterile needle and syringe, preferably affixed with a filtering device, may be effectively employed to transfer solutions from one parenteral product to another (Fig. 8–27). Many hospital pharmacies have established well controlled *I.V. additive* or *admixture* programs to assure additive-solution compatibility, safety and efficacy.[6]

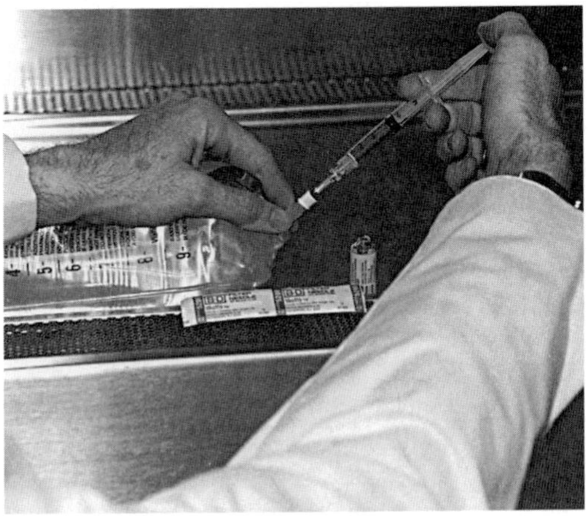

Fig. 8–27. *Utilization of a filter syringe for the aseptic addition of an additive to a large-volume parenteral solution. (Courtesy of William B. French, PhD.)*

Multiple-dose containers are affixed with rubber closures to permit the penetration of a hypodermic needle without the removal or destruction of the closure. Upon withdrawing the needle from the container, the closure reseals and protects the contents from airborne contamination. The needle may be inserted to withdraw a portion of the prepared liquid injection, or it may be used to introduce a solvent or vehicle to a dry powder intended for injection. In either instance, the sterility of the injection may be maintained so long as the needle itself is sterile at the time of entry into the container. It should be recalled that unless otherwise indicated in the monograph, multiple-dose injectables are required to contain added antibacterial preservatives. Also, unless otherwise specified, multiple-dose containers are not permitted to allow the withdrawal of greater than 30 mL in order to limit the number of penetrations made into the closure and thus protect against loss of sterility. The limited volume also guards against an excessive amount of antibacterial preservative being inadvertently coadministered with the drug when unusually large doses of an injection are required, in which case a non-preserved single-dose preparation is advisable. The usual multiple-dose container contains about ten usual doses of the injection, but quantity may vary greatly with the individual preparation and manufacturer.

Because it is impossible in practice to transfer the entire volume of a single-dose container or the last dose in a multiple-dose container into a hypodermic syringe, a slight excess in volume of the contents of ampuls and vials over the labeled "size" or volume of the package is permitted. Table 8–2 presents the recommended "overages" permitted by the USP to allow the withdrawal and administration of the labeled volumes.

The labels on containers of parenteral products must state: (1) the name of the preparation; (2) for a liquid preparation, the percentage content of drug or the amount of drug present in a specified volume, or for a dry preparation, the amount of active ingredient present and the volume of liquid to be added to the dry preparation to prepare a solution or suspension; (3) the route of administration; (4) a statement of storage con-

Table 8–2. Recommended Overages for Official Parenteral Products

Labeled Size, mL	*Excess Volume for Mobile Liquids, mL*	*Excess Volume for Viscous Liquids, mL*
0.5	0.10	0.12
1.0	0.10	0.15
2.0	0.15	0.25
5.0	0.30	0.50
10.0	0.50	0.70
20.0	0.60	0.90
30.0	0.80	1.20
50.0 or more	2%	3%

ditions and an expiration date; (5) the name of the manufacturer or distributor; (6) the manufacturing lot number, which when referred to indicates all manufacturing processes for that preparation. Injections for veterinary use are labeled to that effect. Preparations intended to be used as dialysis, hemofiltration or irrigation solutions should meet the requirements for injections, except those relating to volume present in the containers, and should bear a statement indicating that the solution is not intended for use by intravenous infusion. All containers appropriately labeled should allow a sufficient area of the container to remain free of label for its full length or circumference to permit inspection of the contents. Any injection which upon visual inspection reveals particulate matter other than normally suspended material should be discarded.

Each individual monograph for the official injection states the type of container (single-dose and/or multiple-dose) permitted for the injection, the type of glass preferred for the container, exemptions, if any, to usual package-size limitations, and any special storage instructions. Most injections prepared from chemically pure medicinal agents are stable at room temperature and may be stored without special concern or conditions. However, most biological products—insulin injection and the various vaccines, toxoids, toxins, and related products—are usually stored under refrigeration. Reference should be made to the individual monograph to find the proper storage temperature for a particular injection.

Quality Assurance for Pharmacy-Prepared Sterile Products

In November 1993, the American Society of Hospital Pharmacists published a technical assistance bulletin (TAB) on quality assurance for pharmacy-prepared sterile products.[7] The TAB was developed to help pharmacists establish quality assurance procedures for the component of practice that encompasses the preparation of sterile products. The recommendations of the TAB are appropriate to all practice settings in which pharmacists directly serve patients (e.g., hospitals, community pharmacies, nursing homes, home health care). Note that these are not intended to apply to the manufacturing of sterile pharmaceuticals as defined in state and federal laws and regulations. Nor are they to apply the preparation of medications (i.e., by pharmacists, nurses, physicians) intended for immediate administration (i.e., minimal delay between preparation and administration) to patients.

The term *sterile products* used within the TAB refers to sterile or nutritional substances that are prepared (e.g., compounded or repackaged) by pharmacy personnel, using aseptic technique and other quality assurance procedures.

The objectives of these recommendations are to enable pharmacists to provide:

1. Information to pharmacists on quality assurance and quality control activities that may be applied to the preparation of sterile products in pharmacies, and
2. A scheme to match quality assurance and quality control activities with the potential risks to patients posed by various types of products.

The TAB defines the purpose of these recommendations and encourages pharmacists to participate in quality improvement, risk management, and infection control programs within their organizations. In doing so, pharmacists would be expected to report findings about quality assurance in sterile products to appropriate staffs or committees, and to cooperate with managers of quality improvement, risk management, and infection control to develop optimal sterile product procedures.

In February 1992, the American Society of Hospital Pharmacists had proposed guidelines that formed the basis of TAB.[8] This original document distinguished between quality control (QC) and quality assurance (QA). By definition, *quality control* is the acceptance or rejection of raw materials and packaging components, in-process test materials, and inspections.[9] *Quality assurance* is a systematic method to identify problems in patient care that are resolved via administrative, clinical, or educational actions to ensure that final products and outcomes meet applicable specifications.[9]

The TAB classifies sterile products into three levels based upon risk to the patient. The risk levels range from the least potential risk (level 1) to the greatest potential risk (level 3). It is noteworthy that the classification system is designed only to assist the pharmacist in selecting sterile preparation procedures. Pharmacists must exercise professional judgment in deciding which risk level applies to a specific sterile product or situation. Factors that increase risk (e.g., multiple system breaks, compounding complexities, high-risk administration sites, immunocompromised patients, microbial growth potential of the product, storage conditions) must be weighed by the pharmacist.

There will be situations when the pharmacist must make risk vs. benefit decisions to prepare these products outside of the guidelines (e.g., the preparation of a sterile investigational drug in a compassionate-use protocol for a lifesaving effort). The risk assignments listed in Table 8–3 provide a logical template within which the pharmacist can evaluate risk. These do not, however, preclude the possibility of alternative, logical arrangements that could be based upon scientific information and professional judgment.

Risk level 1 represents the minimum QA guidelines. In risk levels 2 and 3, products must meet or exceed each of the risk level 1 guidelines. In those instances where the risk level assignment might be nebulous, guidelines for the higher risk level should be followed.

The TAB delineates the quality assurance components for each risk level. These include: policies and procedures; personnel education, training, and evaluation; process validation; storage and handling; facilities and equipment; garb; aseptic technique and product preparation; process evaluation; expiration dating; labeling; end-product evaluation; and documentation. Specific recommendations germane to each of these components at each risk level are made in the TAB;

Table 8–3. ASHP Risk Level Classification of Pharmacy-Prepared Sterile Products[7]

Risk Level 1

1. Products
   A. Stored at room temperature and completely administered within 28 hours of preparation; or
   B. Stored under refrigeration for 7 days or less before complete administration to a patient over a period not to exceed 24 hours; or
   C. Frozen for 30 days or less before complete administration to a patient over a period not to exceed 24 hours.
2. Unpreserved sterile products prepared for administration to one patient, or batch-prepared products containing suitable preservatives prepared for administration to more than one patient.
3. Products prepared by closed-system aseptic transfer of sterile, nonpyrogenic, finished pharmaceuticals obtained from licensed manufacturers into sterile final containers (e.g., syringe, minibag, portable infusion-device cassette) obtained from licensed manufacturers.

Risk Level 2

1. Products stored beyond 7 days under refrigeration, or stored beyond 30 days frozen, or administered beyond 28 hours after preparation and storage at room temperature.
2. Batch-prepared products without preservatives that are intended for use by more than one patient. (*Note:* Batch-prepared products without preservatives that will be administered to multiple patients carry a greater risk to the patients than products prepared for a single patient because of the potential effect of product contamination on the health and well-being of a larger patient group.)
3. Products compounded by combining sterile ingredients, obtained from licensed manufacturers, in a sterile reservoir, obtained from a licensed manufacturer, by using closed-system aseptic transfer before subdivision into multiple units to be dispensed to patients.

Risk Level 3 Products Exhibit Either Characteristic 1 or 2

1. Products compounded from nonsterile ingredients or compounded with nonsterile components, containers, or equipment, or
2. Products prepared by combining multiple ingredients—sterile or nonsterile—by using an open-system transfer or open reservoir before terminal sterilization or subdivision into multiple units to be dispensed.

the reader may refer to them for additional information.

Available Injections

There are hundreds of injections on the market of various medicinal agents. Tables 8–4 through 8–7 present some examples of those packaged in small-volume and large-volume containers, the latter for intravenous infusion.

Small Volume Parenterals

Table 8–4 presents some commonly employed injections given in small volume. Some of these injections are solutions and others suspensions.

In recent years, there has been the introduction of manufacturers' premixed intravenous delivery systems. These have simplified the delivery process for small-volume parenterals in particular. A distinct advantage of these ready-to-use systems is that they require little or no manipulation to make them patient specific, and thus a viable alternative to the traditional labor-intensive method of compounding parenteral medications from partial-fill (i.e., individual dose/multiple doses of I.V. medications) vials and an appropriate parenteral solution. Since the introduction of the first ready-to-use systems in the late 1970s, the availability and variety of systems has increased (e.g., Baxter Healthcare Corporation, Kendall McGaw Laboratories, Abbott Laboratories) (refer to Table 8–5).

The traditional method for preparing small-volume parenteral therapy for patient-specific use from a partial-fill drug vial into a minibag can be labor-intensive and costly (e.g., labor supply and inventory costs for materials such as syringes and needles). The savings accrued through ready-to-use systems can be significant and have been documented.[10] Another key advantage of these systems is extended stability dating and reduced wastage. Doses can be put together (but not activated) in cycles, then activated just prior to patient use and delivered to the nursing station by the pharmacy personnel.[10]

The down side of these ready-to-use small parenteral products is that they do not offer flexibility in changing the volume or concentration of the product. This may then pose a problem to the fluid-restricted patient.[10] At present, most small-volume parenterals are available in 50-mL containers, although smaller volumes (i.e., 25 mL) have been advocated. Another disadvantage of the ready-to-use products is that some manufacturers' premixed products require thawing. Microwave use for quick thawing poses stability problems for some of these drug products, and room temperature thawing is a lengthy process. Thus, appropriate planning is required so that large numbers of these products that are thawed in advance are used and recycled efficiently. Otherwise, these small-volume parenteral products potentially increase waste. Finally, getting a prescription label to adhere to a thawed minibag can be a problem.

The available ready-to-use systems have not demonstrated much impact in the pediatric and neonatal population. The unique dosing and fluid requirements of these patients make these systems inappropriate.

Among the most used of the small volume injections are the various insulin preparations described below and presented in Table 8–5. Insulin, the active principle of the pancreas gland, is primarily concerned with the metabolism of carbohydrates, but also influences protein and fat metabolism. Insulin facilitates the cellular uptake of glucose and its metabolism in liver, muscle, and adipose tissue. It increases the uptake of amino acids and inhibits the breakdown of fats and the production of ketones. Insulin is administered to patients having abnormal or absent pancreatic beta cell function to restore glucose metabolism and maintain satisfactory carbohydrate, fat, and protein metabolism. It is used in the treatment of *diabetes mellitus,* in instances in which the condition cannot be controlled satisfactorily by dietary regulation alone or by oral hypoglycemic drugs. Insulin may also be used to improve the appetite and increase the weight in selected cases of nondiabetic malnutrition and is frequently added to intravenous infusions.

Insulin is administered by needle or jet injection (Figs. 8–28, 8–29, and 8–30). A system for the nasal administration of insulin is presently under study.

Since its introduction, U-100 insulin has been suggested as a replacement for the U-40 insulin strength, with the intention of making U-100 the single strength for in-home use by the patient. In December 1991, Eli Lilly announced that it would cease further production of U-40 insulins, and subsequently other insulin manufacturers also decided to cease production of this strength. The basis for this decision was a lack of patient demand (i.e., very low numbers of patient utilizing this strength). Recognizing, however, that lower strengths of insulin (i.e., under 100 U/mL)

Table 8–4. Examples of Some Injections Usually Packaged and Administered in Small Volume

Injection	*Physical Form*	*Category and Comments*
Butorphanol Tartrate Injection	solution	Narcotic Agonist-Antagonist Analgesic; administered IM or IV for relief of moderate to severe pain and as a preoperative or preanesthesia medication.
Cimetidine HCl Injection	solution	Histamine H_2 antagonist; administered IM or IV for patients with pathological GI hypersecretory conditions or intractable ulcers.
Dexamethasone Sodium Phosphate Injection	solution	Glucocorticoid; administered IM or IV for cerebral edema and unresponsive shock. Also used intra-articular, intralesional or soft tissue for joints, bursae, and ganglia.
Digoxin Injection	solution	Cardiotonic given IM (not preferred) or IV with highly individualized and monitored dosage.
Dihydroergotamine Mesylate Injection	solution	Alpha-adrenergic blocking agent specific in migraine, given IM or IV.
Furosemide Injection	solution	Loop diuretic; administered IM or IV [slowly] for edema or acute pulmonary edema.
Heparin Sodium Injection	solution	Anticoagulant administered IV or SubQ, as indicated by activated partial prothrombin time (APTT) or actuated coagulation time (ACT).
Histamine Phosphate Injection	solution	Diagnostic aid given SubQ in the testing of gastric secretion capacity (i.e., achlorhydria).
Hydromorphone HCl Injection	solution	Narcotic analgesic used for the relief of moderate to severe pain; administered subcutaneously or IM or by slow IV injection.
Isoproterenol HCl Injection	solution	Adrenergic (bronchodilator) given IM, SubQ, or IV.
Lidocaine HCl Injection	solution	Cardiac depressant given IV as an antiarrhythmic; also as a local anesthetic, epidurally, by infiltration, and in peripheral nerve block.
Magnesium Sulfate Injection	solution	Anticonvulsant/electrolyte; administered by IM or direct IV injection, IV infusion, or in other IV infusions for management of convulsive toxemia of pregnancy, hyperalimentation therapy, mild magnesium deficiency, or severe hypomagnesemia.
Meperidine HCl Injection	solution	Narcotic analgesic given IM, SubQ, or slow continuous IV infusion.
Metoclopramide Monohydrochloride Injection	solution	Gastrointestinal stimulant; administered IM, direct IV, or slowly as an IV admixture for the prevention of chemotherapy-induced emesis.
Morphine Sulfate Injection	solution	Narcotic analgesic. IM, IV, PCA.
Nalbuphine HCl Injection	solution	Narcotic Agonist-Antagonist Analgesic; administered SC, IM or IV for relief of moderate to severe pain and for preoperative analgesia.
Naloxone HCl Injection	solution	A narcotic antagonist which prevents or reverses the effects of opioids including respiratory depression, sedation and hypotension; administered IV, IM, or subcutaneously.
Oxytocin Injection	solution	Oxytocic, given IM (erratic) or IV obstetrically for the therapeutic induction of labor.
Phenytoin Sodium Injection	solution	Anticonvulsant; administered IM [erratic absorption] as a prophylactic dosage for neurosurgery or IV [slowly] for status epilepticus.
Phytonadione Injection	dispersion	Vitamin K (prothrombogenic) employed in hemorrhagic situations. An aqueous dispersion of phytonadione, a viscous liquid.
Procaine Penicillin G Injection	suspension	Anti-infective; administered IM for moderately severe infections due to penicillin-G sensitive microorganisms.
Prochlorperazine Edisylate Injection	solution	Antidopaminergic; administered IM or IV for control of severe nausea and vomiting associated with adult surgery.
Propranolol HCl Injection	solution	A beta-adrenergic receptor blocking agent indicated in the management of hypertension. Oral dosage (tablets) is usual; intravenous administration is reserved for life-threatening arrhythmias or those occurring under anesthesia.
Sodium Bicarbonate Injection	solution	Electrolyte; administered IV, either undiluted or diluted in other IV fluids for cardiac arrest and in less urgent forms of metabolic acidosis.
Sumatriptan succinate	solution	A selective 5-hydroxytryptamine$_1$ receptor, subtype agonist, used for acute migraine attacks with or without aura. Self-administered SubQ from unit-of-use syringes and *SELFdose* unit.
Verapamil HCl Injection	solution	Calcium channel blocking agent; administered as a slow IV injection over at least 2 minutes for supraventricular tachyarrhythmias

Table 8–5. Some Representative Marketed Premixed Products (Small Volume Parenterals)[a,b]

Drug	Diluent	Storage	Expiration Dating: Frozen (−20 °C)	Expiration Dating: Thawed (5 °C)	Expiration Dating: Thawed (25 °C)	Expiration Dating: Room Temp. (25 °C)
Cefazolin Sodium 500 mg, 1 g	dextrose 5% 50 mL	frozen	18 months	10 days	48 hours	n/a
Ceftazidime Sodium‡ 1 g, 2 g	iso-osmotic in dextrose 50 mL	frozen	9 months	7 days	24 hours	n/a
Ceftriaxone Sodium 1 g, 2 g	iso-osmotic in dextrose 50 mL	frozen	12 months	14 days	72 hours	n/a
Ciprofloxacin 200 mg, 400 mg‖	dextrose 5% 100 mL, 200 mL	room temp.	n/a	n/a	n/a	n/a
Gentamicin Sulfate 40 mg, 60 mg	isotonic 50 mL, 100 mL	room temp.	n/a	n/a	n/a	18 months§
Rantidine ‖ 50 mg	0.45% sodium chloride 100 mL	room temp.	15 months	14 days	24 hours	n/a
Ticarcillin Disodium/ Clavulanate Potassium‡ 3.1 g	iso-osmotic in dextrose 100 mL	frozen	6 months	7 days	24 hours†	n/a
Tobramycin Sulfate ‖ 60 mg, 80 mg	iso-osmotic in dextrose 100 mL	room temp.	n/a	n/a	n/a	

[a] Adapted from Mallekai, et al., *Hosp. Pharm.*, 28:970–971, 975–977, 1993.

[b] The majority of products in this table are co-marketed by Baxter Healthcare Corporation and the various manufacturers of the individual drug. Exceptions are denoted by the symbols § and ‖ following the drug name. Stability information provided by Baxter Healthcare Corporation.

† Stability at 22°C

‡ Available in Galaxy bag.

§ Kendall McGaw's gentamicin in normal saline is stable for 24 months (Baxter Healthcare's preparation of gentamicin is stable for 18 months), metronidazole is stable for 18 months. Both are available in PABR containers and therefore do not require an outer moisture barrier wrap. Information provided by Kendall McGaw.

n/a = not applicable.

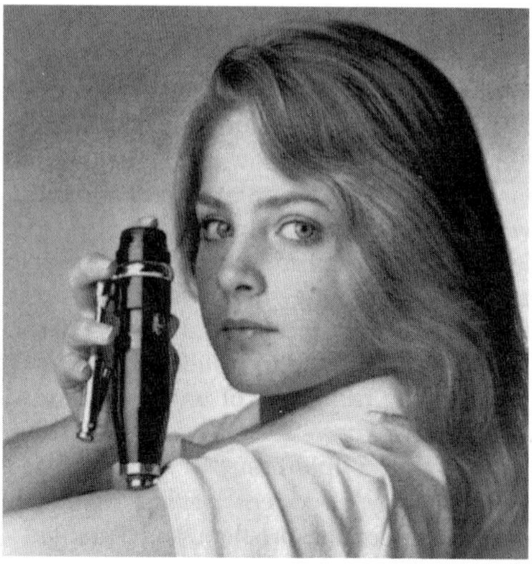

Fig. 8–28. *The Medi-Jector II, an example of a jet injection device. The jet injection method utilizes pressure rather than a needle in providing the subcutaneous distribution of an injectable medication. The device shown can be used with U-100 insulin or a combination of insulins and can deliver 2 to 100 units in half-unit increments. (Courtesy of Derata Corporation.)*

might still be needed (e.g., small children, veterinarian use), Lilly markets a diluting fluid for the Regular, NPH, and Lente insulins of U-100 strength. This fluid can be used to prepare any strength of insulin below 100 U/mL.

Age-associated sight difficulties and the vision deterioration associated with diabetes can inter-

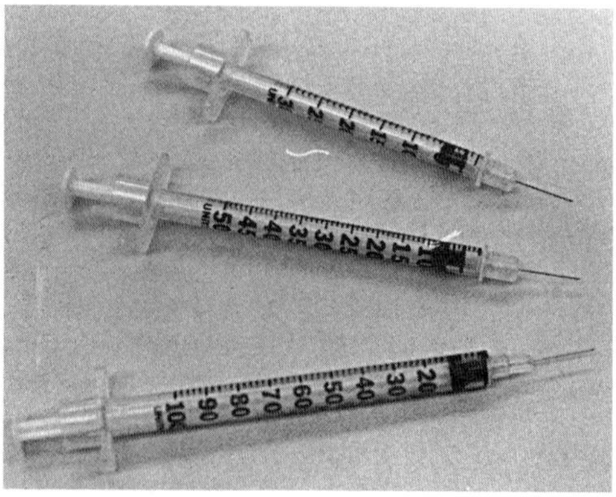

Fig. 8–29. *Examples of insulin syringes calibrated in units. (Courtesy of William B. French, PhD.)*

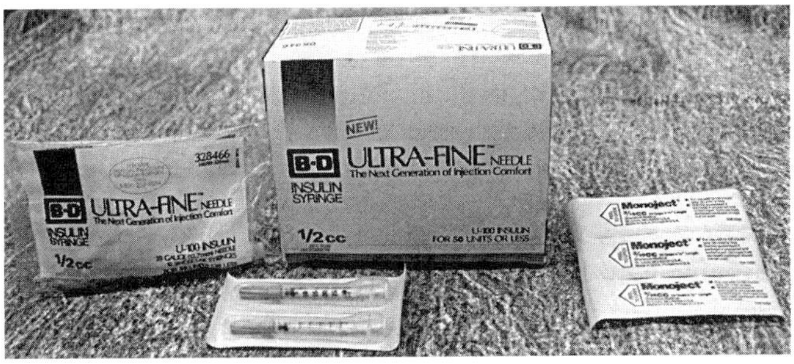

Fig. 8–30. *Example of packaging of disposable sterile insulin syringes and needles. (Courtesy of William B. French, PhD.)*

fere significantly with buying and using insulin products. Therefore, packaging of insulins must make allowances for the visual deficits of patients with diabetes. To facilitate identification of the proper medication at the site of purchase, the arrangement and size of the package lettering must make it easy for the insulin-dependent patient to recognize the insulin type and concentration of the product. In the case of Humulin insulins, an international symbol also appears on the cartons and bottles of all formulations. These symbols help assure that patients with diabetes secure the correct Humulin formulation anywhere in the world.

Insulin Injection (Regular)

Insulin Injection is a sterile aqueous solution of insulin. Commercially, the solution is prepared from beef or pork pancreas or both or through biosynthetic means (Human Insulin), discussed in the next section. The source must be stated on the labeling. In 1980, purified pork insulin [Iletin II, pork (Lilly)] became available for individuals allergic to or otherwise adversely affected by the mixed pork-beef product. The first insulin developed for clinical use was an amorphous insulin. This type has since been replaced by a more purified crystalline insulin composed of zinc-insulin crystals which produces a clear aqueous solution. Originally, insulin injection ("regular insulin") had been produced at a pH of 2.8 to 3.5. This was necessary, because particles formed in the vial when the pH was increased above the acid range. However, changes in the manufacturing methods resulting in the production of insulin of greater purity has allowed for the preparation of insulin injection having a neutral pH. The neutralized product has been shown to exhibit greater stability than the acidic product.

Insulin injection is prepared to contain 100 or 500 USP Insulin Units in each mL. The labeling must state the potency, in USP Insulin Units in each mL and the expiration date, which must not be later than 24 months after the date of distribution from the manufacturer's storage. As an added precaution against the inadvertent use of the incorrect strength of insulin by the patient during self-administration of the drug, the package colors vary, depending upon the strength of the insulin. For instance, all insulins (of the various types) containing 100 units per mL have orange and the 500 units per mL preparation has brown with diagonal white stripes. U-500 insulin is indicated for patients with a marked insulin requirement (more than 200 units per day) because a large unit/dose may be administered subcutaneously in a small volume.

Insulin injection is a colorless to straw-colored solution, depending upon its concentration; that containing 500 Units per mL is straw-colored. It is substantially free from turbidity. A small amount of glycerin (1.4 to 1.8%) is added for stability and 0.1 to 0.25% of either phenol or cresol is added for preservation. Insulin remains stable if stored in a cold place, preferably the refrigerator. However, because the injection of cold insulin is somewhat uncomfortable, the patient may store the vial being used at room temperature (59–86°F or 15–30°C) for up to 1 month. Any insulin remaining in the vial after that time should be discarded. Freezing should be avoided, as this reduces potency.

The various insulin preparations differ as to their rapidity of action (onset of action) after injection, their peak of action, and their duration of action (Table 8–6). Insulin injection, being a solution, is categorized as a prompt-acting insulin preparation. Insulin preparations that are suspensions are slower acting. Only insulin injection may be administered intravenously; all others, as well as insulin injection, are normally given subcutaneously, usually ½ to 2 hours be-

Table 8–6. Insulin Preparations*

Product	*Source*	*Strength, Insulin Units/mL*	*Onset*	*Peak (In Hours)*	*Duration*
Regular Insulins					
Iletin I Regular (Lilly)	beef-pork	U-100	0.5–1	2–5	6–8
Regular (Novo Nordisk)	pork	U-100	0.5–1	2–5	6–8
Velosulin (Novo Nordisk)	pork	U-100	0.5–1	2–5	6–8
Iletin II Regular (Lilly)	pork	U-100, U-500	0.5–1	2–5	6–8
Humulin R (Lilly)	human†	U-100	0.5	2–4	6–8
Humulin BR human† [buffered, regular (Lilly)]	human†	U-100	0.5	2–4	6–8
Novolin R Human (Novo Nordisk)	human, semisynthetic	U-100	0.5	2.5–5	8
Velosulin Human (Novo Nordisk-USA)	human	U-100	0.5	1–3	8
Zinc Suspension, Prompt					
Semilente (Novo Nordisk)	beef	U-100	0.5–1.5	2–10	12–16
Isophane Suspension (NPH)					
Iletin I NPH (Lilly)	beef-pork	U-100	1–2	6–12	18–26
NPH (Novo Nordisk)	beef	U-100	1–1.5	8–12	24
NPH (Novo Nordisk)	pork	U-100	1–1.5	4–12	24
Iletin II NPH (Lilly)	pork	U-100	1–2	6–12	18–26
Insulated (Novo Nordisk)	pork	U-100	1–1.5	8–12	24
Humulin N (Lilly)	human†	U-100	1–2	6–12	18–24
Novolin N (Novo Nordisk)	human, semisynthetic	U-100	1.5	4–12	24
Insulatard, human (Novo Nordisk-USA)	human, semisynthetic	U-100	1.5	4–12	24
Isophane/Regular					
Mixtard (Novo Nordisk)	pork	U-100	0.5–1		24
Novolin 70/30 (Novo Nordisk)	human†	U-100	0.5–1	2–12	24
Humullin N (Lilly)	human	U-100	1–2	6–12	18–24
Humulin 50/50 (Lilly)	human	U-100	0.5	2–12	18–24
Humulin 70/30 (Lilly)	human	U-100	0.5	2–12	18–24
Mixtard Human, 70/30	human	U-100	0.5–1	4–8	24
Zinc Suspension (Lente)					
Iletin I Lente (Lilly)	beef-pork	U-100	1–3	6–12	18–26
Lente (Novo Nordisk)	beef	U-100	1–2.5	8–12	24
Lentard (Novo Nordisk)	beef-pork	U-100	1–2.5	8–12	24
Iletin II Lente (Lilly)	pork	U-100	1–3	6–12	18–26
Humulin L (Lilly)	human†	U-100	1–3	6–12	18–24
Novolin L (Novo Nordisk)	human, semisynthetic	U-100	2.5	4–15	22
Zinc Suspension, Extended					
Ultralente (Novo Nordisk)	beef	U-100	4–8	10–30	36
Humulin U (Lilly)	human	U-100	4–6	8–20	24–28

* Adapted from Drug Information Newsletter, vol. 13, No. 4, 1987, Drug Information Center, Pharmacy Department, and Department of Pharmacology, Medical College of Georgia, and College of Pharmacy, University of Georgia.

† Recombinant DNA origin.

fore a meal so that its physiological effects will parallel the absorption of glucose. The dosage is individually determined, with the usual dosage range being 5 to 100 USP Units. The insulin injection containing 500 units per mL is employed in cases of insulin resistance requiring very large doses.

It is important to emphasize at this point that the pharmacist plays a vital role in the education of the diabetic patient, particularly as it relates to the proper use of insulin. The insulin dosage should always be checked to ensure it is correct. Because it is a solution, Regular Insulin can be used in emergency situations, i.e., ketoacidosis, to effect a rapid decrease in blood glucose levels. However, with the exception of diabetic ketoacidosis, it is rare for a patient to ever require a dose of Regular Insulin greater than 25 units. Typically, diabetic patients combine Regular Insulin with a modified insulin, i.e., NPH, to provide daily coverage using two injections (morning, late-afternoon) or now use available pre-mixed preparations. So it is important that the patient understand how much of each to use and know in what order these should be mixed in the insulin syringe. The unmodified insulin, i.e., Regular Insulin, is drawn up first into the syringe.

In an institutional setting the pharmacist must make sure written insulin orders are correctly transcribed or transmitted. Errors in insulin dosage have occurred because of allied health professional error. Written orders for 6 U of insulin have been interpreted to mean 60 units, an order for 4 U has been read as 4 cc. Each of these occurred because the abbreviation "U" for units was read as a zero or a cc.

The patient should be instructed to rotate the site of insulin injections on a continual basis. Rotation of the site will help to avoid the development of lipohypertrophy, a buildup of fibrous tissue. Otherwise, if there is continual injection into one site, the tissue becomes spongy and avascular. The avascular nature of the site perpetuates the problem because the skin becomes anesthetized and the injection is not felt. This is a particular problem with children who continue to use the same site and do not realize that the absorption of insulin from this site becomes erratic and uncontrollable. Numerous brochures are available from manufacturers of diabetic supplies that demonstrate the appropriate rotation of insulin injection sites over the entire body.

Another encountered problem with insulin injection is the development of lipodystrophy. Generally, this problem appears within 2 months to 2 years following the beginning of insulin therapy and occurs predominantly in women and children. The etiology of the problem has been ascribed to the injection of refrigerated insulin (not giving enough time for it to warm up prior to injection), to a failure to rotate the injection site and to insulin impurities. The result is the formation of a subcutaneous indentation or "pothole" caused by a wasting or atrophy of the lipid tissue. It appears that the greater purity of current insulins significantly have decreased this problem, and a marked improvement in existing atrophic areas has been demonstrated by the injection of highly purified port or human insulin directly into or on the periphery of the atrophic areas.

Prior to use, the patient should be instructed to carefully inspect the insulin. Regular Insulin, a solution, should appear clear, while the other insulins which are suspensions should appear cloudy. With the insulins that are suspensions the patient should be instructed how to prepare the insulin, i.e., the vial is rotated slowly between the palms of the hands several times, prior to drawing the insulin into the syringe. This avoids frothing and bubble formation which would result in an inaccurate dose of insulin. The patient should not shake the insulin vial.

Proper storage should also be encouraged for insulins. These preparations should be stored in a cool place or a refrigerator. The patient should be warned to avoid having the insulin come into contact with extremes of temperature, i.e., freezing [overnight in the car during the wintertime], heat [glove compartment of a car, direct sunlight]. If this occurs, it is preferred that the patient discard the insulin and get a new bottle. Any bottle of insulin that appears "frosted" or "clumped" should be returned to the pharmacy where the purchase took place. Lastly, the patient should use the insulin in a timely fashion, but not beyond the expiration date indicated on the insulin vial.

Human Insulin

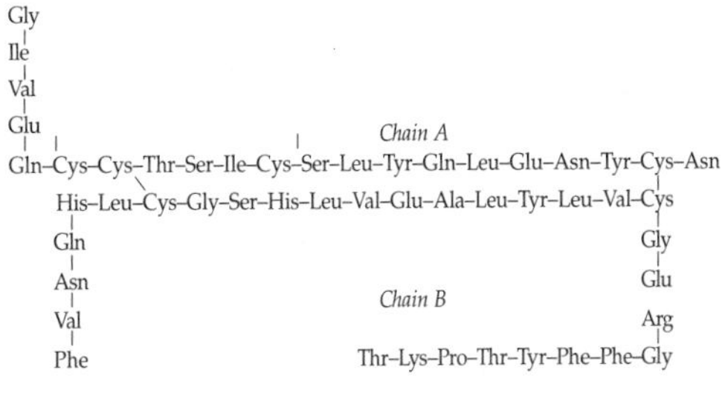

Biosynthetic human insulin was the first drug product developed through recombinant DNA techniques to receive approval by the federal Food and Drug Administration for marketing. This product, HUMULIN, Lilly, became available in 1983. It is produced by utilizing a special nondisease-forming laboratory strain of *Escherichia coli* and recombinant DNA technology. A recombined plasmid DNA coding for human insulin is introduced into the bacteria, and it is then cultured by fermentation to produce the A and B chains of human insulin. These A and B chains are freed and purified individually before they are linked by the specific disulfide bridges to form human insulin. The insulin produced is chemically, physically, and immunologically equivalent to insulin derived from the human pancreas. The biosynthetic insulin is free of contamination with *E. coli* peptides, and, is also free of the pancreatic peptides that are present as impurities in insulin preparations derived from animal pancreatic extraction. These latter impurities include proinsulin and proinsulin intermediates, glucagon, somatostatin, pancreatic polypeptide, and vasoactive intestinal peptide.

Pharmacokinetic studies in some normal subjects and clinical observations in patients indicate that formulations of human insulin have a slightly faster onset of action and a slightly shorter duration of action than their purified pork insulin counterparts. Two formulations of human insulin were initially marketed: Neutral Regular Human Insulin (HUMULIN R, Lilly) and NPH Human Insulin (HUMULIN N, Lilly). Other forms have since been added, as shown in Table 8–6. Neutral Regular human insulin consists of zinc-insulin crystals in solution. It has a rapid onset-of-action and a relatively short duration-of-action (6 to 8 hours). NPH human insulin is a turbid preparation that is intermediate-acting, with a slower onset-of-action and longer duration-of-action (slightly less than 24 hours) than regular human insulin.

Human insulins should be stored as other insulins, in a cold place, preferably a refrigerator. Freezing should be avoided.

Isophane Insulin Suspension (NPH Insulin)

Isophane Insulin Suspension is a sterile suspension, in an aqueous vehicle buffered with dibasic sodium phosphate to between pH 7.1 and 7.4, of insulin prepared from zinc-insulin crystals modified by the addition of protamine so that the solid phase of the suspension consists of crystals composed of insulin, zinc, and protamine. Protamine is prepared from the sperm or the mature testes of fish belonging to the genus *Oncorhynchus* and others. As mentioned earlier during the discussion of the aqueous insulin solutions, suspensions of insulin with a pH on the alkaline side are inherently of a longer duration of action than those preparations that are solutions. Insulin is most insoluble at pH 7.2.

The rod-shaped crystals of isophane insulin suspension should be approximately 30 micrometers in length and the suspension free from large aggregates of crystals following moderate agitation. This is necessary for the insulin suspension to pass freely within the needle used in injection and for the absorption of the drug from the site of injection to be consistent from one manufactured batch of injection to another. When a portion of the suspension is examined microscopically, the suspended matter is largely crystalline with only traces of amorphous material. The official injection is required to contain glycerin and phenol for stability and preservation. The specified expiration date occurring in the labeling is 24 months after the immediate container was filled by the manufacturer. The suspension is packaged in multiple-dose containers having not less than 10 mL of injection. Each mL of the injection contains 100 units of insulin per mL of suspension. The suspension is best stored in a refrigerator, but freezing must be avoided.

As indicated earlier, isophane insulin suspension is an intermediate-acting insulin preparation administered as required mainly as hormonal replacement in diabetes mellitus. The usual dosage range subcutaneously is 10 to 80 USP Units.

The "NPH" used in some produce names stands for "Neutral Protamine Hagedorn," since the preparation is about neutral (pH about 7.2), contains protamine, and was developed by Hagedorn. The term "isophane" is based on the Greek: *iso* and *phane,* meaning "equal" and "appearance" and refers to the equivalent balance between the protamine and insulin.

Isophane Insulin Suspension and Insulin Injection

In years past, patients needing a more rapid onset of insulin and the intermediate duration of activity approximately one day, would routinely mix isophane insulin suspension, an intermediate-acting insulin, with insulin injection, a rapid-acting insulin. Unexpected patient responses (e.g., hypoglycemic episodes) were encountered. It was not uncommon for the patient inadvertently to contaminate one of the vials during the mixing process. Subsequently, a premixed formulation of isophane insulin suspension and insulin injection became available. Currently there are two formulations, a 70/30 combination that consists of 70% isophane insulin suspension and 30% insulin injection, and a 50/50 combination that consists of 50% isophane insulin suspension and 50% insulin injection.

Humulin 50/50, for example, achieves a higher insulin concentration (C_{max}) and higher maximum glucose infusion rates with more rapid elimination than Humulin 70/30. However, as expected, the cumulative amounts of insulin absorbed (AUC) and the cumulative effects over 24 hours following injection are identical. Thus, the 70/30 combination provides an initial insulin response tempered with a more prolonged release of insulin. The 50/50 mixture would be useful in those situations where a greater initial response is required, and in those patients who have been using extemporaneously compounded insulin mixtures in a 50/50 ratio.

The Humulin 70/30 and 50/50 premixed insulins are cloudly suspensions with a zinc content of 0.01–0.04 mg/100 units. These insulins are neutral in pH and phosphate buffered. m-Cresol and phenol are the preservatives employed for both combinations. Protamine sulfate is used as the modifying protein salt.

Patients should not attempt to change the ratio of these products with the addition of NPH or regular insulin. If Humulin N and Humulin R mixtures are prescribed in a different proportion, the individual insulin products should be mixed in the amounts recommended by the physician.

Insulin Zinc Suspension

Insulin for Insulin Zinc Suspension is modified by the addition of zinc chloride so that the suspended particles consist of a mixture of crystalline and amorphous insulin in a ratio of approximately 7 parts of crystals to 3 parts of amorphous material. The sterile suspension is in an aqueous vehicle buffered to pH 7.2 to 7.5 with sodium acetate. In treating insulin with zinc chloride, it is possible to obtain both crystalline and amorphous zinc insulin. The amorphous form has the most prompt hypoglycemic effect, since the particles are the smallest and are absorbed into the system more rapidly after subcutaneous injection than are the zinc insulin crystals. Also, the larger the crystals the less prompt and the longer-acting will be the insulin suspension. By combining the crystalline and amorphous forms into one preparation, an intermediate-acting suspension is obtained. As noted in Table 8–6 the time-activity of insulin zinc suspension is only slightly different than that for isophane insulin suspension. The advantage of the former is that no additional foreign protein (other than the insulin) is present, such as protamine, which may produce local sensitivity reactions. Also, it may be combined as desired with either of the following two suspensions to produce an insulin preparation having the time-activity characteristics that most closely meet the desires and requirements of the individual patient. Suspensions available contain 100 USP Insulin Units per mL packaged in 10-mL vials. The individual crystalline and amorphous particles may be seen microscopically, with the crystals being predominantly between 10 to 40 μm in maximum dimension and the amorphous particles no greater than 2 μm in maximum dimension.

In addition to the sodium acetate as a buffer, the suspension contains about 0.7% sodium chloride for tonicity and 0.10% methylparaben for preservation. The expiration date of the suspension is 24 months after the immediate container was filled. The suspension must be stored in a refrigerator with freezing being avoided. As with all such preparations, the dose depends upon the individual needs of the patient, but generally ranges between 10 and 80 USP Units.

Extended Insulin Zinc Suspension

Extended insulin zinc suspension is a sterile suspension of zinc insulin crystals in an aqueous medium buffered to between pH 7.2 and 7.5 with sodium acetate. Present also are 0.7% sodium chloride for tonicity and 0.1% methylparaben for preservation. Because the suspended matter is composed solely of zinc insulin crystals, which are slowly absorbed, this preparation is classified as a long-acting insulin preparation. Because of the compatibility between the preparations, this suspension may be mixed with either insulin zinc suspension or prompt insulin zinc suspension to achieve the proper time-activity requirements of an individual patient. The usual dosage range is 10 to 80 USP Units. The suspension is commercially available in 10-mL vials providing 100 USP Insulin Units per mL. The suspension must be stored in a refrigerator with freezing being avoided. Under proper storage conditions, the expiration date of the injection is not later than 24 months after the immediate container was filled.

Prompt Insulin Zinc Suspension

The sterile suspension of insulin in Prompt Insulin Zinc Suspension is modified by the addition of zinc chloride so that the solid phase of the suspension is amorphous. The maximum dimension of the shapeless particles of zinc insulin must not exceed 2 micrometers. The suspension is available in 100 USP Insulin Units per mL in vials of 10 mL. This preparation has the same pH and additives as extended insulin zinc suspension, and they may be mixed as desired to achieve a preparation having the desired time-activity characteristics. This is a rapid-acting insulin preparation. It must be stored in a refrigerator and not permitted to freeze. Its expiration date is not greater than 24 months after the immediate container was filled.

Insulin Infusion Pumps

Newly developed insulin infusion pumps allow patients to achieve and maintain blood glucose at near-normal levels on a *constant basis.* Continuous infusion of insulin through use of these pumps eliminates the need for the patient to self-administer daily injections of insulin. This provides patient convenience, better patient compliance, and control over the disease. The main objective of pump therapy is the strict control of the blood glucose level between 70 to 140 mg/dL. This is the primary way to avoid complications in diabetic patients, such as gangrene and diabetic retinopathy.

Early insulin infusion pumps were large bedside units, used mainly in hospitals. Today, portable, battery-operated, and programmable units are available. These systems utilize microcomputers to regulate the flow of insulin from a syringe attached to a catheter (usually 18 gauge) connected to a 27- to 28-gauge needle inserted in the patient. The insulin may be delivered subcutaneously, intravenously, or intraperitoneally.

Patients who use infusion pumps for the continuous subcutaneous administration of insulin may develop hard nodules at the site of injection. Some patients may demonstrate nodules that are tender, develop a rock-hard consistency, and take several months to subside. Although the cause of this nodule formation is unknown, a change in insulin may be beneficial. Speculation as to the cause centers around the development of local trauma or hematoma formation with a subsequent local inflammatory response, stimulation of fibroblast replacement, or dystrophic calcification. The need to rotate sites of injection on a several day basis cannot be overemphasized. For additional information on infusion pumps, the reader is directed to the footnote reference at the end of this chapter.[11]

Large Volume Parenterals (LVPs)

Common examples of large volume parenterals in use today were presented in Table 8–7. These solutions are generally administered by intravenous infusion to replenish body fluids, electrolytes, or to provide nutrition. They are usually administered in volumes of 100 mL to

Table 8–7. Examples of Some Injections Administered in Large Volume by Intravenous Infusion[1]

Injection	*Usual Contents*	*Category and Comments*
Amino Acid Injection	3.5, 5, 5.5, 7, 8.5, 10% crystalline amino acids with or without varying concentrations of electrolytes or glycerin	Fluid and nutrient replenisher.
Dextrose Injection, USP	2.5, 5.0, 10, 20% dextrose, and other strengths	Fluid and nutrient replenisher.
Dextrose and Sodium Chloride Injection, USP	Dextrose varying from 2.5 to 25% and sodium chloride from 0.11 (19 mEq sodium) to 0.9% (154 mEq sodium)	Fluid, nutrient, and electrolyte replenisher.
Mannitol Injection, USP	5, 10, 15, 20 and 25% mannitol	Diagnostic aid in renal function determinations; diuretic. Fluid and nutrient replenisher
Ringer's Injection, USP	0.86% sodium chloride, 0.03% potassium chloride, and 0.033% calcium chloride	Fluid and electrolyte replenisher.
Lactated Ringer's Injection, USP	2.7 mEq calcium, 4 mEq potassium, 130 mEq sodium and 2.45 g lactate per liter	Systemic alkalizer; fluid and electrolyte replenisher.
Sodium Chloride Injection, USP	0.9% sodium chloride	Fluid and electrolyte replenisher; isotonic vehicle.

[1] These solutions may be administered in volumes of 1 liter or more, alone, or with other drugs added.

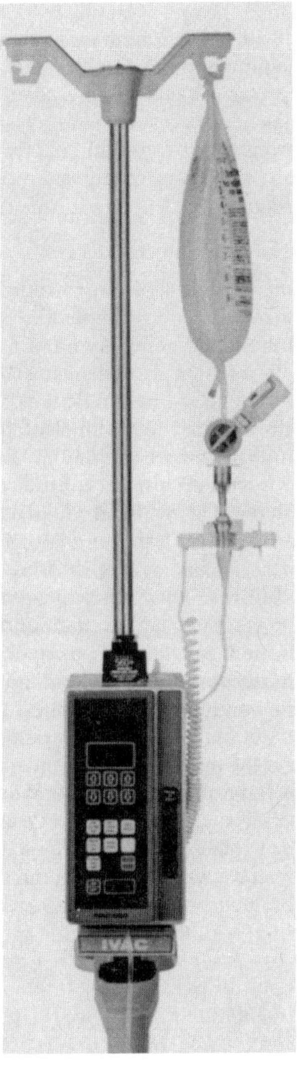

Fig. 8–31. *Accurate delivery of intravenous fluids and medications by use of a controlled rate infusion system (CRIS) for the drug vial and a volumetric infusion pump for the intravenous fluids. (Courtesy of Eli Lilly and Company.)*

liter amounts and more per day by slow intravenous drip with or without controlled-rate infusion systems (Fig. 8–31). Because of the large volumes administered, these solutions must not contain bacteriostatic agents or other pharmaceutical additives. They are packaged in large single-dose containers (Figs. 8–32 and 8–33).

As indicated previously, therapeutic additives as electrolytes, vitamins, and antineoplastics are frequently incorporated into large volume parenterals for coadministration to the patient. It is

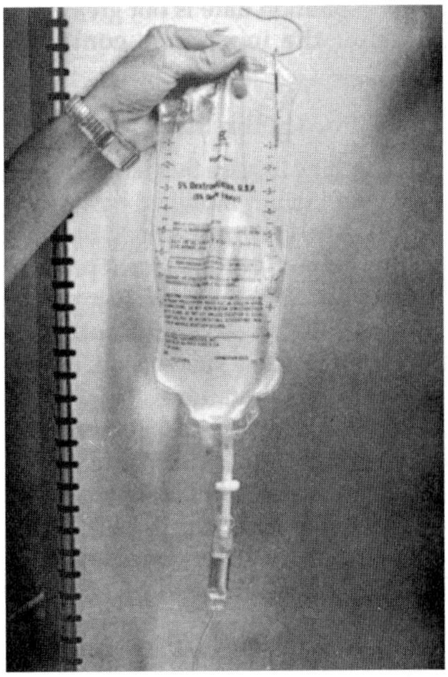

Fig. 8–32. *Intravenous solution packaged in pliable plastic.*

the responsibility of the pharmacist to be knowledgeable of the physical and chemical compatibility of the additive in the solution in which it is placed. Obviously, an incompatible combination which results in the formation of insoluble material or which affects the efficacy or potency of the therapeutic agent of the vehicle is not acceptable.

Large volume parenteral solutions are employed in *maintenance therapy* for the patient entering or recovering from surgery, or for the patient who is unconscious and unable to obtain fluids, electrolytes, and nutrition orally. The solutions may also be utilized in *replacement therapy* in patients who have suffered a heavy loss of fluid and electrolytes.

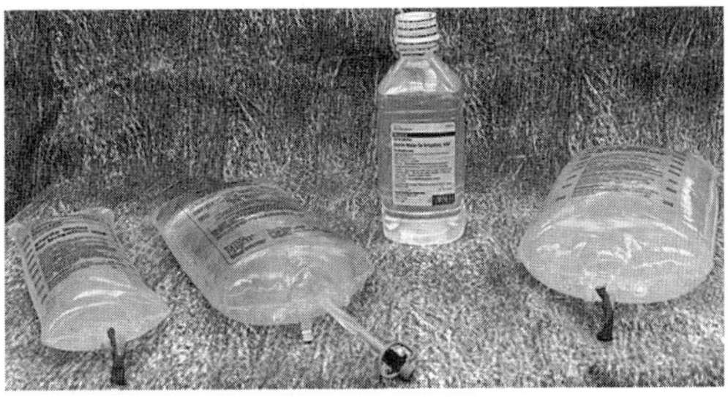

Fig. 8–33. *Examples of peritoneal dialysis and irrigation fluids. (Courtesy of William B. French, PhD.)*

MAINTENANCE THERAPY. When a patient is being maintained on parenteral fluids for only several days, simple solutions providing adequate amounts of water, dextrose, and small amounts of sodium and potassium generally suffice. When patients are unable to take oral nutrition or fluids for slightly longer periods, say 3 to 6 days, solutions of higher caloric content may be used. In instances in which oral feeding must be deferred for periods of weeks or longer, total parenteral nutrition must be implemented to provide all of the essential nutrients to minimize tissue break-down and to maintain normalcy within the body. Total nutrient admixtures (TNA) include all substrates necessary for nutritional support, e.g., carbohydrates, protein, fat, electrolytes, trace elements, that are usually mixed in a single plastic intravenous bag for more convenient administration. These admixtures are very useful for patients undergoing chemotherapy, and for gastrointestinal patients, premature infants, and anorexic patients. When using TNA, the pharmacist must consider the order of substrate mixing, differentiate between various brands of substrate and their physical-chemical properties, determine the type of plastic bag system that is most appropriate to use, determine whether (and by what mode) the TNA should be filtered prior to infusion, determine how the product should be stored, and assess any potential complications that might arise with the use of this method of administering nutritional products. For example, the use of "standard" total parenteral nutrition plastic bags may result in the leaching out of plasticizer into the solution, and be potentially injurious to the patient.

REPLACEMENT THERAPY. In instances in which there is a heavy loss of water and electrolytes, as in severe diarrhea or vomiting, greater than usual amounts of these materials may be initially administered and then maintenance therapy provided. Patients with Crohn's disease, AIDS, burn patients, or those experiencing trauma are candidates for replacement therapy.

WATER REQUIREMENT. In normal individuals, the daily water requirement is that amount needed to replace normal and expected losses. Water is lost daily in the urine, feces, skin and from respiration. The normal daily requirement of water for adults is about 25 to 40 mL/kg of body weight, or an average of about 2,000 mL per square meter of body surface area.[12] Nomograms for the determination of body surface area from body height and weight are presented in Chapter 2, Figure 2–7. Children and small adults need more water per pound of body weight than do larger adults; water requirements correlate more closely with body surface area than with weight. However, in the newborn, the volume administered in the first week or two should be about half that calculated from body surface area.

In water replacement therapy for adults, 70 mL of water per kg per day may be required in addition to the maintenance water requirements; a badly dehydrated infant may require even a greater proportion.[12] Thus, a 50-kg patient may require 3500 mL for replacement plus 2400 mL for maintenance. In order to avoid the consequences of fluid overload, especially in elderly patients, and those with renal or cardiovascular disorders, monitoring of blood pressure is desirable.

Because water administered intravenously as such may cause the osmotic hemolysis of red blood cells, and, since a patient who requires water generally requires nutrition and/or electrolytes, the parenteral administration of water is generally as a solution with dextrose or electrolytes in which the solution has sufficient tonicity (sodium chloride equivalency) to protect the red blood cells from hemolyzing.

ELECTROLYTE REQUIREMENT. Potassium, the primary intracellular cation, is particularly important for normal cardiac and skeletal muscle function. The usual daily intake of potassium is about 100 mEq and the usual daily loss is about 40 mEq. Thus, any replacement therapy should include a minimum of 40 mEq plus the amount needed to replace additional losses. Potassium can be lost through excessive perspiration, repeated enemas, trauma (such as severe burns), uncontrolled diabetes, diseases of the intestinal tract, surgical operations, and the use of such medications as thiazide diuretics. People who suffer from poor nutrition, those using very low-calorie diet products, and victims of anorexia nervosa or acute alcoholism also may have low potassium levels, i.e., hypokalemia, because they are not taking in enough of the mineral. Symptoms of potassium loss include a weak pulse, faint heart sounds, falling blood pressure, and generalized weakness. Severe loss of potassium can lead to death. Too much potassium is not a good thing, either. An excess may cause diarrhea, irritability, muscle cramps, and pain. Hyperkalemia can be caused by kidney failure or consuming excess amounts of potassium-rich foods. Prescribed potassium supplements, potassium-sparing diuretic therapy, and the indiscriminate use of over-the-counter salt-substitute products have also been implicated to induce hyperkalemia.

In cases of severe potassium deficiency, electrolyte replacement through the intravenous administration of potassium is usually employed. The pharmacist who receives a prescription for intravenous potassium chloride must be careful and check the amount of potassium chloride in the prescription and the infusion rate at which the drug is to be administered to the patient. The usual additive dilution of potassium chloride is 40 mEq/liter of intravenous fluid. The maximum desirable concentration is 80 mEq/liter of potassium chloride, although severe emergencies may dictate greater concentrations. The maximum infusion rate should not exceed 40 mEq per hour with a maximum 24-hour dose not exceeding 400 mEq of potassium chloride. Because of its potent ECG effects, when infused it is wise to monitor the patient's ECG, and to check the patient's serum potassium level after the first 50 to 100 mEq of potassium chloride are administered.

Sodium, the principal extracellular cation, is vital to maintain normal extracellular fluids. Average daily intake of sodium is 135 to 170 mEq (8 to 10 g of sodium chloride). The body is able to conserve sodium when this ion is lost or removed from the diet. When there is sodium loss or a deficit, the daily administration of 3 to 5 g of sodium chloride (51 to 85 mEq of sodium) should prevent a negative sodium balance. A low sodium level in the body may result from excessive sweating, the use of certain diuretics, or diarrhea. Fatigue, muscle weakness, apprehension, and convulsions are among the symptoms of excessive sodium loss. Sodium concentrations can increase when a person does not drink enough water, especially in hot weather, or if kidney function is impaired. Dry, sticky mucous membranes, flushed skin, elevated body temperature, lack of tears, and thirst are among the symptoms of sodium excess. In about 20% of individuals who suffer from high blood pressure, sodium has been implicated as a causative factor. Chloride, the principal anion of the extracellular fluid is usually paired with sodium. Chloride is also important for muscle contraction, balancing the fluid levels inside and outside the cells, and maintaining the acid-base balance of the extracellular fluid. An adequate supply of chloride is necessary to prevent bicarbonate, the second most prevalent anion, from tipping the acid-base balance to the alkaline side. (In 1979, a lack of chloride in a brand of infant formula caused metabolic alkalosis in babies who had been exclusively fed that formula. As a result of this episode, Congress passed the Infant Formula Act of 1980, which spells out the nutrients that must be in formulas and establishes quality control procedures for the manufacture of these infant foods.) Although other electrolytes and minerals as calcium, magnesium, and iron are lost from the body, they generally are not required during short-term parenteral therapy.

CALORIC REQUIREMENTS. Generally patients requiring parenteral fluids are given 5% dextrose to reduce the caloric deficit that usually occurs in patients undergoing maintenance or replacement therapy. The use of dextrose also minimizes ketosis and the breakdown of protein. Basic caloric requirements may be estimated by body weight; in the fasting state, the average daily loss of body protein is approximately 80 g/day for a 70 kg man. Daily ingestion of at least 100 g of glucose reduces this loss by half.

PARENTERAL HYPERALIMENTATION. This is the infusion of large amounts of basic nutrients sufficient to achieve active tissue synthesis and growth. It is employed in the long-term intravenous feeding of protein solutions containing high concentrations of dextrose (approximately 20%), electrolytes, vitamins, and in some instances insulin. Among the components utilized in parenteral nutrition solutions are the following, listed in quantities commonly provided per liter of fluid. The individual components and amounts administered to a patient would vary depending upon the patient's needs.

Electrolytes:	
Sodium	25 mEq
Potassium	20 mEq
Magnesium	5 mEq
Calcium	5 mEq
Chloride	30 mEq
Acetate	25 mEq
Phosphate	18 mM
Vitamins:	
Vitamin A	3300 I.U.
Vitamin D	200 I.U.
Vitamin E	10 I.U.
Vitamin C	100 mg
Niacin	40 mg
Vitamin B_2	3.6–4.93 mg
Vitamin B_1	3–3.35 mg

Vitamin B_6	4–4.86 mg
Pantothenic Acid	15 mg
Folic Acid	400 mcg
Vitamin B_{12}	5 mcg
Biotin	60 mcg
Amino Acids: Essential Amino Acids	
L-Isoleucine	590 mg
L-Leucine	770 mg
L-Lysine acetate	870 mg
(free base	620 mg)
L-Methionine	450 mg
L-Phenylalanine	480 mg
L-Threonine	340 mg
L-Tryptophan	130 mg
L-Valine	560 mg
Nonessential Amino Acids	
L-Alanine	600 mg
L-Arginine	810 mg
L-Histidine	240 mg
L-Proline	950 mg
L-Serine	500 mg
Aminoacetic Acid	1.19 g

The large proportion of dextrose increases the caloric value of the solution, while keeping the volume required to be administered to a minimum. The solutions are administered slowly through a large vein, such as the superior vena cava. The superior vena cava is accessed through the subclavian vein, which is located immediately beneath the clavicle and near to the heart. This permits the rapid dilution of the concentrated hyperalimentation fluid and minimizes the risk of tissue or cellular damage due to the hypertonicity of the solution. Generally, final concentrations of dextrose ($\leq$10%) can be given peripherally. Solutions containing dextrose ($>$10%) should be given via the central route, i.e., the superior vena cava.

Figure 8–34 demonstrates a Nutrimix Macro TPN Compounder. This device can pump four nutritional solutions (i.e., dextrose, water, amino acids, fat) simultaneously to compound nutritional admixtures by gravimetric means. The user programs the volume and specific gravity of the fluid to be pumped and the device calculates the weight of the solution that has to be transferred from the source station to the patient bag. The fifth load cell serves as a confirmation of the weights programmed vs. weights delivered.

With the increasing use of parenteral solutions in the pediatric population, including parenteral nutrition solutions, pharmacists are frequently confronted with inquiries concerning the appropriate method of parenteral drug delivery.[11] A dilemma with pediatric patients is that they often have a limited fluid capacity caused by disease (e.g., congestive heart failure, renal insufficiency) and limited vascular access. As a consequence, pharmacists are asked whether a medication can be administered along with a parenteral nutrition solution. Although this practice is to be discouraged, in the pediatric population it may be the only way to ensure that the patient is receiving adequate nutrition as well as appropriate drug therapy. Further, by administering the medication with the PN solution, rather than interrupting the PN to administer medication, rebound hypoglycemia is less likely to develop in the patient. The pharmacist must remember that the practice of administering medication through a central venous line intended for PN solutions is not without risks. Catheter sepsis and occlusion can result.

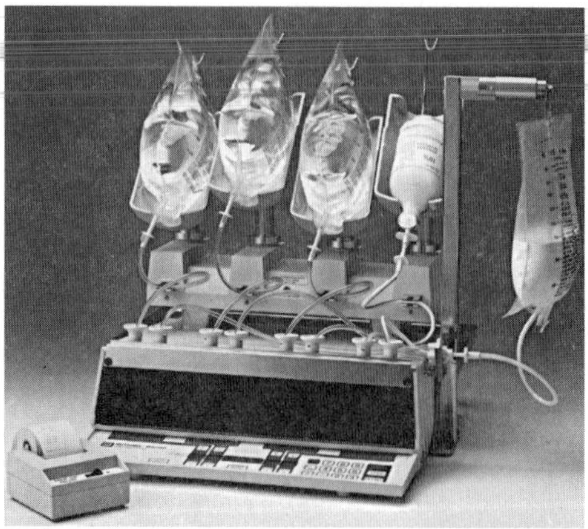

Fig. 8–34. *Nutrimix Macro TPN Compounder. (Courtesy of Abbott Hospital Products Division.)*

Usually, TPNs are prepared 1 liter at a time. However, to conserve pharmacist and nursing time, it is not uncommon to prepare two or three 1-liter bags or one 2- or 3-liter bag (e.g., Viaflex) to be administered over a 24-hour period. The disadvantage is waste, if the physician needs to adjust the formulation dosages downward at times during the day.

The following abbreviations may be used in the hospital in describing the desired order for parenteral nutrition:

TCPN (Total Central Parenteral Nutrition)
PCPN (Partial Central Parenteral Nutrition)

TPPN (Total Peripheral Parenteral Nutrition)
PPPN (Partial Peripheral Parenteral Nutrition)

ENTERAL NUTRITION. As appropriate, hospitalized and home care patients may be provided their nutritional needs through *enteral* rather than *parenteral* means. Enteral nutrition products may be administered orally, via nasogastric tube, via feeding gastrostomy, or via needle-catheter jejunostomy. These products are formulated to contain a variety of vitamins, minerals, carbohydrates, proteins, fats and caloric requirements to meet the specific needs of patients. While parenteral feeding is appropriate for short-term use in a hospital or long-term care facility, or when the gastrointestinal tract is unable to absorb nutrients, enteral feeding is preferable whenever possible. It is just as effective as a source of nutrients, less expensive than parenteral feeding, and has a low potential to cause serious complications.

The defined formula diets may be monomeric or oligomeric (i.e., amino acids or short peptides and simple carbohydrates) or polymeric (more complex protein and carbohydrate sources). Modular supplements are used for individual supplementation of protein (ProMod powder, Propac powder), carbohydrate (Moducal powder), or fat (Lipomul liquid) when formulas do not offer sufficient flexibility. For example, a physician may order a powder reconstituted one-quarter strength, half-strength, or full strength for a particular patient and then have this administered via a nasogastric tube, a feeding gastrostomy, or a needle-catheter jejunostomy.

There is no single classification system for these products, and there are different criteria for evaluating and categorizing them. Caloric density (generally in the range of 1, 1.5, or 2 kcal/mL) influences the density of other nutrients. Protein content is also a major determinant in these products. For those patients who experience diarrhea and cramping, high osmolality formulas may present difficulty. Low-fat-content products should be suggested for patients with significant malabsorption, hyperlipidemia, or severe exocrine pancreatic insufficiency. Medium chain triglycerides (MCT), while providing a useful source of energy in patients with malabsorption, do not provide essential fatty acids.

Originally, enteral feedings contained lactose and presented problems in lactase-deficient individuals. This ingredient has been eliminated from many of the nutritionally complete enteral formulas. For those patients with hepatic or renal disease, the sodium and potassium content of the formulations must be considered. For patients maintained on warfarin therapy, consideration should be focused on the content of Vitamin K in the formulation. Although many products now have less Vitamin K than before, caution is still warranted to avoid hypoprothrombinemic alterations in warfarin therapy.

Specific enteral products are selected according to the patient type they serve. For example, a requirement for less than 2000 calories per day, or increased protein typically involves an elderly, bedfast patient who is not physically active. This level of support is also advocated for postsurgical patients, and those who suffer from infection or fractured bones. While requiring fewer calories, these individuals still need normal nutrients, including protein. Such products as Ensure HN, Sustacal, and Osmolite HN are appropriate in this circumstance. Alternatively, most persons fall within the 2000 to 3000 calorie per day category, inclusive of patients with poor appetite or those suffering from cancer. The last category of patients are those with daily caloric needs which exceed 3000 calories. These individuals usually have high protein losses from severe trauma, e.g., burns, sepsis, multiple trauma. As in the first example there are numerous products for the latter two patient categories.

The pharmacist can be helpful in the selection of these products because these do differ in the amount of their carbohydrate, fat, and protein content, and in fiber. Further, these products differ in taste and consumer acceptability criteria, e.g., "mouth feel," cost. Pharmacists may encounter consumers who wish to self-administer an enteral product. If the intent is to supplement calories or protein in an otherwise healthy individual who simply wishes to assure a balanced dietary intake, a complete formula can be recommended. However, if it is intended to help a person regain weight which has been lost unexpectedly, the individual should be instead referred to a doctor. Sudden weight loss may indicate a serious pathologic problem requiring medical attention.

Pharmacists can also be helpful in cost management associated with these products. Composition (oligomeric or polymeric) and form (ready-to-use vs. powder) of the product influence cost. Generally, the polymeric products are less expensive than the oligomeric products.

While powder forms may be less expensive compared to ready-to-use formulations, there is an indirect cost of labor required in the powder preparation.

INTRAVENOUS INFUSION DEVICES. Since the early 1970s, the use of the intravenous route to administer drugs has become increasingly popular. In 1989, it was estimated that about 40% of all drugs and fluid administered in the hospital setting are done through intravenous administration.[12] This increase has affected the development and use of mechanical infusion devices. Advances in infusion technology and computer technology have resulted in devices with extremely sophisticated drug-delivery capabilities (e.g., multiple-rate programming, pump or controller operation).[13] As a result, these cost-efficient devices provide greater accuracy and reliability of drug delivery than the traditional gravity-flow infusion methods. They also help reduce the fluid volume attributable to the medication infusion and decrease the need for monitoring fluid input (thus, decreased nursing time). Further, multiple-drug dosages can be administered, and incompatible drugs can be administered separately.[12]

There are disadvantages associated with these mechanical devices, however, including the initial capital investment and extensive in-service education. Further, the influence of infusion pump devices on the delivery of a drug has not been fully recognized by clinicians. For example, intrinsic factors (operating mechanisms, flow accuracy, flow continuity, occlusion detection) and an extrinsic factor (backpressure) may alter the rate of drug delivery and the corresponding therapeutic response of the patient.

Pumps are classified by their *mechanism of operation* (peristaltic, piston, diaphragm), *frequency or type of drug delivery* (continuous or intermittent, bolus dosing, single-solution or multiple-solution), or *therapeutic application* (patient-controlled analgesia [PCA]).[14] Current research focuses upon the influence of drug delivery by these devices and the creation of new technologies (e.g., implantable pumps, pumps with chronobiological applications, osmotic-pressure devices, and open- or closed-loop systems).[14]

Biologics

In pharmacy, the broad term *biologics* refers to such pharmaceutical products as vaccines, toxins, toxoids, antitoxins, immune serums, blood derivatives, immunologic diagnostic aids, and other related preparations. The usual intent of the term is to describe materials of biologic origin having *immunologic* effects. In the modern context, immunologic agents may be of biologic and non-biologic origin, as cyclosporine. With current immunologic research and combined with the new biotechnologies, many new immunologic agents will be forthcoming in the future. There is some interest in abandoning the term "biologics" in favor of the term "immunologics." The term "immunobiologics" includes both antigenic substances, as vaccines and toxoids, and antibody-containing preparations, as globulins and antitoxins, from human or animal donors. For the most part, biologics are administered by injection (a notable exception being the oral type of polio vaccine), and for this reason they are presented in this chapter.

Biologics are produced by manufacturers licensed to do so in accordance with the terms of the federal Public Health Service Act of 1944, and each product must meet the specified standards of the Bureau of Biologics of the federal Food and Drug Administration. Generally, each lot of a biologic product must pass rigid control requirements before it may be distributed for general use.

Biologics intended to be administered by injection are packaged and labeled in the same manner as other injections. In addition, however, the label of a biological product must include the name under which the product is licensed under the Public Health Service Act; the name, address, and license number of the manufacturer; the lot number; the expiration date; the recommended individual dose for multiple-dose containers; the preservative used and the amount; the amount of product in the container; the recommended storage temperature; and any other necessary information to assure the safe and effective use of the product.

With a few exceptions most biologics are stored in a refrigerator at between 2°C and 8°C, and freezing is avoided. In many instances it is not the biologic substance that is harmed by freezing, but rather the container which may be broken through the freezing and expansion of an aqueous vehicle so that some of the product is lost. The expiration date for biological products varies with the product and the storage temperatures employed. Generally, most biological products have an expiration date of a year or longer after the date of manufacture or issue. Biologics must be dispensed in their original containers in order to avoid contamination and deterioration. They are sterile when packaged and are injected by aseptic techniques.

As indicated by the listings in Table 8–8 some biologics are diagnostic aids, others are prophylactic, and some are therapeutic. Although it is not within the scope of this book to undertake a discussion of immunity, some brief definitions may assist in the understanding of the use of the official products presented. Also, it is not the intent here to discuss the detailed methods of preparation for these biologics, and only brief descriptions of the products are given. If additional information is desired, the student is encouraged to read other references.

Immunity—The power of the body to resist and overcome infection.

Natural, Innate, or Native Immunity—A constitutional attribute of individuals who because of race, species specificity, endocrine balance, and other factors may be resistant to a particular toxic agent. It is something with which they are born and is not acquired through the use of biologics.

Acquired Immunity—A specific immunity that may be actively acquired (active immunity) or passively acquired (passive immunity).

Active Immunity—Specific immunity developed in an individual in response to the introduction of antigenic substances into his body. This may occur by natural means, as by infection, in which case it is termed *naturally acquired active immunity*, or it may be developed in response to the administration of a specific vaccine or toxoid, in which case it is termed *artificially acquired active immunity*. In either case, the body builds up its own defenses in response to the antigen.

Passive Immunity—Immunity developed by the introduction of already formed antibodies into the body to combat the specific antigen. If the antibodies are passed to the individual naturally, as by the placental transfer of antibodies from the mother to the fetus, the term *naturally acquired passive immunity* applies. However, if the antibodies are passed on to the individual through the injection of a specific antitoxin, the immunity is referred to as *artificially acquired passive immunity*. Passive immunity is not long-lasting.

Vaccines—Agents administered primarily for prophylactic action in the development of active immunity (acquired). Vaccines may contain living, attenuated (weakened), or killed viruses; killed rickettsia; or killed bacteria.

Toxoids—Toxins modified and detoxified by the use of moderate heat and chemical treatment so that the antigenic properties remain. They are employed for the development of active immunity.

Toxins—Poisonous bacterial products that act as antigens and cause the human body to develop specific antibodies to combat their presence. Most toxins are used for diagnostic purposes to determine the susceptibility of the patient to the disease caused by the toxin-containing organism.

Antitoxins—Substances prepared from the blood of animals, usually horses, which have been immunized by repeated injections of specific bacterial toxins. The resulting antitoxins produce passive immunity, or they may be used for curative purposes for persons already known to be infected by the specific antigen.

Antiserums—Serums prepared in the same manner as the antitoxins, except that bacteria or viruses are injected into the animal to stimulate the production of specific antibodies. The antibody-rich blood serum may be employed to produce passive immunity.

Human Immune Serums and Globulins—Serums containing the specific antibodies obtained from the blood of humans and produced as a result of having had the specific disease or having been immunized against it with a specific biologic product. They provide passive immunity.

A recommended immunization schedule for infants and children is presented in Table 8–9.

According to the National Childhood Vaccine Injury Act of 1986, health care-providers who administer certain vaccines and toxoids are required to record permanently and to report adverse effects resulting from the use of one of the biologic products. Among the products included in the law are diphtheria and tetanus toxoids and pertussis vaccine (DTP), pertussis vaccine, measles, mumps and rubella vaccines, tetanus and

Table 8–8. Examples of Official Biologic Products

Biologic Product	*Nature of Contents*	*Route of Administration*[1]	*Use*
Vaccines and Vaccine Combinations			
BCG Vaccine, USP	Dried, living culture of the bacillus Calmette-Guerin strain of *Mycobacterium tuberculosis* var. *bovis.*	Percutaneous via a multiple-puncture device	Active immunizing agent (tuberculosis)
Cholera Vaccine, USP	Suspension of inactivated cholera vibrios (*Vibrio cholerae*).	Intramuscular or subcutaneous	Active immunizing agent
Hepatitis B Vaccine	Originally, biochemically and biophysically inactivated human hepatitis B surface antigen (HBsAg) particles, obtained by plasmapheresis from plasma of screened chronic HBsAG carriers. Currently, only recombinant vaccines derived from HBsAg produced in yeast cells are available in the U.S.	Intramuscular	Active immunizing agent
Influenza Virus Vaccine, USP	Aqueous suspension of inactivated influenza virus prepared from allantoic fluid of influenza virus-infected chick embryo in a phosphate-buffered isotonic sodium chloride injection.	Intramuscular or subcutaneous	Active immunizing agent
Measles Virus Vaccine Live, USP	Live, attenuated Enders' line measles virus derived from attenuated Edmonston strain in chick embryo cell cultures.	Subcutaneous	Active immunizing agent
Measles, Mumps, and Rubella Virus Vaccine Live, USP	Combination of viruses propagated in chick embryo tissue (measles and mumps) and in human diploid cell cultures (rubella).	Subcutaneous	Active immunizing agent
Measles and Rubella Virus Vaccine Live, USP	Live viral vaccine with the measles virus grown on chicken embryo tissue and the rubella virus on duck embryo tissue.	Subcutaneous	Active immunizing agent
Mumps Virus Vaccine Live, USP	Live, attenuated organisms of the Jeryl Lynn (B level) strain of mumps virus propagated in chick embryo tissue cultures.	Subcutaneous	Active immunizing agent
Plague Vaccine, USP	Suspension of inactivated 195/P strain of plague bacilli (*Yersinia pestis*) in 0.9% sodium chloride injection.	Intramuscular	Active immunizing agent
Pneumococcal Vaccine, Polyvalent	A sterile solution containing antigenic capsular polysaccharides extracted from *Streptococcus pneumoniae.* This vaccine contains 23 capsular polysaccharide types. Each 0.5 ml dose of the vaccine contains 25 μg of each type of capsule polysaccharide dissolved in 0.9% sodium chloride injection. The vaccine also contains phenol or thimerosal as a preservative.	Subcutaneous or intramuscular	Active immunizing agent
Poliovirus Vaccine Live Oral, USP	A preparation of one or a combination of the three types of live, attenuated polioviruses, grown separately in primary cultures of monkey kidney tissue.	Oral	Active immunizing agent
Rabies Vaccine, USP	A preparation of inactivated rabies virus harvested from human (HDCV) or rhesus diploid-cell (RDCV) cultures.	HDCV—intramuscular or intradermal; RDCV—intramuscular only	Active immunizing agent
Rubella Virus Vaccine Live, USP	Live rubella (German measles) virus propagated in human diploid cell culture.	Subcutaneous	Active immunizing agent
Rubella and Mumps Viral Vaccine Live, USP	Combination of rubella virus propagated in human diploid cell culture and mumps virus grown on chicken embryo tissue.	Subcutaneous	Active immunizing agent
Smallpox Vaccine, USP	A dried form of living virus of vaccinia that has been grown in the skin of a vaccinated bovine calf.	Percutaneous	Active immunizing agent
Typhoid Vaccine, USP	Parenteral heat/phenol-inactivated *Salmonella typhi* of Ty2 strain or oral form, as enteric-coated capsules, lyophilized, live *S. typhi* of the attenuated Ty21a strain.	Subcutaneous or intradermal; oral	Active immunizing agent
Yellow Fever Vaccine, USP	Dried, frozen, attenuated strain of living yellow fever virus prepared by culturing the virus in the living chick embryo prepared, processed, freeze-dried, and sealed under nitrogen	Subcutaneous	Active immunizing agent

Table 8–8. Continued

Biologic Product	*Nature of Contents*	*Route of Administration*[1]	*Use*
Toxoids			
Diphtheria and Tetanus Toxoids Adsorbed, USP	Suspension prepared by mixing adsorbed diphtheria toxoid and adsorbed tetanus toxoid.	Deep intramuscular	Active immunizing agent
Tetanus Toxoid, USP	Suspension of formaldehyde-treated products of growth of the tetanus bacillus (*Clostridium tetani*).	Intramuscular or subcutaneous	Active immunizing agent
Tetanus Toxoid Adsorbed, USP	Suspension of tetanus toxoid precipitated or adsorbed by the addition of alum, aluminum hydroxide, or aluminum phosphate.	Deep intramuscular	Active immunizing agent
Tetanus and Diphtheria Toxoids Adsorbed for Adult Use, USP	Suspension of tetanus toxoid and diphtheria toxoid adsorbed by addition of alum, aluminum hydroxide, or aluminum phosphate.	Intramuscular	Active immunizing agent
Antitoxins			
Botulism Antitoxin, USP	Solution of refined and concentrated proteins, chiefly globulins, containing antitoxin obtained from the blood serum or plasma of healthy horses immunized against the toxins produced by both type A and B strains of *Clostridium botulinum*.	Intramuscular or intravenous	Passive immunizing agent
Tetanus Antitoxin, USP	Solution of the refined and concentrated proteins, chiefly globulins, containing antitoxic antibodies obtained from the blood serum or plasma of a healthy animal, usually the horse, that has been immunized against tetanus toxoid or toxin.	Intramuscular or subcutaneous (prophylactic) or intravenous (therapeutic)	Passive immunizing agent
Immune Globulin IM (IGIM)	Nonpyrogenic solution of globulins containing many antibodies normally present in adult human blood prepared by cold alcohol fractionation of pooled plasma from venous blood of at least 1000 individuals.	Intramuscular	Passive immunity to hepatitis A and B infections, measles, rubella, varicella zoster, primary immunodeficiency diseases.
Immune Globulin IV (IGIV)	Nonpyrogenic solution of globulins containing many antibodies normally present in adult human blood prepared by cold alcohol fractionation of pooled plasma from venous blood of at least 1000 individuals.	Intravenous	Primary immunodeficiency diseases, HIV infections, idiopathic thrombocytopenia purpura, and beta-cell chronic lymphocytic leukemia.
Rh_o (D) Immune Globulin	Prepared from plasma or serum of adults with a high titer of anti-Rh_o antibody to the red blood cell antigen Rh_o (D). It contains 10–18% protein, of which not less than 90% is immunoglobulin G (gamma globulin, IgG). Commercially available solutions contain glycine as a stabilizing agent and thimerosal as a preservative; pH is adjusted with sodium carbonate or sodium chloride.	Intramuscular	Passive immunizing agent
Vaccinia Immune Globulin, USP	Sterile solution of globulins from blood plasmas of human donors who have been immunized with vaccinia virus smallpox vaccine.	Intramuscular	Passive immunizing agent
Tetanus Immune Globulin, USP	Solution of globulins derived from the blood plasma of adult human donors who have been hyperimmunized with tetanus toxoid.	Intramuscular	Passive immunizing agent

Table 8–8. Continued

Biologic Product	*Nature of Contents*	*Route of Administration*[1]	*Use*
Miscellaneous Biologic Products			
Antivenin (Crotalidae) Polyvalent, USP	A preparation derived by drying a frozen solution of specific venom-neutralizing globulins obtained from the serum of healthy horses immunized against venoms of four species of pit vipers, *Crotalus atrox*, *C. adamanteus*, *C. durissus terrificus*, and *Bothrops atrox*.	Intramuscular or intravenous	To neutralize the toxic effects of venoms of crotalids native to North, Central and South America
Histoplasmin, USP	Liquid concentrate of the soluble growth products developed by the fungus *Histoplasma capsulatum* when grown in the mycelial phase on a synthetic medium.	Intradermal	Diagnostic aid (histoplasmosis)
Plasma Protein Fraction, USP	Solution of selected proteins derived from the blood plasma of adult human donors. It contains about 5% of protein, about 85% of which is albumin, the remainder alpha and beta globulins.	Intravenous	Blood-volume expansion
Tuberculin, USP	Solution of the concentrated, soluble products of growth of the tubercle bacillus, *Mycobacterium tuberculosis*. (Old Tuberculin), or, a soluble partially purified product of growth of the tubercle bacillus prepared in a special liquid medium free from protein (Purified Protein Derivative, PPD).	Intradermal	Diagnostic aid (tuberculosis)

[1] The doses to be administered and the schedule of doses vary widely, depending upon the patient's age, exposure, previous record of immunizations, etc.

diphtheria toxoids, and poliovirus vaccines, both live and inactivated. The health-care provider who observes an adverse effect must permanently record the findings in the patient's medical record and report the incident to the U.S. Department of Health and Human Services as well as to local and state health authorities. Reporting of the adverse effects includes such conditions as anaphylactic shock, encephalitis, and seizures.

Table 8–9. Recommended Immunization Schedule[1]

Age	*Immunizations*
2 months	diphtheria, pertussis, tetanus,[2] polio[3]
4 months	DPT, TOPV
6 months	DPT
15 months	mumps, measles, rubella[4], DPT, TOPV
18 months	Hemophilus b Polysaccharide Vaccine
4–6 years	DPT, TOPV
14–16 years	Td[5] and every 10 years thereafter

[1] Adapted from *Morbidity and Mortality Weekly Report*, Centers for Disease Control, *38*:210, 1989.

[2] May be given combined as DPT: Diphtheria (pediatric) toxoid, tetanus toxoid, and pertussis vaccine.

[3] Usually given as TOPV: trivalent live oral polio vaccine, adsorbed.

[4] May be given as the combined vaccine: MMR.

[5] Combined tetanus and diphtheria (adult) toxoids for anyone over the age of 6.

Other Injectable Products—Pellets or Implants

Historically, pellets or implants were sterile, small, usually cylindrical-shaped solid objects about 3.2 mm in diameter and 8 mm in length, prepared by compression and intended to be implanted subcutaneously for the purpose of providing the continuous release of medication over a prolonged period of time. The pellets, which are implanted under the skin (usually of the thigh or abdomen) with a special injector or by surgical incision, are used for potent hormones. Their implantation provides the patient with an economical means of obtaining long-lasting effects (up to many months after a single implantation) and obviates the need for frequent parenteral or oral hormone therapy. The implanted pellet, which might contain 100 times the amount of drug (e.g., desoxycorticosterone, estradiol, testosterone) given by other routes of administration, release the drug slowly into the general circulation.

Pellets were formulated with no binders, diluents, or excipients, to permit total dissolution and absorption of the pellet from the site of im-

MilliEquivalents

An *equivalent weight* is the atomic weight, in grams, of a material divided by its valence, or charge. MilliEquivalents are related to equivalents, which are also considered measures of combining power, chemical activity, or chemical reactivity. Equivalency, or milliEquivalency, takes into consideration the total number of ionic charges in solution and the valence of the ions. Normally, plasma contains about 155 milliEquivalents of cations and anions in solution. The number of cations is always matched by the number of anions.

A *milliEquivalent* is the quantity, in mg, of a solute equal to 1/1000 of its gram-equivalent weight. Consider the following example.

EXAMPLE 1

What is the milliEquivalent weight of sodium?

1. The atomic weight of sodium is 23.
2. The valence of sodium is +1.
3. The equivalent weight of sodium is (23 g)/(1) = 23 g.
4. The milliEquivalent weight of sodium is (23 g)/1000 = 0.023 g, or 23 mg.
5. Therefore, one milliEquivalent of sodium weighs 23 mg.

MilliEquivalent calculations are commonly required in pharmacy practice today. The following are some examples.

EXAMPLE 2

How many milliEquivalents of potassium chloride are in a solution containing 74.5 mg/mL?

1. The atomic weight of potassium is 39 and chloride is 35.5. The combined molecular weight is 74.5.
2. Since the valence is 1 for both potassium and chloride, the equivalent weight for potassium chloride is 74.5 g and the milliEquivalent weight is 74.5 mg.
3. The solution contains 74.5 mg/mL, and the milliEquivalent weight is 74.5 mg; therefore, there is 1 mEq of potassium chloride in the solution.

EXAMPLE 3

How many milliEquivalents of calcium are in 10 mL of 10% calcium chloride ($CaCl_2.2\ H_2O$) solution?

1. The formula weight for calcium chloride dihydrate is 147.
2. The equivalent weight is 147/2 = 73.5, since calcium is divalent.
3. Therefore, 1 milliEquivalent of calcium chloride weighs 73.5 mg.
4. (10 mL) (10%) = 1 g, or 1000 mg) of calcium chloride dihydrate.
5. (1000 mg)/(73.5 mg) = 13.6 mEq of calcium chloride dihydrate, which also is 13.6 mEq of calcium.

EXAMPLE 4

How many milliEquivalents of sodium are contained in a 1 liter bag of 0.9% sodium chloride solution?

1. (1000 mL) (0.009) = 9 g, or 9000 mg.
2. The formula weight for sodium chloride is 23 + 35.5 = 58.5.
3. The milliEquivalent weight for sodium chloride is 58.5 mg.
4. (9000)/(58.5) = 153.8 mEq, or 154 mEq.

In these cases, since sodium chloride is monovalent, there are 154 mEq of sodium, 154 mEq of chloride, or 154 mEq of sodium chloride.

Osmolality and Tonicity

Biologic systems are compatible with solutions having similar osmotic pressures, i.e., an equivalent number of dissolved species. For example, red blood cells, blood plasma, and 0.9% sodium chloride solution contain approximately the same number of solute particles per unit volume and are termed iso-osmotic and isotonic.

If solutions do not contain the same number of dissolved species i.e., they contain more (hypertonic) or less (hypotonic), then it may be necessary to alter the composition of the solution to bring them into an acceptable range.

An osmol (Osm) is related to a mole (gram molecular weight) of the molecules or ions in solution. One mole of glucose (180 g) dissolved in 1000 g of water has an osmolality of 1 Osm, or 1000 mOsm per kg of water. One mole of sodium chloride (23 + 35.5 = 58.5 g) dissolved in 1000 g of water has an osmolality of almost 2000 mOsm, since sodium chloride dissociates into almost two particles per molecule. In other words, a 1 molal solution of sodium chloride is equivalent to a 2 molal solution of dextrose.

Normal serum osmolality values are in the vicinity of 285 mOsm/kg (often expressed as 285 mOsm/L). Ranges may include values from about 275 to 300 mOsm/L). Pharmaceuticals should be close to this value to minimize discomfort on application to the eyes or nose, or when injected.

Some solutions may be iso-osmotic but not isotonic. This is because the physiology of the cell membranes must be considered. For example, the cell membrane of the red blood cell is not semi-permeable to all drugs. It allows ammonium chloride, alcohol, boric acid, glycerin, propylene glycol, and urea to diffuse freely. In the eye, the cell membrane is semi-permeable to boric acid, and a 1.9% solution of boric acid is an isotonic ophthalmic solution. But even though a 1.9% solution of boric acid is isotonic with the eye and is iso-osmotic, it is not isotonic with blood—since boric acid can freely diffuse through the red blood cells—and it may cause hemolysis.

Pharmacists are often called upon to calculate the quantity of solute that must be added to adjust a hypotonic solution of a drug to isotonic. This can be done using several methods, including the "L," sodium chloride equivalent, and cryoscopic methods.

One of the most frequently used methods for calculating the quantity of sodium chloride necessary to prepare an isotonic solution is the *sodium chloride equivalent method.* A "sodium chloride equivalent" is defined as the amount of sodium chloride that is osmotically equivalent to 1 g of the drug. For example, the sodium chloride equivalent of ephedrine sulfate is 0.23 (i.e., 1 g of ephedrine sulfate would be equivalent to 0.23 g of sodium chloride).

EXAMPLE 1

How much sodium chloride is required to make the following prescription isotonic?

Rx Ephedrine sulfate 2%
Sterile water, qs 30 mL
M. isoton with sodium chloride.

1. (30 mL) (0.009) = 0.270 g sodium chloride would be required if only sodium chloride was present in the 30 mL of solution.
2. (30 mL) (0.02) = 0.6 g ephedrine sulfate is to be present.
3. (0.6 g) (0.23) = 0.138 g is the quantity of sodium chloride "represented" by the ephedrine sulfate present.
4. Since 0.270 g sodium chloride would be required if only sodium chloride is used, and the quantity of sodium chloride that is equivalent to 0.6 g of ephedrine sulfate is 0.138 g, then 0.270 − 0.138 g = 0.132 g of sodium chloride would be required to render the solution isotonic.
5. Therefore, to prepare the solution would require 0.6 grams of ephedrine sulfate, 0.132 grams of sodium chloride, and sufficient sterile water to make 30 mL.

plantation. Recently, a levonorgestrel implant contraceptive system was developed. Rather than dissolute entirely, the surgically implanted capsules are intended to be removed subsequently by surgery after an appropriate amount of time (up to 5 years).

Levonorgestrel Implants

These are a set of six flexible, closed capsules of a dimethylsiloxane/methylvinylsiloxane copolymer, each containing 36 mg of the progestin levonorgestrel.[15] These are found in an insertion kit to facilitate surgical subdermal implantation through a 2 mm incision in the mid-portion of the upper arm about eight to ten cm above the elbow crease. These are implanted in a fan-like pattern, about 15° apart, for a total of 75°. Appropriate insertion facilitates removal by the end of the fifth year. This system provides long-term (up to 5 years) reversible contraception.

Diffusion of the levonorgestrel through the wall of each capsule provides a continuous low dose of progestin. Initially, the dose of levonorgestrel is about 85 mcg/day, followed by a decline to about 50 mcg/day by 9 months, and to about 35 mcg/day by 18 months, with a further decline thereafter to about 30 mcg/day. The resulting blood levels are substantially below those generally observed among users of combination oral contraceptives containing the progestins norgestrel or levonorgestrel. Because of the range of variability in blood levels and variation in individual response, blood levels alone are not predictive of the risk of pregnancy in an individual woman.[15]

Irrigation and Dialysis Solutions

Solutions for irrigation of body tissues and for dialysis resemble parenteral solutions in that they are subject to the same stringent standards. The difference is in their use. These solutions are not injected into the vein, but employed outside of the circulatory system. Since they are generally used in large volumes, they are packaged in large volume containers, generally of the screw-cap type which permits the rapid pouring of the solution.

Irrigation Solutions

Irrigation solutions are intended to bathe or wash wounds, surgical incisions, or body tissues. Examples are presented in Table 8–10.

Dialysis Solutions

Dialysis may be defined as a process whereby substances may be separated from one another

Table 8–10. Examples of Irrigation Solutions

Solution	*Description*
Acetic Acid Irrigation, USP	This solution is employed topically to the bladder as a 0.25% solution for irrigation. It has a pH of between 2.9 and 3.3 and is employed during urologic procedures. It is administered to wash blood and surgical debris away while maintaining suitable conditions for the tissue and permitting the surgeon an unobstructed view.
Neomycin and Polymyxin B Sulfates Solution for Irrigation, USP	This solution is employed as a topical antibacterial in the continuous irrigation of the bladder.
Ringer's Irrigation, USP	This solution contains sodium chloride, potassium chloride, and calcium chloride in purified water, in the same proportions, as is present in Ringer's Injection. The solution is sterile and pyrogen-free. It is used topically as an irrigation and must be labeled "not for injection."
Sodium Chloride Irrigation, USP	This solution contains 0.9% sodium chloride which is isotonic with body fluids. The solution is employed topically to wash wounds and into body cavities where absorption into the blood is not likely. The solution may also be employed rectally as an enema; for simple evacuation, 150 mL is usually employed and for colonic flush, 1500 mL may be used.
Sterile Water for Irrigation, USP	This is water for injection that has been sterilized and suitably packaged. The label must state "for irrigation only" and "not for injection." The water must not contain any antimicrobial or other added agent.

in solution by taking advantage of their differing diffusibility through membranes. *Peritoneal dialysis* solutions, allowed to flow into the peritoneal cavity, are used to remove toxic substances normally excreted by the kidney. In cases of poisoning or kidney failure, or in patients awaiting renal transplants, dialysis is an emergency lifesaving procedure. Solutions are commercially available containing dextrose as a major source of calories, vitamins, minerals, electrolytes, and amino acids or peptides as a source of nitrogen. The solutions are made to be hypertonic (with dextrose) to plasma to avoid absorption of water from the dialysis solution into the circulation.

Peritoneal dialysis involves the principles of osmosis and diffusion across the semipermeable peritoneal membrane and includes the osmotic and chemical equilibration of the fluid within the peritoneal cavity with that of the extracellular compartment. The semipermeable peritoneal membrane restricts the movement of formed elements (e.g., erythrocytes) and large molecules (e.g., protein) but allows the movement of smaller molecules (e.g., electrolytes, urea, water) in both directions across the membrane according to the concentration on each side of the membrane, with net movement occurring in the direction of the concentration gradient. Instillation of dialysis solutions containing physiologic concentrations of electrolytes intraperitoneally allows for the movement of water, toxic substances and/or metabolites across the membrane in the direction of the concentration gradient, resulting in removal of these substances from the body following drainage of the solution from the peritoneal cavity (i.e., outflow).

Hemodialysis is employed to remove toxins from the blood. In this method, the arterial blood is shunted through a polyethylene catheter through an artificial dialyzing membrane bathed in an electrolyte solution. Following the dialysis, the blood is returned to the body circulation through a vein.

Various dialysis solutions are available commercially and the pharmacist may be called upon to provide them or to make adjustments in their composition.

References

1. Rapp, R.P., Bivins, B.A., Littrell, R.A., and Foster, T.S.: Patient-controlled analgesia: A review of effectiveness of therapy and an evaluation of currently available devices. *DICP, The Annals of Pharmacotherapy 23*:899–904, 1989.
2. Kwan, J.W.: Use of infusion devices for epidural or intrathecal administration of spinal opiods. *Am. J. Hosp. Pharm., 47 (Suppl 1)*:S18–S23, 1990.
3. Erstad, B.L. and Meeks, M.L.: Influence of injection site and route on medication absorption. *Hosp. Pharm. 28*:853–856; 858–860; 863–864, 867–868; 871–874; 877–878, 1993.
4. Butler, L.D., Munson, J.M., and DeLuca, P.P.: Effect of inline filtration on the potency of low-dose drugs. *Am. J. Hosp. Pharm. 37*:935–941, 1980.
5. Turco, S., Miele, W.H., and Barnoski, D.: Evaluation of an aseptic technique testing and challenge kit (Attack). *Hosp. Pharm. 28*:11–16, 1993.
6. Crawford, S.Y., Narducci, W.A., and Augustine, S.C.: National survey of quality assurance activities for pharmacy-prepared sterile products in hospitals. *Am. J. Hosp. Pharm. 48*:2398–2413, 1991.
7. American Journal of Hospital Pharmacy.: ASHP technical assistance bulletin on quality assurance for pharmacy-prepared sterile products. *Am. J. Hosp. Pharm. 50*:2386–2398, 1993.
8. ASHP.: Draft guidelines on quality assurance for pharmacy-prepared sterile products. *Am. J. Hosp. Pharm. 49*:407–417, 1992.
9. Erskine, C.R.: Quality assurance and control. *In* Gennaro, A.R. ed., *Remington's Pharmaceutical Sciences*, 18th ed. Easton, PA: Mack Publishing Company, 1990, 1513–1518.
10. Maliekal, J., Bertch, K.E., and Witte, K.W.: An update on ready-to-use intravenous delivery system. *Hosp. Pharm. 28*:970–971, 975–977, 1993.
11. Munzenberger, P.J. and Levin, S.: Home parenteral antibiotic therapy for patients with cystic fibrosis. *Hosp. Pharm. 28*:20–28, 1993.
12. Kwan, J.W.: High-technology IV infusion devices. *Am. J. Hosp. Pharm. 46*:320–335, 1989.
13. KITS: Kit for Infusion Technology Self-Instruction. Marketing Department, Electronic Drug Delivery Systems, Abbott Laboratories, Abbott Park, IL.
14. Keefner, K.R.: Parenteral pumps and controlled-delivery devices. *US Pharmacist 17*(8):H-3–H-16, 1992.
15. Fung, S. and Ferrill, M.: Contraceptive update: Subdermal implants. *California Pharmacist 40*: 35–41, 1992.

9

Biotechnology and Drugs

THE TERM *biotechnology* encompasses any technique that uses living organisms (e.g., microorganisms) in the production or modification of products. Recombinant DNA (rDNA) and monoclonal antibody (MAb) technologies are providing exciting opportunities for new pharmaceuticals development and new approaches to the diagnosis, treatment, and prevention of disease.

It is estimated that by the year 2000 biotechnologic products will have a marked impact upon the practice of pharmacy.[1] Research will continue to generate potent new medications that require custom dosing for the individual patient and concomitant pharmacist expertise in the use of, and familiarity with, sophisticated drug delivery systems.

The revolution in biotechnology is a result of research advancement in intracellular chemistry, molecular biology, recombinant DNA technology, genetics, and immunopharmacology. At present, the first of these novel pharmaceuticals have been proteins, but eventually an increasing number will be smaller molecules, discovered through biotechnologically based methods that will determine just how proteins work. Clearly biotechnology has established itself as a mainstay in pharmaceuticals research and development, and new products will enter the market at an increasing pace during the next decade.

The transition toward molecular medicine has already begun. As biotechnology advances, and growing numbers of cancer-related genes are identified and cloned, therapy with biotechnology products will supplant chemotherapy as the first-line treatment for many malignancies. At the time of this writing, more than 100 gene-therapy trials are in progress, and conjugate molecules, genetically engineered for specific toxicity to cancer cells, are also entering clinical trials.

Worldwide sales of biotechnologic products introduced in 1990 approached $2 billion and were estimated to be $2.5 billion in 1991.[1,2] The U.S. Department of Commerce estimates that the sales of biotechnologic pharmaceutical products will increase 15–20% per year through 1998. More of these products will come to market as drug development continues to escalate. In 1991, the Pharmaceutical Manufacturers Association reported that a total of 58 companies were developing and testing a total of 132 new biotechnology entities–a 63% increase from 1987.[3]

The commercial success of biotechnology has spurred the entry of many additional products into the development pipelines. It is anticipated that patients with hemophilia, serious sepsis infection, skin ulcers, and a number of cancers will benefit over the next several years as drugs in clinical trials secure market approval. This abundant activity has grown out of entrepreneurism among many small, venture-funded, narrowly focused groups. Several of these small companies have by now prospered to the point of becoming fully integrated pharmaceutical companies.

Recombinant DNA (rDNA)

DNA, deoxyribonucleic acid, has been called "the substance of life." It is DNA that constitutes genes, allowing cells to reproduce and maintain life. Of over 1 million kinds of plants and animals known today, no two are exactly alike; however, the similarity within families is the result of genetic information stored in cells, duplicated, and passed from cell to cell and from generation to generation. It is DNA that provides this continuity.

DNA was first isolated in 1869. Its chemical composition was determined in the early 1900s, and by the 1940s it had been proven that the genes within cell chromosomes are made of DNA. It was not until the 1950s, when James D. Watson and Francis H. C. Crick postulated the structure of DNA, that biologists began to comprehend the molecular mechanisms of heredity and cell regulation. Watson and Crick described their model of DNA as a double helix, two strands of DNA coiled about itself like a spiral staircase. It is now known that the two strands of DNA are connected by the bases adenine, guanine, cytosine, and thymine (A, G, C, and T). The order of arrangement of these bases with the two strands of DNA comprise a specific gene for a specific trait. A typical gene has hundreds of bases that are always arranged in pairs. When A occurs on one strand, T occurs opposite it on the other; G pairs with C. A gene is a segment of DNA that has a specific sequence of these chemical base pairs. The pattern constitutes the DNA message for maintaining cells and organisms and building the next generation. To create a new cell, or a whole new organism, DNA must be able to duplicate ("clone") itself. This is done through the unwinding and separation of the two strands and the subsequent attachment to each of new bases from within the cell according to the A-T/C-G rule. The result is two new double strands of DNA, each of the same structure and conformation.

DNA also plays an essential role in the production of proteins needed for cellular maintenance and function. DNA is translated to messenger RNA (ribonucleic acid), which contains instructions for the production of the 23 amino acids from which all proteins are made. Amino acids can be arranged in a vast number of combinations to produce hundreds of thousands of different proteins. In essence, a cell is a miniature assembly plant for the production of thousands of proteins. A single *Escherichia coli* bacterium is capable of making about 2000 proteins.

Through the process of recombinant DNA technology, scientists can utilize nonhuman cells (as a special strain of *E. coli*) to manufacture proteins identical to those produced in human cells. Recombinant DNA is defined as the hybrid DNA produced by joining pieces of DNA from different sources. The process of joining segments of DNA from different organisms for a specific purpose allows the synthesis of specific products from selected host cells. This process has enabled scientists to produce molecules naturally present in the human body in large quantities previously difficult to obtain from human sources. For example, approximately 50 cadaver pituitary glands were required to treat a single growth hormone-deficient child for one year until DNA-produced growth hormone became available through the new technology. Further, the biosynthetic product is more free of viral contamination than the previous cadaver source of the hormone. Human growth hormone and insulin were the first recombinant DNA products to become available for patient use.

DNA probe technology is a new tool utilized to diagnose disease. It utilizes small pieces of DNA to search a cell for viral infection or for genetic defects. DNA probes have application in testing for infectious disease, cancer, genetic defects, and disease susceptibility. Using DNA probes, scientists have acquired the capability of locating a disease-causing gene, which in turn can lead to the development of replacement therapies. In producing a DNA probe, the initial step involves the synthesis of the specific strand of DNA with the sequence of nucleotides that matches those of the gene being investigated. For instance, to test for a particular virus, first the DNA strand is developed to be identical to one in the virus. The second step is to tag the synthetic gene with a dye or radioactive isotope. When introduced into a specimen, the synthetic strand of DNA acts as a probe, searching for a matching or complementary strand. When located, the two hybridize, or join together. When the probe is bound to the virus, the dye reveals the location of the viral gene. If a radioactive isotope was employed on the synthetic DNA strand, it will bind to the viral strand of DNA, and then reveal the virus through x-ray technology.

Products of Biotechnology

The following descriptions provide examples of products of biotechnology that have been approved by the FDA or are being developed for submission for approval (Table 9–1).[4]

Clotting Factors

Hemophiliacs suffer from internal bleeding because of a lack of clotting protein factors. Historically, their treatment has been infusions of protein derived from human blood. Now, through genetic engineering, factors can be created without using donor blood that produce more nearly contaminant-free products and therefore expose the patient to fewer contaminants.

SYSTEMIC ANTIHEMOPHILIC FACTORS—KOGENATE, RECOMBINATE. Recombinant antihemophilic factor (AHF) is indicated for treatment of classi-

Table 9–1. Selected Investigational (U.S.) Biotechnology Products[a]

Generic Name, Synonyms	*Trade Name, Manufacturer*	*Classification*	*Labeled Indications (Potential Indications)*	*Approved (Status)*
Anti-B4-Blocked Ricin	Oncolysin B (ImmunoGen)	Monoclonal Antibody (Linked to Ricin)	B cell leukemias and lymphomas	Phase II/III
Anti-My9-Blocked Ricin	Oncoloysin M (ImmunoGen)	Monoclonal Antibody (Linked to Ricin)	Myelogenous leukemias	Phase I/II
Epidermal Growth Factor (human)	(Chiron/Ethicon)	Recombinant Protein (Modulator)	Wound healing, skin ulcers, burns	Phase II
Basic Fibroblast Growth Factor (human)	(Synergen)	Recombinant Protein (Modulator)	Venous stasis, diabetic leg and foot ulcers	Phase III
Interferon beta	(Biogen)	Recombinant Protein (Communicator)	Multiple Sclerosis	Phase III
Interleukin-1 receptor	(Immunex)	Recombinant Protein (Communicator)	Autoimmune diseases including organ transplant rejection and asthma	Phase I/II
Nebacumab (Centoxin)	HA-1A (Centocor)	Monoclonal Antibody (Human-Therapeutic)	Gram negative sepsis	PLA Filed
Platelet-derived Growth Factor (PDGF)	(Amgen)	Recombinant Protein (Modulator)	Chronic dermal ulcers	Phase I/II
VaxSYN HIV-1	MicroGeneSys	Recombinant Protein (Viral Protein)	Prevention and treatment of AIDS	Phase II

[a] Adapted from: Wordell, C. J. Use of Beta Interferon in Multiple Sclerosis. *Hospital Pharmacy 28*(8):802–807, 1993.

PLA = Product License Application

cal hemophilia A, in which there is a demonstrated deficiency of activity of plasma clotting factor (factor VIII). Human recombinant AHF (rAHF) is a sterile, nonpyrogenic concentrate with biologic and pharmacokinetic activity comparable to that of plasma-derived AHF. Additional clinical trials are being conducted to determine whether antibodies to the recombinant product form more often than that with plasma-derived products.[5]

The recombinant form contains albumin as a stabilizer, as well as trace amounts of mouse, hamster, and bovine proteins. These new products are made by modifying hamster cells through biotechnology processes so that they produce a highly purified version of AHF factor VIII.[5]

Each vial of AHF is labeled with the AHF activity expressed in International Units (IU). The assignment of potency is referenced to the World Health Organization International Standard. One IU of factor VIII activity is approximately equal to the AHF activity of one mL of fresh plasma, and increases the plasma concentration of factor VIII by 2%. The specific Factor VIII activity ranges from 2 to 200 AHF IU per mg of total protein. To determine dosage, the following guidelines may be used:

$$\text{Desired AHF increase (\% of normal)} = \frac{\text{Dose AHF (IU)}}{\text{Body weight (kg)}} \times 2$$

$$\text{Dose of AHF (IU)} = \text{Body weight (kg)} \times \text{Desired AHF increase} \times 0.5$$

Kogenate is available in strengths of 250 IU (with 2.5 mL sterile water for injection provided as diluent), 500 IU (with 5 mL sterile water for injection provided as diluent), and 1000 IU (with 10 mL sterile water for injection provided as diluent). Each strength contains between 2 and 5 mmol of calcium chloride, 100–130 mEq/liter of sodium, 100–130 mEq/liter of chloride, 4 to 10 mg/mL of human albumin, and nanogram quantities of foreign protein (mouse, hamster) per IU. Kogenate is supplied in a single-dose vial, along with a suitable volume of diluent (Sterile Water for Injection, USP), a sterile filter needle, and a sterile administration set.

Recombinate is available in strengths of 250 IU, 500 IU, and 1000 IU, each with 10 mL sterile water for injection provided as diluent. Each strength contains 12.5 mg/mL of human albumin, 180 mEq/l of sodium, 200 mEq/l of calcium, and a small quantity of foreign protein.

Dry concentrates of rAHF should be stored between 2°C and 8°C, and the diluent protected from freezing. Kogenate, however, may be stored at room temperatures not exceeding 25°C for 3 months. After reconstitution, the solution should not be refrigerated.

The diluent and the dry concentrate should be brought to room temperature (approximately 25°C) prior to reconstitution. These may be allowed to warm to room temperature, or in an emergency situation warmed via water bath to a range of 30°–37°C. Once reconstituted, the solution should not be shaken because this could cause the solution to foam. The reconstituted solution should be administered within 3 hours of reconstitution, and any partially used vial discarded. This preparation should be administered alone through a separate line, and without mixing with other intravenous fluids or medications.

Kogenate may be administered intravenously over 5 to 10 minutes, and Recombinate at a rate up to 10 mL per minute. The comfort of the patient should guide the rate at which the recombinant AHF is administered. If a significant increase in pulse rate occurs, the infusion should be slowed or halted until the pulse rate returns to normal. The risk of an allergic reaction to product proteins (mouse, hamster, bovine) may be present in the monoclonal antibody-derived and recombinant AHF products.

Colony Stimulating Factors

Colony stimulating factors (CSFs) are four glycoprotein regulators that bind to specific surface receptors and are able to control the proliferation and differentiation of marrow cells into macrophages, neutrophils, basophils, eosinophils, platelets, or erythrocytes.[6,7] These recombinant human CSFs have potential for wide use in the areas of oncology (e.g., chemotherapy-induced leukopenia, cancer patients having marrow transplants), inherited disorders (e.g., congenital neutropenia) and infectious disease (e.g., AIDS).[8] Patients with low amounts of endogenous CSFs are prone to secondary infections because of diminished resistance associated with some forms of cancer or, more commonly, suppressed marrow function after the use of myelotoxic chemotherapy.

In the absence of pluripotent *stem cells* (an uncommitted cell with the potential to become any cell of the blood), the CSFs cannot be expected to stimulate cell formation and the development of neutrophils. Furthermore, it could be expected that the effectiveness of the CSFs be directly related to the absolute numbers of these potential target cells. For example, cancer patients with bone marrow severely depleted by chemotherapy may not respond as well to CSFs therapy as cancer patients with normal hemopoietic tissues.

If patients with neutropenia develop an infection, they will be unable to defend themselves against it, because neutrophils are the body's initial defense mechanism. If neutrophils are absent, or in very low numbers, the classic signs and symptoms of infection (swelling, pain, redness, heat, purulent discharge) will be absent. Neutrophils cause these signs and symptoms, and if they are not present in sufficient numbers, only a fever—with or without sore throat—may signal a serious infection. Thus, a body temperature that exceeds 100.5°F is a serious occurrence in a patient who has undergone chemotherapy within the past 3–4 weeks.

GRANULOCYTE COLONY STIMULATING FACTOR (G-CSF)—FILGRASTIM. Produced by recombinant DNA technology, this drug stimulates the production of neutrophils within the bone marrow. It is approved for chemotherapy-related neutropenia and is indicated (to decrease the incidence of infection, as manifested by febrile neutropenia) in patients with nonmyeloid malignancies who are receiving myelosuppressive anti-cancer drugs and exhibiting severe neutropenia with fever. This drug can also be used as an adjunct to myelosuppressive cancer chemotherapy to help speed the recovery of neutrophils after treatment and to reduce serious infection risk.

For chemotherapy-induced neutropenia, Filgrastim is administered intravenously (short infusion, 15–30 minutes), as a subcutaneous bolus or continuous intravenous or subcutaneous injection, in a starting dose of 5 $\mu g/kg$ once daily, beginning no earlier than 24 hours after administration of the last dose of cytotoxic chemotherapy. This regimen is continued for up to 2 weeks, until the absolute neutrophil count reaches 10,000/mm^3 following the *nadir* (the lowest neutrophil count, usually occurring 7–10 days after chemotherapy).

Filgrastim injection contains no preservative

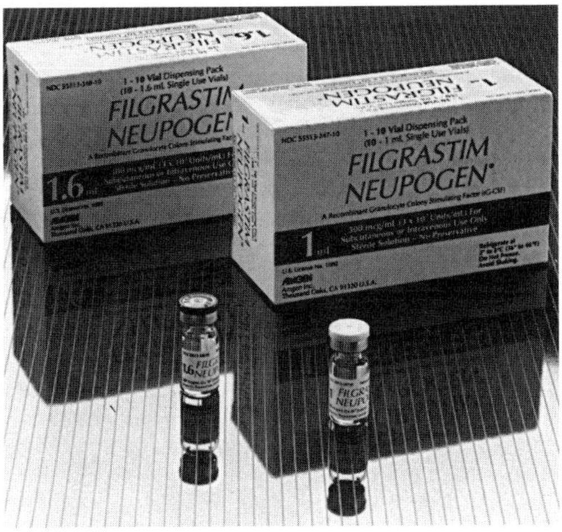

Fig. 9–1. *Example of the product package of Filgrastim (Courtesy of Amgen, Inc.)*

and should be stored between 2°C and 8°C. It is not to be frozen. Before use, the injection may be allowed to reach room temperature for a maximum of 6 hours, after which time it should be discarded. A clear, colorless solution, it should be inspected visually prior to injection. This product is supplied as a 1 mL or 1.6 mL, single-dose vial (Fig. 9–1).

Filgrastim is supplied in boxes containing ten glass vials, which are packaged in a gel-ice insulating container that has a temperature indicator to detect freezing. For convenience, and to minimize the risk of breakage, Filgrastim should be dispensed to the patient in its original packaging, and the patient instructed to refrigerate the product promptly after arriving home.

If the patient has to travel a considerable distance, and/or the outside temperature is high, it may be necessary to place the medication in a small cooler with a gel refrigerant (e.g., blue ice) for transport. It is suggested that the vials be wrapped in a towel to avoid direct contact between the product vials and the blue ice. The drug must be physically separated from the refrigerant to avoid the possibility of freezing. Dry ice should not be used because of the possibility of freezing the product through inadvertent contact.

It is conceivable that, when used as an adjunct to cancer chemotherapy, prescriptions for this product will be written for 7–10 vials. Indeed, patients may have extra vials of this product at home from previous courses of cancer chemotherapy. The pharmacist should question such patients about having any unexpired, properly stored, or unused vials remaining from the previous course of therapy.

Because granulocyte colony stimulating factor (G-CSF) is a protein, it is capable of being denatured if severely agitated. If the vial is shaken vigorously, the solution may foam or appear frothy, making its withdrawal difficult. Thus, the pharmacist should instruct the patient (or guardian) to avoid shaking the vial before use. If mistakenly shaken, the vial should be allowed to stand until the froth diminishes.

The manufacturer of Filgrastim has developed a step-by-step guide to subcutaneous self-injection. However, the pharmacist should always emphasize the use of proper aseptic technique when preparing and administering the drug, to help avoid product contamination and possible infection.

GRANULOCYTE MACROPHAGE COLONY STIMULATING FACTOR (GM-CSF)—SARGRAMOSTIM. Sargramostim is a recombinant human granulocyte-macrophage CSF produced by recombinant DNA technology in a yeast *(Saccharomyces cerevisiae)* expression system. GM-CSF is a hematopoietic growth factor that stimulates proliferation and differentiation of hematopoietic progenitor (i.e., precursor) cells into neutrophils and monocytes. It is a glycoprotein composed of 127 amino acids. The sequence of GM-CSF differs from the natural human GM-CSF at position 23, where leucine is substituted.

This drug is indicated for acceleration of myeloid (i.e., marrow) recovery in patients with non-Hodgkin's lymphoma (NHL), acute lymphoblastic leukemia (ALL), and Hodgkin's disease undergoing autologous bone marrow transplantation (a procedure in which the patient's bone marrow is removed, treated to destroy malignant cells, and later reinfused into the patient). It is also indicated in bone-marrow-transplantation failure or engraftment delay (it takes between 3 and 4 weeks for the new marrow to begin to produce new white blood cells).

GM-CSF accelerates the engraftment process by promoting the production of white blood cells. Health care costs are controlled, because patients treated with it demonstrate significant earlier increases in WBC counts, a reduced need for antibiotics, and a shortened duration of hospitalization. For myeloid reconstitution after autologous bone marrow transplantation, it is administered in a dose of 250 $\mu g/m^2/day$ for 21 days as a 2-hour intravenous infusion beginning 2–4 hours after the autologous bone marrow infusion, and not less than 24 hours after the last dose of chemotherapy and 12 hours after the last dose of radiotherapy. For bone-marrow-transplantation failure or engraftment delay, the dose remains the same, but the duration is 14 days, again using a 2-hour intravenous infusion. The dose can be repeated after 7 days of therapy if engraftment has not occurred.

Sargramostim is manufactured as a powder for injection, lyophilized, in preservative-free, single-use vials of 250 μg or 500 μg. It is reconstituted with one mL of Sterile Water for Injection, USP (without preservative). The reconstituted solution should appear clear and colorless, and will be isotonic with a pH of 7.4 ± 0.3. During the reconstitution procedure, the Sterile Water for Injection, USP, should be directed at the side of the vial and the contents gently swirled to avoid foaming during dissolution. The product must not be shaken or vigorously agitated. The product can also be diluted for IV infusion in 0.9% Sodium Chloride Injection, USP. If the final concentration of GM-CSF is below 10 μg/mL, human albumin (0.1%) should be added to the saline before adding GM-CSF. This addition prevents the adsorption of the drug to the components of the drug delivery system.

Because this product is preservative free, it should be administered as soon as possible, and within 6 hours following reconstitution or dilution for IV infusion.

Erythropoietins

Erythropoietin is a sialic acid-containing protein that enhances erythropoiesis by stimulating the formation of proerythroblasts and the release of reticulocytes from bone marrow. It is secreted by the kidney in response to hypoxemia and transported to the bone marrow through the plasma. It resembles an endocrine hormone more than any other cytokine.[9]

Anemia (a deficiency of red blood cell production) is a frequent complication of cancer and cancer therapy. Although it is easily corrected through blood transfusions, erythropoietins are only available to treat the severest forms of anemia and not to maintain the red blood cell mass required for normal activity and well-being. As anemic patients with solid tumors often have lower serum levels of erythropoietin, correction of the erythropoietin deficiency through erythropoietin therapy may be as beneficial for these cancer patients as it has been for uremic patients.[9]

Kidney disease also impairs the body's ability to produce this substance, and thus results in anemia. In the past, patients received blood transfusions. However, a problem with transfusions was possible exposure to infectious agents (hepatitis, HIV). An exciting alternative is the genetically engineered epoetin alpha, a drug capable of stimulating erythropoiesis. Although expensive (>$1000/month), it may prove beneficial for those patients who require extensive transfusions, because of the high cost of transfusions, the risk of infectious disease, and the consequent additional health care costs.

EPOETIN ALFA—EPOGEN, PROCRIT. Epoetin alfa is a glycoprotein produced by recombinant DNA technology, and contains 165 amino acids in an identical sequence to that of endogenous human erythropoietin. This drug stimulates erythropoiesis by effecting the division and differentiation of committed erythroid progenitor cells. Erythropoietin also effects the release of reticulocytes from the bone marrow into the bloodstream, where these mature into erythrocytes. It is approved for anemia related to cancer chemotherapy, chronic dialysis, and AZT therapy.

Epoetin alfa is administered intravenously or subcutaneously, in a dosage of 50–100 IU/kg body weight three times per week. It is given intravenously to patients with available intravenous access (e.g., patients who undergo hemodialysis), and either intravenously or subcutaneously to other patients. If after 8 weeks of therapy the hematocrit has not increased at least five to six points and is still below the target range of 30–33%, the dosage may be increased.

Epoetin alfa is available in 1 mL, nonpreserved, single-dose vials (Fig. 9–2) in varying

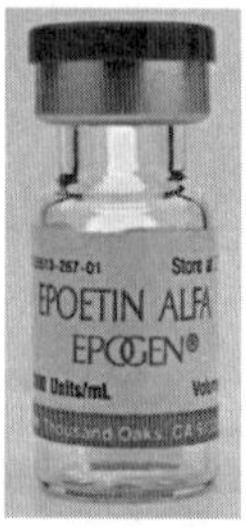

Fig. 9–2. *Example of the product Epogen (Courtesy of Amgen, Inc.)*

strengths of 2000, 3000, 4000, and 10,000 IU/mL. Each 1-mL vial contains human albumin, 2.5 mg, to prevent adsorptive losses. The product should be refrigerated at 2°C to 8°C, and protected from freezing. The vial of epoetin alfa, recombinant injection, should not be shaken because this may denature the glycoprotein and render it biologically inactive. Each vial should be used to administer a single dose only, and any unused portion of the solution must be discarded.

Human Growth Hormone

The pituitary gland secretes human growth hormone (hGH), which stimulates an individual's growth. It is estimated that approximately 15,000 American children suffer from hGH deficiency, and consequently will not achieve normal height as an adult.

In the late 1950s, cadaver pituitaries were harvested to produce hGH and treat these deficient children. Besides the enormous expense, this method exposed the children to the risk of infection from viral contamination of the hormone.[2] Genetic engineering now produces highly purified hGH.

SYSTEMIC GROWTH HORMONE—HUMATROPE, PROTROPIN. Somatrem (Protropin) is a biosynthetic, single polypeptide chain of 192 amino acids, produced by a recombinant DNA procedure in *E. coli*. This drug has one more amino acid (methionine) than the natural occurring human growth hormone. Somatropin recombinant (Humatrope) is biosynthetically produced by another recombinant DNA process and possesses amino acid sequencing identical to the naturally occurring human growth hormone (i.e., 191 amino acids).

This hormone stimulates linear growth by affecting the cartilaginous growth areas of long bones. It also stimulates growth by increasing the number and size of skeletal muscle cells, influencing the size of organs, and increasing red cell mass through erythropoietin stimulation.

Somatrem for injection is initially administered intramuscularly or subcutaneously in a dosage range of 0.025–0.05 mg (0.065–0.13 IU)/kg of body weight every other day, or three times a week. The 5- and 10-mg, single-dose vials (Fig. 9–3) are reconstituted using standard aseptic technique with 1–5 mL of Bacteriostatic Water for Injection, USP (benzyl alcohol preserved) only. Because of the associated toxicity of benzyl alcohol in newborns, when administering to this patient population this product should be reconstituted with Water for Injection. The vial should then be swirled gently to dissolve the contents. If cloudy, the solution should not be used. When prepared with the manufacturer's provided diluent, the reconstituted solution should be stored in the refrigerator and used within 14 days. When Water for Injection is used to reconstitute this product, each vial should only be used for one dose and the unused portion discarded.

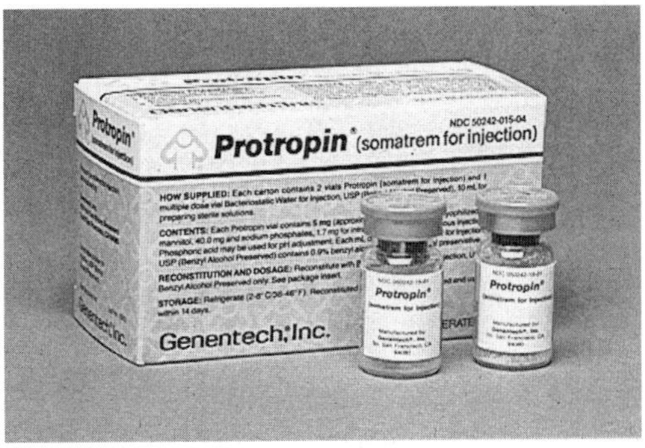

Fig. 9–3. *Example of the product Protropin (Courtesy of Genentech, Inc.)*

Somatropin, recombinant, for injection, is administered intramuscularly or subcutaneously in identical dosage range and duration as Somatrem. The 5 mg vial is reconstituted with water for injection that contains 0.3% m-cresol and 1.7% glycerin. Some brands of Humatrope are packaged with the diluent and somatropin in the same vial, separated by a rubber stopper. Depressing the stopper allows the two components to mix. If, however, the diluent and somatropin are in separate vials, aseptic technique must be used to add the desired amount of diluent (between 1.5 and 5 mL) provided by the manufacturer, or Sterile Water for Injection to a 5 mg vial. Like Somatrem, Somatropin is stable when refrigerated for up to 14 days following reconstitution with the diluent provided by the manufacturer. When Sterile Water for Injection is used to reconstitute this product, each vial should be refrigerated and used within 24 hours.

Interferons

In 1957, two British scientists, Alick Isaacs and Jean Lindenmann, found that infected chick embryo cells released a naturally produced glycoprotein that allowed noninfected cells to resist viral infection. They named this factor *interferon*, because it appeared "to interfere with the transmission of infection." Later, these researchers demonstrated that interferon does not activate viruses directly, but rendered the host cells resistant to viral multiplication. Interferons exert virus-nonspecific but host-specific antiviral activity. By the mid-1970s, it appeared that interferon might also curtail the spread of certain types of cancer (e.g., small cell lung cancer, renal cell carcinoma, basal cell carcinoma).

As a class, interferons are a part of the large immune regulatory network within the body that includes lymphokines, monokines, growth factors, and peptide hormones. Interferons are classified into two types—type I interferons (alpha and beta), which share the same molecular receptor, and type II (gamma or immune), which has a different receptor.[4]

INTERFERON BETA-1b—BETASERON. Interferon beta-1b (IFNB) is a type I interferon made in *E. coli* using recombinant technology; it differs from natural interferon beta only by the substitution of a serine residue for a cysteine at position 17. This manipulation enhances the stability of the drug while retaining the specific activity of the natural interferon beta.

IFNB is effective in the treatment of relapsing-remitting types of multiple sclerosis, an inflammatory demyelinating disease of the CNS, in a dosage of 0.25 mg (8 mIU) injected subcutaneously every other day.[4] This form of disease is characterized by recurrent attacks followed by complete or incomplete recovery.[10]

The lyophilized IFNB (Fig. 9–4), 0.3 mg (9.6 mIU), is reconstituted using a sterile syringe and needle to inject 1.2 mL of supplied diluent (sodium chloride, 0.54% solution) into the vial. The diluent should be added down the side of the vial and the vial then gently swirled, but not shaken, to dissolve the drug completely. After reconstitution with the accompanying diluent, the solution has a strength of 0.25 mg/mL. This product also contains dextrose and albumin (this adjuvant is often used in recombinant protein products to prevent adherence of the product to the glass vial, plastic tubing, or syringe). One mL of reconstituted solution is then withdrawn from the vial into a sterile syringe fitted with a 27-gauge needle and the drug is injected subcutaneously. For purposes of self-injection, the sites may include the arms, abdomen, hips, and thighs.

Because the product has no preservative, the vial is suitable for single use only. Before and after reconstitution, the product should be refrigerated. No more than 3 hours should elapse between reconstitution and use.

IFNB is currently distributed through a nationwide community pharmacy network called PCS Professional Service Network. The advantage of this system is that it eliminates the pharmacy's

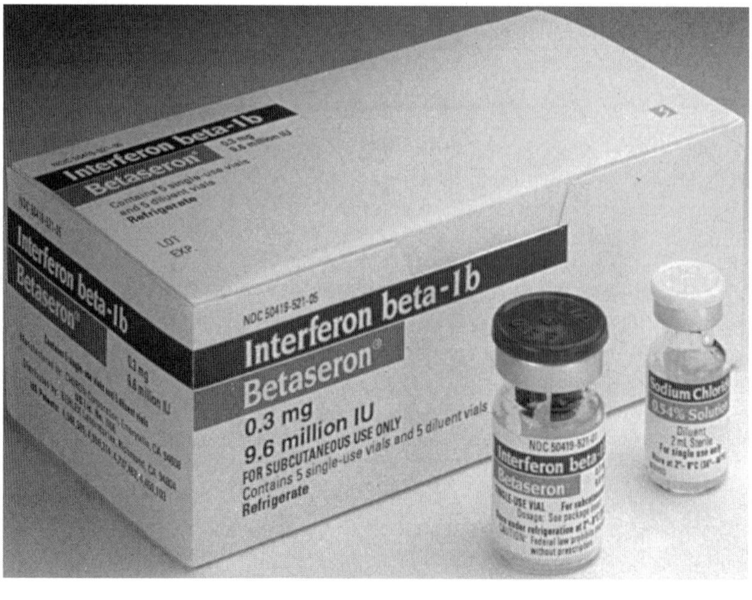

Fig. 9–4. *Example of the product package of Betaseron (Courtesy of Berlex, Inc.)*

inventory and carrying costs, allows the IFNB patient to use a PCS prescription drug card, and pays the participating pharmacy a professional fee for each transaction.[11] The cost of therapy is estimated to be approximately $1000/month.

Interleukins

Originally, these substances were thought to oversee interactions between white blood cells, key components of the immune system. Now, however, it is known that these substances affect a wider variety of cell types. Most clinical interest centers upon Interleukin-1 (IL-1), a substance secreted primarily by the monocyte/macrophage that activates T-cells and B-cells, and Interleukin-2 (IL-2), a substance secreted by the T-cell that supports the growth and differentiation of T-cells and B-cells. There are a total of 14 known interleukins.

IL-1 was discovered in 1972, and within 7 years its structure and function were delineated. It was first manufactured by recombinant-DNA technology in 1984. This substance is a key immune system regulator. It sets into motion a chain reaction that intensifies the immune response. IL-1 responds to the initial presence of an antigen. It activates T-cells to mature, proliferate, and produce other *cytokines* (a generic term for soluble substances produced by cells that communicate with other cells to trigger or suppress cellular activity after interaction with an antigen).

IL-1 also intensifies the production of collagenase, prostaglandins, and antibodies. Because of this activity, excess IL-1 is suspected to be behind many inflammatory disorders (collagenase breaks down connective tissue; prostaglandins are associated with inflammation). The cytokine may also be responsible for the fever, headache, fatigue, and weakness of influenza.

Interleukin-2 (IL-2), like other cytokines, was initially greeted with much enthusiasm. Since that time it has been found to be an essential component in the development of antigen-specific and antigen nonspecific immune responses, but has found few applications.[12] Discovered in 1976, it became available through recombinant-DNA technology in 1984. When applied to white blood cells removed from patients, and then reinfused as "lymphokine activated killer cells" along with a booster injection of IL-2, spectacular remissions occurred in some patients with devastating conditions such as advanced malignant melanoma. Unfortunately, highly toxic side effects occurred because of a lack of knowledge of appropriate dosing. A combination of lower doses and physician experience managing its side effects will make IL-2 safer to use in the future.

Other interleukins are in the research pipeline. IL-11 is being investigated in vitro and in mice to stimulate platelet function. If successful, this substance could help counter the platelet-depleting effects of chemotherapeutic agents. IL-6 (synonymously known as beta-2 interferons) may also be a stimulator of platelet growth, and is being investigated as an antiproliferative treatment for breast, colon, and skin cancer.

ALDESLEUKIN—PROLEUKIN. Aldesleukin is synthetically produced by a recombinant-DNA process involving genetically engineered *Escherichia coli* containing an analog of the human interleukin-2 gene. An expression clone that encodes a modified human interleukin-2 results from genetic engineering techniques used to modify the human interleukin-2 gene. Aldesleukin differs from naturally occurring interleukin-2 in that it is not glycosylated because it is derived from *E. coli,* the molecule has no N-terminal alanine, and the molecule has serine substituted for cysteine at amino-acid position 125.

Designated an orphan drug, aldesleukin is approved for the treatment of metastatic renal carcinoma (about 10,000 cases diagnosed annually) in adults (over 18 years). Because of its life-threatening toxicities (drug-related mortality rate is 4%), the physician should consider the benefit-to-risk ratio for the patient. The dosage of interleukin-2 is usually expressed in units of activity in promoting proliferation in a responsive cell line. Conversion to units from mg of protein varies, depending upon the source of interleukin-2. The strength and dosage of commercially available aldesleukin is expressed in International Units (IU). Eighteen million IU equals 1.1 mg protein.

For metastatic renal carcinoma, high-dose therapy involves an intravenous infusion over a 15-minute period, 600,000 IU/kg of body weight (i.e., 0.037 mg/kg body weight) every 8 hours for a total of 14 doses. Following a rest period of 9 days, the schedule is repeated for another 14 doses, for a maximum of 28 doses per course. The manufacturer of aldesleukin recommends that plastic bags be used as the dilution containers (as opposed to glass bottles and polyvinyl chloride bags) for more consistent drug delivery. In-line filters are not recommended for use during this drug's administration because of the risk of adsorption of aldesleukin to the filter.

Each aldesleukin for injection, single-use vial, contains 22 million IUs (1.3 mg of drug) and is reconstituted for intravenous or subcutaneous injection by adding 1.2 mL of Sterile Water for Injection to the vial. The diluent should be directed to the side of the vial and the contents swirled gently to avoid foaming. The resultant solution should be clear-and-colorless to slightly yellow and will contain 18 million IUs (1.1 mg) per mL. The vial should not be shaken. The appropriate dose is then withdrawn, diluted in 50 mL of 5% Dextrose Injection, and infused over a 15-minute period. Bacteriostatic Water for Injection, or 0.9% Sodium Chloride Injection, should not be used to reconstitute this product because of the increased aggregation of the product.

Because the vial has no preservative, the reconstituted and diluted solutions should be refrigerated. However, it should be brought back to room temperature prior to administration. Reconstituted solutions should be used within 48 hours.

Monoclonal Antibodies

Monoclonal antibodies are ultrasensitive, hybrid, immune-system–derived proteins designed to recognize specific antibodies. They have found use in laboratory diagnostics, site-directed therapies, immunology, and home test kits (e.g., pregnancy, ovulation prediction). Monoclonal antibodies are purified antibodies produced by a single source or clone of cells.[13] These substances are engineered to recognize and bind to a single specific antigen. Thus, when administered, a monoclonal antibody will target a particular protein or cell having the specific matching antigenic feature. When coupled with a drug molecule, radioactive isotope or toxin, a monoclonal antibody theoretically, can target the desired cells or tissues with great precision. To date, however, the majority of the MAb does not reach target tumor cells (less than 0.1% locates in tumor tissue).

Diagnostically, the specificity of monoclonal antibodies helps to detect the presence of endogenous hormones (e.g., luteinizing hormone, human chorionic gonadotropin) in the urine to establish the test results.[14] They are also being used to detect allergies, anemia, and heart disease, and commercial monoclonal antibody diagnostic kits are available for drug assays, tissue and blood typing, and such infectious diseases as hepatitis, AIDS-related cytomegalovirus, streptococcal infections, gonorrhea, syphilis, herpes, and chlamydia. When covalently linked with radioisotopes, contrast agents, or anticancer drugs, monoclonal antibodies can be used to diagnose and treat malignant tumors.

Prior to 1975, when hybridoma technology was fully developed, antibodies for diagnostic, therapeutic, or research use were obtained from the blood of humans or animals. The antibodies, produced through the body's immune system in response to the presence of foreign substances of antigens, were obtained through separation from the blood. It had been difficult to obtain pure antibodies specific to a particular antigen. Today, antibodies are generated in large quantities by laboratory grown hybridomas or hybrid cells. In making monoclonal antibodies, an animal is immunized with the foreign substance or antigen that will yield the antibody desired.[13] The antibody-producing cells are removed and mixed with myeloma cells under conditions that promote cell fusion. The resulting hybrid cells grow indefinitely and produce monoclonal antibodies in large quantities.[15]

MUROMONAB-CD3—ORTHOCLONE OKT3. Muromonab-CD3 is a murine, monoclonal antibody that reacts with a T3 (CD3) molecule that is linked to an antigen receptor on the surface membrane of human T lymphocytes. Thus it blocks both the generation and function of the T cells in response to antigenic challenge, and is indicated for the treatment of organ transplant rejection. Usually it is combined with azathioprine, cyclosporine, and/or corticosteroids to prevent acute rejection of renal transplants. Simultaneously, the amount of immunosuppressive drugs (e.g., azathioprine, prednisone) a patient must receive has been reduced, effecting better patient outcomes.

Muromonab-CD3 injection is administered by intravenous push over a period not less than 1 minute. For acute renal allograft rejection, it is given in a 5 mg/day dosage for 10 to 14 days. To decrease the incidence of reactions resulting from the first injection of muromonab, methylprednisolone sodium succinate, 8 mg/kg, should be intravenously administered 1–4 hours beforehand.

Muromonab-CD3 injection should be drawn into the syringe through a low-protein-binding 0.2–0.22 μm filter. Once withdrawn, the filter should be discarded and the needle for the intravenous bolus injection attached. Because the drug is a protein solution, it may develop a few fine translucent particles that do not affect its potency. This solution has no preservative, and thus the product must be used immediately upon opening and the unused portion discarded. As with other protein products, it must not be shaken.

SATUMOMAB PENDETIDE—ONCOSCINT CR/OV KIT. OncoScint CR/OV-In (Indium In 111 satumomab pendetide) is a diagnostic imaging agent that is indicated for determining the extent and location of extrahepatic malignant disease in patients with known colorectal or ovarian cancer. Clinical studies suggest that this imaging agent should be used after completion of standard diagnostic tests, when additional information regarding disease extent could aid in patient management.

Satumomab pendetide is a conjugate produced from the murine monoclonal antibody, CYT-099 (Mab B72.3). MAb B72.3 is a murine monoclonal antibody of the IgG1, kappa subclass, which is directed to and localizes/binds with a high molecular weight, tumor-associated glycoprotein (TAG-72) that is expressed differentially by adenocarcinomas. (*Note:* Adenocarcinoma is a technical name for a malignant tumor derived from a gland or glandular tissue, or a tumor of which the gland-derived cells form gland-like structures.) In in vitro immunohistologic studies, MAb B72.3 has been reported to be reactive with about 83% of colorectal adenocarcinomas, 97% of common epithelial ovarian carcinomas, and the majority of breast, nonsmall-cell lung, pancreatic, gastric, and esophageal cancers evaluated.

OncoScint CR/OV is prepared by site-specific conjugation of the linker-chelator, glycyltryrosyl-(N,ϵ-diethylenetriaminepentaacetic acid)-lysine hydrochloride, to the oxidized oligosaccharide component of MAb B72.3. Each OncoScint CR/OV kit contains all of the nonradioactive ingredients necessary to produce a single unit dose of OncoScint CR/OV-In for use as an intravenous injection. Each kit contains two vials. A single-dose vial of OncoScint CR/OV, formulated with Water for Injection, contains 1 mg of satumomab pendetide in 2 mL of sodium phosphate–buffered saline solution adjusted to pH 6 with hydrochloric acid. OncoScint CR/OV is sterile, pyrogen-free, clear, colorless, and may contain some translucent particles. A vial of sodium acetate buffer contains 136 mg of sodium acetate trihydrate in 2 mL of water for injection adjusted to pH 6 with glacial acetic acid. It is sterile, pyrogen-free, clear, and colorless. Neither solution contains a preservative. Each kit also contains one sterile 0.22 μm Millex GV filter, prescribing information, and two identification labels. The kit should be stored upright in a refrigerator (2°–8°C), but not frozen.

Proper aseptic technique and precautions for handling radioactive materials should be employed. Waterproof gloves should be worn during the radiolabeling procedure. Consistent with the instructions provided, the sodium acetate buffer solution must be added to the indium In-111 chloride solution to buffer it prior to radiolabeling satumomab pendetide. After radiolabeling with indium-111, the immunoscintigraphic agent, OncoScint CR/OV-In (indium In 111 satumomab pendetide) is formed.

Tissue Plasminogen Activators

These are substances produced in small quantity by the inner lining of blood vessels and by the muscular wall of the uterus. Tissue plasminogen activators prevent abnormal blood clotting by converting plasminogen, a component of blood, to the enzyme plasmin. This latter substance breaks down fibrin, the main constituent of a blood clot.

Genetic engineering has prepared these substances artificially and these are used as *thrombolytic agents* (agents that dissolve blood clots). They are used for conditions such as heart attack, angina, and occluded arteries. Unlike other anticoagulant drugs, tissue plasminogen activator acts only on the site of the clot.

RECOMBINANT ALTEPLASE—ACTIVASE. Alteplase, a tissue plasminogen activator produced by recombinant DNA, is used in the management of acute myocardial infarction. It is a sterile, purified glycoprotein of 527 amino acids. It is synthesized using the complementary DNA (cDNA) for natural human tissue–type plasminogen activator obtained from a human melanoma cell line.

The biological activity of alteplase is determined by an in vitro clot lysis assay. The activity is expressed in International Units as tested against the WHO standard. Its specific activity is 580,000 IU/mg.

Coronary occlusion due to a thrombus is present in the infarct-related coronary artery in approximately 80% of patients experiencing a transmural myocardial infarction evaluated within 4 hours of onset of symptoms. When ad-

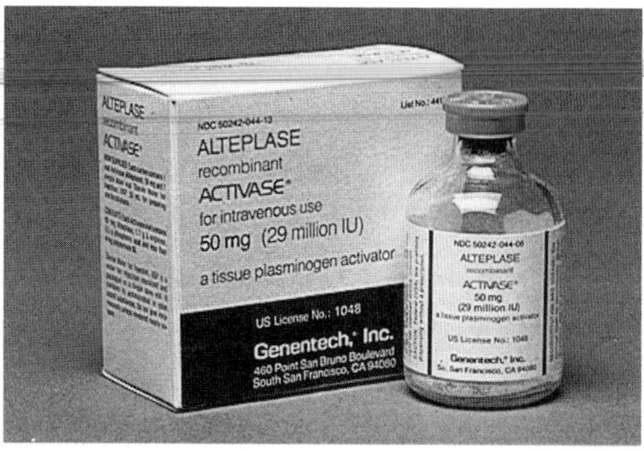

Fig. 9–5. *Example of the product package of Alteplase (Courtesy of Genentech, Inc.)*

ministered into the systemic circulation at pharmacological concentrations, alteplase binds to fibrin in a thrombus and converts the entrapped plasminogen to plasmin. This initiates the lysis of thrombi that are obstructing coronary arteries, thereby improving ventricular function and reducing the incidence of congestive heart failure.

An appropriate volume of the accompanying sterile water for injection (without preservatives) is added to the vial containing the lyophilized powder (i.e., 20 mg or 50 mg) (Fig. 9–5). Reconstitution should be with a large-bore needle (e.g., 18 gauge) and the stream of Sterile Water for Injection directed into the lyophilized cake. A slight foaminess can be expected; when allowed to stand undisturbed, it should dissipate within several minutes. The resultant solution appears as a colorless-to-pale-yellow transparent solution having an approximate pH of 7.3 and containing 1 mg/mL.

There are no antibacterial preservatives in the product, so it should be prepared just before use. The solution may be used for direct intravenous administration within 8 hours following reconstitution when stored between 2° and 30° C. Before diluting or administering the product, it is necessary to inspect it visually for particulate matter and discoloration whenever the solution and container permit.

This product may be administered as reconstituted, i.e., 1 mg/mL. Or the reconstituted solution may be diluted further immediately preceding administration with an equal volume of 0.9% sodium chloride injection or 5% dextrose injection. Alteplase is stable for up to 8 hours in these solutions at room temperature and either polyvinyl chloride bags or glass bottles are acceptable. Light exposure has no influence upon stability.

Vaccines

Genetically engineered vaccines use a synthetic copy of the protein coat of a virus to "fool" the body's immune system into mounting a protective response. This avenue avoids the use of live viruses and minimizes the risk of causing the disease the vaccines were intended to prevent. Further, these vaccines will all but eliminate concern about the natural vaccine, which could be derived from blood-donor carriers who may harbor the AIDS virus.

The first genetically engineered vaccine for use in the United States was approved by the FDA in 1986 for hepatitis B, a widespread liver infection. This vaccine has now replaced the plasma-derived vaccine.

HEPATITIS B VACCINE RECOMBINANT—ENGERIX-B, RECOMBIVAX HB. The plasma-derived hepatitis B vaccine is no longer being produced in the United States, and its use is limited to hemodialysis patients, other immunocompromised patients, and persons with known allergies to yeast. Recombinant hepatitis B vaccine has demonstrated an ability to induce antibody-to–hepatitis B surface antigen (anti-HBs) that is biochemically and immunologically comparable to antibody induced by the plasma-derived hepatitis B vaccine. Studies demonstrate that the two are interchangeable in their use.

Hepatitis B recombinant vaccine is indicated for immunization of persons of all ages against infection caused by all types of hepatitis B virus. A dialysis formulation (Recombivax HB Dialysis Formulation) is indicated for immunization of adult predialysis and dialysis patients. The vaccine should be administered by intramuscular injection into the deltoid muscle (outer aspect of the upper arm) for the immunization of adults and older children. The anterolateral thigh is recommended for infants and younger children. For those patients with a risk of hemorrhage following IM injection, the vaccine may be administered subcutaneously, although the subsequent antibody titer may be lower and there may be an increased risk of a local reaction.

The vaccine is administered in a three-dose schedule, Recombivax HB (at 0, 1 and 6 months). Ideally, immunization with the vaccine for travelers should be 6 months before traveling to allow completion of the full three-dose vaccine series. However, if 6 months of time before travel is not possible, an alternative four-dose schedule, Engerix-B (at 0, 1, 2, and 12 months) may provide better protection if it can be completed before travel ensues. It is assumed that the four-dose schedule provides a more rapid induction of immunity. However, there is no demonstrated evidence that this schedule provides greater protection than the standard three-dose schedule.

Other Drugs

This section includes peptide drugs that are not conveniently classified into the preceding categories of biotechnology drugs. Nonetheless, they are important for the pharmacist to know about. They are all administered nonparenterally to the patient.

GOSERELIN—ZOLADEX. Goserelin is indicated for palliative treatment in advanced prostatic carcinoma. It is a synthetic luteinizing hormone-releasing hormone (LHRH) analog. Administration of this drug stimulates the release of luteinizing hormone (LH) and follicle-stimulating hormone (FSH) from the anterior pituitary, which transiently increases testosterone concentrations in males. However, continual administration of goserelin in the treatment of prostatic carcinoma suppresses the secretion of LH and FSH, causes a fall in testosterone concentrations, and effects "medical castration." This drug offers an alternative treatment of prostatic cancer when *orchiectomy* (removal of one or both testes) or estrogen administration are not indicated or not acceptable to the patient.

Goserelin is also indicated for the management of endometriosis, for pain reduction/relief and reduction of endometriotic lesions during therapy. This drug has been demonstrated to be as effective as danazol in relieving the clinical symptoms (dysmenorrhea, dyspareunia, pelvic pain) and signs (pelvic tenderness) of endometriosis and decreasing the size of endometrial lesions. At present, the duration of therapy is recommended to be no longer than 6 months, because there are no clinical data on the effect of treatment of benign gynecological conditions with goserelin for periods greater than 6 months.

Goserelin is administered as an subcutaneous implant and, along with leuprolide acetate (Lupron Depot) was one of the first polymer systems to receive FDA approval for controlled release of a peptide. This drug is available in a 3.6 mg, biodegradable and biocompatible, sterile, white-to-cream-colored cylinder about the size of a grain of rice, which is implanted every 28 days

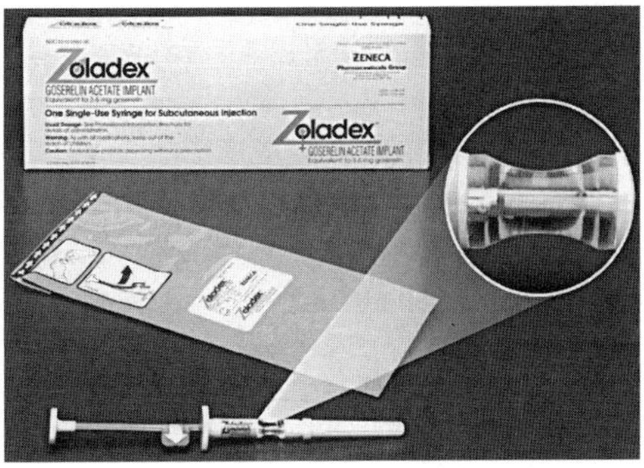

Fig. 9–6. *Example of the product package of Zoladex, which demonstrates the innovative delivery system for the continuous release of goserelin acetate from an injectable pellet (Courtesy of Zeneca Pharmaceuticals Group)*

into the upper abdominal wall (Fig. 9–6). The drug is dispersed in a matrix of D,L-lactic acid and glycolic acids copolymer.

LEUPROLIDE ACETATE—LUPRON. Leuprolide is a synthetic gonadotropin-releasing hormone (GnRH) analog. Like the naturally occurring luteinizing hormone–releasing hormone (LHRH), initial and intermittent administration of this drug stimulates the release of luteinizing hormone (LH) and follicle-stimulating hormone (FSH) from the anterior pituitary. Like goserelin, continuous administration of leuprolide suppresses the secretion of LH and FSH, with a concomitant drop in testosterone concentrations and subsequent "medical castration."

The usual adult dose for prostatic carcinoma is a subcutaneous injection of 1 mg/day. There is also a once-a-month (every 28 to 33 days) depot, intramuscular injection. The 7.5 mg strength is used for prostatic carcinoma. The powder for intramuscular injection is reconstituted with a special diluent composed of D-mannitol, purified gelatin, DL-lactic and glycolic acids copolymer, polysorbate 80, and acetic acid.

Lupron should be refrigerated until dispensed, but patients may store the product at room temperature (no more than 30°C, or 86°F). The product should be protected from light and the vial stored in the carton until use. Following reconstitution, the suspension is stable for 1 day. However, because the product has no preservative, it should be discarded if not used immediately.

RECOMBINANT HUMAN DNASE I—PULMOZYME. In 1989 the cystic fibrosis (CF) gene was discovered, and it has helped to lay the groundwork

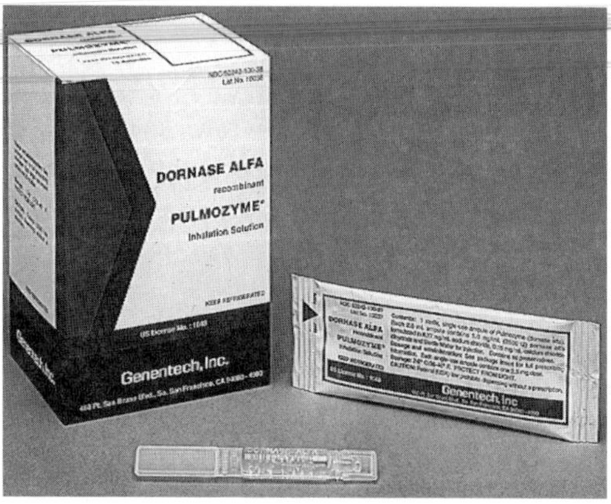

Fig. 9–7. *Example of the product package of Pulmozyme (Courtesy of Genentech, Inc.)*

for new therapies to treat this disease, which is the most common fatal, genetically inherited disease affecting Whites. Cystic fibrosis transmembrane conductance regulator, the protein product of the CF gene, is defective in its ability to facilitate ion transport across the airway epithelial cells in the lung. This defective regulator allows excessive absorption of sodium and adequate amounts of chloride across the cell membrane. Consequently, water from the mucus of the lung gets absorbed into the cell and the mucus becomes dehydrated, resulting in a thick, tenacious mucus that accumulates in the small airways of the lung. This then leads to a domino effect of chronic infection and inflammation, followed by chronic lung disease, pulmonary hypertension, and heart failure.

rhDNase (recombinant human deoxyribonuclease I), or Dornase alfa, is a DNA enzyme indicated for the treatment of symptoms of cystic fibrosis (CF). This enzyme specifically cleaves extracellular DNA, such as that found in the thick, sticky, mucous secretions of CF patients.[16] As a result, airflow in the lung is improved and the risk of bacterial infection may be decreased. This drug offers hope for breaking the cycle of chronic lung infection and inflammation associated with CF disease, and it demonstrates no effect upon the DNA of intact cells.

rhDNase showed very successful efficacy data involving over 1100 patients in Phase II and Phase III testing. The drug improved the quality of life for the CF patient with mild to moderate pulmonary dysfunction by reducing the need for I.V. antibiotics, hospitalizations, and time missed from school, work, and everyday activities. The risk of respiratory infections was reduced by 27% for patients on 2.5 mg once daily in clinical trials, and hospital days were reduced from 7.6 days (untreated patients) to 6.2 days (for treated patients).[17]

Indicated to treat cystic fibrosis in patients age 5 years and older, rhDNase is available in 2.5 mL, single-use polyethylene ampuls for use with compressed air nebulizers (Fig. 9–7). Three nebulizer systems are recommended. These are: Marquest Acorn II nebulizer; Hudson T Updraft II nebulizer powered by a DeVilbiss Pulmo-aide Compressor; and Pari LC nebulizer driven by the Pari Proneb Compressor. Each of these systems delivers approximately 25% of the dose.

Portable jet models and ultrasonic nebulizers should not be used to administer rhDNase. For example, the ultrasonic nebulizers may heat the protein enough to alter its structure. The portable jet nebulizers simply might not be capable of generating enough force or appropriate particle size to ensure optimal delivery of the drug into the lung.

To make administration efficient, it might be tempting to co-administer other compounds (e.g., albuterol, tobramycin) with rhDNase. However, no other medication should be mixed in the nebulizer system with this drug because the possibility exists that, with a pH change, an alteration of the rhDNase protein structure could occur. Bronchodilator and antimicrobial agents that are administered via nebulizer should be administered to patients sequentially, but not mixed together. To date, there is no literature that suggests the optimal sequence for all of these drugs to be administered.

The ampuls will have an 18-month expiration dating when stored in the refrigerator between 2° and 8°C. The product cannot be exposed to room temperatures for more than 24 hours.

The Future of Biotechnology Products

The future will see the development of more protein-based pharmaceuticals as a result of modern biotechnologic strategies, including the development of "artificial" genes. These protein-based drugs will present unique challenges because of intrinsic instability, multifaceted metabolic properties, and limited gastrointestinal absorption.[18] Other problems will include variable tissue penetration (because of the size of the molecules) and toxicity related to the stimulation of an immune or allergic reaction.[18]

A distinct advantage of these biotechnologically derived proteins over proteins from natural sources is enhanced purity. Hepatitis B virus and the human immunodeficiency virus (HIV) are capable of contaminating proteins and enzymes from human plasma. If their presence is known, they can be isolated or neutralized. However, sometimes their presence has been confirmed only after disastrous results. Products derived from recombinant technology will not have co-extracted contaminants.

Research is also directed toward the discovery of new methods of delivery for these agents. Delivery systems being explored include transdermal and nasal routes, other forms of injectables, and oral tablets for smaller proteins. Few protein biopharmaceutical products can be administered orally because of their instability in the strong acid environment of the stomach and the low systemic absorption through gastrointestinal mucosa. A challenge is to deliver regulatory proteins (e.g., insulin, growth hormone) to distant organs or tissue without biotransformation. One strategy that may bear fruit is encapsulating the protein-based compound in lipid complexes (liposomes). *Liposomes* are typically composed of some combination of phosphatidylcholine, cholesterol, phosphatidylglycerol, or other glycolipids or phospholipids. These are water-filled, vesicular structures composed of several phospholipid layers surrounding an aqueous core, and with the outer shell capable of providing direction to specific target cells (e.g., tumors). Typically, liposomes will concentrate the drug in cells of the reticuloendothelial system of the liver and spleen, and will reduce drug intake in the heart, kidney, and gastrointestinal tract. The application of liposome-associated doxorubicin reduces cardiotoxicity, and liposome-associated amphotericin-B reduces nephrotoxicity and other adverse effects.[19]

Liposomes are popular among particulate carriers because of their relatively low toxicity and the versatility of their release characteristics and disposition in vivo by changing preparation techniques and bilayer constituents. Depending upon their size, charge, and bilayer rigidity, among other characteristics, liposomes circulate only for a short period of time (minutes) in the circulation before degradation and uptake by macrophages of the mononuclear phagocyte system. Sometimes, their residence in the systemic circulation can be for hours (and even days) if they are stable and not recognized by macrophages as "foreign bodies."

Insoluble polymers composed of polyethylene glycol can be utilized to form a protective sheath around a drug, thereby inhibiting its degradation.[19] One application of this technology is for the delivery of enzymes that are rapidly cleared from body tissues and fluids. One PEG formulation of the enzyme adenosine deaminase (ADA) has been approved for patients suffering from severe combined immunodeficiency disease (SCID). This condition is caused by a lack of ADA enzyme in lymphocytic WBCs. The polymer affords "protected" delivery of the enzyme to restore lymphocyte function and immunoprotection.

A third strategy delivers extremely toxic proteins to tumor cells. In this approach, antibodies with specific sensitivities (e.g., monoclonal antibodies) are fused to toxic proteins (e.g., ricin, *Pseudomonas* exotoxin) and then administered intravenously.[20] The fused protein is delivered directly to the specified cancer cells, where one released functional molecule can effect cell death. The most widely studied plant toxin is ricin, a natural product of beans from the plant *Ricinus communis*.[21] An example of this strategy is Anti-B4-blocked ricin (Oncolysin B) being tested for B-cell leukemias and lymphomas. Ricin, with a protein structure and a molecular weight of 66 kD, has been the prime target for monoclonal antibody conjugation. This unmodified compound is extremely cytotoxic as it enzymatically blocks intracellular protein synthesis at the ribosomal level. It, as well as other immunotoxins, has demonstrated antitumor activity against cultured melanoma cells and melanoma tumors growing in mice. Unfortunately, to date these complexes still have limited target-cell specificity, and uptake/sequestration by the liver remains a problem. Further, once inside the cell, the toxin must translocate across membranes into the cytosol, where it can inhibit protein synthesis.[21]

It is entirely feasible in the future that protein complexes will be engineered that combine a "transporting" protein with one that encodes the gene sequence to produce a therapeutic protein in the target tissue. In this instance, the gene will become functional only in certain tissue, with a resultant decrease in delivery to an unintended site.

The future will also see the creation of more

products for "in home" testing. Monoclonal antibody-based diagnostic tests that are now restricted to physician use are under development for home testing. These include products for infectious disease processes (e.g., AIDS, chlamydia trachomatis, streptococcal throat infections). In addition, it is anticipated that monoclonal antibody–based tests will also be available to assay blood/plasma concentrations of a number of drugs (e.g., digoxin, phenytoin, theophylline).

To date, monoclonal antibodies have been used in home tests for confirmation of pregnancy or predicting ovulation. Quidel Laboratories has developed a monoclonal antibody product designed to detect pregnanediol glucuronide (a metabolite of progesterone) in female urine and to help avoid pregnancy.[14] Levels of this substance fluctuate during the normal menstrual cycle (low in the follicular phase, high in the luteal phase). The self-test kit will enable a woman to monitor urine levels of pregnanediol to determine when fertilization is possible. A woman could then avoid intercourse during her fertile period and prevent the occurrence of pregnancy.

FDA Office of Biotechnology

The FDA Office of Biotechnology was created in 1989. The office does not evaluate submissions to the FDA for approval of clinical investigations or for product marketing approvals; these functions are executed by the appropriate FDA Centers. Further, this office does not perform laboratory research or mandate research priorities to the FDA centers. Instead, it serves as a central coordinating, problem-solving, and advisory role within the Office of the Commissioner, and it has become an effective point of contact with the FDA for those outside of the agency on issues related to new biotechnology.

The FDA Office of Biotechnology has the following responsibilities: It,

1. advises and assists the Commissioner and other central officials about scientific issues related to biotechnology policy, direction, and long-range goals.
2. represents the Agency of biotechnological issues to other governmental agencies and intergovernmental groups, state and local governments, industry, consumer organizations, Congress, national and international organizations, and the scientific community.
3. provides leadership and direction on scientific and regulatory issues related to biotechnology. This is accomplished through an Agency-wide coordinating group (i.e., the Biotechnology Coordinating Committee) that promotes communication and consistency on biotechnology matters across organizational lines.
4. provides a problem-solving function for individuals, companies, associations, or organizations that have concerns, questions, or complaints about biotechnology policies or procedures, or about product jurisdiction or other aspect of product regulation.
5. coordinates and facilitates guidance on cross-cutting or controversial biotechnology program policies.

Inquiries or requests may be addressed to the Director, Office of Biotechnology, FDA, HF-6, 5600 Fishers Lane, Rockville, MD 20857; (301)443-7573; fax, (301)443-7005.

Patient Information from the Pharmacist

For those products that can be parenterally self-administered, the pharmacist should instruct patients in the use of aseptic technique. Appropriate verbal instruction that reinforces the printed information sheet should also be provided when the product requires reconstitution. It is desirable to perform the first injection under the supervision of an appropriately qualified health care professional to assure patient comprehension and understanding of technique. Some products (e.g., Betaseron) come with a training video that demonstrates reconstitution and self-administration techniques.

Patients who self-administer these products must be educated on how to prepare (Fig. 9–8) and give the injection and how to rotate injection sites (Fig. 9–9). Some products provide a schematic illustration of this on the patient information sheet. Patients should understand that changing sites each time helps avoid injection reactions and gives the site opportunity to "bounce back" from the previous injection. It is important that the patient understand not to administer an injection into the same area as the prior injection, nor within areas that are tender, red, or hard. The pharmacist should provide a method for the patient to record where previous injections have been made. One simple way is

PREPARING THE INJECTION

1. Remove the needle guard of the 1 mL syringe and pull back the plunger to the 1 mL mark.

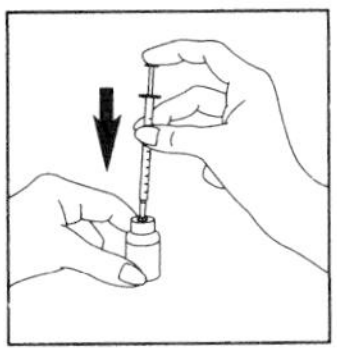

2. Insert the needle of the 1 mL syringe through the stopper of the vial of Betaseron solution.

3. Gently push the plunger all the way down to inject air into the vial (leave the needle in the vial).

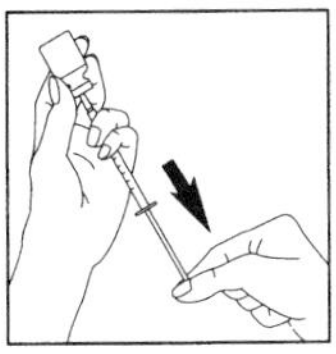

4. Turn the vial of Betaseron (Interferon beta-1b) solution upside down.

NOTE: Keep the needle tip in the liquid.

5. Pull back the plunger to withdraw 1 mL of liquid into the syringe.

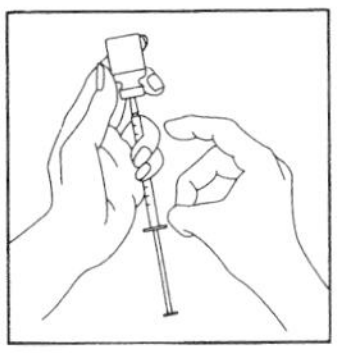

6. Hold the syringe with the needle pointing upward.

7. Tap the syringe gently until any air bubbles that formed rise to the top of the barrel of the syringe.

8. Carefully push in the plunger to eject ONLY THE AIR through the needle.

9. Remove the needle/syringe from the vial.

10. Recap the needle on the syringe.

NOTE: The injection should be administered immediately after mixing (if the injection is delayed, refrigerate the solution and inject it within 3 hours). Do not freeze.

11. Throw away unused portion of the solution remaining in the vial.

Fig. 9–8. *Preparing the Betaseron for injection (Courtesy of Berlex, Inc.)*

to suggest that the patient note the injection site on a calendar.

Patients should be advised about the proper disposal procedures for needles and syringes. In this day of the cost-conscious consumer, patients must be advised against reusing needles and syringes. A puncture-resistant container for disposal of used needles/syringes is very advantageous to provide the patient—along with instruction for the safe disposal of full containers.

The patient should understand that periodic injection-site reactions may occur during therapy. These may be transient (as in the case of interferon beta-1b) and not require discontinuation of the therapy. It is advisable, however, periodically to reevaluate patient understanding and use of aseptic self-administration technique and procedures.

It is very important for the patient to understand that these products should not be agitated or shaken. Otherwise, there is the possibility of product (protein) denaturation and resultant ineffectiveness. Much like the suspension forms of insulin, which should be rolled (or rotated) in the palms of the hands, these products should be gently swirled to dissolve their contents.

Whenever possible, pharmacists must emphasize the need for compliance with dosage regimens. Betaseron, for example, is administered every other day. A calendar reminder system might be helpful for a patient using this medication.

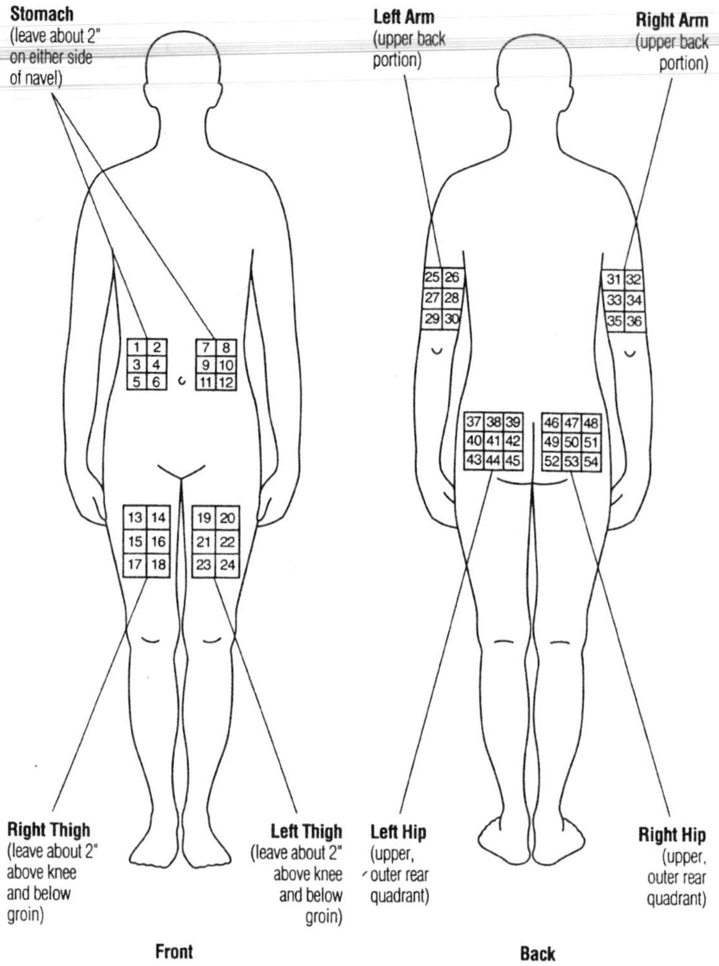

Fig. 9–9. *Schematic for rotation of injection sites (Courtesy of Berlex, Inc.)*

Pharmacist Self Help With Biotechnology Drugs

The advent of biotechnology drugs poses a real dilemma to some pharmacists. They may be reluctant to stock these medications because of their high cost, their special storage and handling requirements, poor understanding of the drug's therapeutics (including side effects and counseling information required), and/or the difficult issue of reimbursement.[22] These products also are comparably far more expensive than "ordinary" pharmaceuticals.

Unfortunately, pharmacists cannot assume that the responsibility for dispensing these products will automatically fall to them.[1] Indeed, the profession's failure to accept responsibility for the radioactive pharmaceutical products used for diagnosis and treatment of disease has resulted in nonpharmacists managing them. Similarly, the profession was not positioned to accept responsibility for patient-controlled analgesia (see Chapter 8) and ultimately lost control to anesthesia departments in many hospitals. Although there are few biotechnological products for chronic conditions currently available in community pharmacies (except insulin, diagnostic tests, vaccines), drugs initially used exclusively in hospitals, as well as newly developed agents (e.g., Betaseron) will soon work their way into community practice.[1]

It is advisable that pharmacists continue their education on these products, and there are numerous programs to do so. Some are available directly from the manufacturer or through professional associations (e.g., APhA–Biotech ℞: Opportunities in Therapy Management) and cover basic biotechnology and/or therapeutic applications of specific products. Pharmacists should realize that various manufacturers of biotechnology products and professional associations provide support services for the profession. Typically, manufacturer services fall into one of three broad categories—professional services, educational materials, reimbursement support. While the professional services may differ among companies, many have toll-free telephone numbers for obtaining information on biotechnology products.

Pharmacists should take advantage of these programs, realizing that complete knowledge of biotechnology drugs' manufacture is not necessary. Pharmacists should, however, understand protein chemistry (as it relates to drug stability and structure) and immunology. Many programs cover basic biotechnology, as well as therapeutic review of individual drugs. Programs can be very helpful—for example, a real danger with these products is that the pharmacist may confuse products with similar names. Many approved and investigational interferons (alfa-n3, alfa-2b, gamma-1b, etc.) differ greatly in activity and indications for use.[22]

That most biotech drugs must be administered parenterally poses a threat to some pharmacists, who are wary of this administration route and cognizant of their limitations/inability to counsel the patients in appropriate technique. Suffice to say, the pharmacist should assume the professional responsibility to secure educational materials (videotapes, print) from the manufacturer. For example, self-injection products contain instruction sheets that offer a step-by-step guide for preparing and administering the injection in the home.

Aside from being knowledgeable about such things as therapeutic use, side effects, precautions, the pharmacist must also be able to identify monitoring parameters that need to be followed to ensure safety and efficacy.[23] Further, the pharmacist should be aware of drugs that are administered in conjunction with these agents to reduce the incidence and severity of side effects (acetaminophen and indomethacin started immediately before aldesleukin therapy to reduce fever; methylprednisolone sodium succinate IV prior to first injection of muromonab-CD3).

Medical and product information services are available from the manufacturers for biotechnology drugs, just as for traditional drugs. In addition to answering conventional questions about drug use, indications, adverse effects, and so on, this service also helps answer difficult questions (e.g., what to do if a product requiring refrigeration has been left at room temperature for an extended period of time) and helps to facilitate quick replacement of defective products.

Reimbursement issues are not relevant here. However, it is important to realize that manufacturers do have support staff who will help the pharmacist deal with third-party payers, particularly if there is a reimbursement issue/problem. Manufacturer reimbursement assurance programs are designed to remove reimbursement barriers when reimbursement has been denied (e.g., if the drug has been used for an unlabeled indication or used in the home rather than in a hospital or physician's office). Many companies also have had a long-standing tradition of providing prescription medications free of charge to those who might not otherwise have access to necessary medicines. Physicians can secure these on behalf of their patients; the pharmacist can *refer* patients and their families to pharmaceutical companies who have cost-sharing or financial assistance programs. The Pharmaceutical Research and Manufacturers of America (PhRMA) has a directory of programs available for patients in need. Up-to-date information can be secured by a health care professional by calling the PhRMA at 1-800-PMA-INFO.

References

1. Wade, D.A. and Levy, R.A.: Biotechnology: An opportunity for pharmacists. *American Pharmacy, NS32*(9):33–37, 1992.
2. Bagley, J.L.: Biotech. *American Druggist, 195*(7): 57–63, 1986.
3. Sindelar, R.E.: Biotech products on the horizon. *American Pharmacy, NS33*(11):27–28, 1993.
4. Wordell, C.J.: Use of beta interferon in multiple sclerosis. *Hospital Pharmacy, 28*(8):802–807, 1993.
5. *FDA Medical Bulletin, 23*(2):4, June, 1993.
6. Sahai, J. and Louis, S.G.: Overview of the immune and hematopoietic systems. *American Journal of Hospital Pharmacy, 50 (Suppl 3)*:S4–S18, 1993.
7. Metcalf, D.: The colony stimulating factors. *Cancer, 65*(10)2185–2195, 1990.
8. Blackwell, S. and Crawford, J.: Colony-stimulating factors: Clinical applications. *Pharmacotherapy, 12*(2, part 2):20S–31S, 1992.
9. Oettgen, H.F.: Cytokines in clinical cancer therapy. *Current Opinion in Immunology, 3*:699–705, 1991.

10. Piascik, P.: A new treatment for multiple sclerosis. *American Pharmacy, NS33*(12):25–26, 1993.
11. Piascik, P.: Administering betaseron for MS *American Pharmacy, NS34*(1):21–22, 1994.
12. Giedlin, M.A. and Zimmerman, R.J.: The use of recombinant human interleukin-2 in treating infectious diseases. *Current Opinion in Biotechnology, 4:* 722–726, 1993.
13. Tami, J.A., et al.: Monoclonal antibody technology. *American Journal of Hospital Pharmacy, 43:* 2816–2826, 1986.
14. Newton, G.D.: Monoclonal antibody-based self-testing products. *American Pharmacy, NS33*(9): 22–23, 1993.
15. Brodsky, F.M.: Monoclonal antibodies as magic bullets. *Pharmaceutical Research, 5*(1):1–9, 1988.
16. Sindelar, R.E.: Biotech products on the horizon. *American Pharmacy, NS33*(11):27–28, 1993.
17. Ramsey, B.: A summary of the results of the phase III multi-center clinical trial: Aerosol administration of recombinant human DNase reduces the risk of respiratory infections and improves pulmonary function in patients with cystic fibrosis. *Pediatric Pulmonology, 9(suppl):*12–153, 1993.
18. Reddy, I.K., and Banga, A.K.: Biotechnology drug delivery: Oral vs. alternate routes. *Pharmacy Times, 59*(11):92–98, 1993.
19. Hudson, R.A. and Black, C.D.: Novel delivery for protein drugs. *American Pharmacy, NS33*(5):23–24, 1993.
20. Houston, L.L.: Targeted delivery of toxins and enzymes by antibodies and growth factors. *Current Opinion in Biotechnology, 4*:739–744, 1993.
21. Houghton, A.N. and Coit, D.G.: Therapy of metastatic melanoma with monoclonal antibodies. *New Perspectives in Cancer Diagnosis and Management, 1* (3):65–70, 1993.
22. Piascik, P.: Getting information about biotechnology products. *American Pharmacy, NS33*(4):18–19, 1993.
23. Fields, S.: Dispensing biotechnology products. *American Pharmacy, NS33*(3):28–29, 1993.

Notes

1. The following reference is directed as a resource guide for faculty within schools/colleges of pharmacy: *Biotechnology Resource Guide,* L. Michael Posey, Editor, PCPS, Philadelphia, PA, 1992. Supported by Amgen Inc.
2. The Pharmaceutical Research and Manufacturers of America periodically disseminates *Biotechnology Medicines in Development,* which demonstrates biotechnology medicines that have reached the clinical marketplace or are currently in development. Those desiring to receive this regularly are asked to write to the Editor, Biotechnology Medicines in Development, Communications Division, Pharmaceutical Research and Manufacturers of America, 1100 15th Street, NW, Washington, DC 20005.

10

Transdermal Drug Delivery Systems, Ointments, Creams, Lotions, and Other Preparations

THIS CHAPTER includes drug delivery systems and dosage forms which are intended to be applied to the skin. Ointments, creams, transdermal drug delivery systems, lotions, and topical solutions represent the most frequently used dermatologic dosage forms; however, other preparations as pastes, liniments, powders, gels, tinctures, and aerosols are also commonly used.

Preparations are applied to the skin either for their physical effects, that is, for their ability to act as skin protectants, lubricants, emollients, drying agents, etc., or for the specific effect of the medicinal agent(s) present. Preparations sold over-the-counter frequently contain mixtures of medicinal substances used in the treatment of such conditions as minor skin infections, itching, burns, diaper rash, insect stings and bites, athlete's foot, corns, calluses, warts, dandruff, acne, psoriasis, and eczema. Skin applications which require a prescription generally contain a single medicinal agent intended to counter a specific diagnosed condition.

Although it is generally desirable in treating skin diseases for the drug in the medicated application to penetrate past the surface and into the skin, it is not generally the intent (except for transdermal medicated systems) that the medication enter the general circulation. However, once past the epidermis, a drug substance finds itself in proximity to blood capillaries feeding the subcutaneous tissues (Fig. 10–1), and absorption into the general circulation is not unlikely. In fact, such absorption commonly results after topical application of certain preparations as evidenced by detectable blood levels of the drug and the urinary excretion of the drug or its metabolic products. However, most of the materials employed for nonsystemic topical use are sufficiently nontoxic in the amounts absorbed so that the effects of absorption are generally unrecognized by the patient.

Percutaneous Absorption

The absorption of substances from outside the skin to positions beneath the skin, including entrance into the blood stream, is referred to as *percutaneous absorption*. In general, the percutaneous absorption of a medicinal substance present in a transdermal therapeutic system, or in a dermatological preparation such as a liquid, gel, ointment, cream, or paste depends not only upon the physical and chemical properties of the medicinal substance but also upon its behavior when placed in the pharmaceutical vehicle and the condition of the skin. It is well known that although a pharmaceutical vehicle may not penetrate the skin to any great extent nor actually carry the medicinal substance through the skin, the vehicle does influence the rate and degree of penetration of a medicinal agent, and the degree and rate vary with different drugs and with different vehicles. Therefore each drug substance-vehicle combination must be examined individually for percutaneous absorption and therapeutic efficacy.

The Skin

Upon the surface of the skin is a film of emulsified material composed of a complex mixture of sebum, sweat, and desquamating horny layer, the latter from the layer of dead epidermal cells, termed the "horny layer" or the "stratum corneum," and situated directly beneath the emulsified film. Beneath the horny layer in order is a "barrier layer," the living epidermis or the stratum germinativum, and the dermis or true skin.

Blood capillaries and nerve fibers rise from the subcutaneous fat tissue into the dermis and up to the epidermis. Sweat glands present in the subcutaneous tissue yield their products by way of sweat ducts which find their way to the surface of the skin. Sebaceous (oil) glands and hair

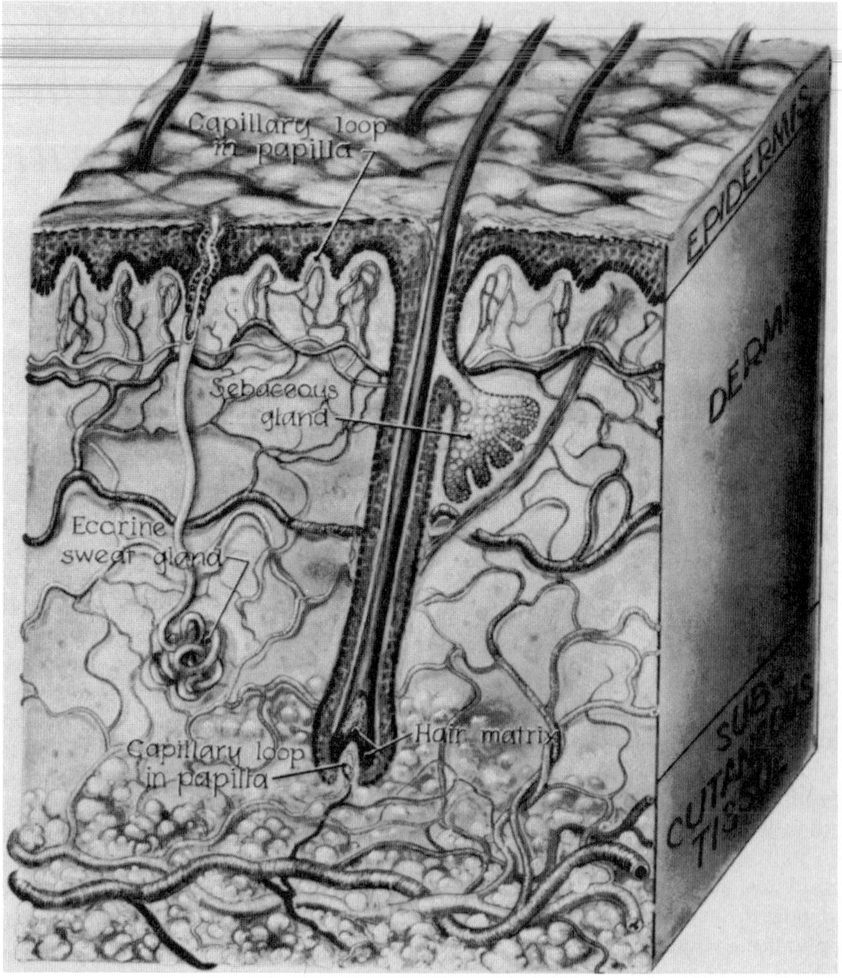

Fig. 10–1. *Stratified organization of the skin. (Pillsbury, D.M. and Heston, Charles, L.: A Manual of Dermatology. 2nd Ed., Courtesy of W.B. Saunders Co., 1979.)*

follicles originating in the dermis and subcutaneous layers also find their way to the surface and are revealed as ducts and hairs respectively.

Penetration of the Skin by Drugs

Drugs may penetrate intact skin after topical application through the walls of the hair follicles, through the sweat glands or the sebaceous glands, or between the cells of the horny layer. Naturally, broken or abraded skin is easily entered by applied substances, but such penetration does not really constitute true percutaneous absorption.

If the skin is intact, the main route for the penetration of drug is generally through the epidermal layers, rather than through the hair follicles or the gland ducts, because the surface area of the latter is rather minute compared to the area of skin containing neither of these anatomical elements. The film covering the horny layer is not generally continuous and presents no real resistance to penetration. Because the composition of the film varies with the proportion of sebum and sweat produced and the degree of their removal through washing and sweat evaporation, the film is not a true barrier to drug transfer, because it has no definite composition, thickness, or continuity.

The percutaneous absorption of a drug generally results from the direct penetration of the drug through the stratum corneum, a 10 to 15 μm thick layer of flat, partially desiccated, nonliving tissue which forms the skin's outermost surface.[1,2] The stratum corneum is composed of approximately 40% protein (mainly keratin) and 40% water, with the balance being lipid, principally as triglycerides, free fatty acids, cholesterol, and phospholipids. The lipid content is concentrated in the extracellular phase of the stratum corneum and forms to a large extent the membrane surrounding the cells. Since a drug's major route of penetration is through the intercellular channels, the lipid component is considered an important determinant in the first step of the absorption process.[3] Once through the stratum corneum, drug molecules may then pass through the deeper epidermal tissues and into the dermis. When the drug reaches the vascularized dermal layer, it becomes available for absorption into the general circulation.

The stratum corneum, being keratinized tissue, behaves as a semipermeable artificial membrane, and drug molecules penetrate by passive diffusion. Thus, the rate of drug movement across this skin layer is dependent on the drug concentration in the vehicle, its aqueous solubility, and its oil/water partition coefficient between the stratum corneum and the vehicle.[4] Substances that possess both aqueous and lipid solubility characteristics are good candidates for diffusion through the stratum corneum as well as through the epidermal and dermal layers.

Although the skin has been divided histologically into the stratum corneum, the living epidermis, and the dermis, collectively it can be considered a laminate of barriers. Permeation of this laminate can occur by diffusion via:[5]

1. *trans*cellular penetration (across the cells)
2. *inter*cellular penetration (between the cells)
3. transappendageal penetration (via hair follicles, sweat and sebum glands, and pilosebaceous apparatus).

Factors Affecting Percutaneous Absorption

Among the factors playing a part in the percutaneous absorption of drugs are the nature of the drug itself, the nature of the vehicle, the condition of the skin, and the presence of moisture. Although general statements applicable to all possible combinations of drug, vehicle, and skin condition are difficult to draw, the consensus of the majority of research findings may be summarized as follows.[1–8]

1. Drug concentration is an important factor. Generally, the amount of drug percutaneously absorbed per unit of surface area per time interval increases as the concentration of the drug substance in the vehicle is increased.
2. More drug is absorbed through percutaneous absorption when the drug substance is applied to a larger surface area.
3. The drug substance should have a greater physiochemical attraction to the skin than to the vehicle in which it is presented in order for the drug to leave the vehicle in favor of the skin. However, some degree of solubility of the drug substance in both lipid and water is thought to be essential for effective percutaneous absorption. In essence, the aqueous solubility of a drug determines the concentration presented to the absorption site and the partition coefficient strongly influences the rate of transport across the absorption site. Solutes with molecular weights below 800 to 100 with adequate solubility in mineral oil and water (>1 mg/mL) can permeate skin.
4. Drug absorption appears to be enhanced from vehicles that easily cover the skin surface, mix readily with the sebum, and bring the drug into contact with the tissue cells for absorption.
5. Vehicles that increase the hydration of the skin generally favor the percutaneous absorption of drugs. Oleaginous vehicles and/or occlusive bandages act as moisture barriers through which the sweat from the skin cannot pass, and the skin therefore remains occluded, generally resulting in an increased hydration of the skin beneath the vehicle.
6. In general, the amount of rubbing in or inunction of the topical application will have a bearing on the amount of drug absorbed; the longer the period of inunction, the greater the absorption.
7. Percutaneous absorption appears to be greater when the drug is applied to skin with a thin horny layer than with one that is thick. Thus, the site of application may have a bearing on the degree of drug absorption, with the absorption from callused or thickened sites as the palms of the hands and soles of the feet being comparatively slow. Studies

have shown that skin in the postauricular area is more permeable to drugs than is skin from the back, chest, forearm, or thigh.[2] In addition to thickness, the properties of the stratum corneum vary at different body sites include differences in number of cell layers, stacking of cells, size of cells, and amount of surface lipid.

8. Generally, the longer the period of time the medicated application is permitted to remain in contact with the skin, the greater will be the absorption. However, changes in the hydration of the skin during the application period or the saturation of the skin with the drug could preclude significant additional absorption with increasing time.
9. Multiple-application dosing (dosing the same site more than once a day) rather than single bolus applications can increase drug bioavailability and absorption.[6]

These general statements on percutaneous absorption apply to skin in the normal state. In injury to the skin or in disease states of varying dimension, differences in drug absorption will occur. Quite clearly, skin that has been abraded, cut, or broken will permit drugs, and for that matter other foreign substances, to gain direct access to the subcutaneous tissues.

The intrinsic permeability of skin shows little variation from a few hours after birth to extreme old age; the ultrastructure of the stratum corneum in a newborn infant is indistinguishable from that of an adult.[2] However, blood levels of drug following topical application may be higher in infants than in adults due to a greater body surface to volume ratio. There is little, if any, difference between the permeability characteristics of human male and female skin. Differences in the drug permeability of skin of different races has not been unequivocally demonstrated.

Percutaneous Absorption Enhancers

There is a continuing interest among pharmaceutical scientists to identify substances that can enhance the percutaneous absorption of therapeutic agents. It is often difficult to determine whether materials used to enhance absorption do so by directly influencing the stratum corneum or by enhancing drug release from the formulation to the skin. However, a number of agents have been credited with enhancing skin penetration including surfactants, azone, dimethylsulfoxide (DMSO), dimethylacetamide, dimethylformamide, alcohol, acetone, propylene glycol, and polythylene glycol.[2,9–12] Proposed mechanisms of action for percutaneous absorption enhancers are: the reduction of the resistance of the stratum corneum by altering its physicochemical properties; alteration of the hydration of the stratum corneum; effecting a change in the structure of the lipids and lipoproteins in the intercellular channels, through solvent action or denaturation; and carrier mechanisms in the transport of ionizable drugs.[2,9–12]

Iontophoresis and Sonophoresis to Enhance Transdermal Drug Delivery

In addition to chemical means, there are some physical methods being studied to enhance transdermal drug delivery and penetration, namely, iontophoresis and sonophoresis.[12–17] *Iontophoresis* involves the delivery of charged chemical compounds across the skin membrane using an applied electrical field. A number of drugs have been the subject of such iontophoretic studies, including lidocaine,[13] amino acids/peptides/insulin,[14–16] verapamil,[16] and propranolol.[17] There is particular interest today in developing alternative routes for the delivery of biologically active peptides. These agents are presently delivered by injection, because of their rapid metabolism and poor absorption following oral delivery. They are also poorly absorbed from the transdermal route, because of their large molecular size, ionic character, and the general impenetrability of the skin.[15] However, iontophoretic-enhanced transdermal delivery has shown promise as a future means for peptide/protein administration. *Sonophoresis,* or high-frequency ultrasound, is also being studied as a means to enhance transdermal drug delivery.[18,19] Among the agents examined have been hydrocortisone, lidocaine, and salicyclic acid in such formulations as gels, creams, and lotions.[18] It is thought that high-frequency ultrasound can influence the integrity of the stratum corneum and thus affect its penetrability.

Percutaneous Absorption Models

Skin permeability and percutaneous absorption have been the subject of numerous studies undertaken to define the underlying principles and to optimize transdermal drug delivery. Although many experimental methods and models have been used, they tend to fall into one of two categories, in vivo or in vitro studies.

In vivo skin-penetration studies may be undertaken for one or more of the following purposes:[20]

1. To verify and quantify the cutaneous bioavailability of a topically applied drug;
2. To verify and quantify the systemic bioavailability of a transdermally delivered drug;
3. To establish bioequivalence of different topical formulations of the same drug substance; and
4. To determine incidence and degree of systemic toxicologic risk following the topical application of a specific drug/drug product.

The most relevant studies are performed in humans; however, animal models may be used insofar as they may be effective as predictors for humans. Animal models include the weanling pig, rhesus monkey, and hairless mouse or rat.[20,21] Biological samples utilized in drug penetration/drug absorption studies include skin sections, venous blood from the application site, blood from the systemic circulation, and excreta (urine, feces, and expired air). Readers interested in the specifics of such studies and methods can turn to the references cited.[20–24]

In vitro penetration studies using human skin are limited because of difficulties of procurement, storage, expense, and variability in permeation.[25] Excised animal skins may also be variable in quality and permeation. Animal skins are generally much more permeable than human skin. One alternative that has been shown to be effective is shed snake skin (*Elaphe obsoleta,* black rat snake), which is nonliving, pure stratum corneum, hairless, and similar to human skin, but slightly less permeable.[25,26] Also, the product Living Skin Equivalent (LSE) Testskin (Organogenesis, Inc.) recently was developed as an alternative for dermal absorption studies. The material is an organotypic coculture of human dermal fibroblasts in a collagen-containing matrix and a stratified epidermis composed of human epidermal keratinocytes. The material may be utilized in cell culture studies or in standard diffusion cells. Diffusion cell systems are employed in vitro to quantify the release rates of drugs from topical preparations.[27] In these systems, skin membranes or synthetic membranes may be employed as barriers to the flow of drug and vehicle, to simulate an in vivo system.

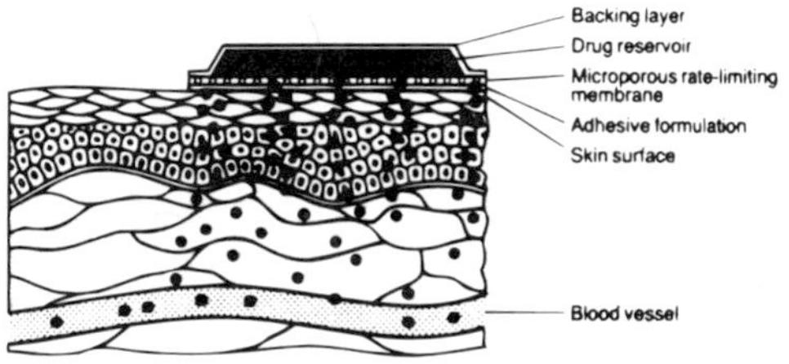

Fig. 10–2. *Depiction of a four-layered therapeutic transdermal system showing the continuous and controlled amount of medication released from the system, permeating the skin and entering the systemic circulation. (Courtesy of Alza Corporation.)*

Transdermal Drug Delivery Systems

Transdermal drug delivery systems are designed to support the passage of drug substances from the surface of the skin, through its various layers, and into the systemic circulation (Fig. 10–2). Physically, these systems are sophisticated patches as shown in Figures 10–3 through

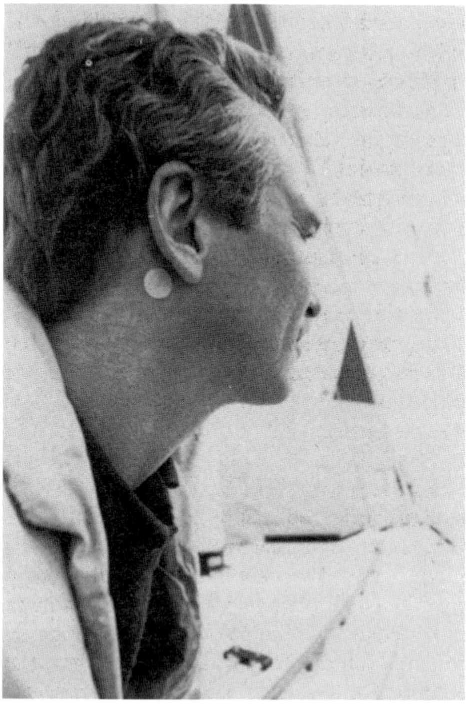

Fig. 10–3. *The Transderm Scōp (scopolamine) disc provides protection from the nausea and vomiting of motion sickness. (Courtesy of Alza Corporation and CIBA Consumer Pharmaceuticals).*

Table 10–1. Examples of Transdermal Drug Delivery Systems[31–41]

Therapeutic Agent	*Product*	*Design/Contents*	*Comments*
Clonidine	Catapres-TTS (Boch-ringer Ingelheim)	Four-layered patch: (1) a backing layer of pigmented polyester film; (2) drug reservoir of clonidine, mineral oil, polyisobutylene, and colloidal silicon dioxide; (3) a microporous polypropylene membrane controlling the rate of drug delivery; and (4) an adhesive formulation of agents noted in (2) above.	Transdermal therapeutic systems designed to deliver a therapeutic dose of the antihypertensive clonidine at a constant rate for 7 days, permitting once-a-week dosing. TTS generally applied to hairless or shaven areas of upper arm or torso.
Estradiol	Estraderm (CIBA)	Four-layered patch: (1) a transparent polyester film; (2) drug reservoir of estradiol and alcohol gelled with hydroxypropyl cellulose; (3) an ethylene-vinyl acetate copolymer membrane; and (4) an adhesive formulation of light mineral oil and polyisobutylene	Transdermal system designed to release 17β-estradiol continuously. The transdermal patch is generally applied twice weekly over a cycle of 3 weeks with dosage frequency adjusted as required. The patch is generally applied to the abdomen, alternating sites with each application.
Fentanyl	Duragesic (Janssen)	Four-layered patch: (1) a backing layer of polyester film; (2) drug reservoir of fentanyl and alcohol gelled with hydroxyethyl cellulose; (3) a rate-controlling ethylene-vinyl acetate copolymer membrane; and (4) a fentanyl-containing silicone adhesive.	Transdermal therapeutic system providing continuous 72-hour systemic delivery of fentanyl, a potent opioid analgesic. The drug is indicated in patients having chronic pain requiring opioid analgesia.
Nicotine	Habitrol (Basel)	Multi-layered round patch: (1) a tan-colored aluminized backing film; (2) a pressure-sensitive acrylate adhesive; (3) methacrylic acid copolymer solution of nicotine dispersed in a pad of nonwoven viscose and cotton; (4) an acrylate adhesive layer; and (5) a protective aluminized release liner that overlays the adhesive layer and is removed prior to use.	Transdermal therapeutic systems providing continuous release and systemic delivery of nicotine as an aid in smoking cessation programs. The patches listed vary somewhat in nicotine content and dosing schedules.
	Nicoderm (Marion Merrell Dow)	Multi-layered rectangular patch: (1) an occlusive backing of polyethylene/aluminum/polyester/ethylene-vinyl acetate copolymer; (2) drug reservoir of nicotine in an ethylene vinyl acetate copolymer matrix; (3) rate-controlling membrane of polyethylene; (4) polyisobutylene adhesive; and (5) protective liner removed prior to application.	
	Nicotrol (Parke-Davis)	Multi-layered rectangular patch: (1) outer backing of laminated polyester film; (2) rate-controlling adhesive, nonwoven material, and nicotine; (3) disposable liner removed prior to use.	
	Prostep (Lederle)	Multi-layered round patch: (1) beige-colored foam tape and acrylate adhesive; (2) backing foil, gelatin and low-density polyethylene coating; (3) nicotine-gel matrix; (4) protective foil with well; and (5) release liner removed prior to use.	
Nitroglycerin	Deponit (Schwarz Pharma)	Nitroglycerin in a matrix of lactose, plasticizer, polyisobutylene, and aluminized plastic.	Transdermal therapeutic systems designed to provide controlled release of nitroglycerin continuously for a 24-hour period. Patches are generally applied to hairless or shaven inner part of upper arm, shoulders, or chest; never to distal part of extremities. Each application is rotated to a slightly different skin area to avoid irritation.
	Minitran (3M Pharmaceuticals)	Nitroglycerin in a hypoallergenic acrylate-based polymer adhesive sealed in a foil/polymer film laminate. The patch is transparent when applied.	
	Nitrodisc (Searle)	Microseal Drug Delivery system consisting of a solid, nitroglycerin-impregnated polymer bonded to a flexible, nonsensitizing adhesive bandage. Inactive ingredients are lactose, isopropyl palmitate, mineral oil, polyethylene glycol, water, silicone rubber, plasticizers, aluminum foil laminate, polyethylene foam, and acrylic adhesive.	

Table 10–1. Continued

Therapeutic Agent	*Product*	*Design/Contents*	*Comments*
Nitroglycerin (cont.)	Nitro-Dur (Key)	Nitroglycerin in a gel-like matrix composed of glycerin, water, lactose, polyvinyl alcohol, povidone and sodium citrate sealed in a polyester-foil-polyethylene laminate.	
	Transderm-Nitro (Summit)	Four-layered patch: (1) backing layer of aluminized plastic; (2) drug reservoir containing nitroglycerin adsorbed on lactose, colloidal silicon dioxide, and silicone medical fluid, (3) an ethylene/vinyl acetate copolymer membrane; and (4) silicone adhesive.	
Scopolamine	Transderm Scōp (CIBA)	Four-layered patch: (1) backing layer of aluminized polyester film; (2) drug reservoir of scopolamine, mineral oil, and polyisobutylene; (3) a microporous polypropylene membrane for rate delivery of scopolamine; and (4) adhesive of polyisobutylene, mineral oil, and scopolamine.	Transdermal therapeutic system for continuous release of scopolamine over a 3-day period as required for the prevention of nausea and vomiting associated with motion sickness. The patch is placed behind the ear. When repeated administration is desired, the first patch is removed and the second patch placed behind the other ear.

10–7, outlined in Table 10–1, and described as follows.

There are two basic types of transdermal dosing systems: (1) *those that control* the rate of drug delivery to the skin, and (2) *those that allow the skin to control* the rate of drug absorption. The second type is useful for drugs for which there is a wide range of plasma concentration over which the drug is effective, but not toxic. For these drugs, transdermal dosage forms may be developed of various sizes and drug concentrations, with the physician increasing the dose and blood level of the drug by increasing the size of the transdermal application until the desired effect is obtained. However, for many drugs, it is important to control more closely and predictably the rate of drug delivery and percutaneous absorption. In these instances, drug delivery systems have been developed that control the rate of drug delivery to the skin for subsequent absorption. Effective transdermal drug delivery systems of this type deliver uniform quantities of drug to the skin over a period of time. The amounts of drug delivered per unit of time are determined to be less than that which is "absorbable" by varied types of skin, and thus, the drug

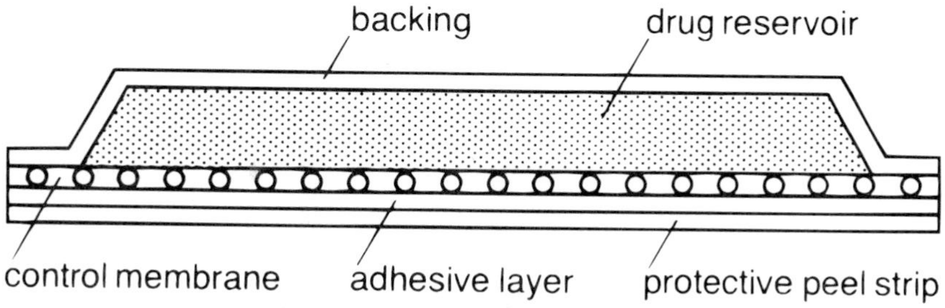

Fig. 10–4. *The Transderm-Nitro Transdermal Therapeutic System (Summit). The patch delivers nitroglycerin through the skin directly into the blood stream for 24 hours. Transderm-Nitro is used to treat and prevent angina. The system consists of a water-resistant backing layer, a reservoir of nitroglycerin, followed by a semipermeable membrane to control precisely and predictably the release of medicine, and an adhesive layer to hold the system onto the skin. The adhesive layer also contains an initial priming dose of nitroglycerin to insure prompt release and absorption of the medication. (Courtesy of Summit Pharmaceuticals.)*

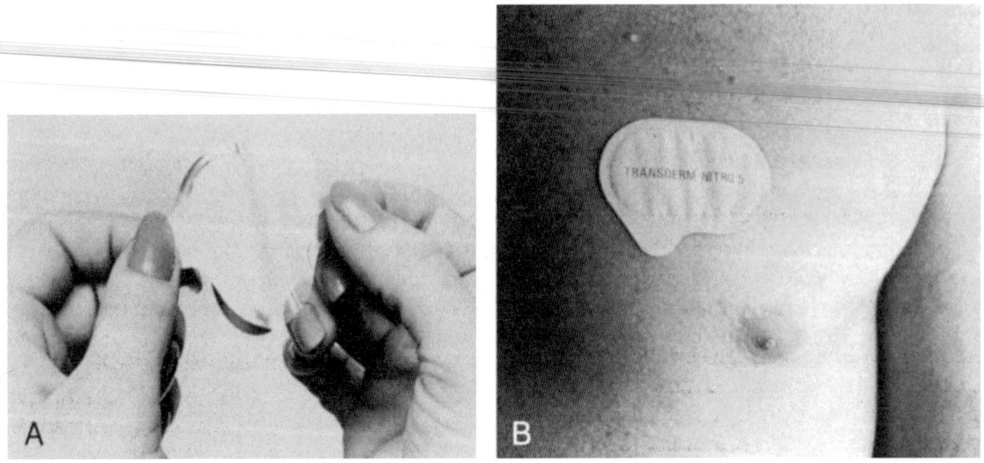

Fig. 10–5 (A,B). *The Transderm-Nitro patch (CIBA). Prior to applying to the skin, a plastic liner is removed exposing the adhesive side of the patch. Transderm-Nitro delivers nitroglycerin at a constant and predetermined rate through the skin directly into the bloodstream. The patch is designed to provide 24-hour protection against angina attacks. (Courtesy of Alza Corporation and CIBA Pharmaceutical Company.)*

delivery system, and not the skin, controls the amount of drug entering the circulation.

Included among the design features and objectives of rate-controlling transdermal drug delivery systems are the following:[1,5,28–30]

1. Deliver the drug substances at a controlled rate, to the intact skin of patients, for absorption into the systemic circulation.
2. The system should possess the proper physicochemical characteristics to permit the ready release of the drug substance and facilitate its partition from the delivery system into the stratum corneum.
3. The system should occlude the skin to ensure the one-way flux of the drug substance.
4. The transdermal system should have a therapeutic advantage over other dosage forms and drug delivery systems.
5. The system's adhesive, vehicle, and active agent should be nonirritating and nonsensitizing to the skin of the patient.

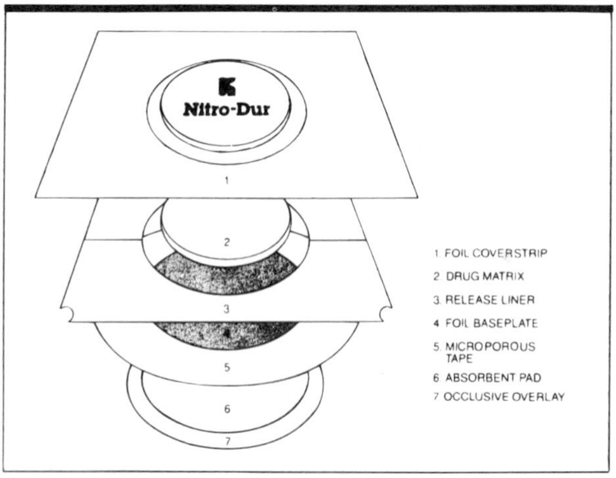

Fig. 10–6. *The Nitro-Dur Transdermal Infusion System, depicting the construction of the product. (Courtesy of Key Pharmaceuticals, Inc.)*

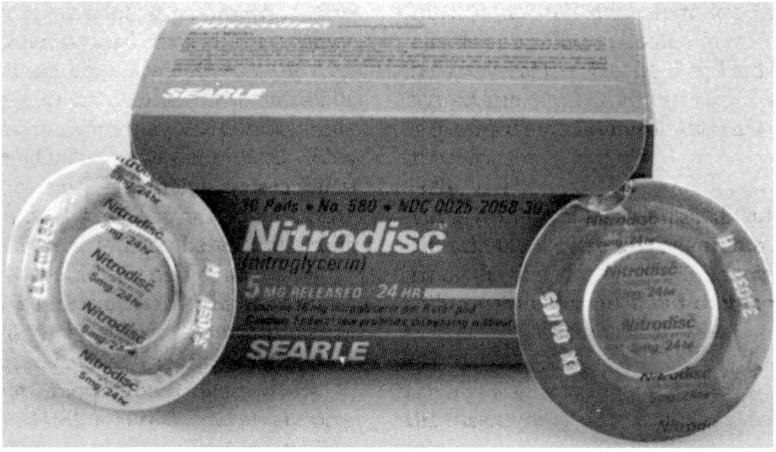

Fig. 10–7. *Example of the product package of the Nitrodisc transdermal nitroglycerin system. The 5 mg/24 hour system contains 16 mg of nitroglycerin over an 8 cm² releasing surface. (Courtesy of G. D. Searle Co.)*

6. The patch should adhere well to the patient's skin and its physical size and appearance and placement on the body should not be a deterrent to use.
7. The system should not permit the proliferation of skin bacteria beneath the occlusion.

Among the advantages of transdermal drug delivery systems are the following:

1. Avoids gastrointestinal drug absorption difficulties caused by gastrointestinal pH, enzymatic activity, drug interactions with food, drink, or other orally administered drugs.
2. Substitutes for oral administration of medication when that route is unsuitable, as in instances of vomiting and/or diarrhea.
3. Avoids *first-pass effect,* that is, the initial pass of a drug substance through the systemic and portal circulation following gastrointestinal absorption (thereby possibly avoiding the drug's deactivation by digestive and liver enzymes).
4. Avoids the risks and inconveniences of parenteral therapy and the variable absorption and metabolism associated with oral therapy.
5. Provides the capacity for multiday therapy with a single application, thereby improving patient compliance over use of other dosage forms requiring more frequent dose administration.
6. Extends the activity of drugs having short half-lives through the reservoir of drug present in the therapeutic delivery system and its controlled release characteristics.
7. Provides capacity to terminate drug effect rapidly (if clinically desired) by removal of drug application from the surface of the skin.
8. Provides ease of rapid identification of the medication in emergencies (e.g., nonresponsive, unconscious, or comatose patient).

Among the disadvantages of transdermal drug delivery systems are the following:

1. The transdermal route of administration is unsuitable for drugs that irritate or sensitize the skin.
2. Only relatively potent drugs are suitable candidates for transdermal delivery due to the natural limits of drug entry imposed by the skin's impermeability.
3. Technical difficulties are associated with the adhesion of the systems to different skin types and under various environmental conditions, and, the development of rate-controlling drug delivery features which are economically feasible and therapeutically advantageous for more than a few drug substances.

Examples of Transdermal Systems in Use

The first transdermal therapeutic system designed to control the delivery of drug to the skin for absorption was developed in 1980 by Alza Corporation. This system was designed to deliver the drug scopolamine to the skin behind the ear for systemic absorption in the control of nausea and vomiting associated with motion sickness (Fig. 10–3).

Transdermal Scopolamine System

Scopolamine has a narrow range of plasma concentration within which it is effective. Dosing levels and intervals which cause peaks and valleys to occur in blood level concentrations of the drug are more likely to produce side effects than when the drug is administered in a steady-state manner. The transdermal drug delivery system which has been developed provides the steady-state drug delivery over a 72 hour (3-day) period. The system obviates the oral route which yields unpredictable absorption, and, utilizes a lower dose which minimizes the incidence of side effects. The system, marketed as Transderm-Scōp by CIBA, is a circular flat adhesive patch designed for the continuous release of scopolamine through a rate-controlling microporous membrane.

The Transderm-Scōp system is a 0.2 mm thick patch having the following four layers:[31] (1) a backing layer of tan-colored, aluminized polyester film; (2) a drug reservoir of scopolamine, mineral oil, and polyisobutylene; (3) a microporous polypropylene membrane that controls the rate of delivery of scopolamine from the system to the skin surface; and (4) an adhesive formulation of mineral oil, polyisobutylene, and scopolamine. Prior to use, a protective peel strip of siliconized polyester which covers layer 4 is removed.

The patch is 2.5 cm^2 in area and contains 1.5 mg of scopolamine. The system is designed to deliver 0.5 mg scopolamine, at an approximately constant rate to the systemic circulation, over the 3-day lifetime of the system. An initial priming dose of 200 mcg of scopolamine, released from the adhesive layer of the system, saturates the skin binding sites for scopolamine and rapidly brings the plasma concentration to the required steady-state level. The continuous controlled release of scopolamine from the drug reservoir through the rate-controlling membrane maintains the plasma level constant. The microporous membrane releases the scopolamine from the drug-reservoir at a rate less than the skin's capability for absorption and thus, the membrane, not the skin, controls the delivery of the drug into the circulation. Because of the small size of the patch, the system is unobtrusive, convenient, and well-accepted by the patient. Patients should be advised to place the adhesive disk behind the ear about 4 hours before the antiemetic effect is required. Only one disk should be worn at a time and may be kept in place for up to 3 days. If continued treatment is desired, the first disk should be removed and discarded, and a fresh disk placed behind the second ear. The most common side effects encountered are dryness of the mouth and/or drowsiness. However, it is known that anticholinergics like scopolamine can also interfere with orientation, cognition and memory, and may cause disruption of global function, i.e., delirium, particularly in the geriatric population. The elderly have a relative deficiency of brain acetylcholine, which can increase their susceptibility to disruption in function because of central-acting anticholinergic drugs. Therefore, the use of transdermal scopolamine,. even in low doses, should be with caution.

Transdermal Nitroglycerin Systems

A second example of a drug used in transdermal drug delivery systems is nitroglycerin. A number of nitroglycerin-containing systems have been developed, including: Deponit (Schwarz) Minitran (3M Pharmaceuticals), Transdermal Nitro (Summit), Nitro-Dur (Key), and Nitrodisc (Searle). As indicated in Table 10–1, these products contain sufficient nitroglycerin to maintain drug delivery for 24 hours.

Nitroglycerin is a drug substance utilized widely in the prophylactic treatment of angina. The drug has a relatively low dose, short plasma half-life, high-peak plasma levels and inherent side-effects when taken sublingually (a popular route for its administration). It is rapidly metabolized by the liver when taken orally, which contributes to its low bioavailability by this route. For these reasons, nitroglycerin is a drug which has been advantageously administered by the transdermal route.

The various commercially available products control the rate of drug delivery to the systemic circulation through a rate-controlling membrane, and/or through controlled drug-release from the drug matrix (the drug-reservoir of the system). One of these products, Transderm-Nitro (Summit), is similar in design to the Transderm-Scōp system, and is depicted in Figures 10–4 and 10–5. The system is a flat unit designed to provide controlled release of nitroglycerin through a semipermeable membrane continuously for 24 hours following application to intact skin. The Transderm-Nitro system comprises four layers:[32] (1) a tan-colored backing layer (aluminized plastic) that is impermeable to nitroglycerin (important since nitroglycerin is a volatile substance which could be lost unless protected); (2) a drug reservoir containing nitroglycerin adsorbed on lactose, colloidal silicon dioxide, and silicone medical fluid; (3) an ethylene/vinyl acetate copolymer membrane that is permeable to nitroglycerin; and (4) a layer of hypoallergenic silicone adhesive. Prior to use, a protective peel strip is removed from the adhesive surface (Fig. 10–5).

When the Transderm-Nitro system is applied to the skin, nitroglycerin is absorbed continuously through the skin into the systemic circulation. This results in active drug reaching the target organs (heart, extremities) before being inactivated by the liver. One-fifth of the total nitroglycerin in the system is delivered transdermally to the patient over 24 hours; the remainder serves as the thermodynamic energy source to release the drug and remains in the system. The rated release of drug is dependent upon the area of the system; 0.02 mg nitroglycerin is delivered per hour for every cm^2 of system size. Systems are rated to release in vivo 2.5, 5, 10, and 15 mg of nitroglycerin over 24 hours in patch sizes of 5, 10, 20, and 30 cm^2 respectively.

Other nitroglycerin transdermal infusion systems have their own unique construction and features. Nitro-Dur (Key) contains 2% of nitroglycerin in a gel-like matrix composed of glycerin, water (purified), lactose, polyvinyl alcohol, povidone and sodium citrate to provide a continuous source of the active ingredient. The transdermal system is available in dosage sizes of 5, 10, 15, 20, and 30 cm^2, containing 20, 40, 60, 80, and 120 mg of nitroglycerin, respectively. Nitro-Dur has a rated release in vivo of approximately 0.5 mg/cm^2/24 hours. Each unit is sealed in a polyester-foil-polyethylene laminate as shown in Figure 10–6.[33] The bandage portion consists of a non-woven, heat sealable, microporous tape.

The Nitro-Dur matrix is in a highly kinetic equilibrium state. Dissolved nitroglycerin molecules are constantly exchanging with adsorbed nitroglycerin molecules bound to the surfaces of the suspended lactose crystals. Sufficient nitroglycerin is adsorbed to the lactose in each matrix to maintain nitroglycerin in the fluid phase (aqueous glycerol) at a stable but saturated level (5 mg nitroglycerin/cm^2 matrix). When the matrix is applied to the surface of the skin, nitroglycerin molecules migrate from solution in the matrix, by diffusion, to solution in the skin. To make up for the molecules lost to the body, there is a shift of equilibrium in the matrix such that more molecules of nitroglycerin leave the crystals than are adsorbed from solution. When balance is restored, the solution is again at a saturated level. Thus, the crystals of lactose act as a "reservoir" of drug to maintain drug saturation in the fluid phase. The Nitro-Dur matrix, in turn, acts as a saturated "reservoir" for diffusive drug input through the skin.

In bioavailability studies, transdermal absorption of nitroglycerin from the gel-like matrix achieved steady rate venous plasma levels comparable to that of sublingual nitroglycerin and maintained these levels for 24 hours. Therapeutic effect is achieved within 30 minutes after application of the unit, and persists about 30 minutes after removal of the unit.[34]

The Nitrodisc (Searle) system consists of a solid, nitroglycerin-impregnated polymer bonded to a flexible, non-sensitizing adhesive bandage. Nitrodisc provides constant and controlled drug delivery over a uniform skin surface area for 24 hours (Fig. 10–7).

Similar to Key's Nitro-Dur system, the core of the Nitrodisc system is a polymeric matrix from which the nitroglycerin is released. However, the matrix of the Nitrodisc system is a solid silicone-based polymer rather than a gel-like matrix. The manufacturing process for the system involves mixing the nitroglycerin and a silicone polymer together as liquids and allowing the polymer to "cure," thereby forming the drug-impregnated solid matrix.

The Nitrodisc system is applied to the skin as a flexible, nonsensitizing foam adhesive bandage. It is available in two strengths which release either 5 mg or 10 mg of nitroglycerin during a 24-hour period. The 5 mg/24 hour system contains 16 mg nitroglycerin over an 8 cm^2 releasing surface. The 10 mg/24 hours system contains 32 mg nitroglycerin over a 16 cm^2 releasing surface.

In clinical studies, transdermal absorption of nitroglycerin from Nitrodisc occurred in a continuous and well-controlled manner for a minimum of 24 hours. Therapeutic plasma levels were attained within 1 hour after the application of the pad and remained in the therapeutic range for 24 hours. Plasma levels of nitroglycerin were still detectable 30 minutes after removal of the system.[35]

Patients should be given explicit instructions regarding the use of transdermal systems. Generally, these patches are placed on the chest, with the back, upper arms or shoulders being used as alternatives. The site selected should be free of hair, clean and dry so that the patch adheres with no difficulty. The use of the extremities below the knee or elbow should be discouraged as should those areas that are abraded or have lesions, cuts, etc. The patient should understand that physical exercise and elevated ambient temperatures, e.g., sauna, may increase the absorption of the nitroglycerin. Further, patients must be told to remove the old patch when the new patch is applied. Because patient preference plays a role in therapy success, the patient should be asked occasionally by the pharmacist about a product's ease of application and removal, adhesiveness, comfort, size, and appearance of the patch. If patient difficulty is encountered with any of these, the patient should be told to discuss this with his/her physician so that the patient can be converted to an acceptable patch that encourages compliance.

Transdermal Clonidine System

In 1985, the first *t*ransdermal *t*herapeutic system for hypertension, Catapres TTS (Boehringer Ingelheim), was marketed. The drug present, clonidine, lends itself to the transdermal delivery system because of its lipid solubility, high volume of distribution, and therapeutic effectiveness in low plasma concentrations. The product, developed jointly by Alza Corporation and Boehringer-Ingelheim provides 7 days of continuous antihypertensive therapy. The product is designed as a four-layered patch to provide the controlled release of clonidine in fixed amounts that yields constant blood levels. The system is 0.2 mm thick with surface areas of 3.5, 7.0, or 10.5 cm^2.[36] The amount of drug released is proportional to the area of the system used. The four areas of the system are: (1) a backing layer of pigmented polyester film; (2) a drug reservoir of clonidine, mineral oil, polyisobutylene, and colloidal silicon dioxide; (3) a microporous polypropylene membrane that controls the rate of delivery of clonidine from the system to the skin surface; (4) an adhesive formulation of clonidine, mineral oil, polyisobutylene, and colloidal silicon dioxide. Prior to use, a protective peel strip of polyester that covers layer 4 is removed.

The 3.5, 7.0 and 10.5 cm^2 systems available respectively deliver 0.1, 0.2, and 0.3 mg clonidine per day. To ensure constant release of drug over 7 days, the total drug content of the system is greater than the total amount of drug delivered. The energy source of drug release derives from the concentration gradient existing between a saturated solution of drug in the system and the much lower concentration prevailing in the skin. Clonidine flows in the direction of the lower concentration at a constant rate, limited by the rate-controlling membrane, so long as a saturated solution is maintained in the drug reservoir.[36]

Following system application to intact skin, clonidine in the adhesive layer saturates the skin sites below the system. Clonidine from the drug reservoir then begins to flow through the rate-controlling membrane and the adhesive layer of the system into the systemic circulation via the capillaries beneath the skin. Therapeutic plasma clonidine levels are achieved 2 to 3 days after initial application of the system. Application of a new system to a fresh skin site at weekly intervals continuously maintains therapeutic plasma concentrations of clonidine. If the patch is removed and not replaced with a new system, therapeutic plasma clonidine levels will persist for about 8 hours and then decline slowly over several days. Over this time period, blood pressure returns gradually to pretreatment levels. If the patient experiences localized skin irritation before completing 7 days of use, the system may be removed and replaced with a new one applied on a fresh skin site.[36]

Transdermal Estradiol System

Another drug developed for transdermal delivery is the estrogen, estradiol. The Estraderm (CIBA) transdermal system is designed to release 17β-estradiol through a rate-limiting membrane continuously upon application to intact skin.[37] Two systems (10 or 20 cm^2) provide delivery of 0.05 or 0.1 mg estradiol per day via skin of average permeability.

The Estraderm system comprises four layers: (1) a transparent polyester film, (2) a drug reservoir of estradiol and alcohol gelled with hydroxypropyl cellulose, (3) an ethylene-vinyl acetate copolymer membrane, and (4) an adhesive formulation of light mineral oil and polyisobutylene. A protective liner of siliconized polyethylene terephthalate film is attached to the adhesive surface and is removed before the system can be used.[37]

Estradiol is indicated for the treatment of moderate-to-severe vasomotor symptoms associated with menopause; female hypogonadism; female castration; primary ovarian failure; and atrophic conditions caused by deficient endogenous estrogen production, such as atrophic vaginitis and kraurosis vulvae.

Orally administered estradiol is rapidly metabolized by the liver to estrone and its conjugates, giving rise to higher circulating levels of estrone than estradiol. In contrast, the skin metabolizes estradiol only to a small extent. Therefore, transdermal administration produces therapeutic serum levels of estradiol with lower circulating levels of estrone and estrone conjugates, and requires smaller total doses than does oral therapy. Research has demonstrated that postmenopausal women receiving either transdermal or oral therapy will obtain the desired therapeutic effects from both dosage forms, e.g., lower gonadotropin levels, lower percentages of vaginal parabasal cells, decreased excretion of calcium, and lower calcium-to-creatinine ratio. Studies have also demonstrated that systemic side effects from oral estrogens can be reduced by using the transdermal dosage form. Because estradiol has a short half-life (~1 hour), transdermal administration of estradiol allows a rapid decline in blood levels after the transdermal system is removed, e.g., in a cycling regimen.[37]

Therapy is usually administered on a cyclic schedule (e.g., 3 weeks of therapy followed by 1 week without) especially in women who have not undergone a hysterectomy. The transdermal system is generally applied to the abdominal skin twice weekly. The woman should be told to place the adhesive side of the patch on a clean dry area of the skin, preferably the abdomen. The system should be applied immediately after opening the pouch and removing the protective liner. The woman should press the patch firmly in place with the palm of the hand for at least 10 seconds and make sure that good contact has been obtained around the edges of the patch. The patch should not be applied to the breast or the waistline because tight clothing may damage or dislodge the system. The area selected should not be oily, damaged, or irritated. The woman should understand the need to remove the old patch when a new patch is applied, and to rotate the application site with an interval at least of 1 week between applications to a particular body area.

Transdermal Nicotine Systems

As shown in Table 10–1, nicotine is prepared in transdermal therapeutic systems for use as an *adjunct* in smoking cessation programs. The once-a-day patch is used in conjunction with psychological reinforcement programs in assisting patients to withdraw from the smoking habit. The transdermally absorbed nicotine is intended to reduce both the craving to smoke and the withdrawal symptoms. The available patches contain from 7 mg to 22 mg of nicotine and are recommended for treatment periods of up to 12 weeks.[38–41] The patch usually is applied to the arm or upper front torso, with patients advised not to smoke when wearing the patch. The patch is replaced daily, with sites alternated. Some of the nicotine replacement programs recommend a gradual reduction in nicotine dosage (patch strength) during the treatment program. Research studies have shown that the nicotine patch is a consistently effective aid to smoking cessation.[42] It is important that the used patches be discarded properly, as the retained nicotine content represents a potential poison to children and pets.

Other Transdermal Therapeutic Systems

A testosterone transdermal system, Testoderm (Alza), is available for hormone replacement in men who have an absence or deficiency of testosterone. The patches contain 10 mg of testosterone for delivery of 4 mg/day and 15 mg of testosterone for delivery of 6 mg/day. The patches are applied to scrotal skin where optimal absorption occurs. According to the manufacturer, scrotal skin is at least five times more permeable to testosterone than other skin sites. Optimum serum levels are reached within 2 to 4 hours following application. The patch is worn 22 to 24 hours daily for 6 to 8 weeks. If patients have not achieved desired results at the end of this treatment period, another form of testosterone replacement therapy is recommended.

A transdermal patch for local application has been introduced for the treatment of viral wart infections. Trans-Ver-Sal (Tsumura Medical) contains 15% salicylic acid in a vehicle consisting primarily of karaya, a substance known for its nonirritating and self-adhesive properties (in ostomy therapy). The system is designed to be applied topically to a wart and provide constant and controlled release of the salicylic acid over an 8-hour treatment period. Each pad is covered with a polyethylene moisture barrier, which creates a desired occlusive effect.

The product is available in two pad sizes, i.e., 6 mm and 12 mm. Preferably the pad is applied at bedtime. The patient should clean the affected area, and then smooth the wart surface as much as possible with the provided cleaning file. The pharmacist should instruct the patient to lift a pad from the clear strip laminate in which it is contained, leaving the top plastic film in place. If the pad is too large for the wart, the patient should trim it to a size that will cover only the wart surface. Prior to application of the pad the patient should wet the wart with a drop of warm water, while ensuring that surrounding healthy skin remains dry. This enhances penetration of the salicylic acid into the wart. With the plastic film side facing up, the patient should apply the sticky bottom side onto the wart. Lastly, the patient uses a strip of tape that is provided to hold the pad in place. The pad is removed by the patient the next morning and discarded. The patient then continues using the Trans-Ver-Sal as the doctor has indicated.

Technology of Transdermal Delivery Systems

Examples of the configuration and composition of transdermal drug delivery systems are described in the text, presented in Table 10–1, and shown in Figures 10–2 through 10–7. Technically, transdermal drug delivery systems may be categorized into two types, monolithic and membrane-controlled systems.

Monolithic systems incorporate a drug matrix layer between backing and frontal layers (Fig. 10–6). The drug-matrix layer is composed of a polymeric material in which the drug is dispersed. The polymer matrix controls the rate at which the drug is released for percutaneous absorption. The matrix may be of two types; that is, with or without an excess of drug with regard to its equilibrium solubility and steady-state concentration gradient at the stratum corneum.[17,30] In types having no excess, drug is available to maintain the saturation of the stratum corneum only as long as the level of drug in the device exceeds the solubility limit of the stratum corneum. As the concentration of drug in the device diminishes below the skin's saturation limit, the transport of drug from device to skin gradually declines.[30,43] In monolithic systems that have an excess amount of drug present in the matrix, a drug reserve is present to assure continued drug saturation at the stratum corneum. In these instances, the rate of drug decline is less than in the type designed with no drug reserve. Nitro-Dur (Key) and Nitrodisc (Searle) are examples of monolithic systems.

In the preparation of monolithic systems, the drug and the polymer are dissolved or blended together, cast as the matrix, and dried.[17] The gelled matrix may be produced in sheet or cylindrical form, with individual dosage units cut and assembled between the backing and frontal layers. Most transdermal drug delivery systems are designed to contain an excess of drug and thus

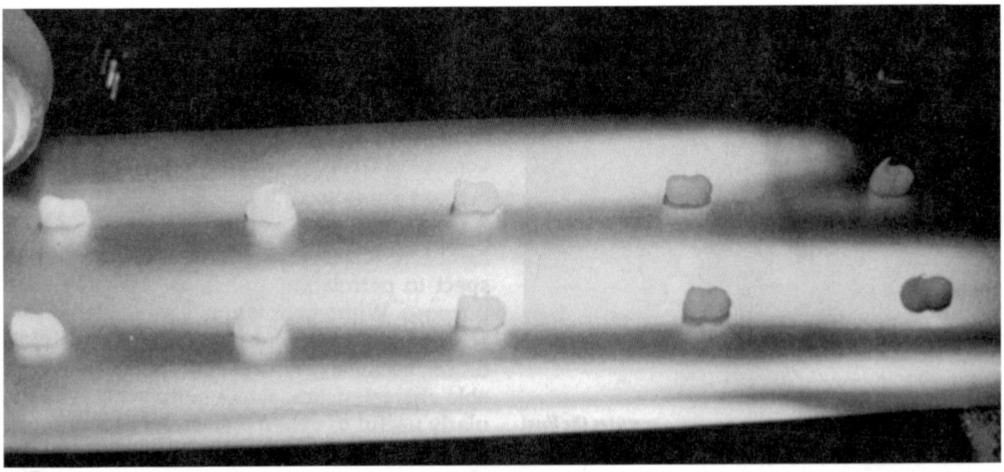

Fig. 10–8. *Measured dose for reservoir, placed on web prior to sealing into the transdermal delivery system. (Courtesy of CIBA Pharmaceutical Company.)*

drug-releasing capacity *beyond the time frame* recommended for replacement. This assures continuous drug availability and absorption as used patches are replaced on schedule with fresh ones.

Membrane-controlled transdermal systems are designed to contain a drug reservoir, usually in liquid or gel form, a rate-controlling membrane, and backing, adhesive, and protecting layers (Fig. 10–4). Transderm-Nitro (Summit) and Transderm-Scōp (CIBA) are examples of this technology. Membrane-controlled systems have the advantage over monolithic systems in that as long as the drug solution in the reservoir remains saturated, the release rate of drug through the controlling membrane remains constant.[18] In membrane systems, a small quantity of drug is frequently placed in the adhesive layer to initiate prompt drug absorption and pharmacotherapeutic effects upon skin placement. Membrane-controlled systems may be prepared by preconstructing the delivery unit, filling the drug reservoir, and sealing, or by a process of lamination, which involves a continuous process of construction, dosing, and sealing. Some steps in the production of transdermal drug delivery systems are shown in Figures 10–8 through 10–11.

In summary, either the drug delivery device or the skin may serve as the rate-controlling mechanism in drug transport from transdermal systems. For example, if the drug is delivered to the stratum corneum at a rate less than the absorption capacity, the *device* is the controlling factor. If, on the other hand, the drug is delivered to the skin area to saturation, the *skin* is the controlling factor to the rate of drug absorption. Thus, in actuality, the rate of drug transport in all transdermal systems, monolithic and membrane, are controlled by either artificial or natural (skin) membranes.

In addition to the drugs currently incorporated into transdermal delivery devices, many others are under study, including: cardiovascular drugs as isosorbide nitrate, propranolol, and mepindolol; and levonorgestrel/estradiol for hormonal contraception.

General Considerations in the Use of Transdermal Drug Delivery Systems

Each transdermal drug delivery system (patch) is accompanied by a product-specific package insert that provides instructions to the patient as to proper use of the product. These instructions should be explained to the patient and reinforced by the pharmacist upon dispensing the prescription.

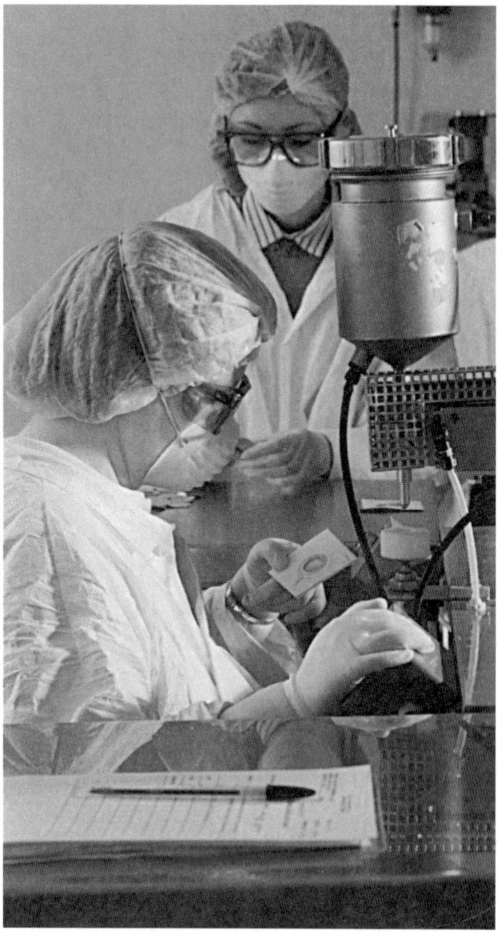

Fig. 10–9. *Pilot scale manufacture of transdermal patches. (Courtesy of Elan Corporation, plc.)*

Some general points applicable to the use of transdermal patches include the following:

1. The site selected for application should be clean, dry, and hairless (but not shaved). Nitroglycerin patches are generally applied to the chest, estradiol to the buttocks or abdomen, scopolamine behind the ear, and nicotine to the upper trunk or upper outer arm. Because of the possible occurrence of skin irritation, the site of application for replacement patches is rotated. Skin sites generally are not reused for a week.
2. The transdermal patch should not be applied

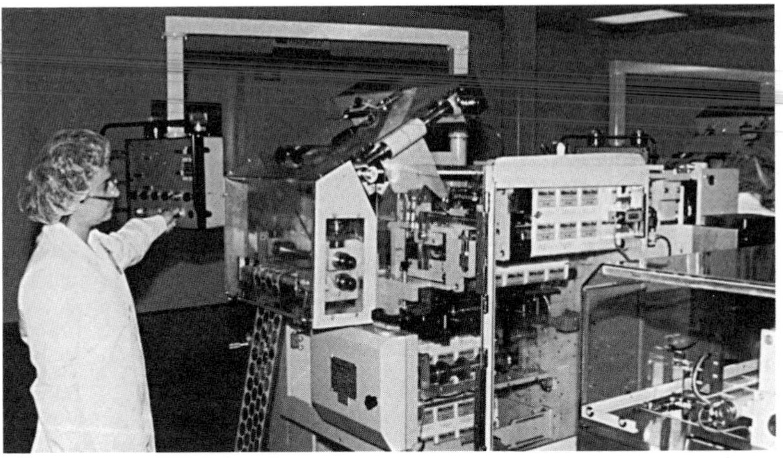

Fig. 10–10. *Equipment utilized in the cutting and packaging of transdermal drug delivery patches. (Courtesy of Schering Laboratories)*

to skin that is oily, irritated, cut, or abraded. This is to assure the intended amount and rate of transdermal drug delivery and absorption.

3. The patch should be removed from its protective package, being careful not to tear or cut it. The patch's protective backing should be removed to expose the adhesive layer, and it should be applied firmly with the palm or heal of the hand until securely in place (about 10 seconds).
4. The patch should be worn for the period of time stated in the product's instructions. Following that period, the patch should be removed and a fresh patch applied as directed. The used patch should be folded in half with the adhesive layer together so that it cannot be reused. The expended patch should be placed in the replacement patch's package pouch and discarded in a manner safe to children and pets.
5. Patches generally may be left on when showering, bathing, or swimming. Should a patch prematurely dislodge, an attempt may be made to reapply it, or it may be replaced with a fresh patch—the latter being worn for a full time period before it is replaced.
6. The patient should be instructed to cleanse the hands thoroughly before and after applying the patch. Care should be taken not to rub the eyes or touch the mouth during handling of the patch.
7. As with all medications, if the patient exhibits sensitivity or intolerance to the drug, or if undue skin irritation results, the patient should seek reevaluation.

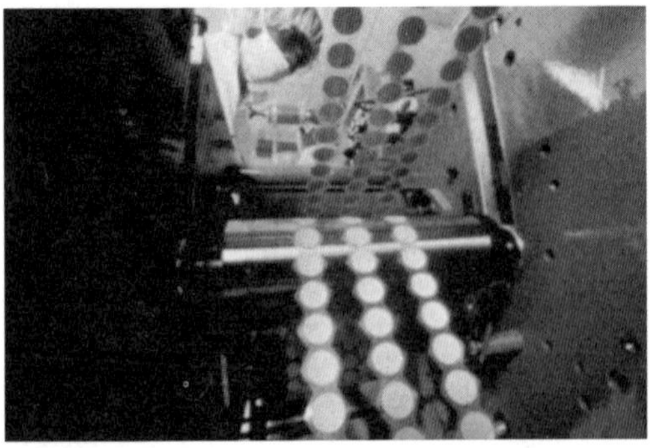

Fig. 11. *A rotary die-cutting pressure executes the final step in manufacturing Transderm Scōp systems prior to packaging. (Courtesy of Alza Corporation.)*

Ointments

Ointments *(unguents)* and semisolid preparations intended for external application. Those intended for application to the eye are specially prepared and are termed *ophthalmic ointments.* They will be taken up in the next chapter. Ointments may be medicated or nonmedicated, the latter type being commonly referred to as *ointment bases* and used as such for their emollient or lubricating effect or used as vehicles in the preparation of medicated ointments.

Ointment Bases

Ointment bases are classified into four general groups: (1) hydrocarbon bases, (2) absorption bases, (3) water-removable bases, and (4) water-soluble bases.

Hydrocarbon Bases

Hydrocarbon bases (oleaginous bases) are water-free, and aqueous preparations may be incorporated into them only in small amounts and then with difficulty. Hydrocarbon bases are used chiefly for their emollient effect. They are retained on the skin for prolonged periods, do not permit the escape of moisture from the skin to the atmosphere, and are difficult to wash off. As such they act as occlusive dressings. They do not "dry out" or change noticeably upon aging.

Petrolatum

Petrolatum, USP, is a mixture of semisolid hydrocarbons obtained from petroleum. Petrolatum is an unctuous mass, varying in color from yellowish to light amber. It melts at temperatures between 38° and 60°C. It may be used alone or in combination with other agents as an ointment base.
Synonyms: Yellow Petrolatum: Petroleum Jelly
Commercial Product: Vaseline (Chesebrough-Pond's)

White Petrolatum

White Petrolatum, USP, is petrolatum that has been decolorized. It differs only in this respect to petrolatum and is used for the same purpose. White petrolatum is more esthetically acceptable to a patient than petrolatum. In addition, because of its occlusive, nonwater-washable characteristics, white petrolatum is particularly useful to treat diaper rash (impervious to urine and protects the baby's skin) and dry skin (helps the skin retain moisture).
Synonym: White Petroleum Jelly
Commercial Product: White Vaseline (Chesebrough-Pond's)

Yellow Ointment

Each 100 g of Yellow Ointment, USP, contains 5g of yellow wax and 95 g of petrolatum. Yellow Wax, is the purified wax obtained from the honeycomb of the bee *(Apis mellifera)*.
Synonym: Simple Ointment

Mineral Oil

Mineral Oil is a mixture of liquid hydrocarbons obtained from petroleum. It is useful as a levigating substance to wet and to incorporate solid substances, e.g., salicylic acid, zinc oxide, into the preparation of ointments that consist of oleaginous bases as their vehicle.
Synonym: Liquid Petrolatum

Absorption Bases

Absorption bases may be of two types: (1) those that permit the incorporation of aqueous solutions, resulting in the formation of water-in-oil emulsions (e.g. *Hydrophilic Petrolatum* and *Anhydrous Lanolin*) and (2) those that are already water-in-oil emulsions *(emulsion bases)* that permit the incorporation of small, additional quantities of aqueous solutions (e.g. *Lanolin* and *Cold Cream*). These bases are useful as emollients although they do not provide the degree of occlusion afforded by the oleaginous bases. Like the oleaginous bases, absorption bases are not easily removed from the skin with water washing. They are also useful pharmaceutically to incorporate aqueous solutions of drugs, e.g., sodium sulfacetamide, into oleaginous bases. For example, an aqueous solution may be first incorporated into the absorption base, and then this mixture added into the oleaginous base. In doing this, an equivalent amount of oleaginous base in the formula is replaced by the absorption base. The classic example of this is in the preparation of occlusive ointment dosage forms of water-soluble drugs, e.g., gentamicin sulfate, for ophthalmic therapy.

Hydrophilic Petrolatum

Hydrophilic Petrolatum is composed of cholesterol, stearyl alcohol, white wax, and white petrolatum. It has the ability to absorb water, with the formation of a water-in-oil emulsion. Aquaphor is a highly-refined variation of Hydrophilic Petrolatum and because it can absorb up to 3 times its weight in water, it has proven useful to pharmacists who have to incorporate extemporaneously a water-soluble drug into an oleaginous base.

Anhydrous Lanolin

Anhydrous Lanolin may contain no more than 0.25% of water. Anhydrous Lanolin is insoluble in water, but mixes without separation with

about twice its weight of water. The incorporation of water results in the formation of a water-in-oil emulsion. Although its rancid odor is offensive, this base finds particular use as a vehicle for the application of compound tincture of benzoin and sucrose to treat decubitus ulcers, i.e., bedsores. The extemporaneous product is rolled onto the lesion with the use of a cotton swab.
Synonym: Refined Wool Fat

Lanolin

Lanolin is a semisolid, fatlike substance obtained from the wool of sheep *(Ovis aries)*. It is a water-in-oil emulsion that contains between 25 and 30% water. Additional water may be incorporated into lanolin by mixing.
Synonym: Hydrous Wool Fat

Cold Cream

Cold Cream is a semisolid, white, water-in-oil emulsion prepared with cetyl esters wax, white wax, mineral oil, sodium borate, and purified water. The sodium borate combines with the free fatty acids present in the waxes to form sodium soaps that act as the emulsifiers. Cold Cream is employed as an emollient and ointment base. Eucerin Creme is a water-in-oil emulsion of petrolatum, mineral oil, mineral wax, wool wax, alcohol and bronopol. It is frequently prescribed as a vehicle for the delivery of lactic acid and glycerin to treat dry skin. Further, the presence of water in the base is useful because the occlusive external phase traps the water onto the skin and enhances skin moisturization.

Water-Removable Bases

Water-removable bases are oil-in-water emulsions that are capable of being washed from skin or clothing with water. For this reason, they are frequently referred to as "water-washable" ointment bases. These bases, which resemble creams in appearance, may be diluted with water or with aqueous solutions. From a therapeutic viewpoint, they have the ability to absorb serous discharges in dermatologic conditions. Certain medicinal agents may be better absorbed by the skin when present in a base of this type than in other types of bases.

Hydrophilic Ointment

Hydrophilic Ointment as the name indicates, is "water-loving." It contains sodium lauryl sulfate as the emulsifying agent, with stearyl alcohol and white petrolatum representing the oleaginous phase of the emulsion and propylene glycol and water representing the aqueous phase. Methylparaben and propylparaben are used to preserve the ointment against microbial growth. The ointment is employed as a water-removable vehicle for medicinal substances.

Water-Soluble Bases

Unlike water-removable bases, which contain both water-soluble and water-insoluble components, water-soluble bases contain only water-soluble components. Like water-removable bases, however, water-soluble bases are water washable. Water-soluble bases are commonly referred to as "greaseless" because of the absence of any oleaginous materials. Because they soften greatly with the addition of water, aqueous solutions are not effectively incorporated into these bases. Rather, they are better used for the incorporation of nonaqueous or solid substances.

Polyethylene Glycol Ointment

The general formula for this base calls for the combining of 400 g of polyethylene glycol 3350 (a solid) and 600 g of polyethylene glycol 400 (a liquid) to prepare 1000 g of base. However, if a firmer ointment is required, the formula may be altered to permit up to equal parts of the two ingredients. If 6 to 25% of an aqueous solution is to be incorporated into the base, the substitution of 50 g of the polyethylene glycol 3350 with an equal amount of stearyl alcohol would be advantageous to render the final product more firm.

Polyethylene glycols are polymers of ethylene oxide and water represented by the formula $HOCH_2(CH_2OCH_2)_nCH_2OH$. The chain length may be varied to achieve polymers having desired viscosity and physical (liquid, semisolid, or solid) form.

Selection of the Appropriate Base

The selection of the base to use in the formulation of an ointment depends upon the careful assessment of a number of factors, including (a) the desired release rate of the particular drug substance from the ointment base, (b) the desirability for enhancement by the base of the percutaneous absorption of the drug, (c) the advisability of occlusion of moisture from the skin by the base, (d) the short-term and long-term stability of the drug in the ointment base, and (e) the influence, if any, of the drug on the consistency or other features of the ointment base. All of these factors, and others, must be weighed one against the other to find the most suitable base. It should be understood that no ointment base is ideal nor possesses all of the desired attributes. For instance, for a drug that hydrolyzes rapidly, a hydrocarbon base would provide the greatest stability, even though from a therapeutic standpoint another base might be preferred. The idea is to find the base that provides the majority of the most desired attributes.

Besides the physical-chemical factors that play a role in the selection of a base, patient factors also play an important role in a base's selection. The condition of the patient's skin, e.g., weeping (oozing) or dry, may dictate an ointment or a cream dosage form. For example, the old rule in dermatology that is still practiced is that if a patient's skin is dry—wet it. If it is wet—dry it. Thus, for example, if a patient's skin is dry, an occlusive ointment base that will retain moisture would be preferable. Therefore, pharmacists must realize that ointment bases and cream bases are not necessarily interchangeable, and that a dermatologist is using the effects of the ointment base as much as the active ingredient within the product to treat the patient's condition.

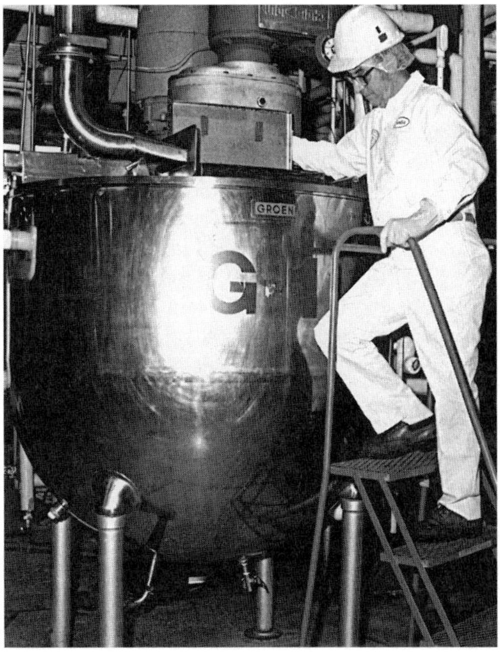

Fig. 10–12. *Creams and ointments in batch sizes up to 1,500 kilos are manufactured in this stainless steel tank, which has counter sweep agitation and a built-in homogenizer. (Courtesy of Lederle Laboratories.)*

Preparation of Ointments

Both on a large and a small scale, ointments are prepared by two general methods: (1) incorporation and (2) fusion. The method for a particular preparation depends primarily upon the nature of the ingredients.

Incorporation

In the incorporation method, the components of the ointment are mixed together by various means until a uniform preparation has been attained. (Fig. 10–12). On a small scale, as in the extemporaneous compounding of prescriptions, the pharmacist may mix the components of an ointment in a mortar with a pestle, or a spatula and an ointment slab (a large glass or porcelain plate) may be used to rub the ingredients together. Some glass ointment slabs are of ground glass to permit greater friction in the rubbing process. Some pharmacists utilize nonabsorbent parchment papers that are large enough to cover the working surface and have the advantage of being disposable, eliminating much of the time-consuming chore of cleaning the ointment slab.

INCORPORATION OF SOLIDS. When preparing an ointment by spatulation, the pharmacist generally works the ointment with a stainless steel spatula with a long, broad blade and periodically removes the accumulation of ointment on the larger spatula with a smaller spatula. If the components of an ointment are reactive with the metal of the spatula (as for example, phenol), hard rubber spatulas may be used. The ointment is prepared by thoroughly rubbing and working the components together on the hard surface with the spatula until the product is smooth and uniform. Generally the ointment base is placed on one side of the working surface, and the powdered components, previously reduced to fine powders and thoroughly blended in a mortar, are placed on the other. Then a portion of the powder is mixed with a portion of the base until uniform, and the process is repeated until all portions of the powder and base are combined. The portions of prepared ointment are then combined and thoroughly blended by continuous movement of the spatula over and through the combined portions of ointment.

When only a small portion of powder is to be added, it may be added in its entirety to a small portion of ointment base. After the two have been thoroughly mixed, another portion is added to this mixture, the process being repeated as in the "geometric method" of diluting until all of the ointment base has been incorporated.

Frequently it is desirable to reduce the particle size of any solid material before incorporation into the ointment base so that the final product will not be gritty. This may be done by *levigating* the powder by mixing it in a vehicle in which it is insoluble to make a smooth dispersion of the material. Most commonly the solid substance is mixed with a levigating agent that is compatible with the base, e.g., mineral oil, glycerin, and then with a portion of the ointment base, using an amount of levigating agent about equal to the material to be levigated, and a mortar and pestle to accomplish the reduction of particle size as well as the dispersion of the substance. After levigation, the dispersion is incorporated with the remainder of the base by spatulation or by using the mortar and pestle.

Solid materials soluble in a common solvent that will affect neither the stability of the drug nor the efficacy of the product may first be dissolved in that solvent, e.g., dissolve salicylic acid crystals in alcohol, and then the solution added to the ointment base by spatulation or by mixing in a mortar and pestle. Generally, the mortar and pestle is preferred when large volumes of liquid are added since the liquid is more captive in the mortar than on an ointment slab.

INCORPORATION OF LIQUIDS. Liquid substances or solutions of drugs, as described above, are added to an ointment only after due consideration of the ointment's nature. For instance, an aqueous solution or preparation would be added with difficulty to an oleaginous ointment, except in very small amounts. However, water-absorbable or hydrophilic ointment bases would be quite suitable for the absorption and incorporation of the aqueous solution. Frequently when adding an aqueous preparation to a base that is hydrophobic in character, the pharmacist replaces a portion of the base with a hydrophilic base, incorporates the solution in the latter, and then mixes the product with the original base. It should be understood, however, that all bases, even if hydrophilic, have their limits of capacity; additional amounts of water render them too soft or semiliquid. Ointments must be semisolid, and sometimes pharmacists may find it necessary to use a drug concentrate or solid dosage form in adding a drug to an ointment base.

Alcoholic solutions of small volume usually may be added quite well to oleaginous vehicles or emulsion bases. Other liquid materials, for instance, natural balsams, are incorporated into ointment bases with difficulty. It is customary to mix a balsam such as Peru balsam with an equal portion of castor oil before incorporating it into the base. This procedure reduces the surface tension of the balsam and provides for the even distribution of the balsam throughout the vehicle.

On a large scale, mechanical ointment roller mills force coarsely formed ointments through moving stainless steel rollers, resulting in the formation of products that are smooth and uniform in composition and texture (Fig. 10–13). Prior to passage through the mills, the ointment may be coarsely prepared in powerful ointment and paste mixers. Small ointment mills are available for the production of small batches of product, and pharmacies that routinely prepare medi-

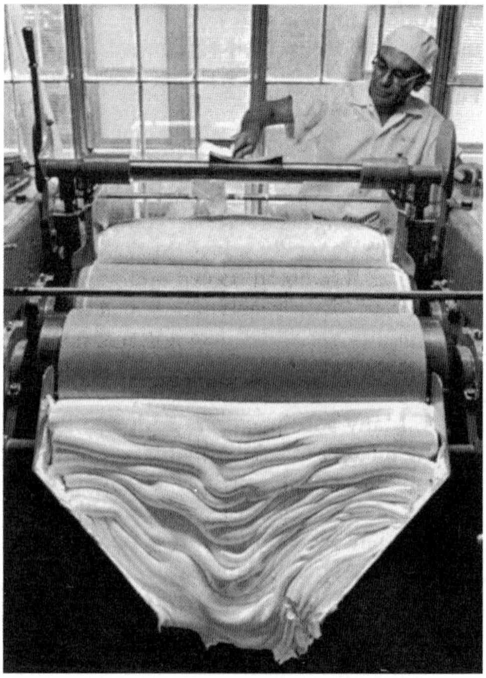

Fig. 10–13. *Day ointment roller mill. Standards of fineness and smoothness require that no grains of material be visible under a ten-power microscope after passage through this machine. (Courtesy of Eli Lilly and Company.)*

cated applications find these small mills useful additions to their equipment.

Fusion

By the fusion method, all or some of the components of an ointment are combined by being melted together and cooled with constant stirring until congealed. Those components not melted are generally added to the congealing mixture as it is being cooled and stirred. Naturally, heat-labile substances and any volatile components are added last when the temperature of the mixture is low enough not to cause decomposition of volatilization of the components. Many substances are added to the congealing mixture in solution, others are added as insoluble powders generally levigated with a portion of the base. On a small scale, the fusion process may be conducted in a porcelain dish or glass beaker; on a large scale, it is generally carried out in large steam-jacketed kettles. Once congealed, the ointment may be passed through an ointment mill (in large-scale manufacture) or rubbed with a spatula or in a mortar (in small-scale preparation) to ensure a uniform texture.

Many medicated ointments and ointment bases containing such components as beeswax, paraffin, stearyl alcohol, and high molecular weight polyethylene glycols, which do not lend themselves well to mixture by incorporation, are prepared by fusion. In preparing an ointment with these types of materials by fusion, it is generally found that the melting points of the individual components are quite varied; therefore, the temperatures required to achieve fusion may also vary from formula to formula. In a given formula, if the item having the highest melting point is melted first and the other components are added to this hot liquid, all of the components will be subjected to this high temperature, irrespective of their own individual melting points, and generally a temperature higher than necessary will have to be employed to achieve fusion. Either by melting the component having the lowest melting point first and adding the components of higher melting points in order of their individual melting points or by melting all of the components together very slowly, a lower temperature is usually sufficient to achieve fusion. This is apparently due to the solvent action exerted by the first melted component on the other components, and if the process is allowed to proceed by using only slowly rising temperatures, the fusion process does not generally require the high temperature normally required to melt the individual component having the highest melting point.

In the preparation of ointments having an emulsion type of formula, the general method of manufacture involves a melting process as well as an emulsification process. Usually, the water-immiscible components such as the oil and waxes are melted together in a steam bath to about 70 to 75°C. Meantime, an aqueous solution of all of the heat-stable, water-soluble components is being prepared in the amount of purified water specified in the formula and heated to the same temperature as the oleaginous components. Then the aqueous solution is slowly added, with constant stirring (usually with a mechanical stirrer), to the melted oleaginous mixture, the temperature is maintained for 5 to 10 minutes to prevent crystallization of waxes, and then the mixture is slowly cooled with the stirring continued until the mixture is congealed. If the aqueous solution were not the same temperature as the oleaginous melt, there would be solidification of some of the waxes upon the addition of the colder aqueous solution to the melted mixture.

Preservation of Ointments

Even though they may not be designed to be sterile, topical preparations are subject to considerations of microbial content.[44,45] It is particularly important that the presence of *Pseudomonas aeruginosa* and *Staphylococcus aureus* be determined and controlled in topical products. Product contamination by these organisms could induce an infectious response in a patient. Some topical products are manufactured to be sterile through the use of microbial filtration of the vehicle, aseptic manufacturing processes, and the filling of containers under laminar-flow hoods. However, the majority of topical products are not intended to be sterile and do not undergo such aseptic procedures, but must still meet acceptable limits for microbial content. Certain preparations, because of the processes involved in their manufacture and/or the nature of their components, may encourage or may discourage microbial contamination and growth. As is the case in the manufacture of all pharmaceutical products, strict adherence to hygienic practices is vital to minimize both the type and number of microorganisms which may be present in a product.

Semisolid pharmaceutical preparations, as ointments, frequently require the addition of chemical antimicrobial preservatives to the formulation to inhibit the growth of contaminating microorganisms. These preservatives include p-hydroxybenzoates, phenols, benzoic acid, sorbic acid, quaternary ammonium salts and other compounds. Semisolid preparations utilizing bases which contain or hold water support microbial growth to a greater extent than those which have little moisture, and thus constitute the greater problem of preservation.

Semisolid preparations must also be protected through proper packaging and storage from the destructive influences of air, light, moisture, and heat, and the possible chemical interactions between the preparation and the container.

Packaging and Storage of Ointments

Ointments are usually packaged either in jars or in tubes. The jars may be made of glass, uncolored, colored green, amber, or blue, or opaque and porcelain-white. Plastic jars are also in use. Opaque and colored-glass containers are useful for ointments containing drugs that are light-sensitive. The tubes are made of tin or of plastic, some of them co-packaged with special tips when the ointment is to be used for rectal, ophthalmic, vaginal, aural, or nasal application. Tubes of ointments for ophthalmic use are most commonly packaged in small, tin or plastic collapsible tubes holding about ⅛ oz (about 3.5 g) of ointment. Tubes of ointments for topical use are more frequently of 5 g to 30 g size. Jars for ointments may vary in size from as little as one half once to one pound or more.

Ointment jars may be filled on a small scale by the pharmacist by packaging the weighed amount of ointment into the jar by means of a flexible spatula and forcing the ointment down and along the sides of the jar to avoid the entrapment of air. In packing an ointment jar, the idea is to attain a level surface of ointment high enough to be near the top of the jar, but not so high as to touch the lid when it is placed on the jar. Through the adept use of the spatula, some pharmacists place a "curl" in the center of the surface of the ointment. Ointments prepared by fusion may be poured directly into the ointment jars for congealing within the jar. These ointments normally assume a finished look. In the large-scale manufacture of ointments, pressure fillers force a specified amount of an ointment into a jar.

Tubes are generally filled by pressure fillers from the open back end (opposite end from the cap end) of the tube (Fig. 10–14), which is then closed and sealed. Ointments prepared by fusion may be poured directly into the tubes. On a small scale, as in the extemporaneous filling of an ointment tube by the community pharmacist, the tube may be filled manually or with a small scale filling machine (Fig. 10–15).

Industrially, automatic tube-filling, closing, crimping, labeling and packaging machines are used for the large-scale production of tube-filled ointments (Figs. 10–16 to 10–18).

Tube-filled ointments predominate over jar-filled ointments primarily because they are more convenient for the patient, with less handling and mess resulting. Also, ointments in tubes are less exposed to air and to potential contaminants and are therefore likely to be more stable and to remain efficacious for longer periods of time than ointments packaged in jars.

Most ointments must be stored at temperatures below 30°C to prevent the softening and even the liquefying of the base.

Creams

Creams are defined as "viscous liquid or semisolid emulsions of either the oil-in-water or the water-in-oil type." Creams are usually employed as emollients or as medicated application to the skin.

The term cream is widely used in the pharmaceutical and cosmetic industry, and many of the commercial products referred to as creams may not actually conform to the above definition. Many products that are creamy in appearance but do not have an emulsion-type base are commonly called creams.

So-called "vanishing creams" are generally oil-in-water emulsions containing large percentages of water and stearic acid. After application of the cream, the water evaporates leaving behind a thin residue film of the stearic acid.

Many patients and physicians prefer creams to ointments. For one thing, they are generally easier to spread, and, in the case of creams of the oil-in-water emulsion-type, easier to remove than many ointments. Pharmaceutical manufacturers frequently market their topical preparations in both cream and ointment bases to satisfy the preference of the patient and physician.

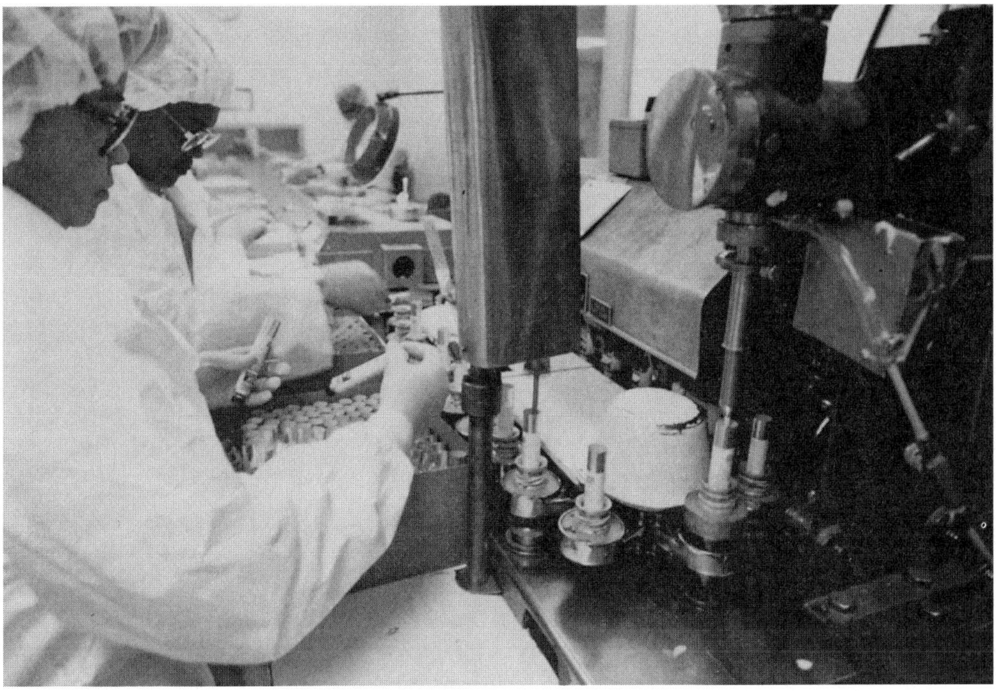

Fig. 10–14. *Empty tubes being prepared for filling. (Courtesy of Abbott Laboratories.)*

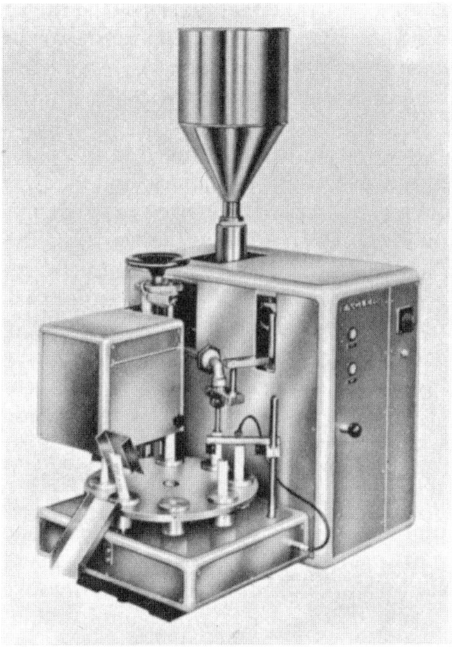

Fig. 10–15. *Example of a small-scale fully automatic filling and crimping machine for collapsible metal tubes. The capacity of the machine is up to 60 units per minute. (Courtesy of Chemical and Pharmaceutical Industry Co.)*

Creams are packaged and preserved in the same manner as discussed previously for ointments. Table 10–2 presents examples of some dermatologic ointments and creams.

Pastes

Pastes, like ointments, are intended for external application to the skin. They differ from ointments primarily in that they generally contain a larger percentage of solid material and as a consequence are thicker and stiffer than ointments. Because of their large percentage of solids, pastes are generally more absorptive and less greasy than ointments prepared with the same components.

Pastes are prepared similarly to ointments. However, when a levigating agent is to be used to render the powdered component smooth, a portion of the base is often used rather than a liquid like mineral oil that would soften the paste.

Because of the stiffness and absorptive qualities of pastes, they remain in place after application with little tendency to soften and flow and are therefore effectively employed to absorb serous secretions from the site of application. Pastes

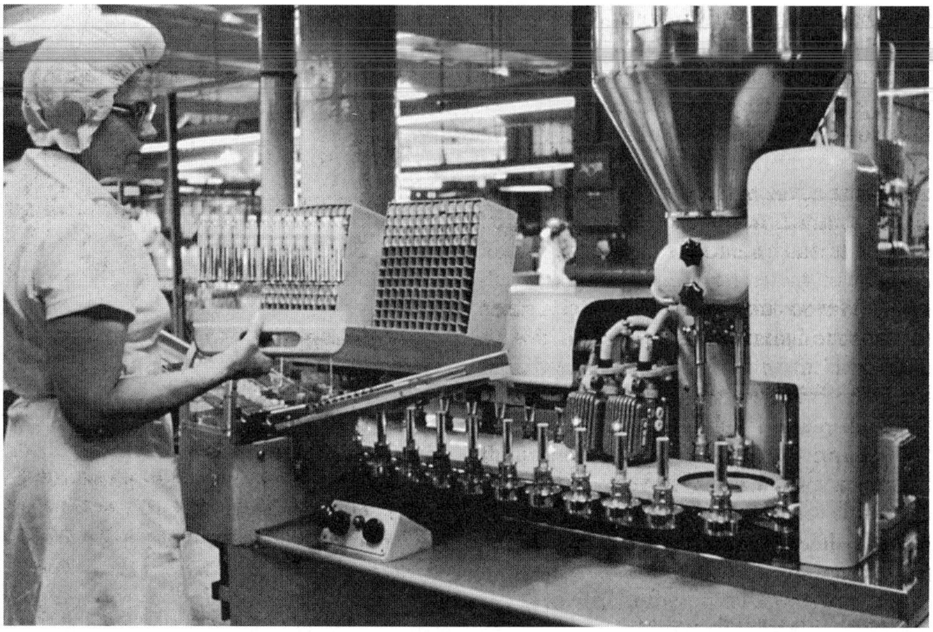

Fig. 10–16. *Arenco tube-filling machine automatically fills 125 tubes a minute with proper amount, tightens cap, orients each tube by electric eye so that label faces forward, then closes and crimps the end. (Courtesy of Eli Lilly and Company.)*

are therefore preferred over ointments for acute lesions that have a tendency toward crusting, vesiculation, or oozing. However, because of their stiffness and impenetrability, pastes are not generally suited for application to hairy parts of the body.

Among the few pastes in use today are Triamicinolone Acetonide Dental Paste, an anti-inflammatory preparation applied topically to the oral mucous membranes and Zinc Oxide Paste.

Zinc Oxide Paste

Zinc Oxide Paste is prepared by levigating and then mixing 25% each of zinc oxide and starch with white petrolatum. The product is very firm and difficult to manipulate with a spatula. It is capable of absorbing moisture to a much greater extent than zinc oxide ointment and is employed as an astringent and protectant. The paste also frequently serves as a vehicle for other medicinal substances, e.g., anthralin therapy for psoriasis. Synonym: Lassar's Plain Zinc Paste

Lotions

Lotions are liquid preparations intended for external application to the skin. Most lotions contain finely powdered substances that are insoluble in the dispersion medium and are suspended through the use of suspending agents and dispersing agents. Other lotions have as the dispersed phase liquid substances that are immiscible with the vehicle and are usually dispersed by means of emulsifying agents or other suitable stabilizers. Most commonly the vehicles of lotions are aqueous. Depending upon the nature of the ingredients, lotions may be prepared in the same manner as suspensions, emulsions, or solutions.

Lotions are intended to be applied to the skin for the protective or therapeutic value of their constituents. Their fluidity permits rapid and uniform application over a wide surface area. Lotions are intended to dry on the skin soon after application, leaving a thin coat of their medicinal components on the skin's surface.

Because the dispersed phase of lotions tends to separate from the vehicle upon standing, they should be shaken vigorously before each use to redistribute any separated matter. Containers of lotions should be labeled to instruct the patient to shake thoroughly before use and also to use externally only.

Examples of medicated lotions are presented

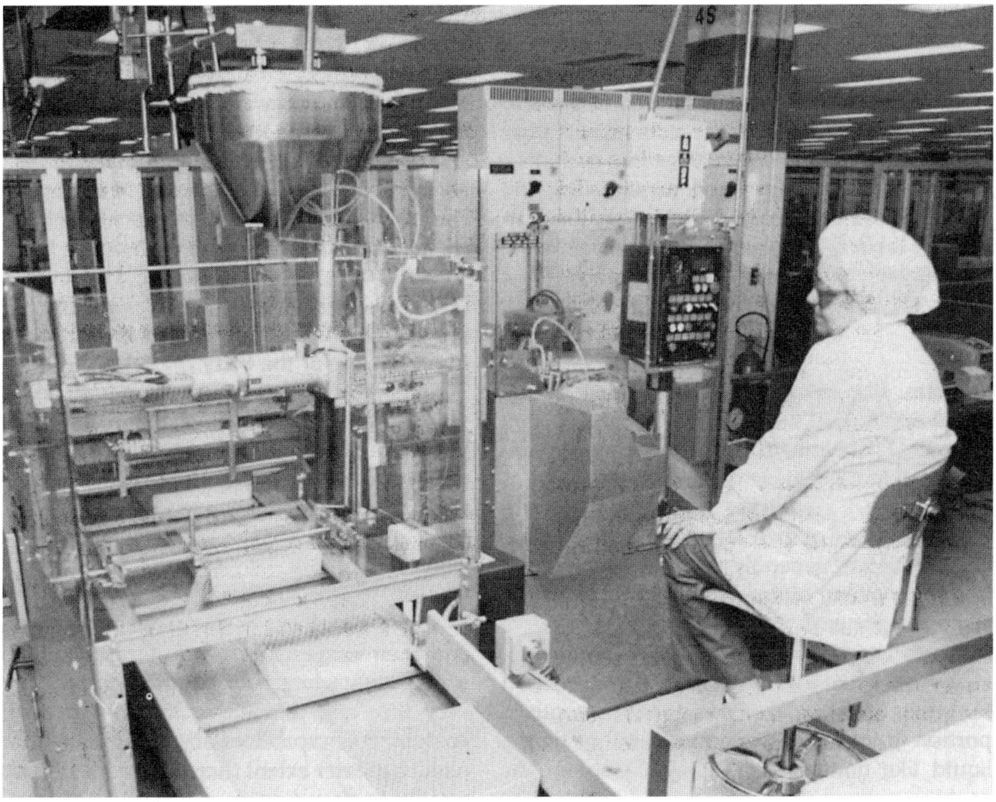

Fig. 10–17. *This glaminate tube filler loads, fills, crimps, codes, and cuts 2-gram, tubes of topical cream. (Courtesy of Lederle Laboratories.)*

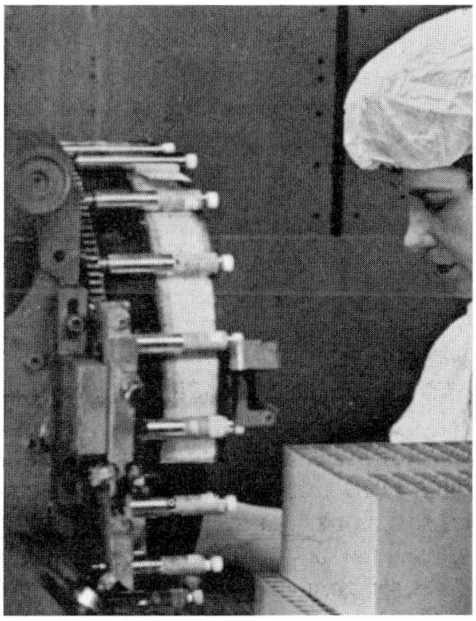

Fig. 10–18. *Industrial scale tube labeling machinery. (Courtesy of Eli Lilly and Company.)*

in Table 10–3. Those lotions of particular pharmaceutical interest are discussed as follows.

Calamine Lotion

Calamine Lotion contains 8% each of zinc oxide and calamine, the latter composed primarily of zinc oxide with a small amount of ferric oxide, which gives calamine its characteristic pink color. In the preparation of the lotion, the two powders are levigated with a small portion of glycerin, the mixture being gradually diluted with a combination of bentonite magma and calcium hydroxide solution and the product made to volume with additional calcium hydroxide solution.

The bentonite magma is used to suspend the zinc oxide and calamine; however, on standing the powders do settle. Calamine is categorized as a protectant and is useful in relieving the itching and pain of sunburn, insect bites, and other minor skin irritations. The pink color helps disguise the presence of the lotion on the skin. Ca-

Table 10–2. Examples of Dermatologic Ointments and Creams by Therapeutic Category

Preparation	*Corresponding Commercial Product*	*Usual Percentage of Active Ingredient*	*Comments*
Adrenocortical Steroids			
Alclomethasone Diproprionate Cream and Ointment	Aclovate Cream and Ointment (Glaxo Dermatology)	0.05% cream and ointment	These preparations are indicated for the relief of the inflammatory manifestations of corticosteroid responsive dermatoses. They are usually applied to affected skin areas once to three times a day.
Betamethasone Valerate Cream and Ointment	Valisone Cream & Ointment (Schering)	0.1% (ointment) and 0.01%, and 0.1% (cream)	
Diflorasone Cream and Ointment	Florone Cream and Ointment (Dermik)	0.05%	
Fluocinolone Acetonide Cream and Ointment	Synalar Cream & Ointment (Syntex)	0.025% and 0.01% (cream) and 0.025% (ointment)	
Hydrocortisone Acetate Cream and Ointment	Cortaid Cream and Ointment (Upjohn)	0.5% and 1%	
Triamcinolone Acetonide Cream and Ointment	Aristocort A Cream and Ointment (Fujisawa)	0.1% (ointment) and 0.1%, 0.025%, and 0.5% (cream)	
Adrenocorticoid/Antifungal Combination			
Betamethasone and Clotrimazole Cream	Lotrisone Cream (Schering)	0.05%/1%	Useful for the relief and treatment of inflammatory and pruritic manifestations of corticosteroid-responsive dermatoses that could be complicated by fungal overgrowth.
Antiacne Drug			
Tretinoin Cream	Retin-A (Ortho)	0.025%, 0.05% and 0.1%	A derivative of vitamin A that is used for the topical treatment of acne vulgaris. It is also approved as a preventive measure for skin aging.
Antianginal Drug			
Nitroglycerin Ointment	Nitro-Bid Ointment (Marion Merrell Dow)	2%	Reduces the workload of the heart by smooth muscle relaxation of peripheral arteries and veins. It is applied by using a specially designed dose-measuring applicator
Antibacterial/Anti-infectives			
Bacitracin Ointment	Baciguent Ointment (Upjohn)	500 units/g	These antibiotic preparations are used in the treatment of skin infections due to susceptible organisms amenable to local treatment.
Gentamicin Sulfate Cream and Ointment	Garamycin Cream and Ointment (Schering)	0.1%	
Neomycin Sulfate Ointment	Myciguent Ointment (Upjohn)	0.5%	
Nystatin Cream and Ointment	Mycostatin Cream and Ointment (Westwood-Squibb)	10,000 units/g	
Meclocycline Sulfosalicylate Cream	Meclan Cream (Ortho)	1%	Topical tetracycline derivative for the treatment of inflammatory acne.
Mupirocin Ointment	Bactroban Ointment (SmithKline Beecham)	2%	Antibacterial agent that possesses activity against organisms most frequently encountered in common, primary bacterial skin infections.

Table 10–2. Continued

Preparation	*Corresponding Commercial Product*	*Usual Percentage of Active Ingredient*	*Comments*
Antifungals			
Nystatin Cream and Ointment	Mycostatin Cream and Ointment (Westwood-Squibb)	100,000 units/g	An antifungal antibiotic for cutaneous and mucocutaneous mycotic infections.
Miconazole Nitrate Cream	Monistat-Derm Cream (Ortho)	2%	For cutaneous candidiasis and treatment of tinea infections caused by *Trichophyton sp.*
Naftidine HCl	Naftin Cream (Allergan)	1%	
Tolnaftate Cream	Tinactin Cream (Schering-Plough)	1%	For topical treatment of tinea pedis, tinea cruris, tinea corporis and tinea manuum.
Antineoplastic			
Fluorouracil Cream	Efudex Cream (Roche Dermatologics)	5%	For treatment of multiple actinic or solar keratoses.
Anesthetics (Local)			
Benzocaine Cream	Various	1% and 5%	Applied to skin to relieve pain and itching of sunburn, insect bites, etc.
Dibucaine Cream and Ointment	Nupercainal Cream and Ointment (CIBA)	0.5% (cream) and 1% (ointment)	
Astringent/Protectant			
Zinc Oxide Ointment	Various	20%	In the extemporaneous preparation of Zinc Oxide Ointment, 20% of zinc oxide is levigated with mineral oil, and the mixture incorporated into white ointment. The ointment is employed topically as an astringent and protective in various skin conditions.
Depigmenting Agents			
Hydroquinone Cream	Eldopaque Cream (ICN Pharmaceuticals)	2% and 4%	Used in the temporary bleaching of hyperpigmented skin blemished due to freckles, old age spots, and cholasma.
Monobenzone Ointment	Benoquin Ointment (ICN Pharmaceuticals)	20%	
Scabicides			
Lindane Cream	Kwell Cream (Reed and Carnrick)	1%	Used in the treatment of scabies and infestations with head lice and crab lice.
Crotamiton Cream	Eurax Cream (Westwood-Squibb)	10%	For eradication of scabies and symptomatic treatment of pruritus.
Sunscreening Agent			
Dioxybenzone and Oxybenzone Cream	Solbar Cream (Person & Covey)	3% each of dioxybenzone and oxybenzone	Protects the skin against burning effects of the sun's ultraviolet rays.

Table 10–3. Examples of Medicated Lotions

Lotion	*Corresponding Commercial Product*	*Percentage Strength of Active Constituent in Commercial Lotion*	*Category and Comments*
Ammonium Lactate Lotion	Lac-Hydrin (Westwood-Squibb)	12%	Promotes hydration and removal of excess keratin dry skin and hyperkeratotic conditions.
Benzoyl Peroxide	Sulfoxyl Lotion Regular and Strong (Stiefel)	5% and 10%	Demonstrates an antibacterial activity against *Propionibacterium acnes,* the predominant organism in sebaceous comedones that cause acne vulgaris.
Betamethasone Diproprionate Lotion	Diprolene	0.05% betamethasone diproprionate	Glucocorticoid indicated for the relief of inflammatory manifestations of corticosteroid-responsive dermatoses.
Betamethasone Valerate Lotion	Betatrex Lotion (Savage)	0.1% betamethasone valerate	Glucocorticoid employed as an anti-inflammatory agent.
Calamine Lotion	. . .	8% each of calamine and zinc oxide	Topical protectant. See text for additional discussion.
Clotrimazole Lotion	Lotrimin Lotion (Schering)	1% clotrimazole	Indicated for the topical treatment of dermal infections tinea pedis, tinea cruris, and tinea corporus.
Lindane Lotion	Kwell Lotion (Reed & Carnrick)	1% gamma benzene HCl	Pediculicide; scabicide. Applied topically to the skin once or twice a week. Contact with eyes or mucous membranes should be avoided.
Hydrocortisone Lotion	Hytone Lotion (Dermik)	1% and 2.5% hydrocortisone	Adrenocortical steroid. Topical anti-inflammatory agent.
Permethrin Rinse	Nix Creme Rinse (Burroughs-Wellcome)	1%	A synthetic pyrethroid which is active against lice, i.e., pediculosis.
Selenium Sulfide Lotion	Selsun and Selsun Blue (Ross)	1% (Selsun Blue) and 2.5% (Selsun) of selenium sulfide	Anti-fungal; antiseborrheic. Used principally in the treatment of dandruff and seborrheic dermatitis. Contact with the eyes should be avoided.
Urea Lotion	Ureacin-10 Lotion (Pedinol)	10%	Promotes hydration and removal of excess keratin dry skin and hyperkeratotic conditions.

lamine lotion must be thoroughly shaken before use.

"Phenolated calamine lotion" contains 1% of liquefied phenol in calamine lotion. Because phenol has anesthetic as well as antiseptic activity, it enhances the antipruritic action of the lotion. Like the plain calamine lotion, it must be shaken thoroughly before use. To maintain the phenol concentration, the container must be tightly closed.

Topical Solutions and Tinctures

Examples of solutions and tinctures intended for application to the skin are presented in Tables 10–4 and 10–5. As shown in these tables, the majority of these preparations are used as anti-infective agents.

Generally, the topical solutions employ an aqueous vehicle, whereas the topical tinctures characteristically employ an alcoholic vehicle. As required, co-solvents or adjuncts to enhance stability or the solubility of the solute are employed.

Most topical solutions and tinctures are prepared by simple solution of the solutes in the solvent. However, certain solutions are prepared by chemical reaction and these in particular are discussed later in this section. Of the tinctures for topical use, one, Compound Benzoin Tincture is prepared by maceration of the natural components in the solvent; the others are prepared by simple solution.

Because of the nature of the active constituents or the solvents, many of the topical solutions and tinctures are self-preserved. Those that are not may contain suitable preservatives. Topical solutions and tinctures should be packaged in containers that make them convenient to use. Those that are used in small volume, as the anti-infectives, are usually packaged in glass bottles having an applicator tip as a part of the cap assembly, or in plastic squeeze bottles which deliver the medication in drops. Many of the anti-infec-

Table 10–4. Examples of Solutions Applied Topically to the Skin

Solution	*Corresponding Commercial Product*	*Percent Active Constituent in Commercial Solution*	*Vehicle*	*Category and Comments*
Aluminum Acetate Topical Solution	. . .	5%	aqueous	Astringent. See text for additional discussion.
Aluminum Subacetate Topical Solution	. . .	Approximately 2.45% aluminum oxide and 5.8% acetic acid	aqueous	Astringent. See text for additional discussion.
Calcium Hydroxide Topical Solution (Limewater)	. . .	0.14%	aqueous	Astringent. See text for additional discussion.
Chlorhexidine Gluconate Solution	Hibiclens Skin Cleanser (Stuart)	4%		Used topically as a skin wound and general skin cleanser, a surgical scrub, and preoperative skin preparation. Effectiveness encompasses gram-positive and gram-negative bacteria such as *Pseudomonas aeruginosa.*
Clindamycin Phosphate Topical Solution	Cleocin T Topical Solution (Upjohn)	1%	isopropyl alcohol/ water	Used in treatment of acne vulgaris.
Clotrimazole Topical Solution	Lotrimin Solution (Schering)	1%	PEG 400	Antifungal
Coal Tar Topical Solution (Liquor Carbonis Detergens; LCD)	. . .	20%	alcoholic	Antieczematic; antipsoriatic. See text for additional discussion.
Erythromycin Topical Solution	Erymax Topical Solution (Allergan Herbert)	2%	polyethylene glycol/ acetone/ alcohol	Used in treatment of acne vulgaris
Fluocinolone Acetonide Topical Solution	Synalar Topical Solution (Syntex)	0.01%	propylene glycol	Adrenocortical steroid (topical anti-inflammatory)
Fluorouracil Topical Solution	Efudex Topical Solution (Roche)	2 and 5%	propylene glycol	Antineoplastic (actinic keratoses).
Hydrogen Peroxide Topical Solution	. . .	3%	aqueous	Topical anti-infective. See text for additional discussion.
Hydroquinone Topical Solution	Melanex Topical Solution (Neutrogena Dermatologics)	3%	water/ alcohol/ propylene glycol	Indicated in the temporary bleaching of hyperpigmented skin in conditions as cholasma and melasma
Minoxidil Solution	Rogaine Topical Solution (Upjohn)	2%	alcohol/ water/ propylene glycol	Long-term topical treatment of male pattern baldness by stimulating hair regrowth.
Povidone-Iodine Topical Solution	Betadine Solution (Purdue Frederick)	7.5 and 10%	aqueous	Topical anti-infective. See text for additional discussion.
Tolnaftate Topical Solution	Tinactin Solution (Schering-Plough)	1%	polyethylene glycol	Topical anti-fungal.

tive solutions and tinctures contain a dye to delineate the area of application to the skin. In contrast to aqueous solutions, when the alcoholic tinctures are applied to abraded or broken skin, they cause a stinging sensation.

All medication intended for external use should be clearly labeled "FOR EXTERNAL USE ONLY" and kept out of the reach of youngsters.

In addition to their listing in Table 10–4, the following topical solutions are discussed because of their particular pharmaceutic interest.

Aluminum Acetate Topical Solution

The solution is colorless and has a faint acetous odor and a sweetish, astringent taste. It is widely applied topically as an astringent wash or wet dressing after dilution with 10 to 40 parts of water. It is frequently used as an ingredient in various types of dermatological preparations, as lotions, creams, and pastes. Commercial premeasured tablets and packets of powders are available for the preparation of this solution.
Synonym: Burow's Solution

Aluminum Subacetate Topical Solution

The requirement for the amount of acetic acid differentiates Aluminum Acetate Topical Solution from Aluminum Subacetate Topical Solution. In the latter solution the ratio of aluminum oxide to acetic acid is 1:2.35, whereas in aluminum acetate topical solution the ratio is 1:3.52. Aluminum Subacetate Topical Solution is the stronger solution and is used in the preparation of the Aluminum Acetate Topical Solution.

The solution, diluted first with 20 to 40 parts of water, is used externally as an astringent wash and wet dressing (modified Burow's Solution).

Calcium Hydroxide Topical Solution

Calcium hydroxide topical solution, commonly referred to as *limewater,* must contain not less than 140 mg of $Ca(OH)_2$ in each 100 mL of solution. Calcium hydroxide is less soluble in hot than in cold water, and, in the preparation of this solution cool purified water is employed as the solvent. The solution is intended to be saturated with solute, and to ensure saturation, an excess of calcium hydroxide, 300 mg for each 100 mL of solution to be prepared, is agitated with the purified water, vigorously and repeatedly, during a period of 1 hour. After this time, the excess calcium hydroxide is allowed to settle and remain at the bottom of the container. This permits the solution to remain saturated should a portion of the dissolved solute at the solution's surface react with the carbon dioxide of the air to form insoluble calcium carbonate:

$$Ca(OH)_2 + CO_2 \rightarrow CaCO_3 + H_2O$$

The calcium carbonate settles to the bottom of the container and by appearance is indistinguishable from the remaining excess of calcium hydroxide. The calcium hydroxide reserve dissolves as calcium is removed from solution in the form of the carbonate and in this way continually maintains the saturation of the solution. After the solution stands for an appreciable length of time, the undissolved material in the bottom of the container is composed of varying proportions of calcium hydroxide and calcium carbonate. Because of the uncertainty of the residue's composition, additional quantities of calcium hydroxide solution may not be prepared by adding more purified water to the solution.

The solution should be stored in well-filled, tightly stoppered containers to deter the absorption of carbon dioxide and should be kept in a cool place to maintain an adequate concentration of dissolved solute. Only the clear supernatant liquid is dispensed. This is best accomplished by the use of a siphoning apparatus assembled so as to avoid the entrainment of the residue in the siphoning tubes.

The solution is categorized as an astringent. For this purpose it is generally employed in combination with other ingredients in dermatological solutions and lotions to be applied topically.

Synonyms: Lime Water; Liquor Calcis

Coal Tar Topical Solution

Coal tar topical solution is an alcoholic solution containing 20% of coal tar and 5% of polysorbate 80. It is prepared by mixing the coal tar with two and a half times its weight of washed sand, adding the polysorbate 80 and most of the alcohol, and then macerating the mixture for 7 days in a closed vessel with frequent agitation followed by filtration and adjustment to the proper volume with alcohol. The final alcoholic content is between 81 and 86% ethyl alcohol.

Coal tar is a nearly black, viscous liquid having a characteristic naphthalene-like odor and a sharp, burning taste. It is the tar obtained as a by-product during the destructive distillation of bituminous coal. It is slightly soluble in water and partially soluble in most organic solvents, including alcohol. In the preparation of the official solution, the coal tar is mixed with the sand in order to distribute it mechanically and create a large surface area of tar exposed to the solvent action of the alcohol. During the period of maceration, or soaking, the alcohol-soluble components of the tar dissolve, leaving the undissolved portion clinging to the sand. Filtration removes the sand and the insoluble tar components from the solution. The container in which the solution was prepared should be rinsed with alcohol, and the washings should be passed through the filter paper in the adjustment of the final volume of the solution.

In the extemporaneous compounding of prescriptions and in the therapeutic application of this preparation onto the skin, the solution is frequently mixed with aqueous preparations or simply diluted with water. Because coal tar is only slightly soluble in water, in instances such as this it would separate from the solution were it not for the presence of the polysorbate 80 in the preparation. This agent, commercially available as Tween 80 (ICI Americas) and as other brandname products, is an oily liquid that is a nonionic surfactant. It is quite effective in dispersing the water-insoluble components of coal tar upon its admixture with an aqueous preparation.

Coal tar is a local antieczematic. The solution is used in the external treatment of a wide variety of chronic skin conditions after dilution with about 9 volumes of water, or in combination with other agents in various lotions, ointments, or solutions.

Synonyms: Liquor Carbonis Detergens: Liquor Picis Carbonis; LCD

Hydrogen Peroxide Topical Solution

Hydrogen Peroxide Topical Solution contains between 2.5 and 3.5% (w/v) of hydrogen peroxide, H_2O_2. Suitable preservatives, totaling not more than 0.05%, may be added.

One method of preparation involves the action of either phosphoric acid or sulfuric acid on barium peroxide:

$$BaO_2 + H_2SO_4 \rightarrow BaSO_4 + H_2O_2$$

Another method involves the electrolytic oxidation of a cold solution of concentrated sulfuric acid to form persulfuric acid, which when hydrolyzed liberates hydrogen peroxide:

$$2H_2SO_4 \rightarrow H_2S_2O_8 + H_2$$

$$H_2S_2O_8 + 2H_2O \rightarrow H_2O_2 + 2H_2SO_4$$

A solution prepared by this method usually contains about 30% of hydrogen peroxide and is capable of liberating 100 times its volume of oxygen. A solution of this strength is commonly referred to as "100 volume peroxide." The dilute solution, which contains about 3% hydrogen peroxide and liberates 10 times its volume of oxygen, may be prepared from the concentrated solution.

The solution is a clear, colorless liquid that may be odorless or may have the odor of ozone. It usually deteriorates upon long standing with the formation of oxygen and water. Preservative agents, as acetanilide, which have been found to retard the solution's decomposition are usually added in the amount stated above. Decomposition is enhanced by light and by heat, and for this reason the solution should be preserved in tight, light-resistant containers, preferably at a temperature not exceeding 35°C (95°F). The solution is also decomposed by practically all organic matter and other reducing agents and reacts with oxidizing agents to liberate oxygen and water; metals, alkalies, and other agents can catalyze its decomposition.

Hydrogen peroxide solution is categorized as a local anti-infective for use topically on the skin and mucous membranes. Its germicidal activity is based on the release of nascent oxygen on contact with the tissues. However, because of the short duration of this release, the chief value of the preparation in the reduction of infection is probably its ability to cleanse wounds by mechanical action through the effervescence and frothing caused by the release of oxygen.

Synonym: "Peroxide"

Chlorhexidine Gluconate Solution

Since 1957 chlorhexidine gluconate has been employed extensively as a broad spectrum antiseptic in clinical and veterinarian medicine. Its spectrum encompasses gram-positive and gram-negative bacteria, including *Pseudomonas aeruginosa*. In a concentration of 4% (Hibiclens, Stuart) it is used as a surgical scrub, hand wash and as a skin wound and general skin cleanser. Procedures are established for all of these purposes to maximize the effectiveness of the chlorhexidine. Experience has demonstrated that irritation, dermatitis and/or photosensitivity associated with the topical use of chlorhexidine are rare.

In 1987, the FDA and the Council of Dental Therapeutics of the American Dental Association approved chlorhexidine gluconate, 0.12% (Peridex, Procter & Gamble) as the first prescription only antiplaque/antigingivitis drug with antimicrobial activity. When used as a mouth rinse, microbiologic sampling of plaque has shown a reduction of aerobic and anaerobic bacteria, ranging from 54 to 97% through 6 months of use. The oral rinse should be used twice daily for 30 seconds, morning and night after toothbrushing. Usually a 15 mL dose of undiluted solution is used, and expectorated after rinsing. The most common side effect of chlorhexidine is the formation of an extrinsic yellow-brown stain on the teeth and tongue, after only a few days use. The amount of stain that appears is dependent upon the concentration of of chlorhexidine and individual susceptibility. Increased consumption of tannin containing substances, e.g., tea, red wine, port wine, will increase the level of discoloration. The developed stain can be periodically removed with a dental prophylaxis.

Povidone-Iodine Topical Solution

The agent povidone-iodine is a chemical complex of iodine with polyvinylpyrrolidone, the latter agent being a polymer having an average molecular weight of about 40,000. The povidone-iodine complex contains approximately 10% of available iodine and slowly releases it when applied to the skin.

The preparation is employed topically as a surgical scrub and nonirritating antiseptic solution with its effectiveness directly attributable to the presence and the release of iodine from the complex.

Commercial Product: Betadine Solution (Purdue Frederick)

Thimerosal Topical Solution

Thimerosal is a water-soluble, organic, mercurial, antibacterial agent used topically for its bacteriostatic and mild fungistatic properties. It is used mainly to disinfect skin surfaces and as an application to wounds and abrasions. In certain instances it has been applied to the eye, nose, throat, and urethra in dilutions of 1:5000. It is also used as a preservative for various pharmaceutical preparations, including many vaccines and other biological products.

Thimerosal Topical Solution contains 0.1% thimerosal. Also present are ethylenediamine solution and sodium borate to maintain the alkalinity (usually pH 9.8 to 10.3) required for the solution's stability. Monoethanolamine is used as an additional stabilizer. The solution is affected by light and must be maintained in light-resistant containers.

Commercial Product: Merthiolate Solution (Lilly)

Topical Tinctures

Examples of tinctures for topical application to the skin are presented in Table 10–5. Those of particular pharmaceutic interest are discussed briefly as follows.

Iodine Tincture

Iodine Tincture is prepared by dissolving 2% of iodine crystals and 2.4% of sodium iodide in an amount of alcohol equal to half the volume of tincture to be prepared and then diluting the solution to volume with sufficient purified water. The sodium iodide reacts with the iodine to form sodium triiodide:

$$I_2 + NaI \rightleftharpoons NaI_3$$

This reaction prevents the formation of ethyl iodide from the interaction between iodine and the alcohol, which would result in the loss of the antibacterial activity of the tincture. An added benefit of the triiodide form of iodine is its water solubility which is important should the tincture, which contains between 44 and 50% alcohol, be diluted with water during use.

The tincture is a popular local anti-infective agent applied topically to the skin in general household first-aid procedures. The reddish-brown color, which produces a stain on the skin, is useful in delineating the application over the affected skin area.

The tincture should be stored in tight containers to prevent loss of alcohol.

Compound Benzoin Tincture

Compound Benzoin Tincture is prepared by the maceration in alcohol of 10% of benzoin and lesser amounts of aloe, storax, and tolu balsam totaling about 24% of starting material. The drug mixture is best macerated in a wide-mouthed container, since it is difficult to introduce storax, a semi-liquid, sticky material into a narrow-mouthed container. Generally, it is advisable to weight the storax in the container in which it will be macerated to avoid possible loss through a transfer of the material from one container to another.

The tincture is categorized as a protectant. It is used to protect and toughen skin in the treatment of bedsores, ulcers, cracked nipples, and fissures of the lips and anus. It is also commonly used as an inhalant in bronchitis and other respiratory conditions, one teaspoonful commonly

Table 10–5. Examples of Tinctures Applied Topically to the Skin

Tincture	*Corresponding Commercial Product*	*Percent Active Constituent in Commercial Tincture*	*Vehicle*	*Category and Comments*
Green Soap Tincture	. . .	65%	alcohol	Detergent. Also contains 2% lavender oil as perfume.
Iodine Tincture	. . .	2%	alcohol-water	Topical anti-infective. See text for additional discussion.
Compound Benzoin Tincture	. . .	10% benzoin; 2% aloe; 8% storax; 4% tolu balsam	alcohol	Topical protectant. Prepared by maceration of the ingredients in alcohol. See text for additional discussion.

being added to a pint of boiling water. The volatile components of the tincture travel with the steam vapor and are inhaled by the patient. Because of the incompatibility of the alcoholic tincture and water, mixture of the two produces a milky product with some separation of resinous material. Alcohol or acetone may be used as necessary to remove the residue from the vaporizer after use.

Compound tincture of benzoin serves as a delivery vehicle of podophyllum in the treatment of venereal warts. It is important that podophyllum not be systemically absorbed after application because the drug can effect peripheral neuropathy characterized by paresthesias, loss of sensation and loss of deep tendon reflexes in the extremities, in addition to neuropathy involving the central nervous system, e.g., lethargy, confusion, coma. Secondly, the podophyllum is teratogenic and should be administered only when the risk to benefit ratio is extremely low in a pregnant woman suffering from venereal warts. Thus, the nonocclusive compound tincture of benzoin is preferred to the occlusive flexible collodion.

Compound Benzoin Tincture is best stored in tight, light-resistant containers. Exposure to direct sunlight or to excessive heat should be avoided.

The tincture originated in the fifteenth or sixteenth century and through the years probably has acquired more synonyms that any other official preparation. A few of these are indicated as follows.

Synonyms: Friar's Balsam; Turlington's Drops; Persian Balsam; Swedish Balsam; Jerusalem Balsam; Wade's Drops; Turlington's Balsam of Life.

Thimerosal Tincture

The same general remarks made during the discussion of Thimerosal Topical Solution apply to Thimerosal Tincture except that sodium chloride and sodium borate are absent from the tincture and the vehicle of the tincture is composed of water, acetone, and about 50% alcohol. A number of metals, notably copper, cause the decomposition of the tincture, and for this reason it must be manufactured and stored in glass or suitably resistant containers. Monoethanolamine and ethylenediamine are used as stabilizers in the official solution and tincture and are thought to be effective because of their chelating action on traces of metallic impurities that may be present at the time of preparation or may later gain access to the preparation.

The commercial preparation is colored orange red and has a greenish fluorescence. The red stain it leaves on the skin defines the area of application. The preparation is a commonly used household antiseptic for application topically on the skin in abrasions and cuts and also in the preoperative preparation of patients for surgery.

Commercial Product: Merthiolate Tincture (Lilly)

Liniments

Liniments are alcoholic or oleaginous solutions or emulsions of various medicinal substances intended for external application to the skin generally with rubbing. Liniments with an alcoholic or hydroalcoholic vehicle are useful in instances in which rubefacient, counterirritant, or penetrating action is desired; oleaginous liniments are employed primarily when massage is desired. By their nature, oleaginous liniments are less irritating to the skin than alcoholic liniments. Liniments are not generally applied to skin areas that are broken or bruised because excessive irritation might result. The vehicle for a liniment should therefore be selected on the basis of the type of action desired (rubefacient, counterirritant, or just massage) and also on the solubility of the desired components in the various solvents. For oleaginous liniments, the solvent may be a fixed oil such as almond oil, peanut oil, sesame oil, or cottonseed oil or a volatile substance such as wintergreen oil or turpentine, or it may be a combination of fixed and volatile oils.

All liniments should bear a label indicating that they are suitable only for external use and must never be taken internally. Liniments that are emulsions or that contain insoluble matter must be shaken thoroughly before use to ensure an even distribution of the dispersed phase, and for these preparations a "Shake Well" label is indicated. Liniments should be stored in tight containers.

Depending upon their individual ingredients, liniments are prepared in the same manner as solutions, emulsions, or suspensions, as the case may warrant.

There are presently no official liniments.

Collodions

Collodions are liquid preparations composed of pyroxylin dissolved in a solvent mixture usually composed of alcohol and ether with or without added medicinal substances. Pyroxylin (soluble gun cotton, collodion cotton) is obtained by the action of a mixture of nitric and sulfuric acids on cotton and consists chiefly of cellulose tetranitrate. It has the appearance of raw cotton when dry but is harsh to the touch. It is frequently available commercially moistened with about 30% alcohol or other similar solvent.

One part of pyroxylin is slowly but completely soluble in 25 parts of a mixture of 3 volumes of ether and 1 volume of alcohol. It is also soluble in acetone and glacial acetic acid. Pyroxylin is precipitated from solution in these solvents upon the addition of water. Pyroxylin, like collodions, is exceedingly flammable and must be stored away from flame in well-closed containers, protected from light.

Collodions are intended for external use. When applied to the skin with a fine camel's hair brush or glass applicator, the solvent rapidly evaporates, leaving a filmy residue of pyroxylin. This provides an occlusive protective coating to the skin, and when the collodion is medicated, it leaves a thin layer of that medication firmly placed against the skin. Naturally, collodions must be applied to dry tissues to effect adhesion to the skin's surface. The products must be clearly labeled "For External Use only" or with words of similar effect.

Collodion

Collodion is a clear or slightly opalescent, viscous liquid prepared by dissolving pyroxylin (4% w/v) in a 3:1 mixture of ether and alcohol. The resulting solution is highly volatile and flammable and should be reserved in tight containers at a temperature not exceeding 30°C remote from fire.

The product is capable of forming a protective film on application to the skin and the volatilization of the solvent. The film is useful in holding the edges of an incised wound together. However, its presence on the skin is uncomfortable due to its inflexible nature. The following product, which is flexible, has greater appeal when a nonpliable film is not required.

Flexible Collodion

Flexible Collodion is prepared by adding 2% of camphor and 3% of castor oil to collodion. The castor oil renders the product flexible, permitting its comfortable use over skin areas that are normally moved, such as fingers and toes. The camphor makes the product waterproof. Physicians frequently apply the coating over bandages or stitched incisions to make them waterproof and to protect them from external stress.

Salicylic Acid Collodion

Salicylic Acid Collodion is a 10% solution of salicylic acid in flexible collodion. It is used for its keratolytic effects, especially in the removal of corns from the toes. Similar preparations are marketed as Compound W (Whitehall) and Freezone (Whitehall). Patients who use these products should be advised about their proper use. The product should be applied one drop at a time onto the corn or wart allowing time to dry before the next drop is added. Because salicylic acid can be irritating to normal, healthy skin every attempt must be made to ensure application directly onto the corn or wart. A useful preventive measure is to line the adjacent healthy skin with some white petrolatum prior to application of the product. Lastly, proper tightening and storage of the product after use is an absolute necessity because of the volatility of the vehicle.

Glycerogelatins

Glycerogelatins may be described as plastic masses intended for topical application and containing gelatin, glycerin, and water, in addition to any added medicinal substance. In dermatologic practice, such medicinal substances as zinc oxide, salicylic acid, resorcinol, and other appropriate agents may be added. Glycerogelatins are melted prior to application, cooled to only slightly above body temperature, and applied to the affected area with a fine brush. After application, the glycerogelatin hardens, is usually covered with a bandage, and is allowed to remain in place for periods up to 6 weeks and longer as is necessary.

Unless otherwise specified, glycerogelatins contain 10% of the medicinal substance prepared according to the formula:

Medicinal Substance	100 g
Gelatin	150 g
Glycerin	400 g
Purified Water	350 g
To make about	1000 g

In preparing a glycerogelatin, the gelatin is first softened in the purified water, being stirred when added, then allowed to stand for about 10 minutes after which time the mixture is heated in a steam bath until the gelatin is dissolved. The medicinal substance is mixed first with the glycerin (either dissolving in it or being dispersed by it) and then with the gelatin solution, the glycerogelatin being stirred until it congeals.

Zinc Gelatin

Zinc Gelatin is a firm, plastic mass containing 10% zinc oxide in a glycerogelatin base. It is used mainly for the treatment of varicose ulcers because of its ability to form a pressure bandage known as a "gelatin boot." The mass is softened in a water bath before being applied to the skin with a soft brush. This coating is then covered with a bandage and allowed to remain in place for up to 6 weeks, depending upon the degree of serous discharge from the lesion.
Synonym: Zinc Gelatin Boot.

Plasters

Plasters are solid or semisolid adhesive masses spread upon a suitable backing material and intended for external application to a part of the body to provide prolonged contact at that site. Among the backing materials used are paper, cotton, felt, linen, muslin, silk, moleskin, or plastic. The plasters are adhesive at body temperature and may be used to provide protection or mechanical support (nonmedicated plasters) or to provide localized or systemic effects (medicated plasters). The backings onto which the masses are placed are cut into different shapes appropriate to the contour and the extent of the body surface to be covered. Commonly used are back plasters, chest plasters, breast plasters, kidney plasters, and corn plasters. Common adhesive tape was formerly official under the title "Adhesive Plaster," the use of this material being well known.

Today, most plasters are prepared industrially. The adhesive material in many of the commercially available plasters consist of either a rubber base or a synthetic resin material.

One plaster in general use is Salicylic Acid Plaster.

Salicylic Acid Plaster

Salicylic Acid Plaster is a uniform mixture of salicylic acid in a suitable base spread on a backing material and is intended to be placed on areas requiring the removal of horny layers of skin. The preparation is employed typically as corn plasters for the toes. The horny layers of skin are removed by virtue of the keratolytic action of salicylic acid. The usual concentration of salicylic acid in the plaster is 10 to 40%.

The effectiveness of these plasters is considerably enhanced when the patient soaks the corn or callus in warm water for a period of time, e.g., 15 to 30 minutes, prior to application of the plaster. Skin hydration enhances the penetration of the salicylic acid into the corn or the callus. Complete removal of the corn or the callus is not always essential because partial removal may provide needed comfort to the patient. Therefore, the FDA restricts the application of over-the-counter salicylic acid disks, pads or plasters to five treatments over a period of not more than 14 days for corns and calluses. Lastly, the patient should be instructed on the proper cutting of the plaster to conform to the size of the corn or callus.

Powders for Application to the Skin

Nonmedicated and medicated powders are frequently applied to the skin. The use of plain talcum powder is common as a topical dusting powder to prevent skin irritation and chafing. Medicated powders are often employed to combat such conditions as diaper rash and athlete's foot.

Powders for topical use are prepared in the same manner as has been described previously in Chapter 5. Powders for use on the skin are generally packaged in paper, metal, or plastic containers having a sifter-type cap. Some commercial powders are also packaged in plastic squeeze bottles in aerosol containers.

Some popular commercial medicated powders in use today include: Tolnaftate (Ting, Fisons) and Miconazole Nitrate (Micatin, Ortho) for athlete's foot, Zinc Undecylenate and Undecylenic Acid (Cruex, Fisons) for jock itch, and Polymyxin B Sulfate and Bacitracin Zinc (Polysporin, Burroughs-Wellcome) for infection prophylaxis in minor skin abrasions. These are generally used in conjunction with corresponding anti-fungal solutions, tinctures, creams or ointments.

Topical Aerosols

Aerosol packages for topical use on the skin are prepared in the same manner as discussed in Chapter 13. Common aerosols used topically include the anti-infective agents: povidone-iodine, tolnaftate and thimerosal; the adrenocortical steroids: betamethasone dipropionate and valerate, dexamethasone, and triamcinolone acetonide; and the local anesthetic dibucaine hydrochloride.

The use of topical aerosols provides to the patient a means of applying the drug in a convenient manner. The preparation may be applied to the desired surface area without the use of the fingertips, thus making the procedure less messy than with most other types of topical preparations. Among the disadvantages to the use of topical aerosols are the difficulty in applying the medication to a small area and the greater expense associated with the aerosol package.

Topical Gels

As described previously in Chapter 7, gels are *semisolid systems* consisting of dispersions of small or large molecules in a liquid vehicle rendered jelly-like through the action of an added substance, as carboxymethylcellulose. A number of topically used drugs are available as gels and are gaining widespread appeal. Examples of such drugs and drug products are: erythromycin and benzoyl peroxide topical gel [Benzamycin Topical Gel (Dermik Laboratories)]; clindamycin topical gel [Cleocin T Topical Gel (Upjohn)], and benzoyl peroxide gel [Desquam-X 10 Gel (Westwood-Squibb)] used in the control and treatment of acne vulgaris; hydroquinone gel [Solaquin Forte Gel (ICN)], a bleach for hyperpigmented skin; salicylic acid gel [Compound W Gel (Whitehall)], a keratolytic; and desoximetasone gel [Topicort Gel (Hoechst-Roussel)], an anti-inflammatory and antipruritic agent.

Tapes and Gauzes

The USP contains monographs setting the standards for a number of topical dressings, including the following:

Adhesive Tape—defined as "fabric and/or film evenly coated on one side with a pressure sensitive adhesive mixture." Standards are set for sterility of those tapes which are labeled to be sterile, as well as for the dimensions, tensile strength, and adhesive strength of the sterile and nonsterile tapes.

Absorbent Gauze—this is cotton or a mixture of cotton and Rayon in the form of a plain woven cloth. Official standards are set for thread count, length, width, weight, absorbency as well as sterility for absorbent gauze that has been rendered sterile.

Gauze Bandage—this is one continuous piece of absorbent gauze, tightly rolled in various widths and lengths and substantially free from loose threads and ravelings. Standards are set for width, length, weight, absorbency, thread count, as well as for sterility for those products labeled to be sterile.

Adhesive Bandage—this is a compress of four layers of absorbent or other suitable material, affixed to a film of fabric coated with a pressure-sensitive adhesive substance. Adhesive bandage is sterile and is protected by a suitable removable covering.

Petrolatum Gauze—this is absorbent gauze saturated with white petrolatum. This gauze is sterile. It is prepared by adding molten, sterile, white petrolatum to dry, sterile absorbent gauze, previously cut to size, ratio of 60 g of petrolatum to each 20 g of gauze. Standards are set for packaging, labeling, and sterility.

Zinc Gelatin Impregnated Gauze—this is absorbent gauze impregnated with zinc gelatin. The gauze is used as a topical protectant.

Miscellaneous Preparations for Topical Application to the Skin

Rubbing Alcohol

Rubbing Alcohol contains about 70% of ethyl alcohol by volume, the remainder consisting of water, denaturants with or without color additives and perfume oils, and stabilizers. In each 100 mL it must contain not less than 355 mg of sucrose octaacetate of 1.4 mg of denatonium benzoate, bitter substances that discourage accidental or abusive oral ingestion. The denaturants employed in rubbing alcohol are according to the Internal Revenue Service, U.S. Treasury Department, Formula 23-H, which is composed of 8 parts by volume of acetone, 1.5 parts by volume of methyl isobutyl ketone, and 100 parts by volume of ethyl alcohol. The use of this denaturant mixture makes the separation of ethyl alcohol from the denaturants a virtually impossible task with ordinary distillation apparatus. This discourages the illegal removal and use as a beverage of the alcoholic content of rubbing alcohol.

The product is volatile and flammable and should be stored in tight containers remote from fire. It is employed as a rubefacient externally and as a soothing rub for bedridden patients, a germicide for instruments, and a skin cleanser prior to injection.

Synonym: Alcohol Rubbing Compound.

Isopropyl Rubbing Alcohol

Isopropyl Rubbing Alcohol is about 70% by volume of isopropyl alcohol, the remainder consisting of water with or without color additives, stabilizers, and perfume oils. It is used externally as a rubefacient and soothing rub. This preparation and a commercially available 91% isopropyl alcohol solution are commonly employed by diabetic patients in preparing needles and syringes for hypodermic injections of insulin and for disinfecting the skin.

Hexachlorophene Liquid Cleanser

The commercial product [pHisoHex (Samofi Winthrop)] is an antibacterial sudsing emulsion containing a colloidal dispersion of hexacholorophene 3% (w/w) in a stable emulsion consisting of entsufon sodium (a synthetic detergent), petrolatum, lanolin cholesterols, methylcellulose, polyethylene glycol, polyethylene glycol monostearate, lauryl myristyl diethanolamide, sodium benzoate and water.

The preparation is a bacteriostatic cleansing agent. It cleanses the skin thoroughly and has bacteriostatic action against staphylococci and other gram-positive bacteria. Cumulative antibacterial action develops with repeated use. The preparation is indicated for use as a surgical scrub and a bacteriostatic skin cleanser.

Hexachlorophene may be absorbed through the skin and its use should be discontinued if signs of absorption (CNS irritation) or sensitivity (dermatoses) occur. Care must be exercised particularly when used on infants and children.

General Considerations in the Application of Topical Medications

Although differences in bioavailability or skin penetration are not a problem associated with a majority of topical products, in the recent past there has been research that has demonstrated differences in bioavailability between topical corticosteroids. Skin penetration is crucial for certain diseases of the skin, e.g., psoriasis, corticosteroid-responsive dermatoses, and vasoconstrictor assay procedures have demonstrated that differences exist in bioavailability between topical ointments and creams which possess an active ingredient in identical strengths. The ability of topical corticosteroids to induce vasoconstriction in normal intact human skin has been used by pharmaceutical companies to predict clinical potency, and more recently by the U.S. FDA to judge the equivalence of generic topical corticosteroids and their brandname counterparts.

When considering brand interchange of a topical steroid product, the pharmacist must be aware that when one product with the same active ingredient and strength is substituted for another, the products may contain adjuvants which differ. Occasionally, an allergic response in a patient may be traced to the adjuvants.

Topical dosage forms, e.g., ointments, creams, are expensive and it is important that the pharmacist ensure the patient use these to maximum benefit. Before these are applied the affected area and adjacent healthy skin should be cleansed with soap and water, unless otherwise directed by the physician or directions on the package. This area should be dried thoroughly before application of the medicine. The patient should gently massage the medicine into the affected area as directed by the prescription.

Creams and ointments should be applied as a thin film onto the skin and spread evenly. Overuse, in general, will merely waste the medication. When using a solution, the patient should place two or three drops at most onto the area and gently massage these to cover the desired area. Powder dosage forms are sprinkled liberally on all areas of need, and for athlete's foot sprinkled into the shoes and socks as well.

How extensive the application of a topical product should be is really a function of the problem being treated. For example, when treating acne vulgaris with a topical product, it is important that patients realize that they should apply the product to the whole face, neck and back, and not merely to just the lesions alone. Application to the entire face is thought to "nip in the bud" forming comedones.

After application of the medicine, especially if it was applied with clean fingertips, the patient should cleanse his/her hands with soap and water. Inadvertent application of contaminated fingertips having residual drug, e.g., benzoyl peroxide, onto mucous membranes, e.g., mouth, eyes, nose, could be quite painful and bothersome.

For any topical product, patients should understand that symptoms should improve within a certain time frame, and that if symptoms persist beyond this time or if irritation develops, they should discontinue use and contact their physician. Patients should also understand not to apply any product to severely broken or abraded skin.

A question that will arise with topical products is the necessity of a bandage or covering. Whenever possible, with the exception of the need for an occlusive dressing with a corticosteroid drug, the wound should be medicated and left open to the atmosphere.

References

1. Black, C.D.: Transdermal Drug Delivery Systems. *US Pharm., 1*:49, 1982.
2. Walters, K.A.: Percutaneous Absorption and Transdermal Therapy. *Pharm. Tech., 10*:30–42, 1986.
3. Hadgraft, J.: Structure Activity Relationships and Percutaneous Absorption. *J. Controlled Release, 25*: 221–226, 1991.
4. Surber, C., et al.: Optimization of Topical Therapy: Partitioning of Drugs into Stratum Corneum. *Pharm. Res., 7*:1320–1324, 1990.
5. Cleary, G.W.: Transdermal Concepts and Perspectives. Key Pharmaceuticals, Miami, FL, 1982.
6. Melendres, J.L., et al.: In Vivo Percutaneous Absorption of Hydrocortisone: Multiple-Application Dosing in Man. *Pharm. Res., 9*:1164, 1992.
7. Barr, M.: Percutaneous Absorption. *J. Pharm. Sci., 51*:395–409, 1962.
8. Idson, B.: Percutaneous Absorption. *J. Pharm. Sci., 64*:901–924, 1975.
9. Idson, B.: Percutaneous Absorption Enhancers. *Drug & Cosmetic Ind., 137*:30, 1985.
10. Ghosh, T.K. and Banga, A.K.: Methods of Enhancement of Transdermal Drug Delivery: Part IIB, Chemical Permeation Enhancers. *Pharm. Tech., 17*: 68–76, 1993.
11. Ghosh, T.K. and Banga, A.K.: Methods of Enhancement of Transdermal Drug Delivery: Part IIA, Chemical Permeation Enhancers,. *Pharm. Tech., 17*: 62–90, 1993.
12. Rolf, D.: Chemical and Physical Methods of Enhancing Transdermal Drug Delivery. *Pharm. Tech., 12*:130–139, 1988.
13. Riviere, J.E., Monteiro-Riviere, N.A., and Inman, A.O.: Determination of Lidocaine Concentrations in Skin after Transdermal Iontophoresis: Effects of Vasoactive Drugs. *Pharm. Res., 9*:211–219, 1992.
14. Green, P.G., et al.: Iontophoretic Delivery of Amino Acids and Amino Acid Derivatives Across the Skin in Vitro. *Pharm. Res., 8*:1113–1120, 1991.
15. Choi, H.K., Flynn, G.L., Amidon, G.L.: Transdermal Delivery of Bioactive Peptides: The Effect of n-Decylmethyl Sulfoxide, pH, and Inhibitors on Enkephalin Metabolism and Transport. *Pharm. Res., 7*:1099–1106, 1990.
16. Ghosh, T.K. and Banga, A.K.: Methods of Enhancement of Transdermal Drug Delivery: Part I, Physical and Biochemical Approaches. *Pharm. Tech. 17*: 72–98, 1993.
17. D'Emanuele, A. and Staniforth, J.N.: An Electrically Modulated Drug Delivery Device. III. Factors Affecting Drug Stability During Electrophoresis. *Pharm. Res., 9*:312–315, 1992.
18. Bommannan, D., et al.: Sonophoresis. I. The Use of High-Frequency Ultrasound to Enhance Transdermal Drug Delivery. *Pharm. Res., 9*:559–564, 1992.
19. Bommannan, D., et al.: Sonophoresis. II. Examination of the Mechanism(s) of Ultrasound-Enhanced Transdermal Drug Delivery. *Pharm. Res., 9*: 1043–1047, 1992.
20. Shah, V.P., et al.: In Vivo Percutaneous Penetration/Absorption. *Pharm. Res., 8*:1071–1075, 1991.
21. Bronaugh, R.L., Stewart, R.F., and Congdon, E.R.: Methods for in Vitro Percutaneous Absorption Studies II. Animal Models for Human Skin. *Tox. and Appl. Pharmacol. 62*:481–488, 1982.
22. Nugent, F.J., and Wood, J.A.: Methods for the Study of Percutaneous Absorption. *Canadian J. Pharm. Sci., 15*:1–7, 1980.
23. Addicks, W., et al.: Topical Drug Delivery from Thin Applications: Theoretical Predictions and Experimental Results. *Pharm. Res., 7*:1048–1054, 1990.

24. Kushla, G.P. and Zatz, J.L.: Evaluation of a Noninvasive Method for Monitoring Percutaneous Absorption of Lidocaine in Vivo. *Pharm. Res., 7:* 1033–1037, 1990.
25. Itoh, T., et al.: A Method to Predict the Percutaneous Permeability of Various Compounds: Shed Snake Skin as a Model Membrane. *Pharm. Res., 7:* 1302–1306, 1990.
26. Itoh, T., et al.: Effects of Transdermal Penetration Enhancers on the Permeability of Shed Snakeskin. Pharm. Res., 9:1168–1172, 1992.
27. Rolland, A., et al.: Influence of Formulation, Receptor Fluid, and Occlusion, on in Vitro Drug Release from Topical Dosage Forms, Using an Automated Flow-Through Diffusion Cell. *Pharm. Res., 9:*82–86, 1992.
28. Fara, J.W.: Short- and Long-term Transdermal Drug Delivery Systems. Drug Delivery Systems. *Pharm. Tech.,* Aster Publishing Corporation, 1983, pp. 33–40.
29. Shaw, J.E. and Chadrasekaran, S.K.: Controlled Topical Delivery of Drugs of Systemic Action. *Drug Metabolism Rev., 8:*223, 1978.
30. Good, W.R.: Transdermal Drug-Delivery Systems. *Medical Device & Diagnostic Ind., 8:*37–42, 1986.
31. *Transderm-Scop* (professional literature). Woodbridge, NJ, CIBA Consumer Pharmaceuticals, 1993.
32. *Transderm-Nitro* (professional literature). Summit, NJ, Summit Pharmaceuticals, 1993.
33. *Nitro-Dur* (professional literature). Kenilworth, NJ, Key Pharmaceuticals, Inc., 1993.
34. Magnuson, D.E., personal communication. Key Pharmaceuticals, 1983.
35. *Nitrodisc* (professional literature). Chicago, IL, G.D. Searle & Co., 1993.
36. *Catapress-TTS,* (professional literature). Ridgefield, CT, Boehringer Ingelheim Pharmaceuticals, Inc., 1993.
37. *Estraderm* (professional literature), Summit, NJ, CIBA Pharmaceutical Company, 1993.
38. *Habitrol* (professional literature), Summit, NJ, Basel Pharmaceuticals, 1993.
39. *Nicoderm* (professional literature), Kansas City, MO, Marion Merrell Dow, 1993.
40. *Nicotrol* (professional literature), Morris Plains, NJ, Parke-Davis, 1993.
41. *PROSTEP* (professional literature), Wayne, NJ, Lederle Laboratories, 1993.
42. Fiore, M.C., Smith, S.S., Jorenby, D.E., and Baker, T.B.: The Effectiveness of the Nicotine Patch for Smoking Cessation. A Meta-Analysis. *JAMA 271:* 1940–1947, 1994.
43. Baker, R.W., and Farrant, J.: Patents in Transdermal Drug Delivery. Drug Delivery Systems. *Pharm. Tech.,* Aster Publishing Corporation, 1987, pp. 26–31.
44. Avallone, H.L.: Microbiological Control of Topicals. *Pharm. Tech., 12:*55–62, 1988.
45. Lee, J.Y.: Sterilization Control and Validation for Topical Ointments. *Pharm. Tech., 16:*104–110, 1992.

11

Ophthalmic, Nasal, Otic, and Oral Preparations Applied Topically

PREPARATIONS APPLIED topically to the eye, ear, nose, and oral cavity include many of the types of pharmaceutic dosage forms previously discussed as solutions, suspensions, and ointments. The purpose of this chapter is to identify more closely the types of dosage forms used with these sites of application and to define the purpose of special formulative components.

Ophthalmic Preparations

Drugs are applied to the eye for the localized effect of the medication on the surface of the eye or on its interior. Most frequently aqueous solutions are employed; however, suspensions, and ophthalmic ointments are also used. Recently, ophthalmic inserts, impregnated with drug, have been developed to provide for the continuous release of medication. These inserts are particularly useful for those drugs requiring frequent daytime and nighttime administration.

Because the capacity of the eye to retain liquid and ointment preparations is limited, they are generally administered in small volume. Liquid preparations are most frequently administered dropwise and ointments by the application of a thin ribbon of ointment to the lid margin. Larger volumes of liquid preparations may be used to flush or wash the eye.

The normal volume of tears in the eye is 7 μL. Whereas a nonblinking eye can accommodate a maximum of 30 μL of fluid, blinking eyes can hold only 10 μL. Excessive liquids, both normally produced and externally added, are rapidly drained from the eye. The usual single drop size of an instilled drug solution may be 50 μL (based on 20 drops/mL) and thus, much of the drop instilled may be lost. The ideal volume of drug solution to administer, based on eye capacity, would be 5 to 10 μL.[1] Since microliter dosing eye droppers are not generally available or used by patients, the loss of instilled medication using standard eye droppers is a common occurrence. Due to the dynamics of the lacrimal system, the retention time of an ophthalmic solution on the eye surface is short, and the amount of drug absorbed is usually only a small fraction of the quantity administered. For example, following the administration of pilocarpine ophthalmic solution, the instilled solution is flushed from the precorneal area within 1 to 2 minutes, resulting in the ocular absorption of less than 1 percent of the administered dose.[2,3] This necessitates the frequent administration of the solution, resulting in patient inconvenience, patient noncompliance, and unevenness in ocular drug levels.[4] If multiple drop therapy is desired, 5-minute intervals between drops is sometimes recommended. This permits the buildup of drug in the cornea while allowing for minimal loss through drainage.[1] Sometimes, use of an ophthalmic solution of greater drug concentration can substitute for multiple drop therapy of a more dilute solution. Pharmaceutical research has been directed toward enhancing ocular bioavailability and the duration of action of pilocarpine and other drugs. A number of drug carriers that slow precorneal drug loss and improve corneal contact time are being studied, including gel systems, liposomes, polymer matrices, mucoadhesive polymers, and absorbable gelatin sponge.[4,5] The Ocusert reservoir system, described later in this chapter, provides continuous and controlled drug release.

Thus, the effective "dose" of medication administered ophthalmically may be varied by the strength of medication administered, the volume administered, the retention time of the medication in contact with the surface of the eye and the frequency of administration. Although the local administration of medications to the eye is the main route of administration employed by the ophthalmologist in the treatment of diseases of the eye, other routes as oral and parenteral may also be used. The use of systemic antibiotic therapy to combat an intraocular infection is an example of this type of therapy.

Ophthalmic Solutions

Considerations in the preparation of ophthalmic solutions includes sterility, preservation, isotonicity, buffering, viscosity, and appropriate packaging.

Sterility and Preservation

All ophthalmic solutions should be sterile when dispensed, and whenever possible, a suitable preservative should be added to ensure sterility during the course of use. Ophthalmic solutions intended to be used during surgery or in the traumatized eye generally do not contain preservative agents, because these are irritating to the tissues within the eye. These solutions are usually packaged in single-dose containers and any unused solution discarded.

Although it is preferable that ophthalmic solutions be sterilized by autoclaving in the final container, the method employed may be dependent upon the thermostability of the particular preparation. With the exception of basic salts of weak acids such as sodium fluorescein or sodium sulfacetamide, solutions of most of the common ophthalmic drugs, prepared in a boric acid vehicle, can be safely sterilized at 121°C for 15 minutes as previously discussed in Chapter 8.

If necessary, a bacterial filter may be used to avoid the use of heat sterilization. Although bacterial filters work with a high degree of efficiency, they are not as trusted sterilizers as is the autoclave. The advantage of filtration, as was pointed out earlier, is the retention of all particulate matter, the removal of which is of prime importance in the manufacture and use of ophthalmic solutions. Figures 11–1 and 11–2 show filtration equipment which may be employed in the extemporaneous filtration of ophthalmic solutions.

Ophthalmic solutions to be used on eyes with intact corneal membranes may be packaged in multiple-dose containers. Even though sterile when dispensed, each of these solutions should contain a rapidly effective, topically nonirritating antibacterial agent or a mixture of such agents to prevent the growth of, or to destroy, microorganisms accidentally introduced into the solution when the container is opened during use. Suitable preservatives and their maximum concentrations for this purpose include (a) benzalkonium chloride, 0.013%; (b) benzethonium chloride, 0.01%; (c) chlorobutanol, 0.5%; (d)

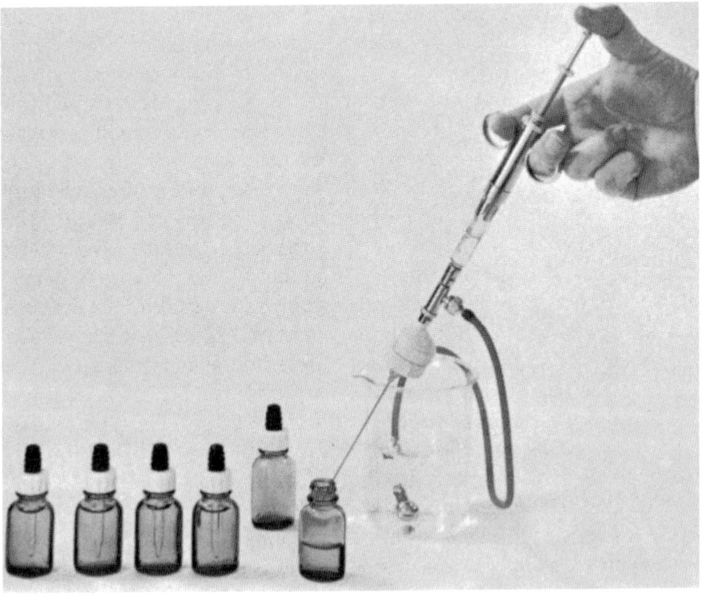

Fig. 11–1. *Sterilization by filtration. The preparation of a sterile solution by passage through a syringe affixed with a microbial filter. (Courtesy of Millipore Corporation.)*

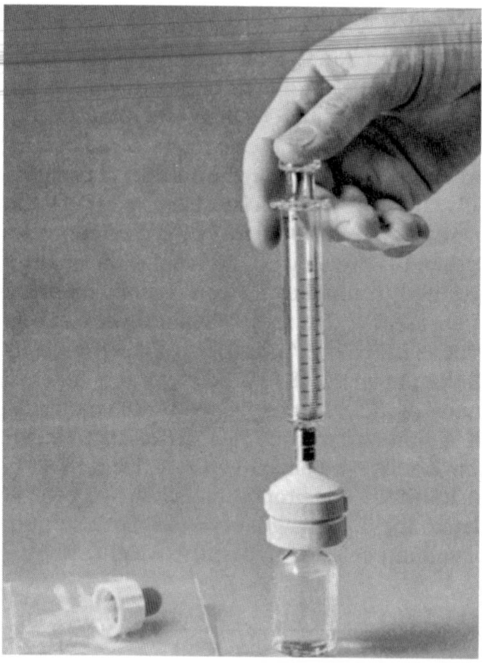

Fig. 11–2. *The preparation of a sterile ophthalmic solution by filtration. (Courtesy of Millipore Corporation.)*

phenylmercuric acetate, 0.004%; (e) phenylmercuric nitrite, 0.004%; and, (f) thimerosal, 0.01%. Each of these has certain limitations with respect to stability, chemical compatibility with other formulative ingredients, and antibacterial activity. For example, chlorobutanol hydrolyzes and decomposes at autoclaving temperatures. Further, the hydrolysis of chlorobutanol may take place under moderate heat or slowly at room temperature with the formation of hydrochloric acid which not only may render the solution susceptible to microorganism growth but may change the pH of an unbuffered solution and affect the stability or the physiologic activity of the active ingredient. Benzalkonium chloride is one of the most reliable ophthalmic solution preservatives, because it has a broad antimicrobial spectrum of activity, but the pharmacist must be aware of its incompatibility with anionic drugs.

In concentrations tolerated by the tissues of the eye, all of the aforementioned preservative agents are ineffective against some strains of *Pseudomonas aeruginosa*, an organism that can invade an abraded cornea and cause ulceration and blindness. It has been found that a preservative mixture of benzalkonium chloride (0.01%) and 1000 USP Units of polymyxin B sulfate, the latter in each mL of solution, is effective against most resistant strains of *Pseudomonas* and is nonirritating to the eye. In some ophthalmic preparations a mixture of benzalkonium chloride (0.01%) and disodium ethylenediaminetetraacetate, 0.01 to 0.1%, is employed for the same purpose. The latter agent is a chelating agent for metals, having the ability to render the resistant strains of *Pseudomonas aeruginosa* more sensitive to the benzalkonium chloride.

Isotonicity Value

If a solution is placed within or behind a membrane that is permeable only to solvent molecules and not to solute molecules (a *semipermeable membrane*), a phenomenon called *osmosis* occurs as the molecules of solvent traverse the membrane. If the solution-filled membrane is placed in a solution of a higher solute concentration than its own, the solvent, which has free passage in either direction, passes into the more concentrated solution. It does this until an equilibrium is established on both sides of the membrane and an equal concentration of solute exists on the two sides. The pressure responsible for this movement is termed *osmotic pressure*.

The concentration of a solution with respect to osmotic pressure is concerned with the number of "particles" of solute in solution. That is, if the solute is a nonelectrolyte (as sucrose), the concentration of the solution will depend solely on the number of molecules present. However, if the solute is an electrolyte (as sodium chloride), the number of particles that it contributes to the solution will depend not only upon the concentration of the molecules present, but also on their degree of ionization. A chemical that is highly ionized will contribute a greater number of particles to the solution than will the same amount of a poorly ionized substance. The effect is that a solution with a greater number of particles, whether they be molecules or ions, has a greater osmotic pressure than does a solution having fewer particles.

Body fluids, including blood and lacrimal fluid, have an osmotic pressure corresponding to that of a 0.9% solution of sodium chloride. Thus, a sodium chloride solution of this concentration is said to be *isosmotic*, or having an equal osmotic pressure, with physiologic fluids. The term *isotonic*, meaning equal tone, is commonly used interchangeably with isosmotic although the former term must be used with reference to some body fluid, and isosmotic actually is a physical chemical term which compares the osmotic pressure of two liquids, one of which may or may not be a physiologic fluid. Solutions with a lower osmotic pressure than body fluids or a 0.9% sodium chloride solution are commonly referred to as *hypotonic,* whereas solutions having a greater osmotic pressure are termed *hypertonic.*

Theoretically, a hypertonic solution added to the body's system will have a tendency to draw water from the body tissues toward the solution in an effort to dilute and establish a concentration equilibrium. In the blood stream, a hypertonic injection could cause the *crenation* (shrinking) of blood cells; in the eye, the solution could cause the drawing of water toward the site of the topical application. Conversely, a hypotonic solution might induce the hemolysis of red blood cells, or the passage of water from the site of an ophthalmic application through the tissues of the eye.

In practice, the isotonicity limits of an ophthalmic solution in terms of sodium chloride, or its osmotic equivalent, may range from 0.6 to 2.0% without marked discomfort to the eye. As indicated, sodium chloride does not have to be used to establish the solution's osmotic pressure. Boric acid in a concentration of 1.9% produces the same osmotic pressure as does 0.9% sodium chloride. All of the ophthalmic solution's solutes, including the active ingredients, contribute to the osmotic pressure of the solution.

The calculations involved in preparing isosmotic solutions may be made in terms of data relating to the colligative properties of solutions.[6] Like osmotic pressure, the other colligative properties of solutions, namely, vapor pressure, boiling point, and freezing point, depend upon the number of particles in solution. These properties, therefore, are related, and a change in any one of them will be accompanied by corresponding changes in the others. Although any one of these properties may be used to determine isosmoticity, a comparison of freezing points between the solutions in question, is most used.

When 1 g molecular weight of a non-electrolyte, such as boric acid, is dissolved in 1000 g of water, the freezing point of the solution is about 1.86°C below the freezing point of pure water. By simple proportion, therefore, the weight may be calculated for any non-electrolyte that should be dissolved in each 1000 g of water to prepare a solution isosmotic with lacrymal fluid and blood serum, which have freezing points of −0.52°C.

Boric acid, for example, has a molecular weight of 61.8, and thus 61.8 g in 1000 g of water should produce a freezing point of −1.86°C. Therefore:

$$\frac{1.86(°C)}{0.52(°C)} = \frac{61.8\ (g)}{\times\ (g)}$$

$$\times = 17.3\ g$$

Hence, 17.3 g of boric acid in 1000 g of water theoretically should produce a solution isosmotic with tears and blood.

The calculation employed to prepare a solution isosmotic (with tears of blood) when using electrolytes is different than when the calculation is made for a non-electrolyte. Since osmotic pressure depends upon the number of particles, substances that dissociate have an effect that increases with the degree of dissociation; the greater the dissociation, the smaller the quantity required to produce a given osmotic pressure. If we assume that sodium chloride in weak solutions is about 80% dissociated, then each 100 molecules yield 180 particles, or 1.8 times as many particles as are yielded by 100 molecules of a non-electrolyte. This dissociation factor, commonly symbolized by the letter *i*, must be included in the proportion when we seek to determine the strength of an isosmotic solution of sodium chloride (molecular weight, 58.5):

$$\frac{1.86\ (°C) \times 1.8}{0.52\ (°C)} = \frac{58.5\ (g)}{x\ (g)} x = 9.09\ g$$

Therefore, 9.09 g of sodium chloride in 1000 g of water should make a solution isosmotic with blood or lachrymal fluid. As indicated previously, a 0.90% (w/v) sodium chloride solution is taken to be isosmotic (and isotonic) with the body fluids.

Simple isosmotic solutions, then, may be calculated by this general formula:

$$\frac{0.52 \times \text{molecular weight}}{1.86 \times \text{dissociation } (i)} = \text{g of solute per 1000 g of water}$$

Although the *i* value has not been determined for every medicinal agent that might be named, the following values may be (generally) used:

Non-electrolytes and substances of slight dissociation	1.0
Substances that dissociate into 2 ions:	1.8
Substances that dissociate into 3 ions:	2.6
Substances that dissociate into 4 ions:	3.4
Substances that dissociate into 5 ions:	4.2

Since 0.9% sodium chloride solution is considered to be isosmotic (and isotonic) with lacrymal fluid, other medicinal substances are compared with regard to their "sodium chloride equivalency." An often used rule states:[6]

quantities of two substances that are tonicic equivalents are proportional to the molecular weights of each multiplied by the i value of the other.

Using the drug atropine sulfate as an example:

Molecular weight of sodium chloride = 58.5; $i = 1.8$

Molecular weight of atropine sulfate = 695; $i = 2.6$

$$\frac{695 \times 1.8}{58.5 \times 2.6} = \frac{1\ (g)}{x\ (g)}$$

$$x = 0.12 \text{ g of sodium chloride represented by 1 g of atropine sulfate}$$

Thus, the *sodium chloride equivalent* for atropine sulfate is 0.12 g. To put it one way, 1.0 g of atropine sulfate equals the "tonic effect" of 0.12 g of sodium chloride. To put it another way, atropine sulfate is 12% as effective as an equal weight of sodium chloride in contributing toward tonicity. When a combination of drugs is used in a prescription or formulation to be rendered isotonic, each agent's contribution to tonicity must be taken into consideration. For instance, consider the following prescription:

Atropine Sulfate	1%
Sodium Chloride	q.s. to isotonicity
Sterile Purified Water, ad	30.0 mL

To make the 30 mL isotonic with sodium chloride; 30 mL × 0.9% = 0.27 g or 270 mg of sodium chloride would be required. However, since 300 mg of atropine sulfate is to be present, its contribution to tonicity needs to be taken into consideration. Since the sodium chloride equivalent for atropine sulfate is 0.12, its contribution is calculated as follows:

$$0.12 \times 300 \text{ mg} = 36 \text{ mg}$$

Thus, 270 mg − 36 mg = 234 mg of sodium chloride would actually be required.

Table 11–1 presents an abbreviated list of sodium chloride equivalents. A more complete list

Table 11–1. Some Sodium Chloride Equivalents

Substance	*Molecular Weight*	*Ions*	*i*	*Sodium Chloride Equivalent*
Atropine sulfate · H_2O	695	3	2.6	0.12
Benzalkonium chloride	360	2	1.8	0.16
Benzyl alcohol	108	1	1.0	0.30
Boric Acid	61.8	1	1.0	0.52
Chlorobutanol	177	1	1.0	0.18
Cocaine hydrochloride	340	2	1.8	0.17
Ephedrine sulfate	429	3	2.6	0.20
Epinephrine bitartrate	333	2	1.8	0.18
Ethylmorphine hydrochloride · $2H_2O$	386	2	1.8	0.15
Naphazoline hydrochloride	247	2	1.8	0.27
Physostigmine salicylate	413	2	1.8	0.14
Pilocarpine hydrochloride	245	2	1.8	0.24
Procaine hydrochloride	273	2	1.8	0.21
Scopolamine hydrobromide · $3H_2O$	438	2	1.8	0.13
Tetracycline hydrochloride	481	2	1.8	0.12
Zinc sulfate · $7H_2O$	288	2	1.4	0.16

may be found in pharmaceutical calculations or physical pharmacy textbooks.

As a convenience, the USP XXI listed precalculated amounts of some common ophthalmic drugs which may be used to prepare isotonic solutions. Some of the drugs and the related values are presented in Table 11–2. The data shown are utilized in the following manner. One gram of each of the drugs listed, when added to purified water, will prepare the corresponding volume of an isotonic solution. For instance, 1 g of atropine sulfate will prepare 14.3 mL of isotonic solution. This solution may then be diluted with an isotonic vehicle to maintain the isotonicity while changing the strength of the active constituent in the solution to any desired level. For instance, if a 1% isotonic solution of atropine sulfate is desired, the 14.3 mL of isotonic solution containing 1 g of atropine sulfate should be diluted to 100 mL (1 g atropine sulfate in 100 mL = 1% w/v solution) with an isotonic vehicle. By utilizing sterile drug, sterile purified water, a sterile isotonic vehicle, and aseptic techniques, a sterile product may be prepared. In addition to being sterile and isotonic, the diluting vehicles generally used are also buffered and contain suitable preservative to maintain the stability and sterility of the product.

Table 11–2. Isotonic Solutions Prepared from Common Ophthalmic Drugs*

Drug (1.0 g)	*Volume of Isotonic Solution Yielded (mL)*
Atropine Sulfate	14.3
Boric Acid	55.7
Chlorobutanol (hydrous)	26.7
Cocaine Hydrochloride	17.7
Colistimethate Sodium	16.7
Dibucaine Hydrochloride	14.3
Ephedrine Sulfate	25.7
Epinephrine Bitartrate	20.0
Eucatropine Hydrochloride	20.0
Fluorescein Sodium	34.3
Homatropine Hydrobromide	19.0
Neomycin Sulfate	12.3
Penicillin G Potassium	20.0
Phenylephrine Hydrochloride	35.7
Physostigmine Salicylate	17.7
Physostigmine Sulfate	14.3
Pilocarpine Hydrochloride	26.7
Pilocarpine Nitrate	25.7
Polymyxin B Sulfate	10.0
Procaine Hydrochloride	23.3
Proparacaine Hydrochloride	16.7
Scopolamine Hydrobromide	13.3
Silver Nitrate	36.7
Sodium Bicarbonate	72.3
Sodium Biphosphate	44.3
Sodium Borate	46.7
Sodium Phosphate (dibasic, heptahydrate)	32.3
Streptomycin Sulfate	7.7
Sulfacetamide Sodium	25.7
Sulfadiazine Sodium	26.7
Tetracaine Hydrochloride	20.0
Tetracycline Hydrochloride	15.7
Zinc Sulfate	16.7

* Adapted from USP XXI, p. 1339.

Buffering

Buffers may be used in an ophthalmic solution for one or all of the following reasons: (1) to reduce discomfort to the patient, (2) to ensure drug stability, and (3) to control the therapeutic activity of the drug substance.

Normal tears, having a pH (see accompanying Physical Pharmacy Capsule) of about 7.4, possess some buffer capacity. The introduction of a medicated solution into the eye stimulates the flow of tears, which attempts to neutralize any excess hydrogen or hydroxyl ions introduced with the solution. Most drugs used ophthalmically, such as alkaloidal salts, are weakly acidic and have only weak buffer capacity. Normally, the buffering action of the tears is capable of neutralizing the ophthalmic solution and is thereby able to prevent marked discomfort. However, a few drugs—notably pilocarpine hydrochloride and epinephrine bitartrate—are quite acid and overtax the buffer capacity of the lacrimal fluid. For maximum comfort, an ophthalmic solution should have the same pH as the lacrimal fluid. However, this is not pharmaceutically possible, since at pH 7.4, many drugs are insoluble in water. Alkaloidal salts, for instance, are likely to precipitate as the free alkaloidal base at pH 7.4.

Most drugs, including many used in ophthalmic solutions, are most active therapeutically at pH levels which favor the undissociated molecule. However, the pH that permits greatest activity may also be the pH at which the drug is least stable. For this reason, a compromise pH is generally selected for a solution and maintained by buffers to permit the greatest activity while maintaining stability. The buffer system of an ophthalmic solution contributes to stability in another way by preventing an increase in the pH

pH and Solubility

pH is one of the most important factors involved in the formulation process. Two areas of critical importance are the effects of pH on solubility and stability. The effect of pH on solubility is critical in the formulation of liquid dosage forms, from oral and topical solutions to intravenous solutions and admixtures.

The solubility of a weak acid or base is often pH dependent. The total quantity of a monoprotic weak acid (HA) in solution at a specific pH is the sum of the concentrations of both the free acid and salt (A^-) forms. If excess drug is present, the quantity of free acid in solution is maximized and constant due to its saturation solubility. As the pH of the solution is increased, the quantity of drug in solution increases because the water-soluble ionizable salt is formed. The expression is:

$$HA \overset{K_a}{\longleftrightarrow} H^+ + A^-$$

where K_a is the dissociation constant.

There may be a certain pH level reached where the total solubility (S_T) of the drug solution is saturated with respect to both the salt and acid forms of the drug, i.e., the pH_{max}. The solution can be saturated with respect to the salt at pH values higher than this, but not with respect to the acid. Also, at pH values less than this, the solution can be saturated with respect to the acid, but not to the salt. This is illustrated in the accompanying figure.

To calculate the total quantity of drug that can be maintained in solution at a selected pH, two different equations can be used, depending upon whether the product is to be in a pH region above or below the pH_{max}. The following equation is used when below the pH_{max}:

$$S_T = S_a\left(1 + \frac{K_a}{[H^+]}\right) \qquad \text{(Equation 1)}$$

The next equation is used when above the pH_{max}:

$$S_T = S_a'\left(1 + \frac{[H^+]}{K_a}\right) \qquad \text{(Equation 2)}$$

where S_a is the saturation solubility of the free acid, and
S_a' is the saturation solubility of the salt form.

EXAMPLE

A pharmacist prepares a 3.0% solution of an antibiotic as an ophthalmic solution and dispenses it to a patient. A few days later the patient returns the eye drops to the pharmacist because the product contains a precipitate. The pharmacist, checking the pH of the solution and finding it to be 6.0, reasons that the problem might be pH-related. The physicochemical information of interest on the antibiotic includes the following:

Molecular weight	285 (salt) 263 (free acid)
3.0% solution of the drug is a	0.1053 molar solution
Acid form solubility (S_a)	3.1 mg/mL (0.0118 molar)
K_a	5.86×10^{-6}

Using Equation 1, the pharmacist calculates the quantity of the antibiotic that would be in solution at a pH of 6.0 (Note: pH of 6.0 = $[H^+]$ of 1×10^{-6})

$$S_T = 0.0118\left(1 + \frac{5.86 \times 10^{-6}}{1 \times 10^{-6}}\right) = 0.0809 \text{ molar}$$

From this the pharmacist knows that, at a pH of 6.0, a 0.0809 molar solution could be prepared. However, the concentration that was to be prepared was a 0.1053 molar solution; consequently, the drug will not be in solution at that pH. What may have occurred was the pH was all right initially but shifted to a lower pH after a period of time, resulting in precipitation of the drug. The question is then asked, At what pH (hydrogen ion concentration) will the drug remain in solution? This can be calculated using the same equation and the information that is available. The S_T value is 0.1053 molar.

pH and Solubility (Continued)

$$0.1053 = 0.0118\left(1 + \frac{5.86 \times 10^{-6}}{[H^+]}\right)$$

$$[H^+] = 7.333 \times 10^{-7}, \text{ or a pH of } 6.135$$

The pharmacist then prepares a solution of the antibiotic, adjusting the pH to greater than about 6.2 using a suitable buffer system, and dispenses the solution to the patient—with positive results.

An interesting phenomenon can be discussed briefly concerning the close relationship of pH to solubility. At a pH of 6.0, only a 0.0809 molar solution could be prepared, but at a pH of 6.13 a 0.1053 molar solution could be prepared. In other words, a difference of 0.13 pH units resulted in:

$$\frac{0.1053 - 0.0809}{0.0809} = \begin{array}{l}\text{30.1\% more drug going into solution at}\\ \text{the higher pH compared to the lower pH}\end{array}$$

In other words, a very small change in pH resulted in about 30% more drug going into solution. According to the figure, the slope of the curve would be very steep for this example drug and a small change in pH (x-axis) results in a large change in solubility (y-axis). From this, it can be reasoned that if one observes the pH: solubility profile of a drug, it is possible to predict the magnitude of the pH change on its solubility.

In recent years, it has been interesting to note that more and more physicochemical information on drugs is being made available to pharmacists in routinely used reference books. This type of information is important for pharmacists in different types of practice, especially those involved in compounding and pharmacokinetic monitoring.

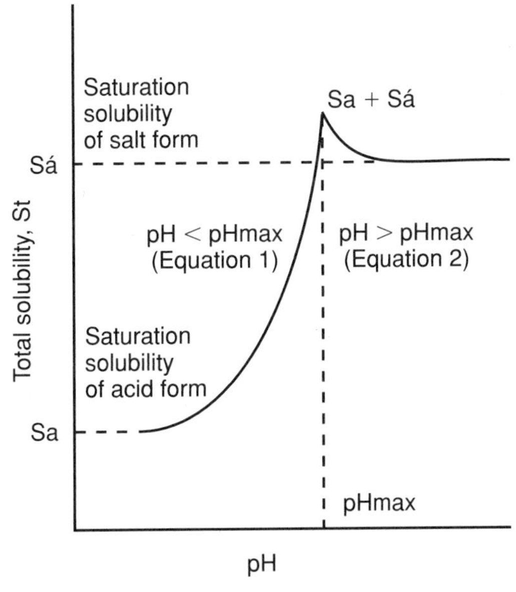

Table 11–3. Isotonic Phosphate Vehicle

Monobasic Sodium Phosphate Solution, mL	*Dibasic Sodium Phosphate Solution, mL*	*Resulting Buffer Solution, pH*	*Sodium Chloride Required for Isotonicity, g/100 mL*
90	10	5.9	0.52
80	20	6.2	0.51
70	30	6.5	0.50
60	40	6.6	0.49
50	50	6.8	0.48
40	60	7.0	0.46
30	70	7.2	0.45
20	80	7.4	0.44
10	90	7.7	0.43
5	95	8.0	0.42

of the solution due to the normal leaching by the solution of alkali from the glass container.

An isotonic phosphate vehicle, prepared at the desired pH (shown in Table 11–3) and adjusted for tonicity, may be employed in the extemporaneous compounding of solutions. The desired solution is prepared through the use of two stock solutions, one containing 8.00 g of monobasic sodium phosphate (NaH_2PO_4) per liter, and the other containing 9.47 g of dibasic sodium phosphate (Na_2HPO_4) per liter, the weights being on an anhydrous basis. The stock solutions are utilized in proportions indicated in Table 11–3.

The vehicles listed in Table 11–3 are satisfactory for many ophthalmic drugs with the exception of pilocarpine, eucatropine, scopolamine and homatropine salts which show instability in the vehicle. The vehicle is used effectively as the diluent for ophthalmic drugs already in isotonic solution, as those prepared according to the method presented in Table 11–2. When drug substances are added directly to the isotonic phosphate vehicle, the solution becomes slightly hypertonic. Generally, this provides no discomfort to the patient. However, if such a solution is not desired, the appropriate adjustment can be made through calculated dilution of the vehicle with purified water.

Viscosity and Thickening Agents

Viscosity is a property of liquids that is closely related to the resistance to flow. The reciprocal of viscosity is *fluidity*. Viscosity is defined in terms of the force required to move one plane surface past another under specified conditions when the space between is filled by the liquid in question. More simply, it can be considered as a relative property with water as the reference material and all viscosities expressed in terms of the viscosity of pure water at 20°C. The viscosity of water is given as one centipoise (actually 1.0087 centipoise). A liquid material ten times as viscous as water at the same temperature has a viscosity of 10 centipoises. The centipoise, abbreviated cp. (*cps.* plural), is a more convenient term than the basic unit, the poise; one poise is equal to 100 centipoises.

Specifying the temperature is important because viscosity changes with temperature; generally, the viscosity of a liquid decreases with increasing temperature. The determination of viscosity in terms of poise or centipoise results in the calculation of *absolute* viscosity. It is sometimes more convenient to use the kinematic scale in which the units of viscosity are *stokes* and *centistokes* (1 stoke equals 100 centistokes). The kinematic viscosity is obtained from the absolute viscosity by dividing the latter by the density of the liquid at the same temperature:

$$\text{kinematic viscosity} = \frac{\text{absolute viscosity}}{\text{density}}$$

Using water as the standard, examples of some viscosities at 20°C are:

Ethyl alcohol	—	1.19	cps
Olive oil	—	100	cps
Glycerin	—	400	cps
Castor oil	—	1000	cps

Viscosity can be determined by any method that will measure the resistance to shear offered by the liquid. For ordinary liquids, it is customary to determine the time required for a given sample of the liquid to flow at a regulated temperature through a small vertical capillary tube and to compare this time with that required to perform the same task by the reference liquid. Many capillary tube viscosimeters have been devised, and nearly all are modifications of the Ostwald type. With an apparatus such as this, the viscosity of a liquid may be determined by the following equation:

$$\frac{\eta_1}{\eta_2} = \frac{\rho_1 t_1}{\rho_2 t_2}$$

where η_1 is the unknown viscosity of the liquid, η_2 is the viscosity of the standard, ρ_1 and ρ_2 are the respective densities of the liquids, and t_1 and t_2 are the respective flow times in seconds.

In the preparation of ophthalmic solutions, a suitable grade of methylcellulose or other thickening agent is frequently added to increase the viscosity and thereby aid in holding the drug in contact with the tissues so as to enhance the therapeutic effectiveness. Generally, methylcellulose of the 4000 cps viscosity type is used in concentrations of 0.25% and the 25 cps type at 1% concentration. Hydroxypropyl methylcellulose and polyvinyl alcohol are also used as thickeners in ophthalmic solutions. Occasionally a 1% solution of methylcellulose without medication is used as a tear replacement. Viscosity for ophthalmic solutions is considered optimal in the range of 15 to 25 cps.

Ocular Bioavailability[1]

As noted previously, the bioavailability of drugs administered to the eye is an important consideration. There are physiologic factors which can affect a drug's ocular bioavailability, including protein binding, drug metabolism, and lacrimal drainage. Protein-bound drugs are incapable of penetrating the corneal epithelium due to the size of the protein-drug complex.[1] Because of the brief time in which an ophthalmic solution may remain present in the eye (due to lacrimal drainage) the protein binding of a drug substance could quickly negate its therapeutic value by rendering it unavailable for absorption. Normally, tears contain between 0.6 and 2.0% of protein content, but disease states (as uvetis) can raise these protein levels.[1]

As in the case with other biological fluids, tears contain enzymes (such as lysozyme) capable of the metabolic degradation of drug substances. However, the full extent to which drug metabolism occurs in the precorneal area is uncertain at this time.

In addition to physiologic factors affecting ocular bioavailability, other factors, as the physicochemical characteristics of the drug substance, and product formulation are important. Because the cornea is a membrane barrier containing both lipophilic and hydrophilic layers, it is permeated most effectively by drug substances having both lipophilic and hydrophilic characteristics.[1] Drugs which can exist in both the ionized state, as the weak bases pilocarpine, atropine, tetracaine, and others, permeate the membrane best. It is advantageous for corneal permeation to adjust the pH of the solution to increase the proportion of unionized drug in the instilled dose. As discussed in Chapter 3, weak bases become more unionized at pHs greater than their pKa, and, weak acids become more ionized at pHs less than their pKa. Drugs which are highly water-soluble do not readily permeate the cornea.

Suspensions of drugs and ophthalmic ointments mix with lacrimal fluids less readily than do solutions, and thus, remain in the cul-de-sac for longer periods of time, enhancing the bioavailability of the drug substance. Ophthalmic solutions of increased viscosity also remain in the cul-de-sac longer than solutions with lower viscosity.

Ophthalmic Suspensions

Ophthalmic suspensions are employed to a lesser extent than are ophthalmic solutions, however, as noted previously, suspensions may be used to increase the corneal contact time of a drug substance and thus provide a more sustained action. Ophthalmic suspensions may be required when the medicinal agent is insoluble in the desired vehicle or unstable in solution form.

Ophthalmic suspensions must possess the same characteristic of sterility as ophthalmic solutions, with proper consideration given also to preservation, isotonicity, buffering, viscosity and packaging. Additionally, ophthalmic suspensions must contain particles of such chemical characteristics and small dimensions that they are non-irritating to the eyes. The ophthalmic suspension must also be of such a quality that the suspended particles do not agglomerate into larger ones upon storage. The suspension must be shaken prior to use and the particles distributed uniformly throughout the vehicle.

Examples of ophthalmic solutions and suspensions are presented in Table 11–4.

Packaging and Use of Ophthalmic Solutions and Suspensions

Ophthalmic solutions and suspensions should be packaged so that they are easily administered and their sterility maintained. Usually they,

Table 11–4. Examples of Some Ophthalmic Agents by Category

Ophthalmic Agent	*Corresponding Commercial Product*	*Concentration of Active Ingredient*	*Comments*
Adrenergic			
Naphazoline HCl	Naphcon-A Ophthalmic Solution (Alcon)	0.025%	Used as a topical ocular vasoconstrictor.
Antiallergic			
Cromolyn Sodium	Opticrom Ophthalmic Solution (Fisons)	4%	For treatment of allergic ocular disorders as vernal conjunctivitis.
Antibacterial			
Chloramphenicol	Ophthochlor Ophthalmic Solution (Parke-Davis)	0.5%	Used for superficial infections of the eye due to susceptible microorganisms.
Ciprofloxacin Hydrochloride	Ciloxan Sterile Ophthalmic Solution (Alcon)	0.35%	
Gentamicin Sulfate	Garamycin Ophthalmic Solution (Schering)	0.3%	
Tetracycline Hydrochloride	Achromycin Ophthalmic Suspension (Lederle)	1%	
Tobramycin	Tobrex Ophthalmic Solution (Alcon)]	0.3%	
Sulfacetamide Sodium	Sodium Sulamyd Ophthalmic Solution (Schering)	10 and 30%	
Antiviral			
Trifluridine	Viroptic Ophthalmic Solution (Burroughs Wellcome)	1%	Indicated in the treatment of herpes simplex keratitis.
Artificial Tears			
Dextran 70, Hydroxypropyl Methylcellulose	Tears Naturale II (Alcon)	. . .	For relief of dry eyes.
Astringent			
Zinc Sulfate	Zincfrin Ophthalmic Solution (Alcon)	0.25%	Used for relief of discomfort and congestion caused by minor irritations to the eyes, such as dust, fatigue, and allergies.
Anti-inflammatory			
Dexamethasone Sodium Phosphate	Decadron Phosphate Sterile Ophthalmic Solution (Merck Sharp & Dohme)	0.1%	Combats inflammation due to mechanical, chemical, or immunologic causes.

Table 11–4. Continued

Ophthalmic Agent	*Corresponding Commercial Product*	*Concentration of Active Ingredient*	*Comments*
Antibacterial/Antiinflammatory Combinations			
Neomycin Sulfate and Dexamethasone Sodium Phosphate	NeoDecadron Ophthalmic Solution (Merck Sharp & Dohme)	0.35% neomycin base equivalent and 0.1% dexamethasone	For steroid-responsive inflammatory ocular conditions where bacterial infection or a risk of bacterial ocular infection exists.
Oxytetracycline and Hydrocortisone Acetate	Terra-Cortril Ophthalmic Suspension (Roerig)	0.5% oxytetracycline equivalent and 1.5% hydrocortisone acetate	
Tobramycin and Dexamethasone	TobraDex Sterile Ophthalmic Suspension (Alcon)]	0.3% tobramycin and 0.1% dexamethasone	
Beta-Adrenergic Blocking Agents			
Betaxolol HCl	Betoptic Sterile Ophthalmic Solution (Alcon)	0.5%	Used for ocular hypertension and chronic open-angle glaucoma.
Timolol Maleate	Timoptic Sterile Ophthalmic Solution (Merck, Sharpe & Dohme)	0.25%, 0.5%	Used in patients with chronic open-angle glaucoma and aphakic patients with glaucoma.
Cholinergic			
Pilocarpine HCl Ophthalmic Solution	Isopto Carpine Ophthalmic Solution (Alcon)	0.25 to 10%	Used as a miotic in treating glaucoma, especially open-angle glaucoma. Also used to neutralize mydriasis following ophthalmoscopy or surgery.
Cholinesterase Inhibitor			
Demecarium Bromide	Humorsol Sterile Ophthalmic Solution (Merck & Co.)	0.125% and 0.25%	Produces intense miosis and ciliary muscle contractions due to inhibition of cholinesterase. Used in open-angle glaucoma when shorter-acting miotics have proved inadequate.

being administered by drop, are packaged in glass or plastic containers with a dropper service. Some plastic packages contain a fixed, built-in dropper that releases the medication when held in the inverted position (Fig. 11–3). The patient must exercise care in protecting the ophthalmic preparation from contamination. Obviously the ophthalmic solution packaged with the fixed dropper is less likely to acquire airborne contaminants than the screw-type bottle which must be opened and the dropper removed when using. However, each type is subject to contamination during use, brought about by the touching of the tip of the dropper to the tissues or to airborne contaminants.

When selecting the packaging material it must be determined that the container does not interfere with the stability or efficacy of the preparation. Ophthalmic solutions used as eye washes are generally copackaged with an eye cup which should be cleaned and dried thoroughly after and prior to each use.

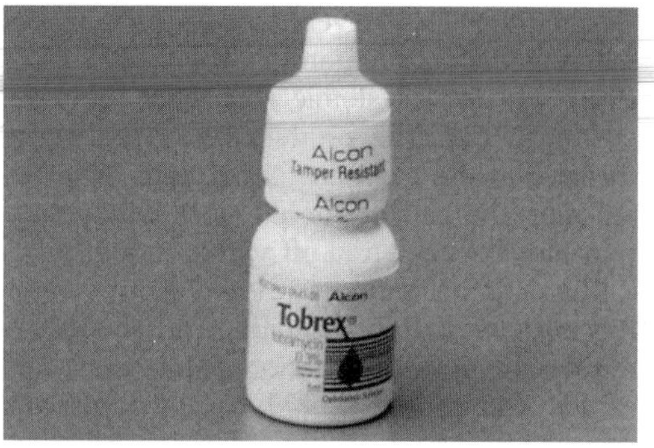

Fig. 11–3. *Commercial package of an ophthalmic solution in plastic container with built-in dropper device. (Courtesy of Alcon.)*

The major types of drugs used ophthalmically are as follows:

Anti-inflammatory Agents: These agents combat inflammation of the eye, such as allergic conjunctivitis. Most prominent among those employed topically are hydrocortisone, prednisolone, and dexamethasone salts.

Antibiotic/Antimicrobial Agents: Antibiotic/antimicrobial agents are used specifically to combat infection of the eye. They are frequently employed both systemically and locally for their effect. Among those applied topically to the eye are gentamicin, sulfacetamide, tetracycline, chloromycetin, ciprofloxacin, erythromycin, polymyxin B sulfate-bacitracin, zinc-neomycin sulfate, terramycin, and tobramycin.

Antiviral Agents: For viral infections, as due to herpes simplex virus, preparations of trifluridine, or vidarabine are employed.

Astringents: These agents are generally used in the treatment of conjunctivitis. Most preparations for this purpose utilize zinc compounds, particularly zinc sulfate, as the astringent.

Beta-Adrenergic Blocking Agents: These are indicated for treatment of intraocular pressure and chronic open-angle glaucoma. Typical preparations include betaxolol HCl, or timolol maleate.

Local Anesthetics: Local anesthetics allow for the relief of pain preoperatively, postoperatively, following trauma, and during ophthalmic examination. Among the local anesthetics used ophthalmically are benoxinate, proparacaine, and cocaine.

Miotics: Miotics are used primarily in the therapy of glaucoma but have been utilized in other conditions as accommodative esotropia, convergent strabismus, and for the local treatment of myasthenia gravis. Many miotics may be absorbed systemically after instillation into the eye and may produce undesirable effects in some patients. Miotics reduce intraocular pressure associated with glaucoma. Among the miotics are pilocarpine, echothiophate iodide, and demecarium bromide. In addition to the miotics, several other types of agents are employed in the treatment of glaucoma, including: carbonic anhydrase inhibitors, as acetazolamide (oral), and betaadrenergic agents, as betaxolol.

Mydriatics and Cycloplegics: Mydriatics allow examination of the fundus through the dilation of the pupil. The stronger mydriatics having a long duration of action are called *cycloplegics.* Among the mydriatics and cycloplegics are atropine, scopolamine, homatropine, cyclopentolate, naphazoline, cocaine, and phenylephrine.

Topical Protectants: These solutions are employed as artificial tears or as a contact lens fluid. Examples of agents used in these solutions are methylcellulose and hydroxypropyl methylcellulose.

Vasoconstrictors: These are intended to soothe, refresh and remove redness due to minor eye irritation. Among these are naphazoline HCl, oxymetazoline HCl, and tetrahydrozoline HCl.

Proper Administration and Use of Eye Drops

Prior to the administration of an ophthalmic solution or suspension, the patient should be advised to wash his/her hands thoroughly with soap and water. If the drops are supplied with a dropper, the patient should inspect the dropper to make sure there are no chips or cracks at the end of it. If the drops are a cloudy suspension, the patient should be told to shake them for about 10 seconds.

The patient should position himself/herself either lying down or tilting the head back. The index finger of one hand should be used to gently pull downward the affected eye to form a pocket or cup. Without touching the dropper to the eye, the prescribed number of drops are then gently placed into the formed pocket. The patient should understand that if the drops are placed directly onto the eyeball (cornea), they may cause a stinging sensation. Once the drops have been instilled, the dropper should be returned to its original container and capped tightly. The dropper should not be rinsed or wiped off.

To allow the drops to remain in the eye and enhance efficacy, the patient should press his/her finger against the inner corner of the eye for 1 minute. This prevents the medication from entering the teardùct and in the case of some drugs prevents systemic absorption from occurring if the drug product passes down the throat into the gastrointestinal tract. After instillation the patient should close the eye and wipe any excess liquid off with a tissue.

The patient should be advised about the correct number of drops to instill, the frequency of application and the duration of treatment necessary. The patient should also be advised to appropriately store the medicine, including out of the reach of children.

Ophthalmic Ointments

Ophthalmic ointments, in contrast to the dermatological ointments discussed in the previous chapter, must be sterile. They are either manufactured from sterilized ingredients and under rigid aseptic conditions, or they are sterilized following manufacture.

The ointment base selected for an ophthalmic ointment must be non-irritating to the eye and must permit the diffusion of the medicinal substance throughout the secretions bathing the eye. Ointment bases utilized for ophthalmics have a melting or softening point close to body temperature. In most instances, mixtures of petrolatum and liquid petrolatum (mineral oil) are utilized as the ointment base. Sometimes a water-miscible agent as lanolin is added. This permits water and water-insoluble drugs to be retained within the delivery system.

The medicinal agent is added to the ointment base either as a solution or as a finely micronized powder. The drug is then intimately mixed with the base, usually by milling.

After preparation the ophthalmic ointments are filled into previously sterilized tin or plastic ophthalmic tubes. These tubes are typically small, holding approximately 3.5 g of ointment and fitted with narrow gauge tips which permit the extrusion of narrow bands of ointment (Fig. 11–4). This is convenient for placement of the ointment onto the margin of the eyelid, the usual site of application. This should be done without touching the applicator tip to the eye.

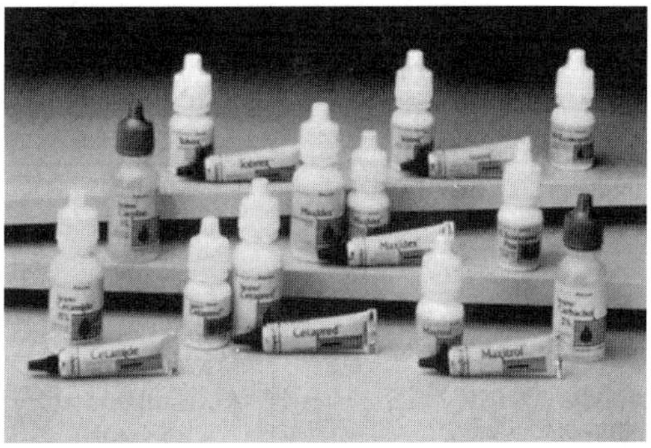

Fig. 11–4. *Examples of ophthalmic product packaging. Liquids are in 5-mL and 15-mL Drop-Tainer dispensers and ointments are in tubes containing 3.5 g of product. (Courtesy of Alcon.)*

The primary advantage of an ophthalmic ointment over an ophthalmic solution is the increased ocular contact time of the drug. Studies have shown that the ocular contact time is two to four times greater when ointments are used than when a saline solution is used.[7] One disadvantage to ophthalmic ointment use is the blurred vision which occurs as the ointment base melts and is spread across the lens.

Examples of ophthalmic ointments are presented in Table 11–5.

Proper Administration of Ophthalmic Ointments

Prior to administration the patient should be advised to wash the hands thoroughly with soap and water. The ointment tube should be held between the thumb and the forefinger and the tube placed as near as possible to the eyelid, without touching it. The patient then tilts the head back, and with the index finger of the opposite hand, the lower lid should be gently pulled downward to form a pocket or cup. A ribbon of medication is then placed into the lower lid. To make this procedure easier, a patient may use a mirror or simply have another person administer the ointment. The patient should then blink gently and with a tissue wipe off any excess ointment from the eyelids and lashes. Lastly, the cap should be replaced onto the ointment tube.

The patient should be advised that when the ointment is instilled into the eye, blurred vision

Table 11–5. Examples of Ophthalmic Ointments

Ophthalmic Ointment	*Corresponding Commercial Product*	*Concentration of Active Ingredient*	*Category*
Chloramphenicol Ophthalmic Ointment	Chloromycetin Ophthalmic Ointment (Parke Davis)	1%	Antibacterial
Dexamethasone Sodium Phosphate Ophthalmic Ointment	Decadron Phosphate Ophthalmic Ointment (Merck Sharp & Dohme)	0.05%	Anti-inflammatory adrenocortical steroid
Gentamicin Sulfate Ophthalmic Ointment	Garamycin Ophthalmic Ointment (Schering)	0.3%	Antibacterial
Isoflurophate Ophthalmic Ointment	Floropryl Sterile Ophthalmic Ointment (Merck)	0.025 isoflurophate	Cholinesterase inhibitor
Neomycin Sulfate and Dexamethasone Sodium Phosphate Ophthalmic Ointment	NeoDecadron Ophthalmic Ointment (Merck)	0.35% neomycin base and 0.05% dexamethasone phosphate equivalents	Antibacterial/ antiinflammatory
Polymyxin B—Bacitracin Ophthalmic Ointment	Polysporin Ophthalmic Ointment (Burroughs Wellcome)	polymyxin B sulfate, 10,000 units and bacitracin zinc, 500 units per g	Antimicrobial
Polymyxin B—Bacitracin—Neomycin Ophthalmic Ointment	Neosporin Ophthalmic Ointment (Burroughs Wellcome)	per g: polymyxin B sulfate, 5000 units; bacitracin, zinc, 400 units; neomycin sulfate, 5 mg	Antimicrobial
Sulfacetamide Sodium Ophthalmic Ointment	Sodium Sulamyd Ophthalmic Ointment (Schering)	10 and 30%	Antibacterial
Sulfisoxazole Diolamine Ophthalmic Ointment	Gantrisin Ophthalmic Ointment (Roche)	4%	Antibacterial
Tetracycline HCl Ophthalmic Ointment	Achromycin Ophthalmic Ointment (Lederle)	1%	Antibacterial
Tobramycin Ophthalmic Ointment	Tobrex Ophthalmic Ointment (Alcon)	0.3%	Antibacterial
Vidarabine Ophthalmic Ointment	Vira-A-Ophthalmic Ointment (Parke Davis)	3%	Antiviral

will occur and not to be alarmed. If the ointment is to be administered one time per day, it is preferable to do so at bedtime where vision impairment will be inconsequential. The patient should be advised about the frequency of application and the length of time the regimen is to be followed. Lastly, it is important to emphasize that the ointment must be kept clean and every effort should be made to avoid touching the tip of the tube against the eye or anything else.

Ophthalmic Inserts

An innovative development in the delivery of medication to the eyes has been that of ophthalmic inserts. One such device, the OCUSERT system (Alza) is shown in Figure 11–5. The insert unit is designed to provide for the release of medication at predetermined and predictable rates permitting the elimination of frequent dosing by the patient, ensuring nighttime medication, and providing a better means of patient compliance.

The insert is elliptical with dimensions of 13.4 by 5.7 mm and 0.3 mm in thickness. The insert is flexible and is a multilayered structure consisting of a drug-containing core surrounded on each side by a layer of copolymer membranes through which the drug diffuses at a constant rate (Fig. 11–6). The rate of drug diffusion is controlled by the polymer composition, the membrane thickness, and the solubility of the drug. The devices are sterile and do not contain preservatives.

Inserts containing pilocarpine are widely used in glaucoma therapy. After placement in the conjunctival sac, the inserts are designed to release medication at the desired rates over a 7-day period at which time they are removed and replaced with new ones.

Another example of an ophthalmic insert is Lacrisert (Merck), a sterile, translucent, rod-

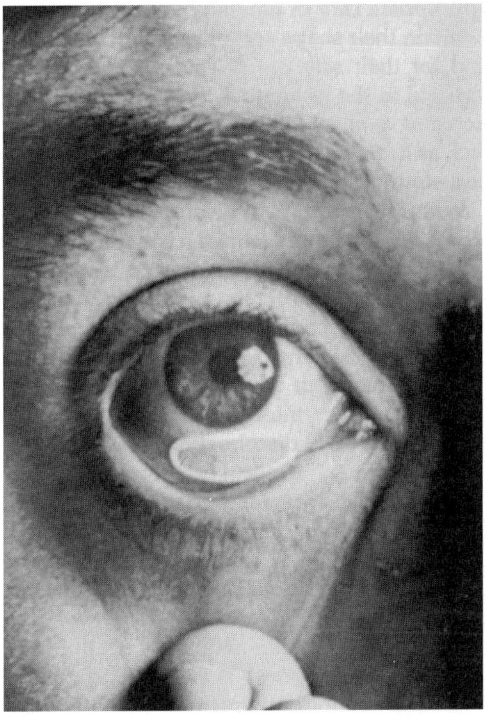

Fig. 11–5. *Ocusert Ocular Therapeutic Systems are thin, flexible wafers placed under the eyelid to provide a week's dosage of pilocarpine in the treatment of glaucoma. Ocusert systems cause less blurring of vision than pilocarpine eyedrops, which must be used 4 times daily. (Courtesy of Alza Corporation.)*

shaped, water-soluble form of hydroxypropyl cellulose. The product is inserted into the inferior cul-de-sac of the eye of patients with dry eye states. The insert acts to stabilize and thicken the precorneal tear film and to delay its breakup. Use of the insert once or twice daily is recommended. Following administration, the inserts soften and slowly dissolve.

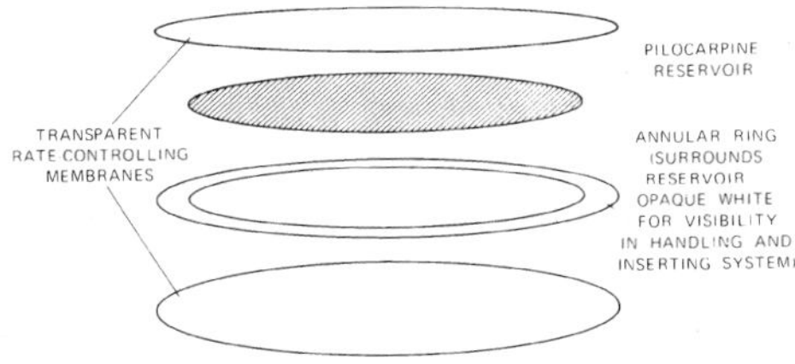

Fig. 11–6. *Construction of the Ocusert Ocular Therapeutic System containing pilocarpine between transparent rate-controlling membranes. (Courtesy of Alza Corporation.)*

Contact Lens Solutions

The number of persons wearing contact lenses grows each year. Their popularity and increased use has fostered the development of new types of lenses and lens care products. In the last decade, many different kinds of soft, hard and rigid gas permeable (RGP) lenses have been tested and marketed. Coupled with this growth has been the emergence of such products as contact lens cleaners and disinfectants.

For the pharmacist it is a responsibility to keep current and know the details of lens cleaning, disinfection, neutralization, rinsing and storage of all lenses. In addition, pharmacists must be knowledgeable about lens lubricating drops and up-to-date about the compatibilities and incompatibilities among all the products that a contact lens wearer might use.[8–10]

The pharmacologic effect of a drug administered topically to the eye may be affected by the presence of contact lenses. For example, soft contact lenses have been shown to be capable of absorbing some topically administered drugs, thereby affecting the drugs' bioavailability.[9] Also, some ophthalmic suspensions may build up between the eye-lens interface, causing undesired effects and discomfort. Some drugs, administered by various routes of administration for systemic effects, may find their way to the lacrimal fluid and produce drug-contact lens interactions such as lens discoloration (e.g., orange staining by rifampin), lens clouding (ribavirin), ocular inflammation (salicylates), refractive changes (acetazolamide), and other effects.[9]

The three basic types of contact lenses are classified by their chemical composition and physical properties, e.g., soft, hard, and rigid gas permeable (RGP).

Hard contact lenses provide durability and clear, crisp vision for the patient. These lenses are termed hard because they are made of a rigid plastic resin, polymethylmethacrylate (PMMA), and as a consequence many people have found them extremely uncomfortable to wear and tolerate. PMMA lenses are practically impermeable to oxygen and moisture (these absorb only about 0.5% water), a disadvantage to corneal epithelial respiration and to patient comfort. Care must be exercised to prevent the hard lens from resting directly on the corneal surface to protect the epithelial tissue from physical damage. To prevent such direct contact, solutions are used that wet the surface of the lens to provide a cushioning layer between the corneal epithelium and the inner surface of the lens.

Soft contact lenses were introduced in 1971 and have become extremely popular in comparison to hard lenses because they are much more comfortable. Soft lenses are made of a hydrophilic transparent plastic, hydroxyethylmethacrylate (HEMA) that contains between 30 and 80% water. This increased water content of the lens improves its permeability to oxygen. There are two types of soft contact lens: daily-wear and extended-wear. As each name suggests, daily-wear lenses must be removed at night before the wearer goes to sleep, whereas the extended-wear lenses are designed to be worn for more than 24 hours. Some of these lenses have been approved for up to 30 days of continuous wear, however, it is advised that a person not leave them in the eye for longer than 4 to 7 days at one time without removal for cleaning and disinfection. Long use without cleaning and disinfection can predispose the wearer to a serious eye infection.

Disposable soft lenses are now available and these do pose an advance for patients. Specifically, disposable lenses do not necessitate lens cleaning and disinfection after a week's wear. These are simply discarded and replaced with a new pair. The problem, however, is that the wearer may be tempted to wear these for longer than suggested with the distinct possibility that a serious eye infection may result. The success of disposable soft lenses will be coupled to a patient's ability to incur the higher cost to use them.

Rigid gas permeable (RGP) contact lenses take advantage of features of the soft and the hard contact lenses. These lenses are constructed of material that is oxygen-permeable but hydrophobic. Thus, they permit the transmission of oxygen through the lens more so than hard lenses, while still providing the durability and ease of handling that hard lenses provide. These lenses have the greater wearing comfort of the soft lenses and usually are intended for daily wear. Some of the newer "super-permeable" RGP lenses are for extended wear.

There are advantages and disadvantages associated with each type of contact lens. Hard contact lenses and RGP lenses provide strength and durability and relatively easy care regimens. These are easy to handle during insertion and removal. Further these are relatively resistant to the absorption of disinfectants, surfactant cleansers, and environmental contaminants. These lenses provide visual acuity superior to soft contact lenses, which is very important to some individuals. On the opposite side of the coin, hard contact lenses and RGP lenses require an adjustment period and may become dislodged or migrate in the eye.

Soft contact lenses are advantageous to wear for longer periods of time, and usually there is little adaptation time associated with them. These lenses make visual adjustment easier for the wearer when it is necessary to switch from contact lenses to eyeglasses. Lastly, soft lenses do not dislodge as easily nor fall out of the eye as readily as the hard contact lenses. Unfortunately, soft contact lenses provide a slight reduction in quality of vision and have a shorter life span. Furthermore, the wearer must ensure that the lenses not dry out because they are extremely fragile.

Color Additives to Contact Lenses

Contact lens manufacturers may produce clear as well as colored lenses. The use of color additives in medical devices, including contact lenses, is regulated by the federal Food and Drug Administration through authority granted by the Medical Device Amendments of 1976. Color additives that come into direct contact with the body for a significant period of time must be demonstrated to be safe for consumer use. This includes colored contact lenses. The FDA permits the use of a specific color additive in contact lenses only after reviewing and approving a manufacturer's official *Color Additive Petition.* The petition must contain the requisite chemical, safety, manufacturing, packaging, and product labeling information for FDA review. Many colored contact lenses are prepared as a reaction product, formed by chemically bonding a dye [e.g. Color Index (C.I.) Reactive Red 180 (Ciba Vision)] to the vinyl alcohol/methyl methacrylate copolymeric lens material.

Care of Contact Lenses

It is important that all contact lenses receive appropriate care in handling and maintenance to retain their shape and optical characteristics, and for their safe use. Wearers should be instructed in the techniques for the proper insertion and removal of the lenses from the eye, as well as in the methods for cleaning, sterilizing, and storing the lenses.

With the exception of disposable soft contact lenses, all soft lenses require a routine care program that includes (1) cleaning to loosen and remove lipid and protein deposits, (2) rinsing to remove the cleaning solution and material loosened by cleaning, and (3) disinfection to kill microorganisms. If these lenses are not maintained at proper intervals, they are prone to deposit build-up, discoloration, and microbial contamination. The moist, porous surface of the hydrophilic lens provides a perfect medium for the growth of bacteria, fungi, and viruses. Thus, disinfection is essential to prevent eye infections and microbial damage to the lens material.

Hard contact lenses require a routine care program that includes (1) cleaning to remove debris and deposits from the lens, (2) soaking the lens in a storage/disinfecting solution while not in use, and (3) wetting the lenses to decrease their hydrophobic characteristics.

To achieve the care needs of lenses there are several solutions employed as follows:

1. Wetting Solutions
2. Cleaning Solutions
3. Soaking Solutions
4. Combination Purpose Solutions

The pharmacist plays a key role in counseling patients about the use of these products as well as other over-the-counter drug products and legend medications. For example, oral medications which are excreted in tear fluid or discolor tears may also affect contact lenses. Most notably, rifampin (orange-colored tears) and sulfasalazine (yellow-colored tears) have been implicated to cause permanent lens staining. Also, those oral or topical drugs that can cause ocular side effects can potentially interfere with contact lens use. For example, drugs with anticholinergic effects, e.g., antihistamines, tricyclic antidepressants, decrease tear secretion and may cause lens intolerance and damage. Isotretinoin, prescribed for severe, recalcitrant acne, can induce marked dryness of the eye, so while acne therapy is being conducted it would be wise for the pharmacist to suggest to the patient to check with his/her ophthalmologist about the advisability to continue wearing contact lenses. Concern must also be expressed when patients are maintained on medicines that promote excessive lacrimation, e.g., reserpine, or ocular or eyelid edema, e.g., primidone, hydrochlorothiazide, chlorthalidone, which may interfere with lens wear.

When the lens wearer is prescribed an ophthalmic ointment, contact lenses should not be worn until the therapy is completed. These dosage forms are capable of discoloring the lens and can interfere with the optimal use of the lens.

It is possible that a lens wearer will consult a pharmacist about the advisability of an OTC ophthalmic product, e.g., topical vasoconstrictor, to relieve eye irritation or redness. These individuals should be counseled to consult their fitter if they experience sharp eye pain, excessive watering of the eyes, persistent irritation or inflammation of the eyes, sudden changes in vision or spectacle blur that does not clear up overnight. Spectacle blur is a phenomenon in which hard lenses worn for a number of hours cause corneal edema. This affects visual acuity from several minutes to hours after lens removal until the eye returns to normal.

It is useful if the pharmacist reinforces several general considerations in the care of contact lens products. Wearers should wash their hands thoroughly before and after handling the lens with a nonabrasive, noncosmetic soap. Wearers should not rub the eyes when the lens are in place, and if irritation develops, the lens should be removed until these symptoms subside. To avoid differences between products produced by different manufacturers it is preferable to use solutions made by the same manufacturer. Cleaning and storing of lenses should be performed in the appropriate solution for that purpose. Lenses should not be stored in tap water, nor should saliva be used to help reinsert a lens into the eye. Saliva is not sterile and contains numerous microorganisms, including *Pseudomonas aeruginosa*.

Because many lens wearers are young women between the ages of 18 to 24, it is appropriate for the pharmacist to counsel these women with regard to cosmetic restriction. Many ophthalmologists advise lens wearers to purchase makeup in the smallest container. Once opened and the longer the container is around the greater the likelihood of bacterial contamination. Further, mascara and pearlized eye shadow should be avoided by women wearing hard lenses because particles of these can get into the eye, and even a small flake can cause much irritation and corneal damage as a possibility. Aerosol hairsprays should be used before the lens is inserted into the eye, and preferably applied in another room. Otherwise airborne particles could attach to the lens during its insertion into the eye and cause irritation. The lenses should be inserted prior to makeup application because oily substances on the fingertips can smudge the lenses when they are handled. For similar reasons, lenses should be removed before removing makeup.

Lastly, it is important that contact lens wearers get their eyes medically checked 3 times per year to make sure that no damage is occurring as a result of wearing contact lenses.

Products for Soft Contact Lenses

CLEANERS. Because of their porous composition, soft lenses tend to accumulate proteinaceous material which forms a film on the lens (decreasing clarity) and serves as a base for microbial growth. The two main categories of cleaners are *surfactants,* which emulsify accumulated oils, lipids and inorganic compounds, and *enzymatic cleaners,* which break down and remove protein deposits. Surfactant materials are utilized either within a mechanical washing device (Opti-Heat) or by simply placing several drops of the solution on the lens surface and gently rubbing the lens back and forth, either by placing the lens on the thumb and rubbing with the forefinger or by placing the lens in the palm of the hand and rubbing gently with a fingertip (about a 20 to 30 second procedure). The ingredients in these cleaners usually include a nonionic detergent, wetting agent, chelating agent, buffers, and preservatives.

Enzymatic cleaning is accomplished by soaking the lenses in a solution prepared from enzyme tablets. This procedure is recommended at least once per week or twice per month in conjunction with regular surfactant cleansing. These tablets contain either papain, pancreatin, or subtilisin, which causes the hydrolysis of protein to peptides and amino acids. Typically these are added to saline solution, but one solution can be prepared using 3% hydrogen peroxide, which combines enzymatic cleaning with disinfection. After the lenses have been soaked for the recommended length of time they should be thoroughly rinsed.

RINSING/STORAGE. Saline solutions for soft lenses should have a neutral pH and be isotonic with human tears, i.e., 0.9% sodium chloride. Besides rinsing the lenses, these solutions are used for storage because saline maintains their curvature and diameter, as well as optical power of the soft lenses. Further, it facilitates lens hydration and prevents the lens from drying out and becoming brittle.

Because they are used for storage, many saline solutions contain preservatives which, while inhibiting bacterial growth, can induce sensitivity reactions or eye irritation. Most notably, thimerosal has been implicated in this regard, and manufacturers have endeavored to create preservative-free saline solutions and package them in aerosol containers or unit-of-use vials. The use of salt tablets to prepare a normal saline solution is discouraged because of the potential of contamination and risk of serious eye infections, e.g., *Acanthamoeba* keratitis.

DISINFECTION AND NEUTRALIZATION. Disinfection can be accomplished by two methods, i.e., thermal (heat) and chemical (no heat). In the past both methods were equally popular, however, with the introduction of hydrogen peroxide systems for chemical disinfection, chemical disinfection has become more popular.

For thermal disinfection, the lenses are placed into a specially designed heating unit with saline solution. The solution is heated sufficiently to kill microorganisms, e.g., for 10 minutes at a minimum of 80°C. It is important that after disinfection the lenses be stored in the unopened case until ready to be worn. Further, the wearer must ensure that the lenses have been thoroughly cleaned prior to using heat disinfection. Otherwise, heating can hasten lens deterioration.

In years past chemical disinfection was conducted with products that contained thimerosal in combination with either chlorhexidine or a quaternary ammonium compound. Unfortunately, many wearers encountered sensitivity reactions and these products fell into disfavor. Subsequently, the introduction of hydrogen peroxide systems for chemical disinfection has revitalized this method of disinfection. It is thought that the "free radicals" chemically released from the peroxide react with the cell wall of the microorganisms. Further, the bubbling action of the peroxide is thought to promote the removal of any remaining debris on the lens.

To prevent eye irritation from residual peroxide after disinfection, it is necessary that the lenses be exposed to one of three types of neutralizing agents. These are the *catalytic type* (an enzyme catalase or a platinum disc), e.g., Lensept Neutralizer (CIBA Vision); a *reactive type* (such as sodium pyruvate or sodium thiosulfate), e.g., Rinsing and Neutralizing Solution (CooperVision); or the *dilution-elution* type, e.g., PureSept Disinfection Solution (Ross).

Chemical disinfection systems may come as two-solution systems, which use separate disinfecting and rinsing solutions, or one-solution systems, which use the same solution for rinsing and storage. It is important that the wearer realize that lenses must not be disinfected by heating when using these solutions.

Products for Hard Contact Lenses

CLEANERS. Hard lenses should be cleaned immediately after their removal from the eye. Otherwise, oils deposits, proteins, salts, cosmetics, tobacco smoke and airborne contaminants can build up, interfere with clear vision and possibly cause irritation. A surfactant cleaner is used by applying the solution or gel onto both surfaces of the lens, and then rubbing the lens in the palm of the hand with the index finger for about 20 seconds. The wearer should realize that too vigorous rubbing can cause scratching or warping of the lens.

SOAKING/STORAGE SOLUTIONS. Although some ophthalmologists advocate dry storage of PMMA lenses, most believe that these lenses should be stored in a soaking solution once they are removed from the eye. To be effective soaking solutions must contain sufficient concentration of disinfecting agent, usually 0.01% benzalkonium chloride and 0.01% edetate sodium, to kill surface bacteria. Overnight soaking is advantageous because it keeps the lenses wettable and the prolonged contact time helps to loosen deposits that remain after routine cleaning.

WETTING SOLUTIONS. These solutions contain surfactants to facilitate the hydration of the hydrophobic lens surface. Wetting solutions enable the tears of the eye to evenly spread across the lens surface by converting the hydrophobic surface of the lens to a temporary hydrophilic surface. These solutions also facilitate a cushion between the lens and the cornea and the eyelid. Typical ingredients include a viscosity-inducing agent, hydroxyethylcellulose, a wetting agent, such as polyvinyl alcohol, preservatives, such as benzalkonium chloride or edetate disodium, and buffering agents/salts to adjust the pH and maintain tonicity.

COMBINATION SOLUTIONS. These solutions serve as cleaning/soaking solutions, wetting/soaking solutions, or cleaning, soaking, and wetting solutions. While patient ease of use is improved with these, combination products may lower the effectiveness of the cleaning function if the concentration of cleaning solution is too low to adequately remove debris from the lens surface. These combination solutions should be reserved for those wearers who have a demonstrated need for simplification of the lens care process.

Products for Rigid Gas Permeable (RGP) Contact Lenses

Wearers of rigid gas permeable contact lenses should know to use only solutions that are compatible with this type of lens. These lenses generally follow the same regimen for care as hard contact lenses, except that specific solutions must be used for this type of lens. One of two cleaning methods may be used, i.e., hand washing or mechanical washing. In the first method, the lens may be cleaned by holding the concave side up in the palm of the hand. The lens should not be held between the fingers because the flexibility of the lens may inadvertently cause the lens to warp or turn inside out. Mechanical washing is advantageous because the possibility of the lens turning inside out or warping during cleaning is minimized.

After cleansing, the RGP lens should then be thoroughly rinsed and soaked in a wetting/soaking solution overnight. After soaking, the next morning the lens is rubbed with fresh wetting/soaking solution and then inserted into the eye. To facilitate removal of stubborn protein deposits, some opthalmologists recommend weekly cleaning with enzymatic, i.e., papain, cleaners.

Nasal Preparations

The vast majority of preparations intended for intranasal use contain adrenergic agents and are employed for their decongestant activity on the nasal mucosa. Most of these preparations are in solution-form, and are administered as nose drops or sprays; however, a few are available as nasal jellies. Examples of products for intranasal use are shown in Figure 11–7 and presented in Table 11–6.

Nasal Decongestant Solutions

Most nasal decongestant solutions are aqueous preparations, rendered isotonic to nasal fluids (approximately equivalent to 0.9% sodium chloride), buffered to maintain drug stability while approximating the normal pH range of the nasal fluids (pH 5.5 to 6.5), and stabilized and preserved as required. The antimicrobial pre-

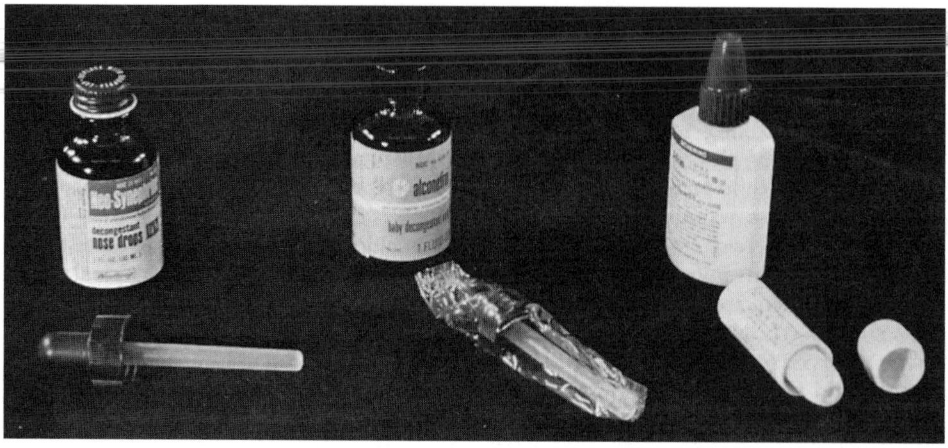

Fig. 11–7. *Examples of commercial packaging of nasal solutions, showing drop and spray containers, and nasal inhaler.*

servatives used are the same as those used in preserving ophthalmic solutions. The concentration of adrenergic agent in the majority of nasal decongestant solutions is quite low, ranging from about 0.05 to 1.0%. Certain commercial solutions which are available for both pediatric and adult use, are generally available in two strengths, the pediatric strength being approximately one-half of the adult strength.

Nasal decongestant solutions are employed in the treatment of rhinitis of the common cold and for vasomotor and allergic rhinitis including hay fever, and for sinusitis. Their frequent use or their use for prolonged periods may lead to

Table 11–6. Examples of Some Commercial Nasal Preparations

Product Name	*Manufacturer*	*Active Ingredient*	*Use/Indications*
Afrin Nasal Spray and Afrin Nose Drops	Schering-Plough	oxymetazole HCl (0.05%)	Nasal adrenergic/decongestant
Beconase AQ Nasal Spray	Allen and Hanburys	beclomethasone diproprionate (0.042%)	Synthetic corticosteroid indicated for the relief of symptoms of seasonal or perennial allergic or vasomotor rhinitis
Diapid Nasal Spray	Sandoz	lopressin (0.185 mg/mL)	Antidiuretic; for control or prevention of diabetes insipidus due to deficiency of endogenous posterior pituitary antidiuretic hormone.
Nasalcrom Nasal Solution	Fisons	cromolyn sodium (4%)	Prevention and treatment of symptoms of allergic rhinitis
Nasalide Nasal Solution	Syntex	flunisolide (0.025%)	Indicated in the treatment of symptoms of seasonal or perennial rhinitis
Neo-Synephrine Nose Drops	Sterling Health	phenylephrine HCl (0.125 to 1.0%)	Nasal adrenergic/decongestant
Neo-Synephrine Maximum Strength 12 Hour	Sterling Health	oxymetrazole (0.05%)	Nasal adrenergic/decongestant
Ocean Mist	Fleming	isotonic sodium chloride	To restore moisture and relieve dry, crusted and inflamed nasal membranes.
Privine HCl Nasal Solution	Ciba	naphazoline HCl (0.05 and 0.1%)	Nasal adrenergic/decongestant
Syntocinon Nasal Spray	Sandoz	oxytocin (40 units/mL)	Synthetic oxytocin hormone. Employed for initial milk let-down preparatory to breast feeding.
Tyzine Pediatric Nose Drops	Kenwood	tetrahydrozoline HCl (0.05%)	Nasal adrenergic/decongestant

chronic edema of the nasal mucosa, i.e., *rhinitis medicamentosa,* aggravating the symptom that they are intended to relieve. Thus, they are best used for short periods of time (no longer than 3 to 5 days) with the patients advised not to exceed the recommended dosage and frequency of use.

The easiest but least comfortable approach to treat rebound congestion is to completely withdraw application of the topical vasoconstrictor. Unfortunately, this approach will promptly result in bilateral vasodilation with almost total nasal obstruction. A more acceptable method is to withdraw application of drug in only one nostril, and have the patient continue using the medication in the other nostril. Once the rebound congestion subsides in the drug-free nostril, about 1 to 2 weeks, a total withdrawal is then instituted. Another approach is the substitution of a topical saline solution or spray *in lieu* of the topical vasoconstrictor. This effectively keeps the nasal mucosa moist and provides psychologic assistance to patients who are dependent upon placing medication into their nostrils.

Most of the adrenergic drugs used in nasal decongestant solutions are synthetic compounds similar in chemical structure, pharmacologic activity, and side effects to the parent compound, naturally occurring epinephrine. Epinephrine as a pure chemical substance was first isolated from suprarenal gland in 1901 and was called both *Suprarenin* and *Adrenalin.* Synthetic epinephrine was prepared just a few years later.

Most solutions for nasal use are packaged in dropper bottles or in plastic spray bottles, usually containing 15 to 30 mL of medication. The products should be determined to be stable in the containers used and the packages tightly closed during periods of nonuse. The patient should be advised that should the solution become discolored or contain precipitated matter, it should be discarded.

The patient should also understand that there is a difference in the duration of the effect of topical decongestants. For example, phenylephrine should be used every 3 to 4 hours, whereas oxymetrazole, which is longer acting, should only be used every 12 hours.

Decongestant Inhalers

Certain nasal decongestants may also be employed in the form of inhalants. For instance the drug propylhexedrine (Benzedrex, Menley & James) is a liquid which volatilizes slowly at room temperature. This quality enables it to be effective as an inhalant. The inhalers in which the drug is held contain cylindrical rolls of fibrous material impregnated with the volatile drug substance. The medication which has an amine-like odor is usually masked with added aromatic agents. The inhaler is placed in the nostril and vapor inhaled to relieve nasal congestion. As with the other nasal adrenergic agents, excessive or too frequent use can result in nasal edema and increased rather than decreased congestion.

The inhalers are effective so long as the volatile drug remains present. To insure that the drug does not escape during periods of nonuse, the caps on the inhalers should be tightly closed.

Proper Administration and Use of Nasal Drops/Sprays

To minimize the possibility of contamination, the pharmacist should point out to the patient that the nasal product only be used by one person and kept out of the reach of children. If the nasal product is intended for a child the directions should be clear to the patient. If an over-the-counter product is used, the parent should note the directions on the label.

Prior to administration, the patient should blow the nose to clear the nostrils and wash his/her hands thoroughly with soap and water. For maximum penetration with drops, a patient should lie down on a flat surface, such as a bed, hanging the head over the edge, and then tilting the head back as far as comfortable. The prescribed number of drops are then gently placed into the nostrils, and to allow the medication to spread in the nose, the patient should remain in this position for a few minutes. After this,the dropper should be replaced in the bottle and tightened.

The patient should be advised to use the drops only as long as prescribed. Long-acting nasal drops, as mentioned, can cause rebound congestion so whenever possible, treatment should not extend beyond 5 days.

If a spray dosage form is utilized by the patient, basically the same suggestions apply with the exception that the patient should not lie on a flat surface. If this is performed there is a chance that the administration would be enhanced by the prone position. It is better to merely have the patient tilt the head back while standing and gently squeeze the medicine container to delivery the medication.

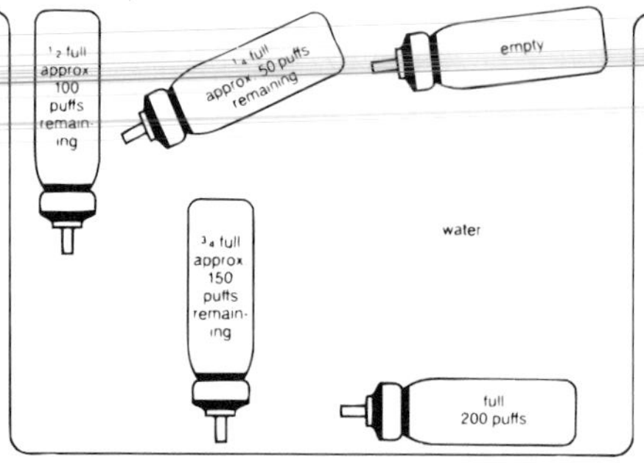

Fig. 11–8. *An easy method of estimating the amount of Vancenase left in an inhaler. The canister is placed in a bowl of water and its position compared with the diagram shown. (Courtesy of Schering Corp.)*

Certain nasal medications (e.g., Vancenase [beclomethasone diproprionate]) are available for administration through aerosol inhalers. A clever method for a patient to estimate the proportion of medication remaining in the inhaler is shown in Figure 11–8.

Nasal Route for Systemic Effects

The nasal route for drug delivery is of current interest because of the need to develop a non-oral, nonparenteral route for newly developed synthetic biologically active peptides and polypeptides.[11–16] Polypeptides, such as insulin, that are subject to destruction by the gastrointestinal fluids are currently administered by injection. However, the nasal mucosa has been shown to be amenable to the systemic absorption of certain peptides, as well as to nonpeptide drug molecules including scopolamine, hydralazine, progesterone, and propranolol.[14,15] The nasal route is advantageous for nonpeptide drugs that poorly absorbed orally.

The adult nasal cavity has about a 20 mL capacity, with a large surface area (about 180 cm^2) for drug absorption afforded by the microvilli present along the pseudostratified columnar epithelial cells of the nasal mucosa.[13,15] The nasal tissue is highly vascularized, providing an attractive site for rapid and efficient systemic absorption. One great advantage to nasal absorption is that it avoids first-pass metabolism by the liver. However, the identification of metabolizing enzymes in the nasal mucosa of certain animal species suggests the same possibility in humans and the potential for some intranasal drug metabolism.[13]

For some peptides and small molecular compounds, intranasal bioavailability has been shown to be comparable to that of injections. However bioavailability decreases as the molecular weight of a compound increases, and for proteins composed of more than 27 amino acids bioavailability may be quite low.[12] Various pharmaceutic techniques and formulation adjuncts, as surface-active agents, have been shown to be capable of enhancing the nasal absorption of large molecules.[12,15]

Pharmaceuticals currently on the market or in various stages of clinical investigation for nasal delivery include lypressin (Diapid, Sandoz), oxytocin (Syntocinon, Sandoz), desmopressin (DDAVP, Rhone-Poulenc Rorer), vitamin B-12 (Ener-B Gel, Nature's Bounty), progesterone, insulin, calcitonin, propranolol, and butorphanol.[11,12]

Topical Oral Preparations

A variety of medicinal substances are employed topically in the oral cavity for a number of purposes and in a wide range of dosage forms. Among the drugs and preparations included in this group are the following:

Benzocaine—Topical anesthetic. Indicated for temporary relief of pain, soreness, and irritation in the mouth associated with teething, orthodontic appliances, new or poorly fitting dentures, and canker sores.

Camphorated Parachlorophenol—Dental anti-infective. A eutectic liquid composed of 65% camphor and 35% parachlorophenol, used in dentistry for the sterilization of deep root canals.

Carbamide Peroxide Topical Solution—Dental anti-infective. Acts as a chemomechanical cleansing and debriding agent through the release of bubbling oxygen. The commercial product (Gly-Oxide Liquid, Smith Kline Beecham) contains 10% carbamide in flavored anhydrous glycerin.

Cetylpyridinium Chloride Solution and Cetylpyridinium Chloride Lozenges—Local anti-infective. Commercial counterparts (Cepacol Mouthwash/Gargle and Cepacol Lozenges, Smith Kline Beecham) contain 1:2000 w/v and 1:1500 w/v of cetylpyridinium chloride respectively. Used primarily as a freshening mouth cleanser.

Lozenges have benzyl alcohol present to act as a local anesthetic in soothing throat irritations.

Erythrosine Sodium Topical Solution and Erythrosine Sodium Soluble Tablets—Diagnostic aid (dental disclosing agent). Solution applied topically to the teeth to reveal plaque left by inadequate brushing. Tablets chewed for the same purpose and are not to be swallowed.

Eugenol—Dental analgesic. Applied topically to dental cavities and dental protectives. Eugenol is a pale yellow liquid having an aromatic odor of clove and a spicy taste.

Lidocaine Oral Spray—Topical dental anesthetic. Applied through metered spray in the amounts of 10 mg per spray; 20 mg per quadrant of gingiva and oral mucosa is usually employed. [Xylocaine Oral Spray (Astra)]

Nystatin Oral Suspension—Antifungal. May be employed for oral fungal infections by retaining in the mouth as long as possible before swallowing.

Saliva Substitutes—These contain electrolytes in a carboxymethylcellulose base and are indicated for the relief of dry mouth and throat in xerostomia.

Sodium Fluoride Oral Solution, and Sodium Fluoride Tablets—Dental caries prophylactic. Solution applied to the teeth or, when drinking water does not contain adequate fluoride, a dilute solution may be swallowed. Tablets containing 1.1 or 2.2 mg of sodium fluoride are chewed or swallowed as required.

Sodium Fluoride and Phosphoric Acid Gel and Sodium Fluoride and Phosphoric Acid Topical Solution—Dental caries prophylactic. Gel and solution applied to the teeth; each contains 1.23% of fluoride ion and 1% of phosphoric acid.

Triamcinolone Acetonide Dental Paste—Topical anti-inflammatory agent. Applied to the oral mucous membranes as a 0.1% paste.

Zinc Oxide-Eugenol Mixture—A temporary filling mix available over-the-counter, i.e., DenTemp, so that a consumer can prepared and use the mixture when a dental filling falls out or dislodges.

In addition to the above-named drugs and preparations, a host of other products for oral use are commercially available. Some of these products are medicated, as teething lotions and toothache drops, whereas others are used for hygienic purposes, as dentrifrices, denture products, and many of the mouthwashes. Among the variety of products is a like variety of physical forms, as solutions, emulsions, ointments, pastes, aerosols, etc., with the manufacture of each following the same general procedures as has been previously outlined in this text. One type of dosage form for oral use, the lozenge, has not been previously described.

Lozenges

Lozenges, also called *troches,* are disk-shaped solid dosage forms containing a medicinal substance and generally flavoring and sweetening agents, intended to be dissolved slowly in the oral cavity for localized effects. Commercially, lozenges may be made by compression, using a tablet machine and large, flat punches. The tablet machines are operated at high compression to produce troches that are harder than ordinary tablets so that they slowly dissolve or disintegrate in the mouth. The use of adhesives such as mucilages or natural gums, added to effect the adhesion of the powders used, also contributes to the hardness of the resulting lozenges.

Medicinal substances that are heat stable may be prepared into hard, sugar candy lozenges by candy-making machines that process a warm, highly concentrated, flavored syrup as the base. These lozenges dissolve slowly, and because of their high sugar content are especially soothing to the throat. Most of the commercially available cough drops are of a hard candy base.

Historically, lozenges have been employed to relieve minor sore throat pain and irritation and have conveniently delivered topical anesthetics and antibacterials for this purpose, e.g., phenol, sodium phenolate, cetylpyridinium chloride. In recent years there has been an emergence of other lozenge/troche products. Clotrimazole (Mycelex Troche (Miles)] and nystatin [Mycostatin Pastilles (Bristol-Myers)] are marketed in troche dosage forms and intended to treat oropharyngeal candidiasis. Lozenge/troche dosage forms are also a convenient means to deliver drugs, e.g., dextromethorphan [Hold DM (Menley & James)], to treat cough and cold symptoms.

When patients are prescribed medications that employ the troche dosage form, the pharmacist should recommend that the patient allow the troche/lozenge to dissolve slowly in the mouth. Further, the intent of the product and the duration of treatment should be emphasized to the patient.

Ear Preparations

Ear preparations are sometimes referred to as *otic* or *aural* preparations. Solutions are most frequently used in the ear, with suspensions and ointments also finding some application. Ear preparations are usually placed in the ear canal by drops or in small amounts for the removal of excessive cerumen (ear wax) or for the treatment of ear infections, inflammation, or pain. Because the outer ear is a skin-covered structure and susceptible to the same dermatologic conditions as other parts of the body's surface, skin conditions which arise are treated using the variety of topical dermatological preparations previously discussed in Chapter 10.

Cerumen-Removing Preparations

Cerumen is a combination of the secretions of the sweat and sebaceous glands of the external auditory canal. The secretions, if allowed to dry, form a sticky semisolid which holds shed epithelial cells, fallen hair, dust and other foreign bodies that make their way into the ear canal. Excessive accumulation of cerumen in the ear may cause itching, pain, impaired hearing and is a deterrent to otologic examination. If not removed periodically, the cerumen may become impacted and its removal made more difficult and painful.

Through the years, light mineral oil, vegetable oils, and hydrogen peroxide have been commonly used agents to soften impacted cerumen for its removal. Recently, solutions of synthetic surfactants have been developed for their *cerumenolytic* activity in the removal of ear wax. One of these agents, triethanolamine polypeptide oleate-condensate, commercially formulated in propylene glycol, is used to emulsify the cerumen thereby facilitating its removal [Cerumenex Drops (Purdue Frederick)]. Another commercial product utilizes carbamide peroxide in glycerin/propylene glycol [Debrox Drops (Marion Merrell Dow)]. On contact with the cerumen, the carbamide peroxide releases oxygen which disrupts the integrity of the impacted wax, allowing its easy removal.

In removing cerumen, the procedure usually involves placing the otic solution in the ear canal with the patient's head tilted at a 45° angle, inserting a cotton plug to retain the medication in the ear for 15 to 30 minutes, followed by gentle flushing of the ear canal with lukewarm water using a soft rubber ear syringe.

Anti-infective, Anti-inflammatory, and Analgesic Ear Preparations

Drugs used topically in the ear for their anti-infective activity include such agents as chloramphenicol, colistin sulfate, neomycin, polymyxin B sulfate, and nystatin, the latter agent used to combat fungal infections. These agents are generally formulated into ear drops (solutions or suspensions) in a vehicle of anhydrous glycerin or propylene glycol. These viscous vehicles permit maximum contact time between the medication and the tissues of the ear. In addition, their hygroscopicity causes them to draw moisture from the tissues thereby reducing inflammation and diminishing the moisture available for the life process of the microorganisms present. To assist in relieving the pain which frequently accompanies ear infections, a number of anti-infective otic preparations also contain analgesic agents as antipyrine and local anesthetics as lidocaine, dibucaine, and benzocaine.

Topical treatment of ear infections is frequently considered adjunctive, with concomitant systemic treatment with orally administered antibiotics also undertaken.

Liquid ear preparations of the anti-inflammatory agents hydrocortisone and dexamethasone sodium phosphate are prescribed for their effects against the swelling and inflammation which frequently accompany allergic and irritative manifestations of the ear as well as for the inflammation and pruritus which sometimes follow treatment of ear infections. In the latter instance, some physicians prefer the use of corticosteroids in ointment form, packaged in ophthalmic tubes. These packages allow the placement of small amounts of ointment in the ear canal with a minimum of waste. Many of the commercially available products used in this manner are labeled "eye-ear" to indicate their dual use.

Aside from the antibiotic-steroid combinations that are used to treat otitis externa, which is known synonymously as swimmer's ear, acetic acid (2%) in aluminum acetate solution and boric acid (2.75%) in isopropyl alcohol are used. These drugs help to re-acidify the ear canal and the vehicles serve to help dry the ear canal. By drying the ear canal, the growth medium for the offending microorganisms, usually *Pseudomonas aeruginosa*, is kept in check. Pharmacists may also be called upon to extemporaneously prepare a solution of acetic acid, 2 to 2.5% in rubbing alcohol (70% isopropyl alcohol or ethanol), propylene glycol or anhydrous glycerin. The source of the acetic acid can be glacial acetic acid but usually distilled white vinegar (5% acetic acid) is used. Boric acid, 2 to 5%, dissolved in either ethanol or propylene glycol has also been recommended for use in the ear. This substance, however, may be absorbed from broken skin and be toxic. Thus, its use is usually limited, especially in children with burst ear drums.

Pain in the ear frequently accompanies ear infection or inflamed or swollen ear tissue. Frequently, the pain is far out of proportion to the actual condition. Because the ear canal is so narrow, even a slight inflammation can cause intense pain and discomfort for the patient. Topical analgesic agents generally are employed together with internally administered analgesics, as aspirin, and other agents, as anti-infectives, to combat the cause of the problem.

Topical analgesics for the ear are usualy solutions and frequently contain the analgesic antipyrine and the local anesthetic benzocaine in a vehicle of propylene glycol or anhydrous glycerin (e.g., Auralgan Otic Solution, Wyeth-Ayerst). Again, these hygroscopic vehicles reduce the swelling of tissues (and thus some pain) and the growth of microorganisms by drawing moisture from the swollen tissues into the vehicle. These preparations are commonly employed to relieve the symptoms of acute otitis media. Examples of some commercial otic preparations are presented in Table 11–7.

As determined on an individual product basis, some liquid otic preparations require preservation against microbial growth. When preservation is required, such agents as chlorobutanol (0.5%), thimerosal (0.01%), and combinations of the parabens are commonly used. Antioxidants, as sodium bisulfite, and other stabilizers are also included in otic formulations, as required.

Ear preparations are usually packaged in small (5 to 15 mL) glass or plastic containers with a dropper.

Pharmacists must be aware that there may be subtle differences in the formulation of otic drops that could be potentially bothersome to the patient. This is especially so as it relates to inactive or inert ingredient differences between formulations from manufacturers which are considered equivalent on the basis of active ingredient(s) and strength. For example, several generic suspension combinations of polymyxin B sulfate, neomycin sulfate and hydrocortisone have been shown to be more acidic, i.e., pH 3.0 to 3.5, com-

Table 11–7. Examples of Some Commercial Otic Preparations

Product Name	*Manufacturer*	*Active Ingredient*	*Vehicle*	*Use/Indications*
Americaine Otic	Fisons	benzocaine	glycerin, polyethylene glycol 300	Local anesthetic for relief of ear pain and puritis in otitis media, swimmer's ear, and similar conditions
Auralgan Otic Solution	Ayerst-Wyeth	antipyrine, benzocaine	dehydrated glycerin	Acute otitis media
Cerumenex Drops	Purdue Frederick	triethanolamine polypeptide oleate-condensate	propylene glycol	Cerumenolytic agent to remove impacted earwax
Chloromycetin Otic	Parke-Davis	chloramphenicol	propylene glycol	Antiinfective
Cortisporin Otic Solution	Burroughs Wellcome	polymyxin B sulfate, neomycin sulfate, hydrocortisone	glycerin, propylene glycol, water for injection	Superficial bacterial infections
Debrox Drops	Marion Merrell Dow	carbamide peroxide	anhydrous glycerin	Ear wax removal
PediOtic Suspension	Burroughs-Wellcome	polymyxin B sulfate, neomycin sulfate, hydrocortisone	mineral oil, propylene glycol, water for injection	Superficial bacterial infections
Metreton Ophthalmic/Otic Solution	Schering	prednisolone sodium phosphate	aqueous	Antiinflammatory
Otobiotic Otic Solution	Schering	polymyxin B sulfate, hydrocortisone	propylene glycol, glycerin, water	Superficial bacterial infections
VoSol Otic Solution	Wallace	acetic acid	propylene glycol	Antibacterial/antifungal

pared to the standard brand name, i.e., Cortisporin Otic Suspension, which possesses a higher pH range, i.e., 4.8 to 5.1. Consequently, there is a risk that when the generic drops are legally substituted, a burning and stinging sensation can occur when the drops are introduced into the ear of young children, especially those with tympanostomies. Further, it has been demonstrated that with time, the pH of these formulations, including Cortisporin, becomes more acidic, e.g., pH 3.0. Thus, if stored on the shelf for a period of time, it is conceivable that if used again, the acidity could cause irritation to the ear canal. For this reason, Burroughs-Wellcome has specially formulated this antibiotic-hydrocortisone combination into a new suspension product, i.e., PediOtic, which has a minimum pH of 4.1, which is less acidic than the parent Cortisporin Otic Suspension.

Proper Administration and Use of Otic Drops

When ear drops are prescribed, it is important for the pharmacist to first determine how the drops are to be used. For example, ear wax removal drops should be instilled and then removed by the patient with an ear syringe. Alternatively, drops intended to treat external otitis infection are intended to be instilled and left in the ear.

The pharmacist should make sure the patient or parent understands that administration is intended for the ear and the frequency of application. To facilitate patient acceptance the pharmacist should point out that the bottle or container of medication should first be warmed in the hands, and if the product is a suspension, shaken prior to withdrawal into the dropper. The pharmacist should also explain the need to store the mediation in a safe place out of the reach of children and away from extremes of temperature.

When instilled into the ear, to allow the drops to run in deeper, the earlobe should be held up and back. For a child, the earlobe should be held down and back. For convenience it is probably easier to have someone other than the patient to administer the drops.

Some ear drops by virtue of their formulation, i.e., low pH, may cause stinging upon administration. Thus, parents and children should be forewarned especially if a child, for example, has tympanostomy tubes in the ear. The patient should also understand the length, in days, to use the product. For antibiotic ear drops it is not necessary to finish the entire bottle because therapy could last 20 to 30 days depending upon the dosage regimen. Therefore, patients should be instructed to continue using the drops for 3 days beyond the time ear symptoms disappear. Products for otitis externa may take up to 7 to 10 days to demonstrate efficacy.

If a child is prone to develop ear infections as a result of swimming or showering, it might be advisable to recommend the parents to consult a physician for prophylactic medication to use during swimming season, and consider using form-fitting ear plugs that fit snugly in the ear when swimming or showering. Further, after the child emerges from the water or shower, the parents can be advised to use a home hair blow dryer on a low setting to dry out the ear. It will dry out the ear quickly without trauma. The dryer should not be placed too close to the child's ear.

References

1. Akers, H.J.: Ocular Bioavailability of Topically Applied Ophthalmic Drugs. *Am. Pharm., NS23*:33–36, 1983.
2. Lee, V.H.L. and Robinson, J.R.: Mechanistic and Quantitative Evaluation of Precorneal Pilocarpine Distribution in Albino Rabbits. *J. Pharm. Sci., 68*: 673–684, 1979.
3. Shell, J.W.: Pharmacokinetics of Topically Applied Ophthalmic Drugs. *Surv. Ophthalmol. 26*:207–218, 1982.
4. Nadkarni, S.R. and Yalkowski, S.H.: Controlled Delivery of Pilocarpine. 1. In Vitro Characterization of Gelfoam Matrices. *Pharm. Res., 10*:109–112, 1993.
5. Davies, N.M., et al.: Evaluation of Mucoadhesive Polymers in Ocular Delivery. II. Polymer-Coated Vesicles. *Pharm. Res., 9*:1137–1144, 1992.
6. Stoklosa, M.J., and Ansel, H.C.: *Pharmaceutical Calculations*, 9th ed. Malvern, PA: Lea & Febiger, 1991, pp. 174–186.
7. Fraunfelder, F.T. and Hanna, C.: Drug Delivery Systems. *Surv. Ophthalmol. 18*:292–298, 1974.
8. Hind, H.W. and Zuccaro, V.S.: *Pharmacist's Handbook of Contact Lenses and Contact Lens Solutions.* Sunnyvale, CA: Barnes-Hind, Inc., 1986.
9. Engle, J.P.: Assessing and Counseling Contact Lens Wearers. *Am. Pharm, NS33*:39–45, 1993.
10. Engle, J.P.: Contact Lens Solutions. *Drug Topics, 132*:56–66, 1988.
11. Nudelman, I.: Nasal Delivery: A Revolution in Drug Administration. *Drug Delivery Systems.* Eugene, OR: Aster Publishing Corp., 1987, pp. 43–48.
12. Longenecker, J.P.: New Drug Delivery Systems. Intranasal Delivery: A Novel Route for Protein Therapeutics. *Wellcome Trends in Pharmacy, 11*:7–9, 1989.
13. Sarkar, M.A.: Drug Metabolism in the Nasal Mucosa. *Pharm. Res. 9*:1–9, 1992.

14. Fu, R.C.C., Whatley, J.L., and Fleitman, J.S.: Intranasal Delivery of RS-93522, a Dihydropyridine-Type Calcium-Channel Antagonist. *Pharm. Res., 8*: 134–138, 1991.
15. Donovan, M.D., Flynn, G.L., and Amidon, G.L.: The Molecular Weight of Nasal Absorption: The Effect of Absorption Enhancers. *Pharm. Res., 8*: 808–815, 1990.
16. Schipper, N.G.M., Verhoef, J.C., and Merkus, F.W.H.M.: The Nasal Mucociliary Clearance: Relevance to Nasal Drug Delivery. *Pharm. Res., 8*: 807–814, 1991.

12

Suppositories and Other Rectal, Vaginal, and Urethral Preparations

Suppositories

SUPPOSITORIES ARE solid dosage forms intended for insertion into body orifices where they melt, soften, or dissolve and exert localized or systemic effects. The derivation of the word *suppository* is from the Latin *supponere,* meaning "to place under," as derived from *sub* (under) and *ponere* (to place).[1] Thus, suppositories are meant both linguistically and therapeutically to be placed "under" the body, as into the rectum.

Suppositories are commonly employed rectally, vaginally, and occasionally urethrally. They have various shapes and weights (Fig. 12–1). The shape and size of a suppository must be such that it is capable of being easily inserted into the intended body orifice without causing undue distension, and once inserted, it must be retained for the approporiate period of time. Rectal suppositories are generally inserted with the fingers, but certain vaginal suppositories, particularly the vaginal "inserts" or vaginal tablets prepared by compression, may be inserted high in the vaginal tract with the aid of a special insertion appliance.

Rectal suppositories are usually about 32 mm (1½ inches) in length, are cylindrical, and have one or both ends tapered. Some rectal suppositories are shaped like a bullet, a torpedo, or the little finger. Depending upon the density of the base and the medicaments present in the suppository, the weight of rectal suppositories may vary. Adult rectal suppositories weigh about 2 g when cocoa butter (theobroma oil) is employed as the suppository base. Rectal suppositories for use by infants and children are about half the weight and size of the adult suppositories and assume a more pencil-like shape. Vaginal suppositories, also called *pessaries,* are usually globular, oviform, or cone-shaped and weigh about 5 g when cocoa butter is the base. However, depending upon the base and the individual manufacturer's product, the weights of vaginal suppositories may vary widely. Urethral suppositories, also called *bougies,* are slender, pencil-shaped suppositories intended for insertion into the male or female urethra. Male urethral suppositories may be 3 to 6 mm in diameter and approximately 140 mm in length, although this may vary. When cocoa butter is employed as the base, these suppositories weigh about 4 g. Female urethral suppositories are about half the length and weight of the male urethral suppository, being about 70 mm in length and weighing about 2 g when of cocoa butter.

Local Action

Once inserted, the suppository base melts, softens, or dissolves, distributing the medicaments it carries to the tissues of the region. These medicaments may be intended for retention within the cavity for localized drug effects, or they may be intended to be absorbed for the exertion of systemic effects. Rectal suppositories intended for localized action are most frequently employed to relieve constipation or the pain, irritation, itching, and inflammation associated with hemorrhoids or other anorectal conditions. Antihemorrhoidal suppositories frequently contain a number of components, including local anesthetics, vasoconstrictors, astringents, analgesics, soothing emollients, and protective agents. A popular laxative, glycerin suppositories, promote laxation by the local irritation of the mucous membranes, probably by the dehydrating effect of the glycerin on those membranes. Vaginal suppositories or inserts intended for localized effects are employed mainly as contraceptives, antiseptics in feminine hygiene, and as specific agents to combat an invading pathogen. Most commonly, the drugs employed are nonoxynol-9 for contraception, and trichomonacides to combat vaginitis caused by *Trichomonas vaginalis, Candida (Monilia) albicans,* and other microorgan-

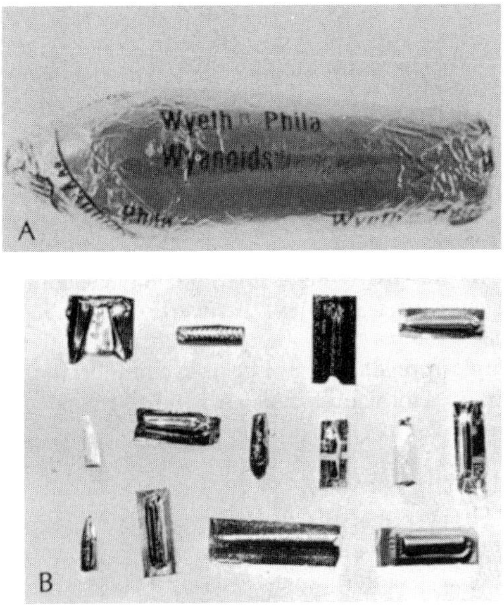

Fig. 12–1. *A. Close-up of a commercially prepared and packaged rectal suppository (Courtesy of Wyeth-Ayerst Laboratories); B. Examples of a variety of commercially available rectal and vaginal suppositories wrapped in paper, foil, and plastic.*

isms. Urethral suppositories may be used as antibacterials and as a local anesthetic preparative to urethral examination.

Systemic Action

For systemic effects, the mucous membranes of the rectum and vagina permit the absorption of many soluble drugs. Although the rectum is utilized quite frequently as the site for the systemic absorption of drugs, the vagina is not as frequently used for this purpose.

Among the advantages over oral therapy of the rectal route of administration for achieving systemic effects are these: (a) drugs destroyed or inactivated by the pH or enzymatic activity of the stomach or intestines need not be exposed to these destructive environments; (b) drugs irritating to the stomach may be given without causing such irritation; (c) drugs destroyed by portal circulation may bypass the liver after rectal absorption (drugs enter the portal circulation after oral administration and absorption); (d) the route is convenient for administration of drugs to adult or pediatric patients who may be unable or unwilling to swallow medication; and (e) it is an effective route in the treatment of patients with vomiting episodes.

Examples of drugs administered rectally in the form of suppositories for their systemic effects include (a) prochlorperazine and chlorpromazine for the relief of nausea and vomiting and as a tranquilizer; (b) oxymorphone HCl for narcotic analgesia; (c) ergotamine tartrate, for the relief of migraine syndrome and (d) indomethacin, a non-steroidal antiinflammatory analgesic and antipyretic.

Some Factors of Drug Absorption from Rectal Suppositories

The dose of a drug administered rectally may be greater than or less than the dose of the same drug given orally, depending upon such factors as the constitution of the patient, the physicochemical nature of the drug and its ability to traverse the physiologic barriers to absorption, and the nature of the suppository vehicle and its capacity to release the drug and make it available for absorption.

The factors affecting the rectal absorption of a drug administered in the form of a suppository may be divided into two main groups: (1) physiologic factors and (2) physicochemical factors of the drug and the base.[2,3]

Physiologic Factors

The human rectum is approximately 15 to 20 cm in length. When empty of fecal material, the rectum contains only 2 to 3 mL of inert mucous fluid. In the resting state, the rectum is nonmotile; there are no villi or microvilli on the rectal mucosa.[3] However, there is abundant vascularization of the submucosal region of the rectum wall with blood and lymphatic vessels.

Among the physiologic factors affecting drug absorption from the rectum are the colonic contents, circulation route, and the pH and lack of buffering capacity of the rectal fluids.

COLONIC CONTENT. When systemic effects are desired from the administration of a medicated suppository, greater absorption may be expected from a rectum that is void than from one that is distended with fecal matter. A drug will obviously have greater opportunity to make contact with the absorbing surface of the rectum and colon in the absence of fecal matter. Therefore, when deemed desirable, an evacuant enema may be administered and allowed to act before the administration of a suppository of a drug to be absorbed. Other conditions such as diarrhea, colonic obstruction due to tumorous growths, and tissue dehydration can all influence the rate and degree of drug absorption from the rectal site.

CIRCULATION ROUTE. Drugs absorbed rectally, unlike those absorbed after oral administration, bypass the portal circulation during their first pass into the general circulation, thereby enabling drugs otherwise destroyed in the liver to exert systemic effects. The lower hemorrhoidal veins surrounding the colon receive the absorbed drug and initiate its circulation throughout the body, bypassing the liver. Lymphatic circulation also assists in the absorption of rectally administered drugs.

PH AND LACK OF BUFFERING CAPACITY OF THE RECTAL FLUIDS. Because rectal fluids are essentially neutral in pH (7–8) and have no effective buffer capacity, the form in which the drug is administered will not generally be chemically changed by the rectal environment.

The suppository base employed has a marked influence on the release of active constituents incorporated into it. While cocoa butter melts rapidly at body temperature, because of its immiscibility with fluids, it fails to release fat-soluble drugs readily. For systemic drug action, it is preferable to incorporate the ionized rather than the unionized form of a drug in order to maximize bioavailability. Although unionized drugs partition out of water-miscible bases such as glycerinated gelatin and polyethylene glycol more readily, the bases themselves tend to dissolve slowly and thus retard the release of the drug.

Physicochemical Factors of the Drug and Suppository Base

Physicochemical factors include such properties as the relative solubility of the drug in lipid and in water and the particle size of a dispersed drug. Physicochemical factors of the base include its ability to melt, soften, or dissolve at body temperature, its ability to release the drug substance, and its hydrophilic or hydrophobic character.

LIPID-WATER SOLUBILITY. The lipid-water partition coefficient of a drug (discussed in Chapter 3) is an important consideration in the selection of the suppository base and in anticipating drug release from that base. A lipophilic drug that is distributed in a fatty suppository base in low concentration has less of a tendency to escape to the surrounding aqueous fluids than would a hydrophilic substance present in a fatty base to an extent approaching its saturation. Water-soluble bases—for example, polyethylene glycols—which dissolve in the anorectal fluids, release for absorption both water-soluble and oil-soluble drugs. Naturally, the more drug a base contains, the more drug will be available for potential absorption. However, if the concentration of a drug in the intestinal lumen is above a particular amount, which varies with the drug, the rate of absorption is not changed by a further increase in the concentration of the drug.

PARTICLE SIZE. For drugs present in the suppository in the undissolved state, the size of the drug particle will influence its rate of dissolution and its availability for absorption. As indicated many times previously, the smaller the particle size, the more readily the dissolution of the particle and the greater the chance for rapid absorption.

NATURE OF THE BASE. As indicated earlier, the base must be capable of melting, softening, or dissolving to release its drug components for absorption. If the base interacts with the drug inhibiting its release, drug absorption will be impaired or even prevented. Also, if the base is irritating to the mucous membranes of the rectum, it may initiate a colonic response and prompt a bowel movement, negating the prospect of a thorough drug release and absorption.

In a study of the bioavailability of aspirin from five brands of commercial suppositories, it was shown that the absorption rates varied widely, and that even with the best product only about 40% of the dose was absorbed when the retention time in the bowel was limited to 2 hours. Thus, the absorption rates were considered exceedingly low, especially when compared to orally administered aspirin, and of dubious dependability.[4]

Because of the possibility of chemical and/or physical interactions between the medicinal agent and the suppository base, which could affect the stability and/or bioavailability of the drug, the absence of any drug interaction between the two agents should be ascertained before or during formulation.

Suppository Bases

Analogous to the ointment bases, suppository bases play an important role in the release of the medication they hold and therefore in the availability of the drug for absorption for systemic effects or for localized action. Of course, one of the first requisites for a suppository base is that it remains solid at room temperature but softens, melts, or dissolves readily at body temperature so that the drug it contains may be made fully available soon after insertion. Certain bases are more efficient in drug relase than others. For instance, cocoa butter (theobroma oil) melts quickly at body temperature, but because the resulting oil is immiscible with the body fluids, fat-soluble drugs tend to remain in the oil and have little tendency to enter the aqueous physiologic fluids. For water-soluble drugs incorporated in cocoa butter, the reverse is generally true, and good release results. Fat-soluble drugs seem to be released more readily from bases of glycerinated gelatin or polyethylene glycol, both of which dissolve slowly in body fluids. When irritation or inflammation is to be relieved, as in the treatment of anorectal disorders, cocoa butter appears to be the superior base because of its emollient or soothing, spreading action.

Classification of Suppository Bases

For most purposes, it is convenient to classify suppository bases according to their physical characteristics into two main categories and a third miscellaneous group: (1) fatty or oleaginous bases, (2) water-soluble or water-miscible bases, and (3) miscellaneous bases, generally combinations of lipophilic and hydrophilic substances.

FATTY OR OLEAGINOUS BASES. Fatty bases are perhaps the most frequently employed suppository bases, principally because cocoa butter is a member of this group of substances. Among the other fatty or oleaginous materials used in suppository bases are many hydrogenated fatty acids of vegetable oils such as palm kernel oil and cottonseed oil. Also, fat-based compounds containing compounds of glycerin with the higher molecular weight fatty acids, such as palmitic and stearic acids, may be found in fatty suppository bases. Such compounds as glyceryl monostearate and glyceryl monopalmitate are examples of this type of agent. The suppository bases in many commercial products employ various and varied combinations of these types of materials to achieve a base possessing the desired hardness under conditions of shipment and storage and the desired quality of submitting to the temperature of the body to release their medicaments. In some instances, suppository bases are prepared with the fatty materials emulsified or with an emulsifying agent present to prompt emulsification when the suppository makes contact with the aqueous body fluids. These types of bases are arbitrarily placed in the third, or "miscellaneous," group of suppository bases.

Cocoa Butter, NF, is defined as the fat obtained from the roasted seed of *Theobroma cacao.* At room temperature it is a yellowish, white solid having a faint, agreeable chocolate-like odor. Chemically, it is a triglyceride (combination of glycerin and one or different fatty acids) primarily of oleopalmitostearin and oleodistearin. Because cocoa butter melts between 30° to 36°C, it is an ideal suppository base, melting just below body temperature and yet maintaining its solidity at usual room temperatures. However, because of its triglyceride content, cocoa butter exhibits marked *polymorphism,* or the property of existing in several different crystalline forms. Because of this, when cocoa butter is hastily or carelessly melted at a temperature greatly exceeding the minimum required temperature and then quickly chilled, the result is a metastable crystalline form (α crystals) with a melting point much lower than the original cocoa butter. In fact, the melting point may be so low that the cocoa butter will not solidify at room temperature. However, since the crystalline form represents a metastable condition, there is a slow transition to the more stable β form of crystals having the greater stability and the higher melting point. This transition may require several days. Consequently if suppositories that have been prepared by melting cocoa butter for the base do not harden soon after molding, they will be useless to the patient and a loss of time, materials, and prestige to the pharmacist. Cocoa butter must be slowly and evenly melted, preferably over a water bath of warm water, to avoid the formation of the unstable crystalline form and ensure the retention in the liquid of the more stable β crystals that will constitute nuclei upon which the congealing may occur during chilling of the liquid.

Substances such as phenol and chloral hydrate have a tendency to lower the melting point of cocoa butter when incorporated with it. If the melting point is lowered to such an extent that it is not feasible to prepare a solid suppository using cocoa butter alone as the base, solidifying agents like cetyl esters wax (about 20%) or beeswax (about 4%) may be melted with the cocoa butter to compensate for the softening effect of the added substance. However, the additions of hardening agents must not be so excessive as to prevent the melting of the base after the suppository has been inserted into the body, nor must the waxy material interfere with the therapeutic agent in any way so as to alter the efficacy of the product.

WATER-SOLUBLE AND WATER-MISCIBLE BASES. The main members of this group are bases of glycerinated gelatin and bases of polyethylene glycols.

Glycerinated gelatin suppositories may be prepared by dissolving granular gelatin (20%) in glycerin (70%) and adding a solution or suspension of the medication (10%). A glycerinated gelatin base is most frequently used in the preparation of vaginal suppositories, where the prolonged localized action of the medicinal agent is usually desired. The glycerinated gelatin base is slower to soften and mix with the physiologic fluids than is cocoa butter and therefore provides a more prolonged release.

Because glycerinated gelatin-based suppositories have a tendency to absorb moisture due to the hygroscopic nature of glycerin, they must be protected from atmospheric moisture in order for them to maintain their shape and consistency. Due also to the hygroscopicity of the glycerin, the suppository may have a dehydrating effect and be irritating to the tissues upon insertion. The water present in the formula for the suppositories minimizes this action; however, if necessary, the suppositories may be moistened with water prior to their insertion to reduce the initial tendency of the base to draw water from the mucous membranes and irritate the tissues.

Urethral suppositories may be prepared from a glycerinated gelatin base of a formula somewhat different from the one indicated above. For urethral suppositories, the gelatin constitutes about 60% of the weight of the formula, the glycerin about 20%, and the medicated aqueous portion about 20%. Urethral suppositories of glycerinated gelatin are much more easily inserted than suppositories with a cocoa butter base, owing to the brittleness of cocoa butter and its rapid softening at body temperature.

Polyethylene glycols are polymers of ethylene oxide and water, prepared to various chain lengths, molecular weights, and physical states. They are available in a number of molecular weight ranges, the more commonly used being polyethylene glycol 200, 400, 600, 1000, 1500, 1540, 3350, 4000, 6000, and 8000. The numerical designations refer to the average molecular weights of each of the polymers. Polyethylene glycols having average molecular weights of 200, 400, and 600 are clear, colorless liquids. Those having average molecular weights of greater than 1000 are wax-like, white solids with the hardness increasing with an increase in the molecular weight. Various combinations of these polyethylene glycols may be combined by fusion, using two or more of the various types to achieve a suppository base of the desired consistency and characteristics.

Pharmacists have been called upon in recent years to prepare progesterone vaginal suppositories extemporaneously. These suppositories, used in premenstrual syndrome, are commonly prepared by molding using a polyethylene glycol base. Formulas for these suppositories are presented later in this chapter.

Polyethylene glycol suppositories do not melt at body temperature but rather dissolve slowly in the body's fluids. Therefore, the base need not be formulated to melt at body temperature. Thus it is possible, and in fact routine, to prepare suppositories from polyethylene glycol mixtures having melting points considerably higher than that of body temperature. Not only does this property permit a slower release of the medication from the base once the suppository has been inserted, but it also permits the convenient storage of these suppositories without need of refrigeration and without danger of their softening excessively in warm weather. Their solid nature also permits them to be inserted slowly without the fear that they will melt in the fingertips (as cocoa butter suppositories sometimes do). Because they do not melt at body temperature, but mix with mucous secretions upon their dissolution, polyethylene glycol-based suppositories do not "leak" from the orifice as do many cocoa butter-based suppositories. If the polyethylene glycol suppositories do not contain at least 20% of water to avoid the irritation of the mucous membranes after insertion, they should be dipped in water just prior to use. This procedure prevents moisture being drawn from the tissues after insertion and the "stinging" sensation.

MISCELLANEOUS BASES. In the miscellaneous group of bases are included those which are mixtures of the oleaginous and water-soluble or water-miscible materials. These materials may be chemical or physical mixtures. Some are preformed emulsions, generally of the w/o type, or they may be capable of dispersing in aqueous fluids. One of these substances is polyoxyl 40 stearate, a surface-active agent that is employed in a number of commercial suppository bases. Polyoxyl 40 stearate is a mixture of the monostearate and distearate esters of mixed polyoxyethylene diols and the free glycols, the average polymer length being equivalent to about 40 oxyethylene units. The substance is a waxy, white to light tan solid that is water-soluble. Its melting point is generally between 39°C and 45°C. Other surface active agents useful in the preparation of suppository bases also fall into this broad grouping. Mixtures of many fatty bases (including cocoa butter) with emulsifying agents capable of forming w/o emulsions have been prepared. These bases have the ability to hold water or aqueous solutions and are sometimes referred to as "hydrophilic" suppository bases.

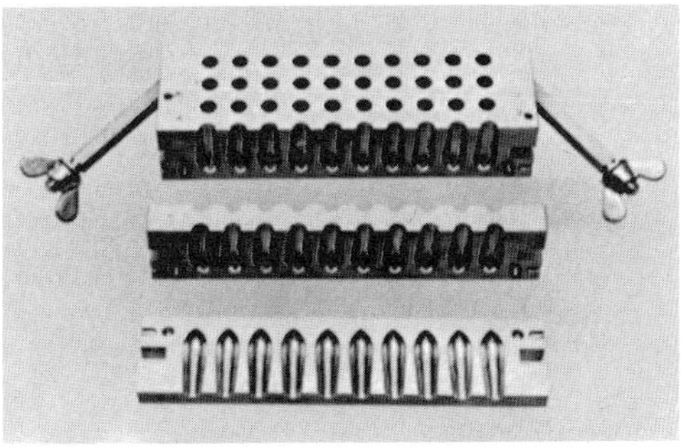

Fig. 12–2. *Partially opened suppository mold capable of producing 50 torpedo-shaped suppositories in a single molding. (Courtesy of Chemical and Pharmaceutical Industry Co., Inc.)*

Preparation of Suppositories

Suppositories are prepared by three methods: (1) *molding* from a melt, (2) *compression*, and (3) *hand rolling* and *shaping*. The method most frequently employed in the preparation of suppositories both on a small scale and on an industrial scale is molding.

Preparation by Molding

Basically, the steps in molding include (a) the melting of the base, (b) incorporating of any required medicaments, (c) pouring the melt into molds, (d) allowing the melt to cool and congeal into suppositories, and (e) removing the formed suppositories from the mold. Suppositories of cocoa butter, glycerinated gelatin, polyethylene glycol, and most other suppository bases are suitable for preparation by molding.

SUPPOSITORY MOLDS. Suppository molds are commercially available with the capability of producing individual or large numbers of suppositories of various shapes and sizes. Individual plastic suppository molds may be obtained to form a single suppository. Other molds, as those most commonly found in the community pharmacy, are capable of producing 6, 12, or more suppositories in a single operation (Fig. 12–2). Industrial molds produce hundreds of suppositories from a single batch (Figs. 12–3 and 12–4).

Molds in common use today are made from stainless steel, aluminum, brass, or plastic. The molds, which separate into sections, generally longitudinally, are opened for cleaning before and after the preparation of a batch of suppositories, closed when the melt is poured, and opened again to remove the cold, molded suppositories. Care must be exercised in cleaning the molds, as any scratches on the molding surfaces will take away from the desired smoothness of the resulting suppositories. Plastic molds are especially prone to scratching.

Although satisfactory molds are commercially available for the preparation of suitable rectal, vaginal, and urethral suppositories, if necessary in the extemporaneous preparation of suppositories, temporary molds may be successfully formed by pressing heavy aluminum foil about an object having the shape of the desired suppository, then carefully removing the object, and filling the shaped foil with the melt. For instance, glass stirring rods may be used to form molds for urethal suppositories, cylindrical pencils or pens may be used to form molds for rectal suppositories, and any cone-shaped object may be used to form vaginal supporitories.

LUBRICATION OF THE MOLD. Depending upon the formulation, suppository molds may require lubrication before the melt is poured to facilitate the clean and easy removal of the molded suppositories. Lubrication is seldom necessary when the suppository base is cocoa butter or polyethylene glycol, as these materials contract sufficiently on cooling within the mold to separate from the inner surfaces and allow their easy removal. Lubrication is usually necessary when glycerinated gelatin suppositories are prepared. A thin coating of mineral oil applied with the finger to the molding surfaces usually suffices to provide the necessary lubrication. It should be stressed, however, than any materials which might cause irritation to the mucous membranes should not be employed as a mold lubricant.

CALIBRATION OF THE MOLD. Each individual

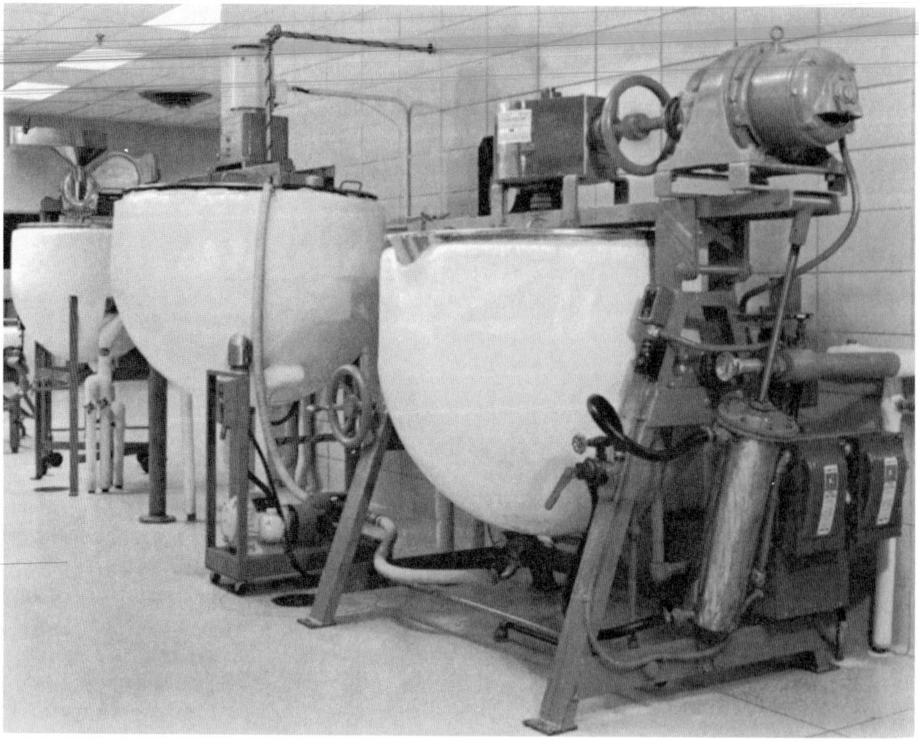

Fig. 12–3. *Large, heated tanks for the preparation of the melt in the commercial production of suppositories by molding. (Courtesy of Wyeth-Ayerst Laboratories.)*

mold is capable of holding a specific volume of material in each of its openings. If the maerial is cocoa butter, the weight of the resulting suppositories will differ from the weight of suppositories prepared in the same mold with a mixture of polyethylene glycols as the base because of the difference in the densities of the materials. Similarly, any added medicinal agent would further alter the densities of the bases, and the weights of the resulting suppositories would be different from those prepared with base material alone.

It is important that the pharmacist calibrate each of his suppository molds for the suppository bases that he generally employs (usually cocoa butter and a polyethylene glycol base) in order that he may prepare medicated suppositories each having the proper quantity of medicaments.

The first step in the calibration of a mold is to prepare molded suppositories from base material alone. After removal from the mold, the suppositories are weighed, and the total weight and the average weight of each suppository are recorded (for the particular base used). To determine the volume of the mold, the suppositories are then carefully melted in a calibrated beaker, and the volume of the melt is determined for the total number as well as for the average of one suppository.

DETERMINATION OF THE AMOUNT OF BASE REQUIRED. In his prescriptions for medicated suppositories to be prepared extemporaneously by the pharmacist, the prescribing physician generally indicates the amount of a medicinal substance that he desires in each suppository, but he leaves the amount of base to the discretion of the pharmacist. Generally, in filling such prescriptions, the pharmacist calculates the amounts of materials needed for the preparation of one or two more suppositories than the number prescribed to compensate for the inevitable loss of some material and to ensure having enough material to prepare the last required suppository.

In determining the amount of base to be incorporated with the medicaments, the pharmacist must be certain that the required amount of drug is provided in each suppository. Because the vol-

Fig. 12–4. *Highly automated large-scale production of molded suppositories. Molding operation (at the right) is followed by the removal of the suppositories from the molds, dropping them onto a conveyor belt and into a collection basket. (Courtesy of Wyeth-Ayerst Laboratories.)*

ume of the mold is known (from the determined volume of the melted suppositories formed from the base), the volume of the drug substances subtracted from the total volume of the mold will give the volume of base required. In instances in which the added amounts of medicaments are slight, they may be considered to be negligible, and no deduction from the total volume of base may be deemed necessary. However, if considerable quantities of substances are to be incorporated into the suppository, the volumes of these materials are important and should be used to calculate the amount of base actually required to completely fill the mold. The total volumes of these materials are subtracted from the volume of the mold, and the appropriate amount of base is added. Since the suppository bases are solids at room temperature, the volume of base determined may be converted to weight from the density of the material. For example, if 12 mL of cocoa butter are required to fill a suppository mold and if the medicaments in the formula have a collective volume of 2.8 mL, then 9.2 mL of the cocoa butter will be required. By multiplying 9.2 mL times the density of cocoa butter, 0.86 g/mL, it may be calculated that 7.9 g of cocoa butter will be required. After adjusting for the preparation of an extra suppository or two, the calculated amount is weighed.

Another method for the determination of the amount of base in the preparation of medicated suppositories requires the following steps: (a)

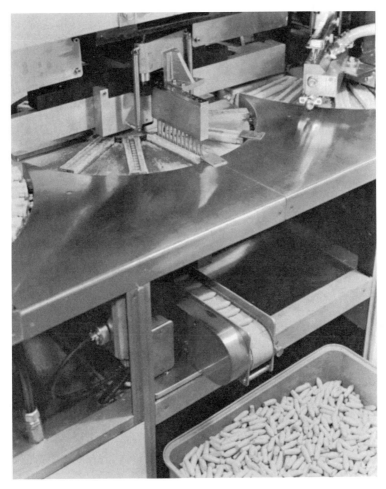

weigh the active ingredient for the preparation of a single suppository; (b) dissolve it or mix it (depending upon its solubility in the base) with a portion of melted base insufficient to fill one cavity of the mold, and add the mixture to a cavity; (c) add additional melted base to the cavity to fill it completely; (d) allow the suppository to congeal and harden; and (e) remove the suppository from the mold and weigh it. The weight of the active ingredients present, subtracted from the weight of the suppository, yields the weight of the amount of base used. This amount of base multiplied by the number of suppositories to be prepared in the mold is the total amount of base required.

A third method involves the placing of all of the required medicaments for the preparation of the total number of suppositories (including one extra) in a calibrated beaker. To this is added a portion of the melted base and the drug substances incorporated. Then sufficient additional melted base is added until the volume of mixture is reached that is required for the preparation of the necessary suppositories, based on the original calibration of the volume of the mold.

PREPARING AND POURING THE MELT. Using the least possible heat, the weighed suppository base material is melted, generally over a water bath, since a great deal of heat is not usually required. A porcelain casserole, which is a dish having a pouring lip and a handle, is perhaps the best utensil to use, since it later permits the convenient pouring of the melt into the cavities of the mold. Medicinal substances are usually incorporated into a portion of the melted base by mixing on a glass or porcelain tile with a spatula. After incorporation, this material is added with stirring to the remaining base which has been allowed to cool almost to its congealing point. Any volatile materials or heat labile substances should be incorporated at this point with thorough stirring.

It is generally best to chill the mold in the refrigerator before pouring the melt. Then, the melt is added carefully and continuously in the filling of each cavity in the mold. If any undisolved materials in the mixture are of greater density than the base so that they have a tendency to settle, constant stirring, even during pouring, is required, else the last filled cavity will contain a disproportionate share of the undissolved materials. The solid materials remain suspended if the pouring is performed just above the congealing point and not when the base is too fluid. The chilled mold encourages prompt congealing and discourages any settling of the materials within the mold's cavities. If the melt is not near the congealing point when poured, the solids may settle within each cavity of the mold to reside at the tips of the suppositories, with the result that the suppositories may be broken when removed from the mold. In filling each suppository cavity, the pouring must be continuous to prevent *layering,* which may lead to a product easily broken on handling. To ensure a completely filled mold upon congealing, the melt is poured excessively over each opening, actually rising above the level of the mold. The excessive material may actually form a continuous ribbon along the top of the mold above the cavities. This use of extra suppository material prevents the formation of recessed dips in the ends of the suppositories and justifies the preparation of extra suppository melt. When solidified, the excess material is evenly scraped off of the top of the mold with a spatula. The mold is usually placed in the freezer section of the refrigerator to hasten the hardening of the suppositories.

When the suppositories are hard, the mold is removed from the freezer, and slight pressure is exerted with the thumb on the ends of each suppository to loosen it in the mold. Then the sections of the mold are separated, and the suppositories are dislodged with the pressure being exerted principally on their ends and only if needed on the tips. Generally, little, if any, pressure is required, and the suppositories simply fall out of the mold when it is opened.

A summary of density calculations for the preparation of suppositories by molding is found in the accompanying Physical Pharmacy Capsule.

Preparation by Compression

Suppositories may be prepared by forcing the mixed mass of the suppository base and the medicaments into special molds using suppository-making machines. In preparation for compression into the molds, the suppository base and the other formulative ingredients are combined by thorough mixing, the friction of the process causing the base to soften into a pastelike consistency. On a small scale, mortar and pestle may be used. If the mortar is heated in warm water before use and then dried, the softening of the base and the mixing process is greatly facilitated. On a large scale, a similar process may be used, employing mechanically operated kneading mixers and a warmed mixing vessel.

Density (Dose Replacement) Calculations for Suppositories

In the preparation of suppositories, it is generally assumed that if the quantity of active drug is less than 100 mg, then the volume occupied by the powder is insignificant and need not be considered. This is usually based on a 2 gram suppository weight. Obviously, if a suppository mold of less than 2 grams is used, the powder volume may need to be considered.

The density factors of various bases and drugs need to be known to determine the proper weights of the ingredients to be used. Density factors relative to cocoa butter have been determined. If the density factor of a base is not known, it is simply calculated as the ratio of the blank weight of the base and cocoa butter. Density factors for a selected number of ingredients are shown in Table 1.

Three different methods of calculating the quantity of base that the active medication will occupy and the quantities of ingredients required will be illustrated here: (1) dosage replacement factor, (2) density factor, and (3) occupied volume methods.

DETERMINATION OF THE DOSAGE REPLACEMENT FACTOR METHOD

$$f = \frac{100\,(E - G)}{(G)(X)} + 1$$

where E = the weight of the pure base suppositories, and
G = the weight of suppositories with X% of the active ingredient.

Cocoa butter is arbitrarily assigned a value of 1 as the standard base. Examples of other dosage replacement factors are shown in Table 2.

EXAMPLE 1

Prepare a suppository containing 100 mg of phenobarbital (f = 0.81) using cocoa butter as the base. The weight of the pure cocoa butter suppository is 2.0 g. Since 100 mg of phenobarbital is to be contained in an approximately 2.0 g suppository, it will be about 5% phenobarbital. What will be the total weight of each suppository?

$$0.81 = \frac{100\,(2 - g) + 1}{(g)(5)}$$

$$g = 2.019$$

DETERMINATION OF DENSITY FACTOR METHOD

1. Determine the average blank weight, A, per mold using the suppository base of interest.
2. Weigh the quantity of suppository base necessary for 10 suppositories.
3. Weigh 1.0 g of medication.
   The weight of medication per suppository, B, is then equal to 1 g/10 supp = 0.1 g/supp.
4. Melt the suppository base and incorporate the medication, mix, pour into molds, cool, trim, and remove from the molds.
5. Weigh the 10 suppositories and determine the average weight (C).
6. Determine the density factor as follows:

   $$\text{Density factor} = \frac{B}{A - C + B}$$

   where A = average weight of blank,
   B = weight of medication per suppository, and
   C = average weight of medicated suppository.
7. Take the weight of the medication required for each suppository and divide by the density factor of the medication to find the replacement value of the suppository base.
8. Subtract this quantity from the blank suppository weight.
9. Multiply by the number of suppositories required to obtain the quantity of suppository base required for the prescription.
10. Multiply the weight of drug per suppository by the number of suppositories required to obtain the quantity of active drug required for the prescription.

Density (Dose Replacement) Calculations for Suppositories (Continued)

EXAMPLE 2

Prepare 12 acetaminophen 300 mg suppositories using cocoa butter, where the average weight of the cocoa butter blank is 2 g and the average weight of the medicated suppository is 1.8 g.

$$\mathrm{DF} = \frac{0.3}{2 - 1.8 + 0.3} = 0.6$$

From step 7: (0.3 gm)/0.6 = 0.5 (the replacement value of the base)
From step 8: 2.0 gm − 0.5 g = 1.5 g
From step 9: 12 × 1.5 g = 18 g cocoa butter required
From step 10: 12 × 0.3 g = 3.6 g acetaminophen

DETERMINATION OF OCCUPIED VOLUME METHOD

1. Determine the average weight per mold (blank) using the suppository base of interest.
2. Weigh the quantity of suppository base necessary for 10 suppositories.
3. Divide the density of the active drug by the density of the suppository base to obtain a ratio.
4. Divide the total weight of active drug required for the total number of suppositories by the ratio obtained in step 3 (this will give the amount of suppository base displaced by the active drug).
5. Subtract the amount obtained in step 4 from the total weight of the prescription (number of suppositories multiplied by the weight of the blanks) to obtain the weight of suppository base required.
6. Multiply the weight of active drug per suppository times the number of suppositories to be prepared to obtain the quantity of active drug required.

EXAMPLE 3

Prepare 10 suppositories, each containing 200 mg of a drug with a density of 3.0. The suppository base has a density of 0.9 and a prepared blank weighs 2.0 g. Using the "determination of occupied volume method," prepare the requested suppositories.

From step 1: The average weight per mold is 2.0 g.
From step 2: The quantity required for 10 suppositories would be 2 g × 10 supp = 20 g.
From step 3: The density ratio is 3.0/0.9 = 3.3.
From step 4: The amount of suppository base displaced by the active drug is 2.0 g/3.3 = 0.6 g.
From step 5: The weight of the suppository base required is 20 g − 0.6 g = 19.4 g.
From step 6: The quantity of active drug required is 0.2 g × 10 = 2.0 g.

The required weight of the suppository base is 19.4 g and the active drug is 2 g.

Table 1 Density Factors for Cocoa Butter Suppositories

Alum	1.7	Cocaine HCl	1.3	Potassium iodide	4.5
Aminophylline	1.1	Digitalis leaf	1.6	Procaine	1.2
Aspirin	1.3	Glycerin	1.6	Quinine HCl	1.2
Barbital	1.2	Ichthammol	1.1	Resorcinol	1.4
Belladonna extract	1.3	Iodoform	4.0	Sodium bromide	2.3
Benzoic Acid	1.5	Menthol	0.7	Spermaceti	1.0
Bismuth carbonate	4.5	Morphine HCl	1.6	Sulfathiazole	1.6
Bismuth salicylate	4.5	Opium	1.4	Tannic acid	1.6
Bismuth subgallate	2.7	Paraffin	1.0	White wax	1.0
Bismuth subnitrate	6.0	Peruvian Balsam	1.1	Witch hazel fluidextract	1.1
Boric Acid	1.5	Phenobarbital	1.2	Zinc oxide	4.0
Castor oil	1.0	Phenol	0.9	Zinc sulfate	2.8
Chloral hydrate	1.3	Potassium bromide	2.2		

Density (Dose Replacement) Calculations for Suppositories (Continued)

Table 2 Dosage Replacement Factors for Selected Drugs

Balsam Peru	0.83	Chloral hydrate	0.67	Resorcin	0.71
Bismuth subgallate	0.37	Ichthammol	0.91	Silver protein, mild	0.61
Bismuth subnitrate	0.33	Phenobarbital	0.81	Spermaceti	1.0
Boric Acid	0.67	Phenol	0.9	White/yellow wax	1.0
Camphor	1.49	Procaine HCl	0.8	Zinc oxide	0.15–0.25
Castor oil	1.0	Quinine HCl	0.83		

The process of compression is especially suited for the making of suppositories containing medicinal substances that are heat labile and for suppositories containing a great deal of substances insoluble in the base. In contrast to the molding method, there is no likelihood of insoluble matter settling during the preparation of suppositories by compression. The disadvantage to the process is that the special suppository machine is required and there is some limitation as to shapes of suppositories that can be made from the available molds.

In preparing suppositories with the compression machine, the suppository mass is placed into a cylinder which is then closed, and pressure is applied from one end, mechanically, or by turning a wheel, and the mass is forced out of the other end into the suppository mold or die. When the die is filled with the mass, a movable end plate at the back of the die is removed and when additional pressure is applied to the mass in the cylinder, the formed suppositories are ejected. The end plate is returned, and the process is repeated until all of the suppository mass has been used. Various sizes and shapes of dies are available. It is possible to prepare suppositories of uniform circumference by extrusion through a perforated plate and by cutting the extruded mass to the desired length.

Preparation by Hand Rolling and Shaping

With the ready availability of suppository molds of accommodating shapes and sizes, there is little requirement for today's pharmacist to shape suppositories by hand. Hand rolling and shaping is a historic part of the art of the pharmacist; a description of the method may be found in the third edition of this text.

Rectal Suppositories

Examples of rectal suppositories are presented in Table 12–1. As noted earlier, drugs as aspirin given for pain, ergotamine tartrate for treating migraine headaches, theophylline as a smooth muscle relaxant in treating asthma, and chlorpromazine and prochlorperazine, which act as antiemetics and tranquilizers, are intended to be absorbed into the general circulation to provide systemic drug effects. The rectal route of administration is especially useful in instances in which the patient is unwilling or unable to take medication by mouth.

Suppositories are also intended to provide local action within the perianal area. Local anesthetic suppositories are commonly employed to relieve *pruritus ani* of various causes, and the pain sometimes associated with hemorrhoids. Many of the commercial hemorrhoidal suppositories contain a number of medicinal agents including astringents, protectives, anesthetics, lubricants, and others, intended to relive the discomfort of the conditon. Cathartic suppositories are contact-type agents which act directly on the colonic mucosa to produce normal peristalsis. Because the contact action is restricted to the colon, the motility of the small intestine is not appreciably affected. Cathartic suppositories are more rapid-acting than orally administered medication. Suppositories of bisacodyl are usually effective in 15 minutes to an hour, and glycerin suppositories usually within a few minutes following insertion.

Some commercially prepared suppositories are available for both adult and pediatric use. The difference is in the shape and drug content. Pediatric suppositories are more narrow and pencil-shaped than the typical bullet-shaped

Table 12–1. Examples of Rectal Suppositories

Suppository	Corresponding Commercial Product	Active Constituent per Suppository	Type of Effect	Category and Comments
Bisacodyl Suppositories	Dulcolax Suppositories (Ciba Consumer)	10 mg	Local	Cathartic. See text for additional discussion. Base: hydrogenated vegetable oil.
Chlorpromazine Suppositories	Thorazine Suppositories (SmithKline Beecham)	25 and 100 mg	Systemic	Anti-emetic; tranquilizer. Base: glycerin, glyceryl monopalmitate and monostearate, and hydrogenated fatty acids of coconut and palm kernel oils.
Ergotamine Tartrate and Caffeine Suppositories	Cafergot Suppositories (Sandoz); Wigraine Suppositories (Organon)	2 mg ergotamine tartrate and 100 mg caffeine	Systemic	Ergotamine is an alpha adrenergic blocking agent with a direct stimulating effect on the smooth muscle of peripheral and cranial blood vessels. Caffeine is also a cranial vasoconstrictor. The product is used to abort or prevent vascular headaches such as migraine. Base: cocoa butter.
Hydrocortisone Suppositories	Anusol-HC Suppositories (Parke-Davis)	25 mg	Local	For use in prutitis ani, inflamed hemorrhoids, and other inflammatory conditions of the anorectum. Base: hydrogenated glycerides.
Indomethacin Suppositories	Indocin Suppositories (Merck & Co.)	50 mg	Systemic	Nonsteroidal antiinflammatory analgesic indicated in various forms of arthritis. The rate of rectal absorption from suppositories is more rapid than from orally administered capsules. Base: polyethylene glycols 3350 and 8000.
Prochlorperazine Suppositories	Compazine Suppositories (SmithKline Beecham)	2.5, 5, and 25 mg	Systemic	Anti-emetic. Base: glycerin, glyceryl monopalmitate and monostearate, and hydrogenated fatty acids of coconut and palm kernel oils.
Promethazine HCl Suppositories	Phenergan Suppositories (Wyeth-Ayerst)	12.5, 25, and 50 mg	Systemic	Antihistaminic, antiemetic and sedative actions: used to manage conditions of allergic origin; for preoperative or postoperative sedation or nausea and vomiting; and for motion sickness. Base: cocoa butter and white wax.

adult suppository. Glycerin suppositories are commonly available in each type.

A formula for Glycerin Suppositories is as follows:

Glycerin	91 g
Sodium Stearate	9 g
Purified Water	5 g
To make about	100 g

In the preparation of this suppository, the glycerin is heated in a suitable container to about 120°F. Then the sodium stearate is dissolved with stirring in the hot glycerin, the purified water added, and the mixture immediately poured into the suppository mold. It is recommended that if the mold is of metal, that it also be heated prior to the addition of the glycerin mixture. After cooling to solidification, the suppositories are removed. From the above formula, about fifty adult suppositories may be prepared.

Glycerin, a hygroscopic material, contributes to the laxative effect of the suppository by drawing water from the intestine and also from its irritant action on the mucous lining. The sodium stearate, a soap, is the solidifying agent in the suppository and may also contribute to the laxative action. Because of the hygroscopic nature of glycerin, the suppositories attract moisture and should be maintained in tight containers, preferably at temperatures below 25°C.

The pharmacist should relate several helpful items of information about the proper use of suppositories. If they must be stored in the refrigerator, suppositories should be allowed to warm to room temperature before insertion. The patient should be advised to rub cocoa butter suppositories gently with the fingers to melt the surface to provide lubrication for insertion. Glycerinated gelatin or polyethylene glycol suppositories should be moistened with water to enhance lubrication. If the polyetheylene glycol suppository formulation does not contain at least 20% water, dipping it into water just prior to insertion prevents moisture from being drawn from rectal tissues after insertion and decreases subsequent irritation. The shape of the suppository determines how it will be inserted. Bullet-shaped rectal suppositories should be inserted point-end first. When the patient is instructed to use one-half suppository, the patient should be told to cut the suppository in half lengthwise with a clean razor blade. Most suppositories are dispensed in paper, foil, or plastic wrappings, and the patient must be instructed to remove the wrapping thoroughly before insertion.

Vaginal Suppositories

Examples of vaginal suppository and tablets are presented in Table 12–2. These preparations are employed principally to combat infections occurring in the female genitourinary area, to restore the vaginal mucosa to its normal state, and for contraception. In combating vaginal infections, the usual pathogenic organisms involved are *Trichomonas vaginalis, Candida (Monilia) albicans* or other species, and *Hemophilus vaginalis.* Among the anti-infective agents found in commercial vaginal preparations are: nystatin, clotrimazole, butoconazole nitrate, terconazole, and miconazole (antifungals) and triple sulfas, sulfanilamide, povidone-iodine, clindamycin phosphate, metronidazole and oxytetracycline (antibacterials). Nonoxynol-9, a spermicide, is employed for vaginal contraception. Estrogenic substances as dienestrol are found in vaginal preparations to restore the vaginal mucosa to its normal state.

In the preparation of vaginal suppositories, the most commonly used base consists of combinations of the various molecular weight polyethylene glycols. To this base is frequently added surfactants and preservative agents, commonly the parabens. Many of the vaginal suppositories and other types of vaginal dosage forms are buffered to an acid pH, usually around pH 4.5 which resembles that of the normal vagina. This acidity discourages pathogenic organisms and at the same time provides a favorable environment for eventual recolonization by the acid-producing bacilli normally found in the vagina.

The polyethylene glcyol-based vaginal suppositories are water-miscible and are generally sufficiently firm for the patient to handle and insert without great difficulty. However, to make the task even easier, many manufacturers provide plastic insertion devices with their products which are used to hold the suppository or vaginal tablet during insertion for proper placement within the vagina (Fig. 12–5).

As noted earlier, pharmacists frequently are called upon to prepare progesterone vaginal suppositories. Formulas for the extemporaneous preparation of these suppositories have been presented in the professional literature.[5,6] Micronized progesterone powder is generally utilized in a base of polyethylene glycol, although in some formulas cocoa butter is employed. The suppositories are prepared by mixing the progesterone to a melt of the base and molding. Some representative formulas are:

Table 12–2. Examples of Vaginal Suppositories and Tablets

Product/Manufacturer	*Active Constituents*	*Category and Comments*
AVC Suppositories (Marion Merrell Dow)	sulfanilamide, 1.05 Gm	For the treatment of *Candida albicans* infections.
Betadine Medicated Vaginal Suppositories (Purdue Federick)	povidone-iodine, 10%	For relief of vaginitis due to *Candida albicans, Trichomonas,* and *Gardnerella vaginalis*
Gyne-Lotrimin Vaginal Inserts (Schering-Plough)	clotrimazole, 100 mg	Treatment of vulvovaginal yeast (Candida) infections.
Monistat 7 Suppositories (Ortho)	miconazole nitrate, 200 mg	Antifungal for treatment of localized vulvovaginal candidiasis (moniliasis).
Semicid Vaginal Contraceptive Inserts (Whitehall)	nonoxynol-9, 100 mg	Non-systemic reversible method of birth control
Sultrin Vaginal Tablets (Ortho)	sulfathiazole, sulfacetamide and sulfabenzamide, 500 mg total	Treatment of *Haemophilus vaginalis* vaginitis.
Terazol 3 Vaginal Suppositories (Ortho)	terconazole, 80 mg	Treatment of vulvovaginal candidiasis (moniliasis)

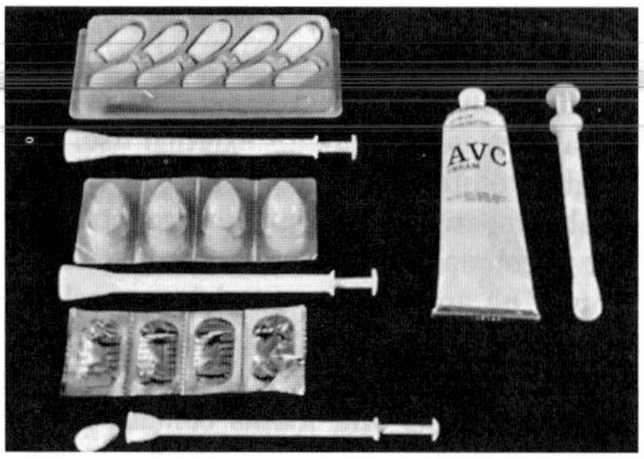

Fig. 12–5. *Dosage forms used intravaginally, including suppositories (top and middle), vaginal tablets packaged in foil (bottom), vaginal cream, and corresponding insert devices.*

Progesterone, micronized powder	q.s.
Polyethylene Glycol 400	60%
Polyethylene Glycol 8000	40%

Progesterone, micronized powder	q.s.
Polyethylene Glycol 1000	75%
Polyethylene Glycol 3350	25%

Progesterone, micronized powder	q.s.
Cocoa Butter	100%

The amount of progesterone prescribed per suppository ranges from 25 to 600 mg. The suppositories are used in treating luteal phase defect, premenstrual syndrome, luteal phase spotting, and in the preparation of the endometrium for implantation.[6]

The pharmacist should share several helpful hints with a woman who is about to use a vaginal suppository product. She should first be told to read the patient instructions included with the product. Throughout the entire course of therapy, the suppository should be inserted high into the vagina with the provided applicator. The patient should not discontinue therapy when the symptoms abate. Further, she should notify her physician if burning, irritation, or any signs of an allergic reaction occur. When vaginal inserts (i.e., compressed tablets) are prescribed, the pharmacist should instruct the woman to dip the tablet into water quickly before insertion. Because these dosage forms are usually administered at bedtime and can be somewhat messy if formulated into an oleaginous base, the pharmacist should suggest that the woman wear a sanitary napkin to protect her nightwear and bed linens.

Packaging and Storage

Glycerin suppositories and glycerinated gelatin suppositories are generally packaged in tightly closed glass containers to prevent a moisture change in the content of the suppositories. Suppositories prepared from a cocoa butter base are usually individually wrapped or otherwise separated in compartmentalized boxes to prevent contact and adhesion. Suppositories containing light-sensitive drugs are generally individually wrapped in an opaque material such as a metallic foil. In fact, most commercially available suppositories are individually wrapped in either foil or a plastic material. Some are packaged in a continuous strip with suppositories being separated by tearing along perforations placed between suppositories. Suppositories are also commonly packaged in slide boxes or in plastic boxes.

Since suppositories are adversely affected by heat, it is necessary to maintain them in a cool place. Suppositories having cocoa butter as the base must be stored below 30°F, preferably in a refrigerator. Glycerinated gelatin suppositories are best stored at temperatures below 35°F. Suppositories made from a base of polyethylene glycol may be stored at usual room temperatures without the requirement of refrigeration.

Suppositories stored in environments of high humidity may absorb moisture and tend to become spongy, whereas suppositories stored in places of extreme dryness may lose moisture and become brittle.

Other Dosage Forms Used Rectally, Vaginally, and Urethrally

Tablets and Capsules

Vaginal tablets are more widely used nowadays than are vaginal suppositories. The tablets are easier to manufacture, more stable, and less messy to handle in use. Vaginal tablets, frequently referred to as *vaginal inserts,* are usually ovoid in shape and are accompanied in their packaging with a plastic inserter, a device for easy placement of the tablet within the vagina. Vaginal tablets contain the same types of antiinfective and hormonal substances as the vaginal suppositories. They are prepared by tablet compression, and are commonly formulated to contain lactose as the base or filler, a disintegrating agent, as starch, a dispersing agent, as polyvinylpyrrolidine, and a tablet lubricant, as magnesium stearate. The tablets are intended to disintegrate within the vagina releasing their medication. Examples of vaginal tablets are presented in Table 12–2.

Some vaginal inserts are capsules of gelatin containing medication to be released intravaginally. Capsules may also be used rectally, especially in pediatrics to administer medication to children unwilling or unable to tolerate the drug orally. Their insertion into the rectum is facilitated by first lightly wetting the capsule with water. Drugs are absorbed from the rectum, but frequently at unpredictable rates and in varying amounts as has been previously noted in this chapter. Drugs which do not dissolve rapidly and which are irritating to mucous membranes should not be placed in direct contact with such membranes.

BIOADHESIVE VAGINAL TABLETS. In recent years, bioadhesive vaginal tablets have been developed as a new type of drug delivery system for the controlled release of drugs having both topical and systemic effects.[7] Because of their prolonged presence in the vagina, bioadhesive vaginal tablets forms have the advantage over other forms in that they require less frequent dosing. Mucosa-adhesive tablets hydrate and become gel-like in an aqueous environment producing a barrier that can reduce the rate of drug release from the formulation. The drug release rate from bioadhesive tablets is governed by several factors, including the composition and construction of the tablet matrix, the drug's solubility, and its partition coefficient. Among the tableting excipients found to impart the desired bioadhesive qualities are polymers of polyacrylic acid, hydroxypropylmethylcellulose, and carboxymethylcellulose.[7,8]

Ointments, Creams, and Aerosol Foams

Rectal and vaginal ointments and vaginal creams are in common use. Rectal ointments are used primarily to allay local conditions as pruritus ani and to relieve the pain and discomfort associated with hemorrhoids. The drugs present are generally the same as previously discussed for rectal suppositories, including local anesthetics, analgesics, protectives, and anti-inflammatory agents. To facilitate the insertion of ointment into the rectum, each rectal ointment tube is accompanied with a special rectal insertion and delivery tip. This tip replaces the ordinary ointment cap prior to use. After placement of the rectal tip on the ointment tube, the tip is slowly and carefully inserted into the anus. The ointment tube is depressed to release the medication through the rectal tip and into the anal canal. After use, the tip should be removed from the ointment tube and replaced with the original cap. The rectal tip should be thoroughly cleaned following each use. During the product selection process, either by the physician or the patient with assistance from the pharmacist, consideration should be given to the product formulation base. Water-soluble bases are easier and less messy to clean from applicator tips than oleaginous bases.

Patients should be advised by the pharmacist not to interchange rectal tips from one product to another. Unfortunately, this is the means that some patients use to rectally insert, for example, over-the-counter hydrocortisone ointments that are really intended only for external use.

Vaginal ointments and creams are typically available containing anti-infective agents, estrogenic hormonal substances, and contraceptive agents. The anti-infective and hormonal substances used are the same as have previously been discussed for vaginal suppositories. Contraceptive creams and foams contain spermicidal agents such as nonoxynol-9 and octoxynol and are used alone or in combination with a cervical diaphragm to prevent conception. When used with a diaphragm, the cream is placed on the diaphragm surface in contact with the cervix and around the edges of the diaphragm. When used alone, the cream is first squeezed into the special inserter-applicator tube provided. This applicator is then inserted well into the vagina, the plunger of the applicator depressed and the cream deposited. The contraceptive creams are utilized just prior to intercourse.

Aerosol foams are commercially available containing estrogenic substances and contraceptive agents. The foams are used intravaginally in the same manner as that employed for creams. The aerosol package contains an inserter device which is filled with foam and the contents placed in the vagina through activation of the plunger. The foams are generally oil-in-water emulsions, resembling light creams. They are water-miscible and non-greasy.

There are some commercial preparations of rectal foams available which utilize rectal inserters for the presentation of the foam to the anal canal. One such product, ProctoFoam (Reed & Carnrick), contains pramoxine hydrochloride

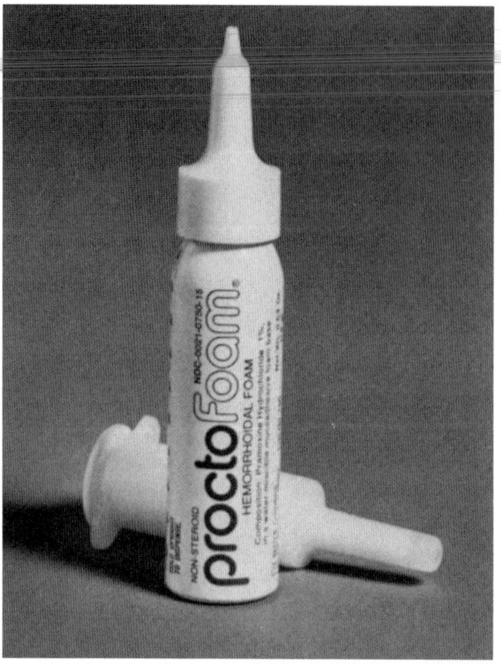

Fig. 12–6. *A product-example of a foam for anal and perianal use. To fill the applicator, the foam container is shaken vigorously, held upright, and the applicator tip placed on the container opening. With the plunger of the applicator drawn out all the way, pressure is exerted on the container cap and foam fills the applicator tube. (Courtesy of Reed & Carnrick.)*

and is used in relieving inflammatory anorectal disorders (Fig. 12–6).

Jellies and Gels

Jellies are a class of gels in which the structural coherent matrix contains a high proportion of liquid, usually water. Pharmaceutical jellies are usually formed by adding a thickening agent as tragacanth or carboxymethyl cellulose to an aqueous solution of a drug substance. The resultant product is usually clear and of a uniform semisolid consistency.

There are a number of commercially available contraceptive jellies and gels containing the same types of spermicidal agents and used intravaginally in the same manner as previously discussed for contraceptive creams. Also, a number of antispetic, antifungal, anesthetic, and nonmedicated lubricant jellies are available, primarily for use by physicians in their rectal, urethral, and vaginal examination procedures.

Jellies are subject to bacterial contamination and growth and thus most are preserved with antimicrobial preservatives. The tubes of jellies should be tightly closed when not in use, as they have a tendency to lose water to the air and dry out.

Contraceptive Sponge

A vaginal contraceptive sponge (Today, Whitehall) passed the FDA new drug review process for safety and efficacy in 1983 and was placed on the market as an over-the-counter drug. The product, shown in Figure 12–7, consists of a resilient, hydrophilic, polyurethane foam sponge, impregnated during manufacture with nonoxynol-9, a spermicidal agent. Contraception occurs by the action of the spermicidal agent, sperm absorption on the sponge, and by physical blockage by the sponge of the cervix.[9]

The contraceptive sponge is manufactured in a slightly concave, rounded form designed to fit snugly in the upper vagina (see Fig. 12–8). During manufacture, approximately 1 g of the spermicide nonoxynol-9 is incorporated into its structure. The spermicide is activated when the sponge is moistened with water and inserted into the vagina. The sponge is designed to provide contraceptive protection for a 24-hour period. The sponge is intended to remain in place for at least 6 hours following intercourse. A ribbon loop attached to the interior scrim facilitates removal.

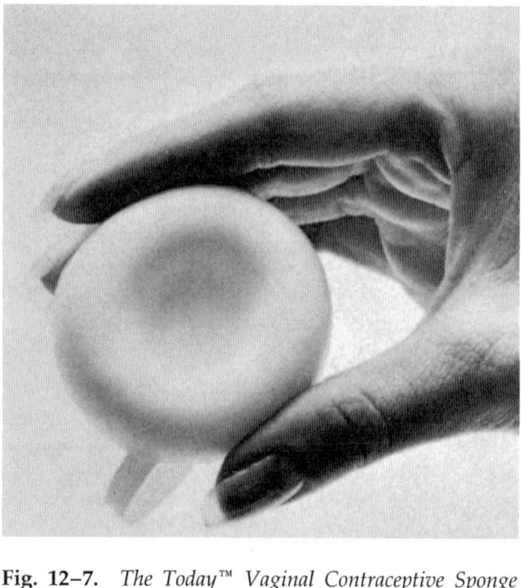

Fig. 12–7. *The Today™ Vaginal Contraceptive Sponge (Courtesy of Whitehall Laboratories).*

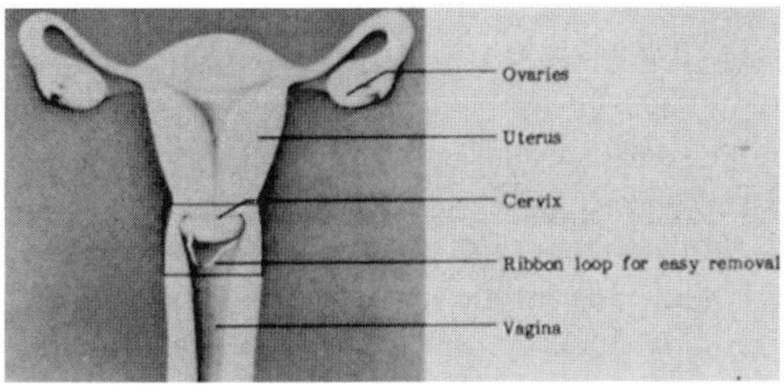

Fig. 12–8. *Placement of the Today™ Vaginal Contraceptive Sponge (Courtesy of Whitehall Laboratories).*

Intrauterine Progesterone Drug Delivery System

The Progestasert System (Alza Corporation) shown in Figures 12–9 and 12–10 slowly releases an average of 60 μg of progesterone per day for a period of 1 year after insertion. The continuous release of progesterone into the uterine cavity provides a local rather than a systemic action. Two hypotheses for the contraceptive action have been offered: progesterone-induced inhibition of sperm capacity or survival; and, alteration of the uterine milieu so as to prevent nidation.[10] The intrauterine device contains 38 mg of progesterone, a much smaller amount than would

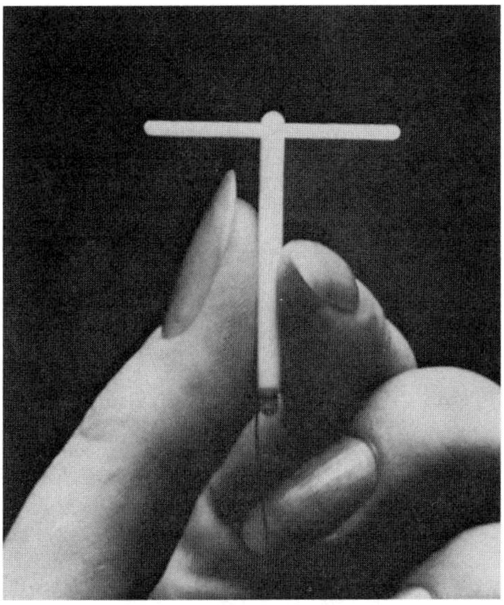

Fig. 12–9. *Progestasert Intrauterine Progesterone Contraceptive System enables the prevention of pregnancy in women for a year or more after each insertion. This small, flexible unit releases the natural hormone progesterone directly into the uterus. (Courtesy of Alza Corporation.)*

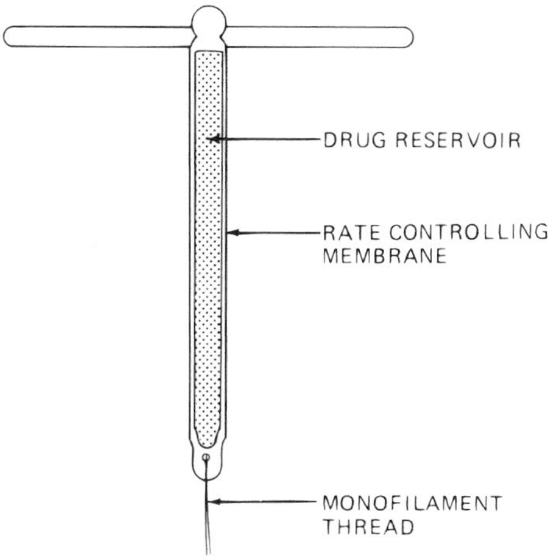

Fig. 12–10. *Schematic of the Progestasert intrauterine drug delivery system. (Courtesy of Alza Corporation.)*

otherwise be taken by other routes over a year period for the same purpose. The intrauterine device is replaced annually for the maintenance of contraception.

Powders

Powders are used to prepare solutions for vaginal *douche,* that is, for the irrigative cleansing of the vagina. The powders themselves may be prepared and packaged in bulk or as unit packages. A unit package is designed to contain the appropriate amount of powder to prepare the specified volume of douche solution. The bulk powders are utilized by the teaspoonful or tablespoonful amounts in the preparation of the desired solution. The user simply adds the prescribed amount of powder to the appropriate volume of warm water and stirs until dissolved. Among the components of douche powders are the following:

a. Boric acid or sodium borate.
b. Astringents, as potassium, alum, ammonium alum, zinc sulfate.
c. Antimicrobials, as oxyquinoline sulfate, povidone-iodine.
d. Quaternary ammonium compounds, as benzethanium chloride.
e. Detergents, as sodium lauryl sulfate.
f. Oxidizing agents, as sodium perborate.
g. Salts, as sodium citrate, sodium chloride.
h. Aromatics, as menthol, thymol, eucalyptol, methyl salicylate, phenol.

Douche powders are generally employed for their hygienic effects. A few douche powders, containing specific therapeutic anti-infective agents as those mentioned previously in the discussion of vaginal suppositories, are employed against Monilial and Trichomonal infections.

Solutions

Vaginal Douches—Solutions may be prepared from powders as indicated above or from liquid solutions or liquid concentrates. In using liquid concentrates, the patient is instructed to add the prescribed amount of concentrate (usually a teaspoonful or bottle-capful) with a certain amount of warm water (frequently a quart). The resultant solution then contains the appropriate amount of chemical agents in proper strength. The agents present are similar to the ones described above for douche powders. Examples are shown in Figure 12–11.

RETENTION ENEMAS. A number of solutions are administered rectally for the local effects of the medication (e.g., hydrocortisone) or for systemic absorption (e.g., aminophylline). In the case of aminophylline, the rectal route of administration minimizes the undesirable gastrointestinal reactions associated with oral therapy. Clinically effective blood levels of the agents are usually obtained within 30 minutes following rectal instillation.

Corticosteroids are administered as retention enemas or continuous drip as adjunctive treatment of some patients with ulcerative colitis.

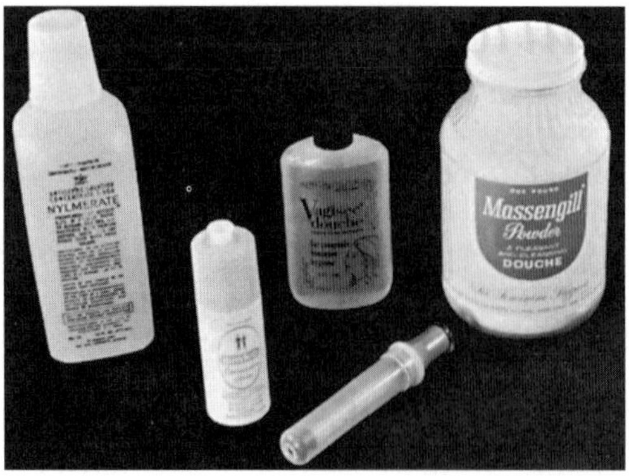

Fig. 12–11. *Products for vaginal use, including solution concentrates, powder, and aerosol foam with insert device.*

EVACUATION ENEMAS. Rectal enemas are employed to cleanse the bowel. Commercially, many enemas are available in disposable plastic squeeze bottles containing a premeasured amount of enema solution. The agents present are solutions of sodium phosphate and sodium biphosphate, glycerin and docusate potassium, and light mineral oil.

Patient instruction from a pharmacist is advantageous to ensure that the patient correctly uses these products. The patient should be advised to gently insert the rectal tip of the product with steady pressure and be told that it is not absolutely necessary to squeeze all of the contents out of the disposable plastic bottle. Lastly, the patient should be told that the product will most probably work within 5 to 10 minutes.

Suspensions

Barium Sulfate for Suspension, USP, previously discussed in Chapter 7, may be employed orally or rectally for the diagnostic visualization of the gastrointestinal tract. Mesalamine (i.e., 5-aminosalicylic acid) suspension was introduced onto the market in 1988 as Rowasa (Solvay) for treatment of Crohn's disease, distal ulcerative colitis, proctosigmoiditis, and proctitis.

References

1. Merkus, F.W.H.M.: The Correct Application of Suppositories. Editorial. *Pharmacy International,* December 1980.
2. Anschel, J. and Lieberman, H.A.: Suppositories. *Drug & Cosmetic Ind., 97:*341, 1965.
3. Moolenaar, F. and Schoonen, A.J.M.: Biopharmaceutics of the Rectal Administration of Drugs. *Pharmacy International 1:*444–146, 1980.
4. Gibaldi, M. and Grundhofer, B.: Bioavailability of Aspirin from Commercial Suppositories. *J. Pharm. Sci., 64:*1064–1066.
5. Roffe, B.D., Zimmer, R.A., and Derewicz, H.J.: Preparation of Progesterone Suppositories. *Am. J. Hosp. Pharm., 34:*1334, 1977.
6. Allen, L.V., and Stiles, M.L.: Progesterone Suppositories. *U.S. Pharmacist, 13:*16–19, 1988.
7. Gursoy, A. and Bayhan, A.: Testing of Drug Release from Bioadhesive Vaginal Tablets. *Drug Devel. Ind. Pharm., 18:*203–211, 1992.
8. Smart, J.D.: Some Formulation Factors Influencing the Rate of Drug Release from Bioadhesive Matrices. *Drug Devel. Ind. Pharm., 18:*223–232, 1992.
9. Product literature, *Today* Vaginal Contraceptive Sponge, Whitehall Laboratories, New York, 1993.
10. Product literature, Alza Corp., Palo Alto, CA, 1993.

13

Aerosols, Inhalations, and Sprays

Pharmaceutical Aerosols

PHARMACEUTICAL AEROSOLS are pressurized dosage forms containing one or more active ingredients which upon actuation emit a fine dispersion of liquid and/or solid materials in a gaseous medium. *See Physical Pharmacy Capsule, page 445.* Pharmaceutical aerosols are similar to other dosage forms in that they require the same types of considerations with respect to formulation, product stability, and therapeutic efficacy. However, they differ from most other dosage forms in their dependence upon the function of the container, its valve assembly, and an added component—the propellant—for the physical delivery of the medication in proper form.

The term *pressurized package* is commonly used when referring to the aerosol container or completed product. Pressure is applied to the aerosol system through the use of one or more liquefied or gaseous propellants. Upon activation of the valve assembly of the aerosol, it is the pressure exerted by the propellant which forces the contents of the package out through the opening of the valve. The physical form in which the contents are emitted is dependent upon the formulation of the product and the type of valve employed. Aerosol products may be designed to expel their contents as a fine mist, a coarse, wet or a dry spray, a steady stream, or as a stable or a fast-breaking foam. The physical form selected for a given aerosol is based on the intended use of that product. For instance, an aerosol intended for inhalation therapy, as in the treatment of asthma or emphysema, must present particles in the form of a fine liquid mist or as finely divided solid particles if the product is to be efficacious. It has been generally accepted that particles less than 6 μm will reach the respiratory bronchioles, and those less than 2 microns will reach the alveolar ducts and alveoli (see Fig. 13–1). In contrast, the particle size for a dermatologic spray intended for deposition on the skin would be more coarse and generally less critical to the therapeutic efficacy of the product. Some dermatologic aerosols present the medication in the form of a powder, a wet spray, a stream of liquid (usually a local anesthetic), or an ointment-like product. Other pharmaceutical aerosols include vaginal and rectal foams.

Aerosols used to provide an airborne mist are termed *space sprays*. Room disinfectants, room deodorizers, and space insecticides characterize this group of aerosols. The particle size of the released product is generally quite small, usually below 50 μm, and must be carefully controlled so that the dispersed droplets or particles remain airborne for a prolonged period of time. A one-second burst from a typical aerosol space spray will produce 120 million particles, a substantial number of which will remain suspended in the air for an hour.

Aerosols intended to carry the active ingredient to a surface are termed *surface sprays* or *surface coatings*. The dermatologic aerosols can be placed in this group. Also included are a great many nonpharmaceutical aerosol products, as personal deodorant sprays, cosmetic hair lacquers and sprays, perfume and cologne sprays, shaving lathers, toothpaste, surface pesticide sprays, paint sprays, and various household products such as spray starch, waxes, polishes, cleaners, and lubricants. A number of veterinary and pet products have been put into aerosol form as have been such food products as dessert toppings and food spreads. Some of these products are sprays; others, foams; and a few, paste-like products.

Advantages of the Aerosol Dosage Form

Some features of pharmaceutical aerosols that may be considered advantages over other types of dosage forms are as follows:

1. A portion of medication may be easily withdrawn from the package without contamination or exposure to the remaining material.

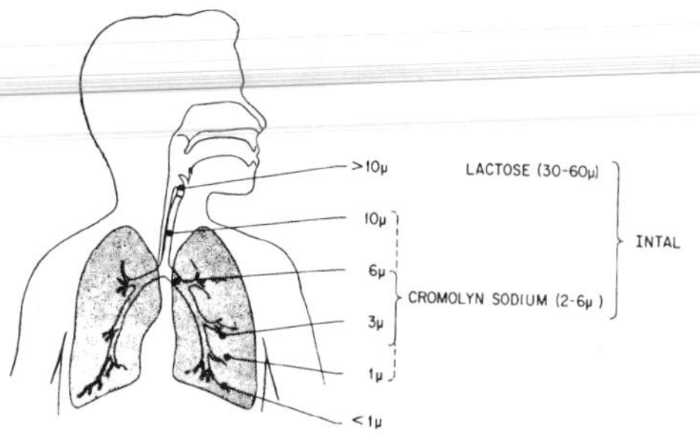

Fig. 13–1. *Relationship of INTAL (cromolyn sodium, Fisons) particle size to airway penetration. (Courtesy of Fisons Corporation.)*

2. By virtue of its hermetic character, the aerosol container protects medicinal agents adversely affected by atmospheric oxygen and moisture. Being opaque, the usual aerosol container also protects drugs adversely affected by light. This protection persists during the use and the shelf-life of the product. If the product is packaged under sterile conditions, sterility may also be maintained during the shelf-life of the product.
3. Topical medication may be applied in a uniform, thin layer to the skin, without touching the affected area. This method of application may reduce the irritation that sometimes accompanies the mechanical (fingertip) application of topical preparations. The rapid volatilization of the propellant also provides a cooling, refreshing effect.
4. By proper formulation and valve control, the physical form and the particle size of the emitted product may be controlled which may contribute to the efficacy of a drug; e.g., the fine controlled mist of an inhalant aerosol. Through the use of *metered valves*, dosage may be controlled.
5. Aerosol application is a "clean" process, requiring little or no "wash-up" by the user.

The Aerosol Principle

An aerosol formulation consists of two component parts, the *product concentrate* and the *propellant*. The product concentrate is the active ingredient of the aerosol combined with the required adjuncts, such as antioxidants, surface-active agents, and solvents, to prepare a stable and efficacious product. When the propellant is a liquefied gas or a mixture of liquefied gases, it frequently serves the dual role of propellant and solvent or vehicle for the product concentrate. In certain aerosol systems, nonliquefied compressed gases, as carbon dioxide, nitrogen, and nitrous oxide, are employed as the propellant.

For many years, the liquefied gas propellants most used in aerosol products were the chlorofluorocarbons (CFCs). However these propellants are being phased out and will be prohibited for nonessential use under federal regulations due to scientific recognition that they reduce the amount of ozone in the stratosphere, which results in an increase in the amount of ultraviolet radiation reaching the earth, an increase in the incidence of skin cancer, and other adverse environmental effects. Under the law, the FDA has the authority to exempt from the prohibition specific products under the agency's jurisdiction when there is sufficient evidence showing that: (1) there are no technically feasible alternatives to the use of a chlorofluorocarbon propellant in the product; (2) the product provides a substantial health or other public benefit unobtainable without the use of the chlorofluorocarbon; and (3) the use does not involve a significant release of chlorofluorocarbons into the atmosphere or, if it does, the release is warranted by the benefit conveyed. A number of metered-dose pharmaceutical products for oral inhalation have received such essential-use exemptions. Among the chlorofluorocarbons used as propellants in pharmaceuticals were dichlorodifluoromethane, dichlorotetrafluoroethane, and trichloromonofluoromethane (see Table 13–1).

Fluorinated hydrocarbons are gases at room temperature. They may be liquefied by cooling below their boiling point or by compressing the gas at room temperature. For example, dichlorodifluoromethane ("Freon 12") gas will form a liquid when cooled to −22°F or when compressed to 70 psig (pounds per square inch gauge) at 70°F. Both of these methods for liquefying gases are employed in aerosol packaging as will be discussed later in this section.

When a liquefied gas propellant or propellant mixture is sealed within an aerosol container with the product concentrate, an equilibrium is quickly established between that portion of propellant which remains liquefied and that which vaporizes and occupies the upper portion of the aerosol container (Fig. 13–2). The vapor phase exerts pressure in all directions—against the walls of the container, the valve assembly, and the surface of the liquid phase, which is composed of the liquefied gas and the product con-

Partial Pressure and Aerosol Formulation

Aerosols generally contain an active drug in a liquefied gas propellant, in a mixture of solvents with a propellant, or in a mixture with other additives and a propellant. The gas propellants can be formulated to provide desired vapor pressures for enhancing the delivery of the medication through the valve and actuator, in accordance to the purpose of the medication. Aerosols are used as space sprays, surface sprays, aerated foams, and for oral inhalation.

Various propellants have properties including molecular weight, boiling point, vapor pressure, liquid density, and flash point that can be of importance. An example of a calculation to determine the vapor pressure of a certain mixture of hydrocarbon propellants follows.

EXAMPLE 1

What is the vapor pressure of a 60:40 mixture of propane and isobutane. Information on the two propellants is as follows:

Property	*Propane*	*Isobutane*
Molecular formula	C_3H_8	C_4H_{10}
Molecular weight	44.1	58.1
Boiling point (°F)	−43.7	10.9
Vapor pressure (psig @ 70°F)	110	30.4
Liquid density (g/mL @ 70°F)	0.50	0.56
Flash point (°F)	−156	−117

1. Assume an ideal solution.
2. For Raoult's Law, we need to determine the number of moles of each propellant:

   $n_{propane} = 60/44.1 = 1.36$
   $n_{isobutane} = 40/58.1 = 0.69$
3. From Raoult's Law, the partial pressure exerted by the propane is:

   $P_{propane} = [(n_{propane})/(n_{propane} + n_{isobutane}) P_{propane}$
   $P_{propane} = [(1.36)/(1.36 + 0.69)]\ 110 = 72.98$ psi
4. The partial pressure exerted by the isobutane is:

   $P_{isobutane} = [(0.69)/(1.36 + 0.69)]30.4 = 10.23$ psi
5. The vapor pressure exerted by both gases, P_T, is:

   $P_T = 72.98 + 10.23 = 83.21$ psi at 70°F

The vapor pressure required for a specific application can be calculated in a similar manner and different ratios of propellants may be used to obtain that pressure.

centrate. It is this pressure which upon actuation of the aerosol valve forces the liquid phase up the dip tube and out of the orifice of the valve into the atmosphere. As the propellant meets the air, it immediately evaporates due to the drop in pressure, leaving the product concentrate as airborne liquid droplets or dry particles, depending upon the formulation. As the liquid phase is removed from the container, equilibrium between the propellant remaining liquefied and that in the vapor state is reestablished. Thus even during expulsion of the product from the aerosol package, the pressure within remains virtually constant, and the product may be continuously released at an even rate and with the same propulsion. However, when the liquid reservoir is depleted, the pressure may not be maintained, and the gas may be expelled from the container with diminishing pressure until it is exhausted.

Aerosol Systems

The pressure of an aerosol is critical to its performance. It can be controlled by (1) the type and amount of propellant and (2) the nature and amount of material comprising the product concentrate. Thus, each formulation is unique unto

Table 13–1. Physical Properties of Some Fluorinated Hydrocarbon Propellants

Chemical Name	*Chemical Formula*	*Numerical Designation*[a]	*Vapor Pressure (psia*[b]*) 70°F*	*Boiling Point (1 ATM) °F*	*Liquid Density (g/mL) 70°F*
Trichloromonofluoromethane	CCl_3F	11	13.4	74.7	1.485
Dichlorodifluoromethane	CCl_2F_2	12	84.9	−21.6	1.325
Dichlorotetrafluoroethane	$CClF_2CClF_2$	114	27.6	38.4	1.468
Chloropentafluoroethane	$CClF_2CF_3$	115	117.5	−37.7	1.29
Monochlorodifluoroethane	CH_3CClF_2	142b	43.8	15.1	1.119
Difluoroethane	CH_3CHF_2	152a	76.4	−11.2	0.911
Octafluorocyclobutane	$CF_2CF_2CF_2CF_2$	C318	40.1	21.1	1.513

[a] The numerical designations for fluorinated hydrocarbon propellants have been designed within the refrigeration industry to simplify communications when referring to these agents. The numerical designations are arrived at by the following method: (1) the digit at the extreme right refers to the number of fluorine atoms in the molecule; (2) the second digit from the right represents one *greater* than the number of hydrogen atoms in the molecule; (3) the third digit from the right is one *less* than the number of carbon atoms in the molecule; if this number is zero, it is omitted and a two-digit number is used; (4) a capital letter "C" is used before a number to indicate the cyclic nature of a compound; (5) the small letters following a number are used to indicate decreasing symmetry of isomeric compounds, with the "b" indicating less symmetry than the "a," and so forth. The number of chlorine atoms in a molecule may be determined by subtracting the total number of hydrogen and fluorine atoms from the total number of atoms which may be added to the carbon chain.

[b] psia is pounds per square inch absolute, which is equal to psig + 14.7.

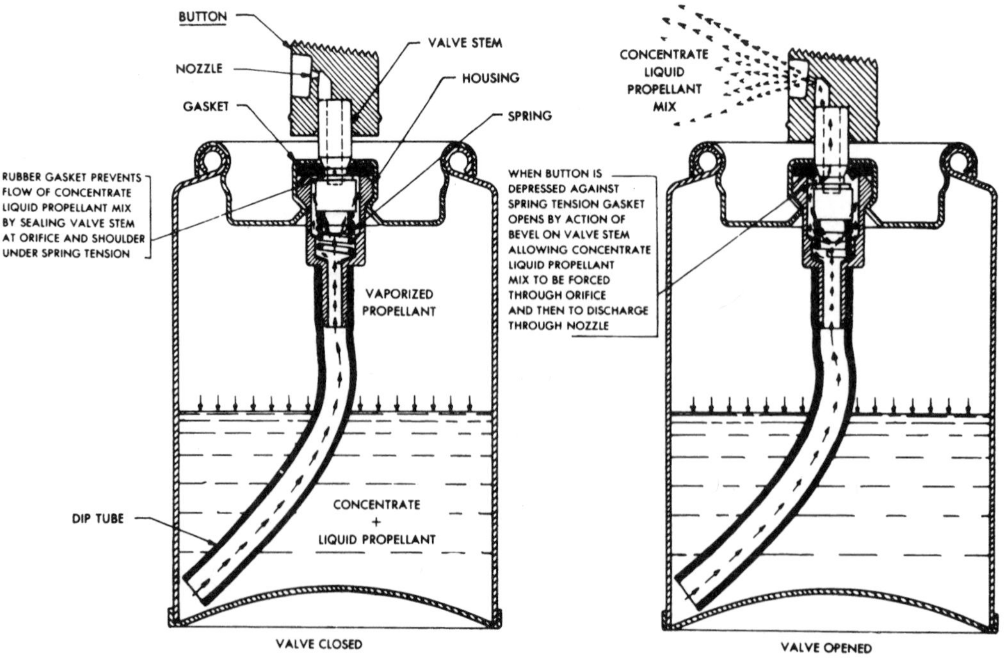

Fig. 13–2. *Cross section sketches of contents and operation of a typical two-phase aerosol system. (Courtesy of Armstrong Laboratories, Inc., Division of Aerosol Techniques, Inc.)*

itself, and a specific amount of propellant to be employed in aerosol products cannot be firmly stated. However, some general statements may be made within the context of this discussion. Space sprays generally contain a greater proportion of propellant than do aerosols intended for surface coating, and thus they are released with greater pressure, and the resultant particles are projected more violently from the valve. Space aerosols usually operate at pressures between 30 and 40 psig at 70°F and may contain as much as 85% propellant. Surface aerosols commonly contain 30 to 70% propellant with pressures between 25 and 55 psig at 70°F. Foam aerosols usually operate between 35 and 55 psig at 70°F and may contain only 6 to 10% propellant.

Foam aerosols may be considered to be emulsions, in that the liquefied propellant is partially emulsified with the product concentrate rather than being dissolved in it. Because the fluorinated hydrocarbons are nonpolar organic solvents having no affinity for water, the liquefied propellant does not dissolve in the aqueous formulation. The utilization of surfactants or emulsifiers in the formulation encourages the mixing of the two components to enhance the emulsion. Shaking of the package prior to use further mixes the propellant throughout the product concentrate. When the aerosol valve is activated, the mixture is expelled to the atmosphere where the propellant globules vaporize rapidly, leaving the active ingredient in the form of a foam.

Blends of the various liquefied gas propellants are generally used in pharmaceutical aerosols to achieve the desired vapor pressure and to provide the proper solvent features for a given product. Some propellants are eliminated from use in certain products because of their reactivity with other formulative materials, or with the proposed container or valve components. For instance, trichloromonofluoromethane tends to form free hydrochloric acid when formulated with systems containing water or ethyl alcohol, the latter a commonly used cosolvent in aerosol systems. The free hydrochloric acid not only affects the efficacy of the product, but also exerts a corrosive action on some container components.

The physiologic effect of the propellant must also be considered in formulating an aerosol to assure safety of the product in its intended use. Even though an individual propellant or propellant blend and the active ingredient of a formulation are nontoxic when tested individually, the use of the combination in aerosol form may have undesirable features. For instance, when an active ingredient ordinarily used in a nasal or oral spray is placed in a fine aerosol mist, it may reach deeper into the respiratory tract than desired and may result in irritation. In other instances, as with new dermatologic, vaginal, and rectal aerosol products, the influence of the aerosol form of the drug on the recipient tissue membranes must be evaluated for irritating effects and changes in the absorption of the drug from the site of application. The absorption pattern of a drug may change due to an increased rate of solubility of the fine particles usually produced in aerosol products.

Although the fluorinated hydrocarbons have a relatively low order of toxicity and are generally nonirritating, certain individuals, who may be sensitive to the propellant agent and who utilize an inhalation aerosol, may exhibit cardiotoxic effects following rapid and repeated use of the aerosol product.[1]

TWO-PHASE SYSTEMS. As noted previously, the two-phase aerosol system is comprised of the liquid phase, containing the liquefied propellant and product concentrate, and the vapor phase.

THREE-PHASE SYSTEMS. This system is comprised of a layer of water-immiscible liquid propellant, a layer of highly aqueous product concentrate, and the vapor phase. Because the liquefied propellant usually has a greater density than the aqueous layer, it generally resides at the bottom of the container with the aqueous phase floating above it. As with the two-phase system, upon activation of the valve, the pressure of the vapor phase causes the liquid phase to rise in the dip tube and be expelled from the container. To avoid expulsion of the reservoir of liquefied propellant, the dip tube must extend only within the aqueous phase (product concentrate) and not down into the layer of liquefied propellant. The aqueous product is broken up into a spray by the mechanical action of the valve. If the container is shaken immediately prior to use, some liquefied propellant may be mixed with the aqueous phase and be expelled through the valve to facilitate the dispersion of the exited product or the production of foam, depending upon the formulation. The vapor phase within the container is replenished from the liquid propellant phase.

COMPRESSED GAS SYSTEMS. Compressed rather than liquefied, gases may be used to prepare aerosols. The pressure of the compressed gas contained in the headspace of the aerosol container forces the product concentrate up the dip tube and out of the valve. The use of gases that are insoluble in the product concentrate, as is nitrogen, will result in the emission of a product in essentially the same form as it was placed in the container. An advantage of nitrogen as a propellant is its inert behavior toward other formulative components and its protective influence on products subject to oxidation. Further, nitrogen is an odorless and tasteless gas and thus does not contribute adversely to the smell or taste of a product.

Other gases, such as carbon dioxide and nitrous oxide, which are slightly soluble in the liquid phase of aerosol products, may be employed in instances in which their expulsion with the product concentrate is desired to achieve spraying or foaming.

Unlike aerosols prepared with liquefied gas propellants, there is no reservoir of propellant in compressed gas filled aerosols. Thus higher gas pressures are generally required in these systems, and the pressure in these aerosols progressively diminishes as the product is used.

The Aerosol Container and Valve Assembly

The effectiveness of a pharmaceutical aerosol is dependent upon achieving the proper combination of formulation, container, and valve assembly. The formulation must not chemically interact with the container or valve components so as to interfere with the stability of the formulation or with the integrity and operation of the container and valve assembly. The container and valve must be capable of withstanding the pressure required by the product, it must be corrosive-resistant, and the valve must contribute to the form of the product to be emitted.

CONTAINERS. Various materials have been used in the manufacture of aerosol containers, including (1) glass, uncoated or plastic coated; (2) metal, including tin-plated steel, aluminum, and stainless steel; and (3) plastics. The selection of the container for an aerosol product is based on its adaptability to production methods, compatibility with formulation components, ability to sustain the pressure intended for the product, the interest in design and aesthetic appeal on the part of the manufacturer, and cost.

Were it not for their brittleness and danger of breakage, glass containers would be preferred for most aerosols. Glass presents fewer problems with respect to chemical compatibility with the formula than do metal containers and is not subject to corrosion. Glass is also more adaptive to creativity in design. On the negative side, glass containers must be precisely engineered to provide the maximum in pressure safety and impact resistance. Plastic coatings are commonly applied to the outer surface of glass containers to render them more resistant to accidental breakage, and in the event of breaking, the plastic coating prevents the scattering of glass fragments. When the total pressure of an aerosol system is below 25 psig and no more than 50% propellant is used, glass containers are considered quite safe. When required, the inner surface of glass containers may be coated to render them more chemically resistant to formulation materials.

At the present time, tin-plated steel containers are the most widely used metal containers for aerosols. Because the starting material used is in the form of sheets, the completed aerosol cylinders are seamed and soldered to provide a sealed unit. When required, special protective coatings are employed within the container to prevent corrosion and interaction between the container and formulation. The containers must be carefully examined prior to filling to ensure that there are no flaws in the seam or in the protective coating that would render the container weak or subject to corrosion.

Most aluminum containers are manufactured by extrusion or by other methods that make them seamless. They have the advantage over the seam type of container in that there is greater safety against leakage, incompatibility, and corrosion. Stainless steel is employed to produce containers for certain small volume aerosols in which a great deal of chemical resistance is required. The main limitation of stainless steel containers is their high cost.

Plastic containers have met with varying success in the packaging of aerosols due to their inherent problem of being permeated by the vapor within the container. Also, certain drug-plastic interactions have been found to occur which affect the release of drug from the container and reduce the efficacy of the product.

VALVE ASSEMBLY. The function of the valve assembly is to permit the expulsion of the contents of the can in the desired form, at the desired rate, and, in the case of metered valves, in the proper amount or dose. The materials used in the manufacture of valves must be inert toward the formulations and must be approved by the Food and Drug Administration. Among the materials used in the manufacture of the various valve parts are plastic, rubber, aluminum, and stainless steel.

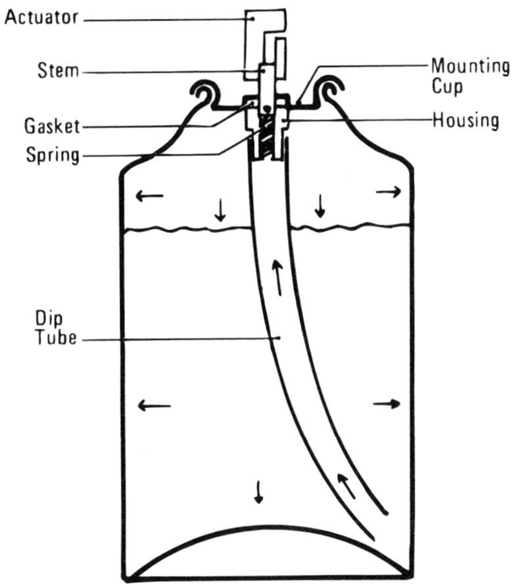

Fig. 13–3. *Sketch showing valve assembly components.*

The usual aerosol valve assembly is composed of the following parts (Fig. 13–3):

1. *Actuator*—The actuator is the button which the user presses to activate the valve assembly for the emission of the product. The actuator permits the easy opening and closing of the valve. It is through the orifice in the actuator that the product is discharged. The design of the inner chamber and size of the emission orifice of the actuator contribute to the physical form (mist, coarse spray, solid stream, or foam) in which the product is discharged. The combination of the type and quantity of propellant used, and the actuator design and dimensions control the particle size of the emitted product. Larger orifices (and less propellant) are used for products to be emitted as foams and solid streams than for those intended to be sprays or mists.
2. *Stem*—The stem supports the actuator and delivers the formulation in the proper form to the chamber of the actuator.
3. *Gasket*—The gasket, placed snugly with the stem, serves to prevent leakage of the formulation when the valve is in the closed position.
4. *Spring*—The spring holds the gasket in place and also is the mechanism by which the actuator retracts when pressure is released, thereby returning the valve to the closed position.
5. *Mounting cup*—The mounting cup, which is attached to the aerosol can or container, serves to hold the valve in place. Because the underside of the mounting cup is exposed to the formulation, it must receive the same consideration as the inner part of the container, with respect to meeting criteria of compatibility. If necessary, it may be coated with an inert material (as an epoxy resin or vinyl) to prevent an undesired interaction.
6. *Housing*—The housing, located directly below the mounting cup, serves as the link between the dip tube and the stem and actuator. With the stem, its orifice helps to determine the delivery rate and the form in which the product is emitted.
7. *Dip tube*—The dip tube, which extends from the housing down into the product, serves to bring the formulation from the container to the valve. The viscosity of the product and its intended delivery rate dictate to a large extent the inner dimensions of the dip tube and housing for a particular product.

The actuator, stem, housing, and dip tube are generally made of plastic, the mounting cup and spring of metal, and the gasket of rubber or plastic predetermined to be resistant to the formulation.

Metered Dose Inhalers (MDIs)

Metering valves are employed when the formulation is a potent medication, as in inhalation therapy (Fig. 13–4). In these metered valve systems, the amount of material discharged is regulated by an auxiliary valve chamber by virtue of its capacity or dimensions. A single depression of the actuator causes the evacuation of this chamber and the delivery of its contents. The integrity of the chamber is controlled by a dual valving mechanism. When the actuator valve is in the closed position, a seal is effected between the chamber and the atmosphere. However, in this position the chamber is permitted to fill with the contents of the container to which it is open. Depression of the actuator causes a simultaneous reversal of positions sealed; the chamber becomes open to the atmosphere, releasing its contents, and at the same time becomes sealed from the contents of the container. Upon release of the actuator, the system is restored for the next dose. The USP contains a test to determine quantita-

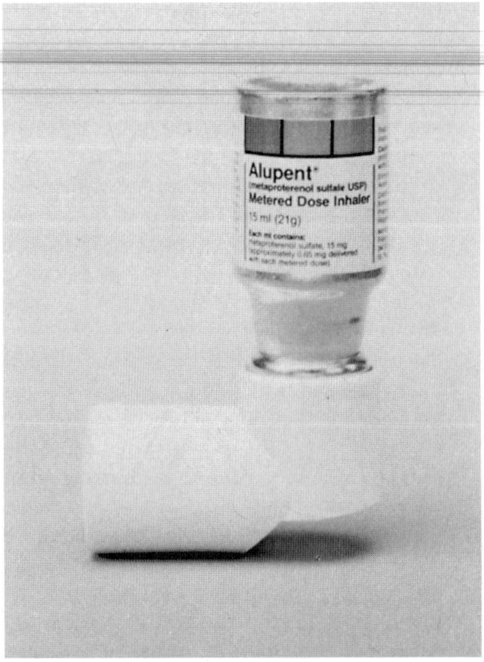

Fig. 13–4. *Example of metered dose inhaler. Each metered dose is delivered through the mouthpiece upon actuation of the aerosol unit's valve. (Courtesy of Boehringer Ingelheim.)*

tively the amount of medication from a metered valve.

As noted previously, the effectiveness in delivering medication to the lower reaches of the lungs for local or systemic effects depends in part on the particle size of the inhaled drug. Breathing patterns and the depth of respiration also play important roles in the deposition of inhaled aerosols into the lungs. Analysis of dose uniformity,[2] particle size distribution patterns,[3–5] and the "respirable" fractions of aerosol-delivered particles,[6,7] are areas of current research interest in developing aerosol products for optimal oral inhalation therapy.

A unique translingual aerosol formulation of nitroglycerin has been developed (Nitrolingual Spray, (Rhône-Poulenc Rorer) that permits a patient to spray droplets of nitroglycerin onto or under the tongue for acute relief of an attack, or for prophylaxis, of angina pectoris due to coronary artery disease. The product is not to be inhaled. At the onset of an attack, two metered spray emissions, each containing 0.4 mg of nitroglycerin, are administered. The product contains 200 doses of nitroglycerin in a propellant mixture of dichlorodifluoromethane and dichlorotetrafluoroethane.

Filling Operations

As explained earlier, fluorinated hydrocarbon gases may be liquefied by cooling below their boiling points or by compressing the gas at room temperature. These two features are utilized in the filling of aerosol containers with propellant.

COLD FILLING. In the cold method, both the product concentrate and the propellant must be cooled to temperatures of −30° to −40°F. This temperature is necessary to liquefy the propellant gas. The cooling system may be a mixture of dry ice and acetone or a more elaborate refrigeration system. After the chilled product concentrate has been quantitatively metered into an equally cold aerosol container, the liquefied gas is added. The heavy vapors of the cold liquid propellant generally displace the air present in the container. However, in the process, some of the propellant vapors are also lost. When sufficient propellant has been added, the valve assembly is immediately inserted and crimped into place. Because of the low temperatures required, aqueous systems cannot be filled by this process, since the water turns to ice. For nonaqueous systems, some moisture usually appears in the final product due to the condensation of atmospheric moisture within the cold containers.

PRESSURE FILLING. By the pressure method, the product concentrate is quantitatively placed in the aerosol container (Fig. 13–5), the valve assembly is inserted and crimped into place, and the liquefied gas, under pressure, is metered into the valve stem from a pressure burette (Fig. 13–6). The desired amount of propellant is allowed to enter the container under its own vapor pressure. When the pressure in the container equals that in the burette, the propellant stops flowing. Additional propellant may be added by increasing the pressure in the filling apparatus through the use of compressed air or nitrogen gas. The trapped air in the package may be ignored if it does not interfere with the quality or stability of the product, or it may be evacuated prior to filling or during filling, using special apparatus. After filling the container with sufficient propellant, the valve actuator is tested for proper function. This spray testing also rids the dip tube of pure propellant prior to consumer use.

Pressure filling is used for most pharmaceutical aerosols. It has the advantage over the cold filling method in that there is less danger of mois-

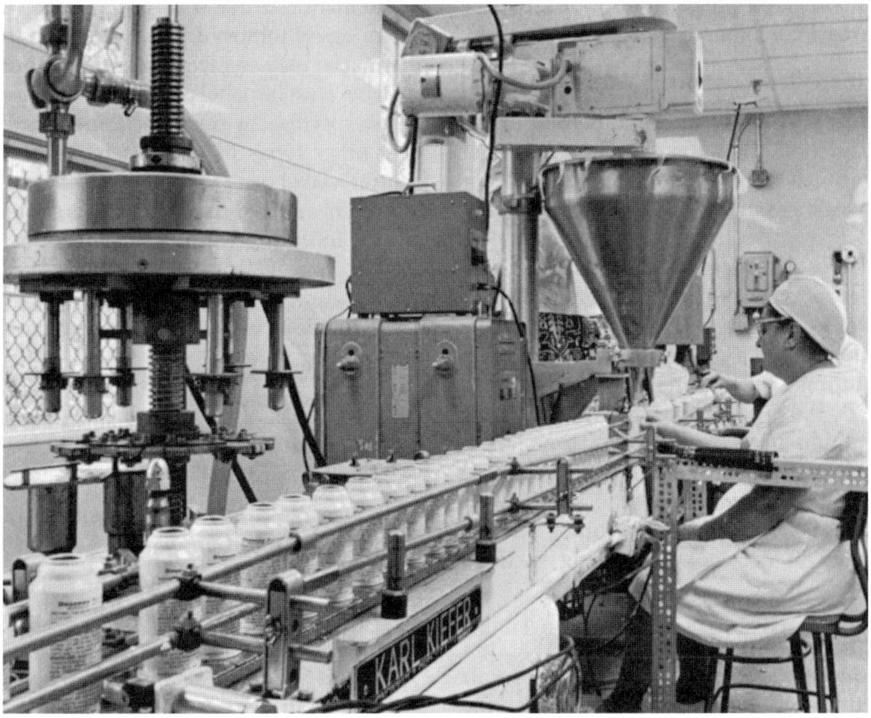

Fig. 13–5. *Filling the empty aerosol cans with the drug mixture. (Courtesy of Pennwalt Corp.)*

Fig. 13–6. *Pressure filling of aerosol containers. (Courtesy of Pennwalt Corp.)*

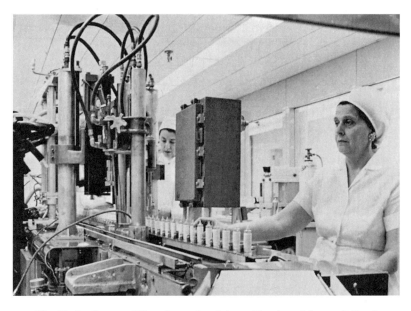

ture contamination of the product, and also less propellant is lost in the process.

When compressed gases are employed as the propellant in aerosol systems, the gas is transferred from large steel cylinders into the aerosol containers. Prior to filling, the product concentrate is quantitatively placed in the container, the valve assembly is crimped into place, and the air is evacuated from the container by a vacuum pump. The compressed gas is then passed into the container through a pressure reducing valve attached to the gas cylinder; when the pressure within the aerosol container is equal to the predetermined and regulated delivery pressure, the gas flow stops, and the aerosol valve is restored to the closed position. For gases like carbon dioxide and nitrous oxide, which are slightly soluble in the product concentrate, the container is manually or mechanically shaken during the filling operation to achieve the desired pressure in the headspace of the aerosol container.

Testing the Filled Containers

After filling by either the cold method or the pressure method, the aerosol container is tested under various environmental conditions for leaks or weakness in the valve assembly or container.

Filled aerosol containers are also tested for the proper function of the valve. The *valve discharge rate* is determined by discharging a portion of the contents of a previously weighed aerosol during a given period of time, and calculating, by the difference in weight, the grams of contents discharged per unit of time. As is deemed desirable, aerosols may be tested for their spray patterns, for particle size distribution of the spray, and for accuracy and reproducibility of dosage when using metered valves.

Packaging, Labeling, and Storage

A unique aspect of pharmaceutical aerosols compared to other dosage forms is that the product is actually packaged as part of the manufacturing process. With most other dosage forms, the product is completely manufactured and then placed in the appropriate container.

Most aerosol products have a protective cap or cover that fits snugly over the valve and mounting cup. This protects the valve against contamination with dust and dirt. The cap, which is generally made of plastic or metal, also serves a decorative function.

Medicinal aerosols that are to be dispensed only upon prescription usually may be labeled by the manufacturer with plastic peel-away labels or easily removed paper labels so that the pharmacist may easily replace the manufacturer's label with his label containing the directions for use specified by the prescribing practitioner. Most other types of aerosols have the manufacturer's label printed directly on the container or on firmly affixed paper.

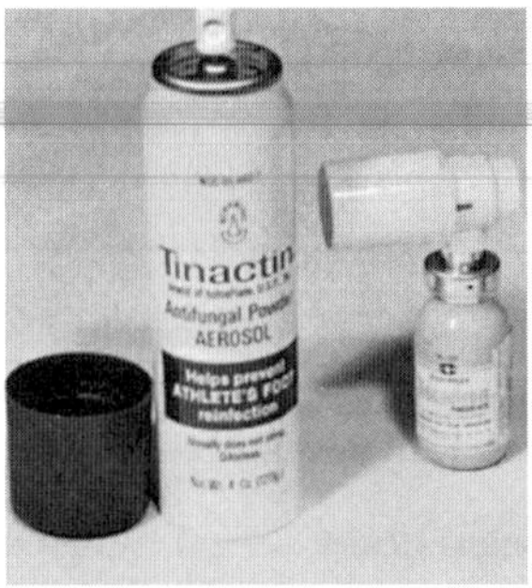

Fig. 13–7. *Examples of some pharmaceutical aerosols.*

In addition to the usual labeling requirements for pharmaceutical products, aerosols have special requirements related to their use and storage. For example, for safety, labels must warn users not to puncture pressurized containers, not to use or store them near heat or an open flame, and not to incinerate. Exposure to temperatures above 120°F may cause an aerosol container to burst. Most medications in aerosol containers are intended for use at ambient room temperatures. When the canisters are cold, less than the usual spray may result. This may be particularly important to users of metered dose inhalation sprays. These products are generally recommended for storage between 15°C and 30°C (36°F and 86°F). Pharmaceutical aerosols are labeled with regard to shaking before use, holding at the proper angle and/or distance from the target; there are special detailed instructions for inhaler devices.

Aerosols should be maintained with the protective caps in place to prevent accidental activation of the valve assembly or its contamination by dust and other foreign materials.

Examples of pharmaceutical aerosols are shown in Figure 13–7 and presented in Table 13–2.

Proper Administration and Use of Pharmaceutical Aerosols

The pharmacist should make every attempt to educate the patient about aerosol dosage forms, particularly for oral or nasal administration, be-

Table 13–2. Examples of Inhalation Aerosols

Aerosol	*Some Representative Commercial Products*	*Category and Comments*
Albuterol Inhalation Aerosol	Proventil Inhalation Aerosol (Schering) Ventolin Inhalation Aerosol (Allen & Hanburys)	Beta-adrenergic agonist indicated for the prevention and relief of bronchospasm in patients with reversible obstructive airway disease and for the relief of exercise-induced bronchospasm.
Beclomethasone Dipropionate Inhalation Aerosol	Beclovent Inhalation Aerosol (Allen & Hanburys) Vanceril Inhaler (Schering)	Adrenocortical steroid; aerosol for oral inhalation for control of bronchial asthma in patients requiring chronic treatment with corticosteroids with other therapy, e.g., xanthines, sympathiomimetics.
	Beconase Nasal Inhaler (Allen & Hanburys) Vancenase Pockethaler Nasal Inhaler (Schering)	Adrenocortical steroid; aerosol for intranasal relief of symptoms of seasonal or perennial rhinitis in those cases poorly responsive to conventional treatment.
Cromolyn Sodium Inhalation Aerosol	Intal Inhaler (Fisons)	An antiasthmatic, antiallergic and mast cell stabilizer; metered-dose aerosol for oral administration for prevention of exercise-induced bronchospasm, and for prevention of acute bronchospasm induced by environmental pollutants and known allergens.
Ipratropium Bromide Inhalation Aerosol	Atrovent Inhalation Aerosol (Boehringer Ingelheim)	Anticholinergic (parasympatholytic) agent used as a bronchodilator in the treatment of bronchospasm.
Isoetharine Mesylate Inhalation Aerosol	Bronkometer (Sanofi Winthrop)	Sympathomimetic for the temporary relief of bronchial asthma and other conditions of bronchospasm.
Metaproterenol Sulfate Inhalation Aerosol	Alupent Inhalation Aerosol (Boehringer Ingelheim)	Sympathomimetic for the relief of bronchospasm in patients with reversible obstructive airway disease.
Nedocromil Sodium Inhalation Aerosol	Tilade Inhaler (Fisons)	Maintenance therapy of patients with mild to moderate bronchial asthma.
Salmeterol Xinafoate Inhalation Aerosol	Serevent Inhalation Aerosol (Allen & Hanburys)	Beta-adrenergic agonist used in the long-term maintenance treatment of asthma and prevention of bronchospasm in patients with reversible obstructive airway disease.
Terbutaline Sulfate Inhalation Aerosol	Brethaire (Geigy)	Beta-adrenergic agonist indicated for the relief of bronchospasm.
Triamcinolone Acetonide Oral Inhaler	Azmacort (Rhone-Poulenc Rorer)	Indicated in patients who require chronic treatment with corticosteroids for the control of symptoms of bronchial asthma.
Triamcinolone Acetonide Topical Aerosol	Kenalog Spray (Westwood-Squibb)	Anti-inflammatory; applied topically to the affected area.

cause these are only effective when properly used. To complement verbal instructions the pharmacist should provide the patient with the written instructions found within the product package. It is difficult to predict what percentage of patients will read or even understand the printed instruction. Thus, the pharmacist must verbally transmit instruction for proper use. Using the oral, metered aerosols as a model, the pharmacist should demonstrate how the inhaler is assembled, stored and cleaned. The patient should be told whether the inhaler requires shaking before use and how to hold it between the index finger and thumb so that the aerosol canister is up-side-down. The patient should understand that coordination must be achieved between inhalation (after exhaling as completely as possible) and pressing down the inhaler to release one dose. The patient should be instructed to hold his breath for several seconds or as long as possible to gain the maximum benefit from the medication. The patient is told to then remove the inhaler from the mouth and exhale slowly through pursed lips.

Some patients are unable to use metered-dose inhalers properly. Thus, after a new prescription is dispensed, it is advisable for the pharmacist to follow up with the patient to make sure the patient is capable of using the inhaler. If the patient confides an inability to use the inhaler, it is advisable for the pharmacist to recommend to the patient or the patient's physician the use of an extender device with the inhaler. Extender devices or "spacers" were originally developed for patients who could not learn to coordinate release of the medication with inhalation. These are now considered an important therapeutic aid because they can effectively assist the delivery of medication despite improper patient inhalation technique. By placing an extender device between the metered-dose inhaler's mouthpiece and the patient's mouth, the patient is permitted to separate activation of the aerosol from inhalation by up to 3 to 5 seconds (a valve in the spacer opens when the patient inhales). Another advantage of the extender device is that aerosol velocity is reduced, and droplet size is decreased because there is time for evaporation of the fluorohydrocarbon propellant. Thus, extender devices also cause less deposition of medication in the oropharynx. Extender devices are available that can be used with most pressurized canisters, e.g., Brethancer Inhaler (Geigy) and InspirEase (Schering).

To ensure continuity of therapy it is wise for the pharmacist to share with the patient ways to assess how much medication is left in the canister (see Fig. 11–8, p. 418). This is important to ensure continuity of therapy, especially for those who suffer from respiratory illness and may need their medication on a moment's notice.

For topical administration of aerosol dosage forms, the patient should be told to first clean the affected area gently and to pat it dry. Holding the canister with the nozzle pointing toward the body area and about 6 to 8 inches away, the patient should press down the button to deliver enough medication to cover the area. The patient should allow the spray to dry and not cover the area with a bandage or dressing unless instructed to do so by the physician. The patient should avoid accidentally spraying the product into the eyes or mouth. If it is necessary to apply the product to a facial area, the patient should spray the product into the palm of the hand and apply it by this means.

Inhalations

Inhalations are drugs or solutions of drugs administered by the nasal or oral respiratory route. The drugs may be administered for their local action on the bronchial tree or for their systemic effects through absorption from the lungs. Certain gases, as oxygen and ether, are administered by inhalation as are finely powdered drug substances and solutions of drugs administered as fine mists. Sterile Water for Inhalation, USP and Sodium Chloride Inhalation, USP may be used as vehicles for inhalation solutions.

As noted in Table 13–2, a number of drug substances are administered through pressure packaged *inhalation aerosols,* as the type shown in Figure 13–4. In order for the inhaled drug substance or solution to reach the bronchial tree, the inhaled particles must be just a few microns in size.

A unique form of powder administration involves the inhalation of a micronized powder directly into the lungs using a special breath-activated device (Fig. 13–8). The drug present in the inhaled powder is cromolyn sodium, an agent used in the management of patients with severe perennial asthma. The drug is supplied to the patient in hard gelatin capsules as a powder mixture with the inert substance lactose. The particles of lactose are designed to be larger (30 to 60 μ) than the particles of cromolyn sodium powder (1 to 10 μ) and upon inhalation the cromolyn sodium passes deeply into the respiratory tract, whereas the lactose particles are retained in the

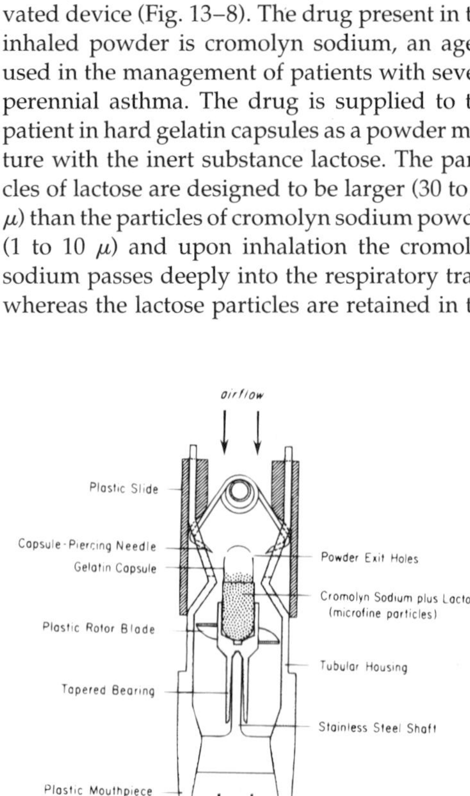

Fig. 13–8. *Cross section of the SPINHALER turbo inhaler, used in the administration of INTAL (cromolyn sodium, Fisons). (Courtesy of Fisons Corporation.)*

upper airways (Fig. 13–1). The powder in the capsule is prepared for inhalation by placing it in the special inhaler device. When ready for medication the patient makes two perforations in the capsule by a piercing mechanism present in the inhaler-device. When the mouth is placed on the mouth-piece and air inhaled, the turbo-vibratory action of the propeller causes the powdered drug to be dispensed into the inspired air through the perforations in the capsule wall.

A widely used instrument capable of producing fine particles for inhalation therapy is the *nebulizer.* This apparatus, shown in Figure 13–9, contains an atomizing unit within a curved, glass, bulb-like chamber. A rubber bulb at the end of the apparatus is depressed and the medicated solution is drawn up a narrow glass tube and broken into fine particles by the passing airstream. The fine particles produced range between 0.5 and 5 microns. The larger, heavier droplets of the mist do not exit the apparatus but fall back into the reservoir of medicated liquid. The lighter particles do escape with the airstream and are inhaled by the patient who operates the nebulizer with the exit orifice in his mouth, inhaling as he depresses the rubber bulb.

The pharmacist should advise the patient on the proper technique to use the nebulizer and provide additional patient instructions, e.g., do not exceed physician's instructions and use the smallest amount of product necessary to afford relief. The pharmacist could also advise on how to cope with dryness of the mouth that might occur. Further, the pharmacist should emphasize the need to clean the nebulizer after its use and explain how to do it.

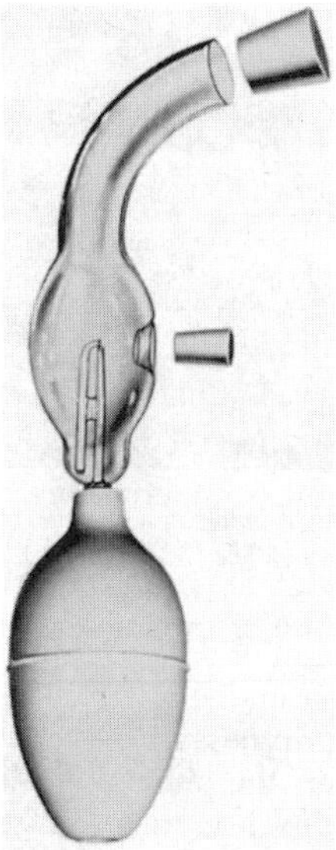

Fig. 13–9. *An example of a nebulizer used in inhalation therapy. See text for description of operation. (Courtesy of The DeVilbiss Co.)*

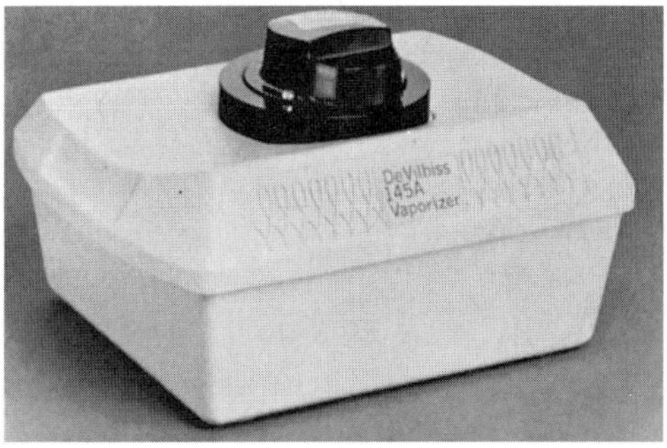

Fig. 13–10. *An example of commercially available vaporizer. (Courtesy of The DeVilbiss Co.)*

The common household *vaporizer,* as the one depicted in Figure 13–10, produces a fine mist of steam that may be used to humidify a room. When a volatile medication is added to the water in the chamber or to a special medication cup present in some models, the medication volatilizes and is also inhaled by the patient. *Humidifiers,* as shown in Figure 13–11, are employed to provide a cool mist to the air in a room. Moisture in the air is important to prevent mucous membranes of the nose and throat from becoming dry and irritated. Vaporizers and humidifiers are commonly used in the adjunctive treatment of colds, coughs, and chest congestion.

The pharmacist can help a patient select a va-

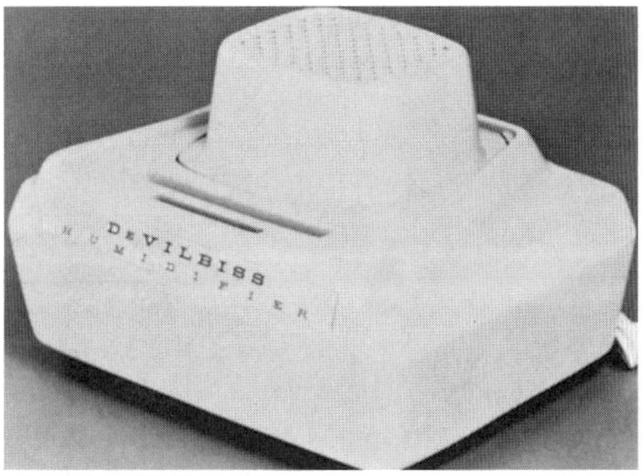

Fig. 13–11. *An example of a commercially available humidifier. (Courtesy of The DeVilbiss Co.)*

porizer or humidifier depending upon one's needs. Both devices have advantages and disadvantages. Manufacturing guidelines and legal regulations, e.g., lock tops, have made vaporizers more safe today than in the years past. So the possibility of scalding due to an overturned vaporizer is less with newer models. Further, the heat generated in a vaporizer kills the mold and bacteria that may be in the water tank. Humidifiers are more costly, but use less electricity than vaporizers. In addition, compared to vaporizers, humidifiers are noisier during operation, can leave a deposition of minerals on woodwork and furniture, and can effectively cool down a room by 1° to 3° (a problem with young children). The patient should learn about these subtle differences from the pharmacist.

Ultrasonic humidifiers are also available, and while they are effective and operate at an almost noiseless level, they apparently pose a health problem. While these are highly efficient at nebulizing water into fine droplets, they are also efficient at nebulizing up to 90% of water contaminants as well. These contaminants include mold, bacteria, lead, and dissolved organic gases, which could ultimately cause acute respiratory irritation to chronic lung problems in unsuspecting patients. Thus, patients should either be advised to run water through a high-grade demineralization filter before filling their ultrasonic humidifier, or buy a humidifier with a built-in filter that works.

Examples of Medicated Inhalations

As noted previously, a number of inhalations are pressure packaged as inhalation aerosols and were listed in Table 13–2. Several other inhalations used in medicine are solutions intended to be administered by nebulizer or other apparatus. Among these are: isoetharine inhalation solution (Bronkosol, Sanofi Winthrop) and isoproterenol inhalation solution (Isuprel Solution, Sanofi Winthrop), both used for the relief of bronchial spasms in the treatment of bronchial asthma and related conditions.

Inhalants

Inhalants are drugs or combinations of drugs that by virtue of their high vapor pressure can be carried by an air current into the nasal passage where they exert their effect. The device in which the drug or drugs is contained and from which they are administered is termed an *inhaler.*

Amyl Nitrite Inhalant

Amyl nitrite is a clear, yellowish, volatile liquid that acts as a vasodilator when inhaled. The drug is prepared in sealed glass vials which are covered with a protective gauze cloth (Fig. 13–12). Upon use, the glass vial is broken in the fingertips and the cloth soaks up the liquid which is then inhaled. The vials generally contain 0.3 mL of the drug substance. The effects of the drug are rapid and are used in the treatment of anginal pain.

Propylhexedrine Inhalant

Propylhexedrine is a liquid adrenergic (vasoconstrictor) agent that volatilizes slowly at room temperature. This quality enables it to be effectively used as an inhalant. The official inhalant consists of cylindrical rolls of suitable fibrous material impregnated with propylhexedrine, usually aromatized to mask its amine-like odor, and contained in a suitable inhaler. The vapor of the drug is inhaled into the nostrils when needed to relieve nasal congestion due to colds and hay fever. It may also be employed to relieve ear block and the pressure pain in air travelers.

Each plastic tube of the commercial product contains 250 mg of propylhexedrine with aromatics. The containers should be tightly closed after each opening to prevent loss of the drug vapors. The counterpart commercial product is Benzedrex Inhaler (Menley & James).

Sprays

Sprays may be defined as aqueous or oleaginous solutions in the form of coarse droplets or as finely divided solids to be applied topically, most usually to the nasal-pharyngeal tract or to the skin. Many commercially available sprays are used intranasally to relieve nasal congestion and inflammation and to combat infection and contain antihistamines, sympathomimetic agents, and antibiotic substances. Because of the noninvasive nature and quickness with which nasal sprays can deliver medication systemically, the future will demonstrate the administration of several drugs by this route that typically have been administered by other routes of administration. Most notably, insulin and glucagon will be administered in this fashion. Research has

Fig. 13–12. *Silking operation in the production of amyl nitrate Vaporole. (Courtesy of Burroughs Wellcome Company.)*

demonstrated that the administration of glucagon, for example, via a nasal spray can relieve hypoglycemic symptoms within 7 minutes, a definite advantage over conventional emergency intravenous glucose or intramuscular glucagon.

Other sprays are employed against sunburn and heat burn and contain local anesthetics, antiseptics, skin protectants, and antipruritics. Throat sprays containing antiseptics, deodorants, and flavorants may be effectively employed to relieve conditions such as halitosis, sore throat, or laryngitis. Other sprays may be employed to treat athlete's foot and other fungal infections. Numerous other medicinal and cosmetic uses of sprays are commonly available in pharmacies.

To achieve the breaking up of a solution into small particles so that it may be effectively sprayed or to facilitate the spraying of a powder, several mechanical devices have been developed and are commonly employed. The plastic spray bottle, which is gently squeezed to issue a spray

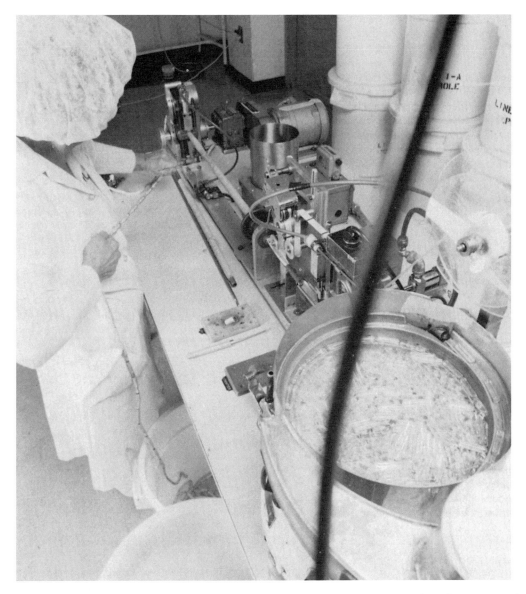

of its contents, is familiar to most persons. It is commonly used for nasal decongestant sprays as well as cosmetically, especially for body deodorant products. Recently, one-way pump sprays have been developed to deliver medication into the nose. These sprays are used for both legend, e.g., Nasalide (Syntex), and nonlegend, e.g., Nostrilla (Boehringer Ingelheim), medicines. The advantage of these over the conventional sprays is that its design prevents drawback contamination of nasal fluids into the bottle after administration, a definite advantage for someone trying to cope with viruses associated with the common cold. Pharmacists are familiar with medicinal *atomizers*, which are employed for the issuance of a medicated solution to the patient in the form of fine droplets (Fig. 13–13). One type of atomizer operates by the squeezing of a rubber bulb at the end of the apparatus, which causes a flow of air partially to enter the glass reservoir in which the solution is held and partially to exit from the opposite end of the system. The air forced into the reservoir causes the liquid to rise in a small dip tube, which is maintained below the level of the liquid, forcing the solution up and into the stream of air exiting the system. The air and the solution are forced through a jet opening and the liquid is broken up into a spray, the droplets being carried by the airstream. In other similar apparatuses, the stream of air caused by the depression of the bulb does not enter the reservoir of solution, but passes swiftly over it, creating a pressure change that causes a sucking up of the liquid into the dip tube and into the airstream in which it exits the system. In instances in which powdered substances are employed rather than solutions, a *powder blower* or a powder *insufflator* may be employed to produce a powder spray. Such an apparatus is similar to the atomizer for liquids; the squeezing of the rubber bulb causes a turbulence within the reservoir of powder, forcing some up the dip tube

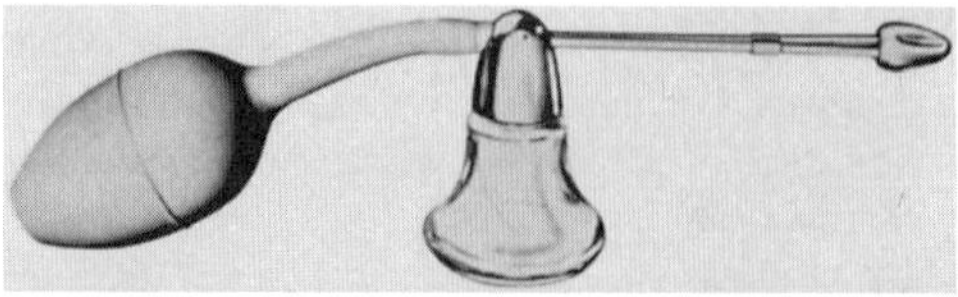

Fig. 13–13. *A common type of atomizer for the administration of a spray of liquid medication. The model shown has an adjustable tip for directing the spray upward or downward to reach otherwise inaccessible areas of the throat. (Courtesy of The DeVilbiss Co.)*

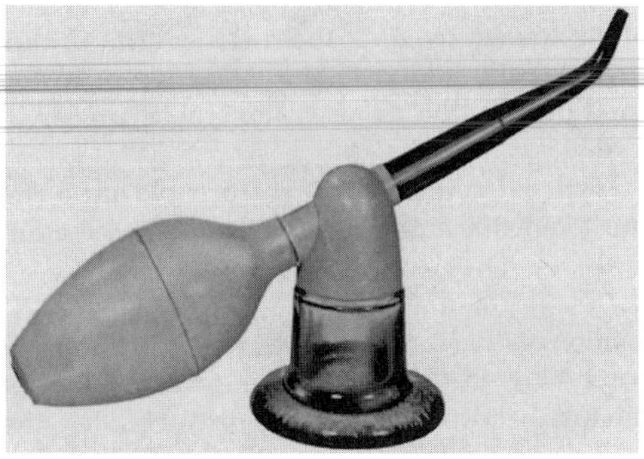

Fig. 13–14. *A general purpose insufflator, used in the application of powdered substances to the nose, throat, ear, tooth sockets, or to body surfaces. (Courtesy of The DeVilbiss Co.)*

and out of the tip of the apparatus by the exiting airstream (Fig. 13–14).

Proper Administration and Use of Nasal Sprays

Before using the drops the patient should be advised to gently blow the nose to clear the nostrils. The patient should be told not to shake the plastic squeeze bottle for use, but be sure to remove the plastic cap. While holding the head upright the patient should insert the nose-piece into the nostril, pointing it slightly backward, and close the other nostril with one finger. The patient should then spray the prescribed or recommended amount, squeezing the bottle sharply and firmly while sniffing through the nose. Sprays should always be administered with the patient in an upright position. Spraying medicine into the nostrils should not be performed with the head over the edge of a bed (the preferred procedure for administration of nasal drops) because it could result in the systemic absorption of the drug, rather than a local effect.

The patient should be advised not to overuse the product. For example, some decongestant medicines such as oxymetazoline and xylometazoline can predispose the patient to rebound congestion if used for more than three to five consecutive days. The patient should also understand the normal time frame in which to see results and be advised that after a certain number of days if relief is not achieved to consult the physician. Lastly, patients should realize not to share their medicated spray with another person to prevent the possibility of cross-contamination between individuals.

Examples of Medicated Sprays

A number of nasal solutions are commercially packaged in plastic spray-bottles for use as sprays. Among these are:

Flunisolide Nasal Solution [Nasalide (Syntex)]
Oxymetrazoline Hydrochloride Nasal Solution, USP [Afrin Nasal Spray (Schering-Plough)]
Phenylephrine Hydrochloride Nasal Solution, USP [Neo-Synephrine Hydrochloride Nasal Spray (Sterling Health)]
Sodium Chloride Nasal Solution [Salinex Solution (Muro)]
Xylometazoline Hydrochloride Nasal Solution [Sine-Off (SmithKline Beecham Consumer)]

References

1. Chiou, W.L.: Aerosol Propellants: Cardiac Toxicity and Long Biological Half-Life. *JAMA, 227*:658, 1974.
2. Cyr, T.D., et al.: Low First-Spray Drug Content in Albuterol Metered-Dose Inhalers. *Pharm. Res., 8:* 658–660, 1991.
3. Miller, N.C., et al.: Assessment of the Twin Impinger for Size Measurement of Metered-Dose Inhaler Sprays. *Pharm. Res., 9:*1123–1127, 1992.
4. Ranucci, J.A. and Chen, F.C.: Phase Doppler Anemometry: A Technique for Determining Aerosol Plume-Particle Size and Velocity. *Pharm. Tech., 17:* 62–73, 1993.
5. Ranucci, J.A., Cooper, D., and Sethachutkul, K.: Effect of Actuator Design on Metered-Dose Inhaler Plume-Particle Size. *Pharm. Tech., 16:*84–92, 1992.
6. Martonen, T.B., and Katz, I.M.: Deposition of Aerosolized Drugs Within Human Lungs: Effects of Ventilatory Parameters. *Pharm. Res., 10:*871–878, 1993.
7. Martonen, T.B., et al.: Use of Analytically Defined Estimates of Aerosol Respirable Fraction to Predict Lung Deposition Patterns. *Pharm. Res., 9:*1634–1639, 1992.

14

Radiopharmaceuticals and Miscellaneous Preparations

Radiopharmaceuticals

A RADIOPHARMACEUTICAL is a chemical containing a radioactive isotope for use in humans for the purpose of diagnosis, mitigation, or treatment of a disease. It should be recalled from general chemistry that substances that have the same number of protons but have varying numbers of neutrons are called *isotopes*. Isotopes may be stable or unstable; those that are unstable are radioactive because their nuclei undergo a rearrangement while changing to a stable state, and energy is given off.

All of the atoms of an unstable isotope do not completely rearrange at the same instant. The time required for a radioisotope to decay to 50% of its original activity is termed its radioactive half-life. Isotopes vary widely in their half-life; carbon-14 has a radioactive half-life of some 5730 years, whereas that for sodium-24 is only 15 hours.

The activity of a radiactive material is expressed as the number of nuclear transformations per unit time.

The half-life ($T_{1/2}$) may be calculated by the equation:

$$T_{1/2} = \frac{0.69315}{\lambda}$$

where λ is the transformation or decay constant, which has a characteristic value for each radionuclide.

The fundamental unit of radioactivity is the *curie* (Ci), defined as 3.700×10^{10} nuclear transformations per second. The *millicurie* (mCi), *microcurie* (μCi), and *nanocurie* (nCi) are commonly used subunits:

$$1 \text{ millicurie} = 10^3 \text{ curie}$$

$$1 \text{ microcurie} = 10^6 \text{ curie}$$

$$1 \text{ nanocurie} = 10^9 \text{ curie}$$

The Becquerel (Bq) is the international unit of radiactivity and is equal to one disintegration per second, i.e., 1 mCi = 37 MBq (megabecquerels). The amount of radiation absorbed by body tissue in which a radioactive substance resides is called the "radiation dose." Traditionally, this is measured in units of rads (i.e., *r*adiation *a*bsorbed *d*ose); 1 rad = 100 ergs of energy absorbed by 1 g of tissue. The Gray is the international unit of absorbed dose and equal to 1 joule of energy absorbed in 1 kg of tissue (i.e., 1 Gy = 100 rads).

The three types of radiation most frequently emitted from radioactive nuclei are *alpha, beta,* and *gamma* radiations. Alpha particles, which constitute alpha radiation, consist of two protons and two neutrons, thus being identical with the helium nucleus. As an alpha particle loses energy, its velocity decreases. It then attracts electrons and becomes a helium atom. Most alpha particles are unable to pierce the outer layers of skin or penetrate a thin piece of paper. Beta particles may be either electrons with negative charge, *negatrons*, or positive electrons, *positrons*. These two particles, β and β^+, have a range of over 100 feet in air and up to about 1 mm in tissue. Nuclear medicine depends mostly on radiopharmaceuticals that decay by gamma (γ) emission. Gamma rays are electromagnetic vibrations comparable with light but of much shorter wavelength. Because of their short wavelength and high energy, they are very penetrating.

The optimum dosage of radiopharmaceuticals is that which allows the acquisition of the desired information with the least amount of radiation dose or exposure to the patient. Thus, the clinical utility of a radiopharmaceutical is determined by the radionuclide's physical properties (e.g., radiation, energy, half-life). Thus, the best diagnostic images at the lowest radiation dose are attained if the radionuclide has a short half-life and emits only gamma radiation of low energy. Technetium-99m is a prime example of a radionuclide with these properties. Its half-life is 6 hours and gamma emission is of the nature of 140 keV, efficiently detected by the gamma camera. For therapeutic use, however, radionuclides should emit particulate radiation (i.e., beta particles), which deposits the radiation within the target organ. Iodine-131 is a prime example and used for hyperthyroidism and eradication of metastatic disease of the thyroid gland. But because iodine-131 emits both beta and gamma radiation, it can be used diagnostically (gamma rays) and therapeutically (beta rays).

The majority of radiopharmaceuticals are produced by the process of nuclear activation in a nuclear reactor. In such a reactor, stable atoms are bombarded with excess neutrons present in the reactor. The resulting neutron additions to the stable atoms produce unstable atoms and radioactive isotopes. The facilities for the production, use, and storage of radioactive pharmaceuticals are subject to licensing by the Nuclear Regulatory Commission, or in certain instances to appropriate state agencies. As for all pharmaceuticals, the Federal Food and Drug Administration enforces strict adherence to good manufacturing practice and proper labeling and use of the products. The Federal Department of Transportation regulates the conditions of shipment of the radiopharmaceuticals, as do state and local agencies.

Radiopharmaceuticals are used to diagnose the presence of disease or evaluate the progression of disease following specific therapy intervention. Radiopharmaceuticals can also be used to evaluate drug-induced toxicity, and to a less extent have been utilized to treat diseased tissue with radiation.

The distribution pattern of radiopharmaceuticals can be used for imaging purposes to attain diagnostic information about organs or various body systems.[1] Imaging procedures are classified either as *dynamic* or *static*. The dynamic study provides useful information through the rate of accumulation and removal of the radiopharmaceutical from a specific organ. A static study merely provides morphological information, i.e., organ size, shape, position, presence of space occupying lesions.

Every radiopharmaceutical is formulated with the intent to localize it within a target organ. Sodium iodide, I-131, is actively taken up by thyroid cells following its absorption into the bloodstream after oral administration from either a capsule or a solution dosage form. The extent of the uptake of the dose by the gland helps assess thyroid function, or an image of the gland can be obtained after administration to visualize, i.e., static imaging, thyroid morphology. Alternatively, if I-131 is labeled to orthoiodohippuric acid and intravenously injected, kidney tubules will actively secrete this agent into urine. Measuring the time course of activity over the kidney with a gamma camera and plotting the rate of radioactivity accumulation and removal *versus* time, yields a measure of kidney function. Such a dynamic study is termed a *renogram*, a particularly useful procedure to assess renal function in patients with transplanted kidneys.

Radiopharmaceuticals also are useful to evaluate a patient's response to drug therapy and surgery. These agents can detect early changes in physiologic function which come before morphologic or biochemical endpoints. An example is perfusion lung imaging using Tc-99 macroaggregated albumin particles to detect pulmonary embolism. Once the embolism is confirmed and thrombolytic and/or anticoagulant therapy initiated, this lung perfusing agent can be readministered to evaluate its resolution with drug therapy. Cardiac radionuclide ventriculograms utilizing Tc-99m labeled red blood cells are performed to assess left ventricular function (e.g., ejection fraction, regional wall motion) to evaluate the effect of surgery (e.g., coronary artery bypass graft, valve repair) or the response to drug therapy (e.g., beta-blocking agents, calcium channel blocking agents).

Radiopharmaceuticals also find utility to help monitor drug therapy inclusive of toxicity. For example, the ability of doxorubicin to cause irreversible drug-induced heart failure is well known and the cumulative dosage of this drug should not exceed 550 mg/m^2. Because there is much variability in the individual response to this drug, serial determinations of left ventricular ejection fraction using Tc-99m radiopharmaceuticals are useful to determine on an individual basis the risk of developing doxorubicin-induced heart failure.

To a limited degree, radiopharmaceuticals can be used therapeutically. Thyroid disease can be treated with sodium iodide, I-131, polycythemia vera can be treated with sodium phosphate, P-32, and peritoneal effusions can be treated with chromic phosphate, P-32. The intent is to use the beta radiation of the radiopharmaceutical to selectively destroy diseased tissue in which it resides. Thus, a minimum, sufficient dosage must be administered. In the case of I-131, the therapeutic dosage is between 1000 to 10000 times greater than the diagnostic dosage used to assess organ function. The major indications for radioiodine therapy include hyperthyroidism (e.g., diffuse toxic goiter [Graves' disease], toxic multinodular goiter) and eradication of metastatic disease (i.e., thyroid cancer).

A number of new areas of nuclear medicine are emerging, including the use of radiolabeled monoclonal antibodies (MAbs) in the imaging and treatment of targeted cancer cells. For example, Cytogen Corporation, a biotechnology company, has developed linker payload systems with the attachment of diagnostic (OncoScint Colorectal and OncoScint Ovarian) or therapeutic substances (cancer-cell-killing yttrium in OncoRad Ovarian and OncoRad Prostate systems) on the carbohydrate region of monoclonal antibodies. After injection, the monoclonal antibodies bind to the targeted tumor antigen to facilitate diagnosis or treatment. Peptides are being investigated to succeed antibodies as delivery vehicles for linked diagnostic or therapeutic agents. Peptides would have the advantage over MAbs of being more rapidly cleared from the body with a potentially lower level of toxicity.

Radiopharmaceuticals

Examples of some radiopharmaceuticals are presented below. The category for each indicates the types of cells or tissues for which the isotope has an affinity.

- Cyanocobalamin Co 57 Capsules—Diagnostic aid (pernicious anemia)
- Iodinated I 125 Serum Albumin Injection—Diagnostic aid (blood volume determination)
- Iodohippurate Sodium I 131 Injection—Diagnostic aid (renal function)
- Sodium Chromate Cr 51 Injection—Diagnostic aid (blood volume determination)
- Sodium Iodide I 131 Capsules—Diagnostic aid (thyroid function); thyroid inhibitor
- Sodium Iodide I 131 Solution—Diagnostic aid (thyroid function); thyroid inhibitor
- Sodium Pertechnetate Tc 99m Injection—Diagnostic aid (brain scanning; thyroid scanning)
- Sodium Phosphate P 32 Solution—Antipolycythemic; diagnostic aid (ocular tumor localization)
- Technetium Tc 99m Albumin Aggregated Injection—Diagnostic aid (lung scanning)
- Technetium Tc 99m Sulfur Colloid Injection—Diagnostic aid (liver scanning)
- Technetium Tc-99m labeled red blood cells—Diagnostic aid (cardiac blood pool imaging)
- Technetium Tc-99m methylene diphosphonate (MDP)—Diagnostic aid (bone imaging)
- Technetium Tc-99m pyrophosphate (PYP)—Diagnostic aid (cardiac infarct imaging)
- Technetium Tc-99m sulfur colloid cooked in scrambled eggs—Diagnostic aid (gastric emptying imaging)

Positron Emission Tomography

An interesting new area within nuclear pharmacy is positron emission tomography (PET).[2,3] It is a method for quantitative imaging of regional function and chemical reactions within various organs of the living human body. Basically, this procedure allows the physician and pharmacist to obtain a patient image that is essentially a low-resolution "autoradiograph" showing the regional concentration of a positron-emitting nuclide inside of the living body. In fact no other technology can image body chemistry with such sensitivity, so that the moment-to-moment change in concentration of a tracer in the blood or tissue can be determined in absolute units. Other imaging modalities, such as x ray computed tomography (CT) and magnetic resonance imaging (MRI), provide predominantly anatomic information. CT scanning is based on the portrayal of the distribution of attenuation of x rays passing through the body. MRI exploits the variation in regional concentrations of hydrogen and nuclear relaxation parameters to generate image contrast and to provide information about free water content, relative blood flow and the concentration of contrast agents.

Chemical changes occur prior to anatomic changes in most disease states, and PET offers the advantage of being capable to detect functional abnormalities before anatomic changes have occurred. It has already been introduced in epilepsy, Huntington's disease, cerebrovascular disease, coronary artery disease and recently as a means to assess estrogen receptors in primary and metastatic breast cancers. In epilepsy, PET and surface electroencephalography (EEG) are used in concert with clinical assessment of symptoms and signs to try to localize areas of the brain that are the foci of epileptic seizures when surgical intervention is the only remaining method to prevent the seizures.

In tissue, a positron travels only about 1 mm before it encounters a negative electron. Their interaction results in the simultaneous emission of two photons, each having a specific energy and emitted at an angle of exactly 180° from each other. Thus, if two scintillation detectors are placed, one on either side of the tissue in which the isotope is located, and detectors connected to a coincident circuit which provides an output only when a certain level of gamma ray radiation can be simultaneously detected by both, the result is a low background detector, highly specific for the particular isotope used and also giving excellent resolution.

The major production source of isotopes for PET are in-house cyclotrons, a very expensive proposition. Thus, PET is conducted primarily in large medical centers. Another consideration is that PET nuclides have short half-lives (e.g., 2 to 20 minutes) which makes their availability from commercial sources almost nonexistent. By the time the nuclear pharmacist would receive the nuclide it would already be gone. Out of necessity the production facility must be on site and after rapid synthesis, the pharmaceutical needs to be purified. Thus, research at present focuses upon noncyclotron, e.g., radionuclide generators, sources of PET nuclides that would allow PET technology in community-based nuclear medicine/pharmacy environments.

It is anticipated that studies of new drug entities in the future will include pharmacokinetic determination using PET technology. Further, PET will allow the manufacturer actually to quantify how much of the drug reaches a specific drug receptor. Thus, comparative PET studies will shed light on which drug, for example, within a therapeutic category attains the most optimal distribution and concentration at the intended receptor site. It is also conceivable that PET technology will open new vistas for the interpretation of drug interactions, particularly where there is competition by two drugs for one receptor site.

The following is an abbreviated listing of some positron-emitting radiopharmaceuticals used for common PET imaging procedures:

- [^{15}O]-O_2—Cerebral oxygen extraction and metabolism
- [^{11}C]-n-butanol—Cerebral blood flow
- [^{11}C]-glucose—Cerebral glucose metabolism
- [^{13}N]-ammonia—Cerebral and myocardial blood flow
- [^{18}F]-fluorodeoxyglucose—Cerebral and myocardial glucose metabolism
- [^{18}F]-16-alpha-fluoro-17-beta-estradiol—Estrogen receptor binding
- [^{68}Ga]-citrate/transferrin—Plasma volume

The Practice of Nuclear Pharmacy

Nuclear pharmacy is a patient-oriented service that embodies the scientific knowledge and professional judgment required to improve and promote health through the assurance of the safe and efficacious use of radioactive drugs for diagnosis and therapy. The pharmacist is expected to understand nuclear medicine procedures, their advantages and disadvantages, when used for diagonstic or therapeutic purposes. The practice is composed of the following general areas: the procurement of radiopharmaceuticals, the compounding of radiopharmaceuticals, the performance of routine quality control procedures, the dispensing and distribution of radiopharmaceuticals, the implementation of basic radiation protection procedures and practices, the consultation and education to the nuclear medicine community, e.g., patients, health professionals, general public, and research and development of new formulations.

In a typical nuclear pharmacy environment the daily routine of the nuclear pharmacist begins with the elution of the Technetium Tc-99m generator, preparation of Tc-99m labeled radiopharmaceuticals for the day's studies, performing quality control tests on these agents and on radiation measuring instruments and receiving prepared radiopharmaceuticals from commercial manufacturers. Because most radiopharmaceuticals are administered intravenously, the nuclear pharmacist must also take precaution to ensure the sterility of these products against microbial and foreign contamination, as well as for personal protection against radiation exposure.

Prior to administration to the patient, the nuclear pharmacist reviews the prescription or hospital order that has been signed by the authorized nuclear medicine physician. Radioactive decay calculations are made, and the required dosage is prepared and radioassayed to assure the correct amount of radioactivity. The drug product is then labeled and appropriately shielded prior to release for patient use.

The nuclear pharmacist must also be prepared to handle encountered questions about the clinical use of radiopharmaceuticals. Much like inquiries about non-radioactive drugs questions center on the pharmacokinetic properties of radiopharmaceuticals, adverse effects encountered with radiopharmaceuticals, dosing questions (e.g., pediatric, pregnancy), and alternative routes of administration.

Nuclear pharmacy was the first specialty in pharmacy recognized by the Board of Pharmaceutical Specialties (BPS).

Miscellaneous Preparations

Tinctures, Fluidextracts, Extracts

Certain pharmaceutical preparations are prepared by the process of *extraction*—that is, by the withdrawal of desired constituents from crude drugs through the use of selected solvents in which the desired constituents are soluble. *Crude drugs* are vegetable or animal drugs that have undergone no other processes than collection, cleaning, and drying. Because each crude drug contains a number of constituents that may be soluble in a given solvent, the products of extraction, termed *extractives,* do not contain just a single constituent but rather varying numbers of constituents, depending upon the drug used and the conditions of the extraction. *Tinctures, fluidextracts* and *extracts* are the pharmaceutical products most commonly prepared from extractives.

Plant materials are composed of heterogeneous mixtures of constituents, some of which are pharmacologically active and others that are pharmacologically inactive and considered inert. Among the varied plant constituents are sugars, starches, mucilages, proteins, albumins, pectins, cellulose, gums, inorganic salts, fixed and volatile oils, resins, tannins, coloring materials, and a number of very active constituents such as alkaloids and glycosides. The solvent systems used in extraction are selected on the basis of their capacity to dissolve the maximum amount of desired active constituents and the minimum amount of undesired constituents.

In many instances the *active* constituents of a plant drug are of the same general chemical type, have similar solubility characteristics and can be simultaneously extracted with a single solvent or a single solvent-mixture. The process of extraction concentrates the active constituents of a crude drug and removes from it the extraneous matter. In drug extraction, the solvent or solvent-mixture is referred to as the *menstruum,* and the plant residue, which is exhausted of active constituents, is termed the *marc.*

The selection of the menstruum to use in the extraction of a crude drug is based primarily upon the relative solubility in it of the active constituents. Although water and alcohol and, to a lesser extent, glycerin are probably the most frequently employed solvents in drug extraction, acetic acid and organic solvents like ether may be used for special purposes.

Because of its ready availability, cheapness, and good solvent action for many plant constituents, water has some use in drug extraction, particularly in combination with other solvents. However, as a sole solvent it has many disadvantages and is infrequently used alone. For one thing, most active plant constituents are complex organic chemical compounds that are less soluble in water than in alcohol. Although water has a great solvent action on such plant constituents as sugars, gums, starches, coloring principles, and tannins, most of these are not particularly desirable components of an extracted preparation. Water also tends to extract plant principles which upon standing in the extractive later separate leaving an undesired residue. Finally, unless preserved, aqueous preparations serve as excellent growth media for molds, yeasts, and bacteria. When water alone is employed as the menstruum, alcohol is frequently added to the extractive or to the final preparation as an antimicrobial preservative.

Hydroalcoholic mixtures are perhaps the most versatile and most widely employed menstruums. They combine the solvent effects of both water and alcohol, and the complete miscibility of these two agents permits a flexible combining of the two agents to form solvent mixtures most suited to the extraction of the active principles from a particular drug. A hydroalcoholic menstruum generally provides inherent protection against microbial contamination and helps to prevent the separation of extracted material on standing. Alcohol is used alone as a menstruum only when necessary because it is more expensive than hydroalcoholic mixtures.

Glycerin, a good solvent for many plant substances, is occasionally employed as a cosolvent with water or alcoholic menstruums because of its ability to extract and then prevent inert materials from precipitating upon standing. It is especially useful in this regard in preventing the separation of tannin and tannin oxidation products in extractives. Because glycerin has preservative action, depending upon its concentration in the final product, it may contribute to the stability of a pharmaceutical extractive.

Methods of Extraction

The principal methods of drug extraction are maceration and percolation. Generally, the method of extraction selected for a given drug depends on several factors, as the nature of the crude drug, its adaptability to each of the various extraction methods, and the interest in obtaining complete or near-complete extraction of the drug.

Frequently a combination of maceration and percolation is actually employed in the extraction of a crude drug. The drug is macerated first to soften the plant tissues and to dissolve much of the active constituents, and the percolation process is then conducted to achieve the separation of the extractive from the marc.

MACERATION. The term *maceration* comes from the Latin *macerare,* meaning "to soak." It is a process in which the properly comminuted drug is permitted to soak in the menstruum until the cellular structure is softened and penetrated by the menstruum and the soluble constituents are dissolved.

In the maceration process, the drug to be extracted is generally placed in a wide-mouth container with the prescribed menstruum, the vessel is stoppered tightly, and the contents are agitated repeatedly over a period usually ranging from 2 to 14 days. The agitation permits the repeated flow of fresh solvent over the entire surface area of the comminuted drug. An alternative to this repeated shaking is to place the drug in a porous cloth bag that is tied and suspended in the upper portion of the menstruum, much the same as a tea bag is suspended in water in the preparation of a cup of tea. As the soluble constituents dissolve in the menstruum, they tend to settle to the bottom because of an increase in the specific gravity of the liquid due to its added weight. Occasional dipping of the drug bag may facilitate the speed of the extraction. The extractive is separated from the marc by expressing the bag of drug and washing it with additional fresh menstruum, the washings being added to the extractive. If the maceration is performed with an unbagged drug, the marc may be removed by straining and/or filtration, with the marc being washed free of extractive by the additional passage of menstruum through the strainer or filter into the total extractive.

For drugs containing little or no cellular material, such as benzoin, aloe and tolu, which dissolve almost completely in the menstruum, maceration is the most efficient method of extraction.

Maceration is usually conducted at a temperature of between 15° to 20°C for a period of 3 days or until the soluble matter is dissolved.

PERCOLATION. The term *percolation,* from the Latin *per,* meaning "through," and *colare,* meaning "to strain," may be described generally as a process in which a comminuted drug is extracted of its soluble constituents by the slow passage of a suitable solvent through a column of the drug. The drug is packed in a special extraction apparatus termed a *percolator,* with the extractive collected called the *percolate.* Most drug extractions are performed by percolation.

In the process of percolation the flow of the menstruum over the drug column is generally downward to the exit orifice, drawn by the force of gravity as well as the weight of the column of liquid. In certain specialized and more sophisticated percolation apparatus, additional pressure on the column is exerted with positive air pressure at the inlet and suction at the outlet or exit.

Percolators for drug extraction vary greatly as to their shape, capacities, composition, and, most important, their utility. Percolators employed in the large-scale industrial preparation of extractives are generally made of stainless steel or are glass-lined large metal vessels that vary greatly in size and in operation. Percolators used to extract leaves, for instance, may be 6 to 8 feet in diameter and 12 to 18 feet high (Fig. 14–1). Percolators employed to extract other vegetable parts like seeds that are greater in density than leaves and would pack too tightly in percolators of such large dimensions are extracted in much smaller percolators. Some special industrial percolators are designed to percolate with hot menstruums; in others pressure is utilized to force the menstruum through the drug columns.

Percolation on a small scale generally involves

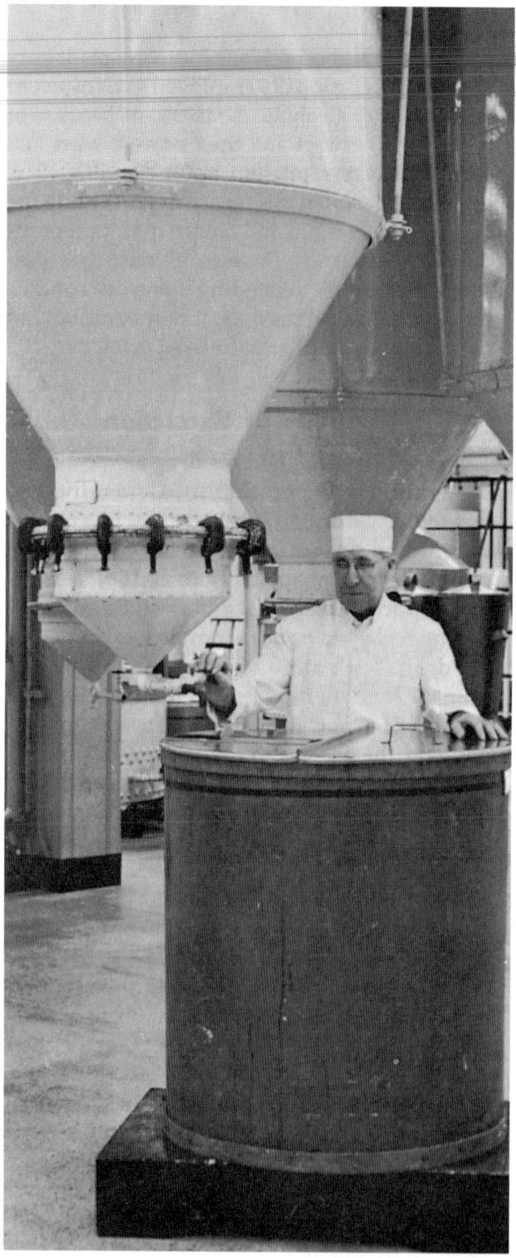

Fig. 14–1. *Large industrial percolators used in extracting crude drugs to make fluidextracts, tinctures, and powdered extracts. (Courtsey of the Upjohn Company.)*

the use of glass percolators of various shapes for extraction of small amounts (perhaps up to 1000 g) of crude drug. The shape of percolators in common laboratory and small-scale use are generally (a) cylindrical, with little if any taper except for the lower orifice; (b) cylindrical-like, but with a definite taper downward; and (c) conical, or funnel-shaped. Each type has a special utility in drug extraction.

The cylindrical percolator is particularly suited to the complete extraction of drugs with a minimal expenditure of menstruum. By the passage of the menstruum over the drug contained in a high, narrow column (rather than in a lower, wider column), each drug particle is more repeatedly exposed to passing solvent. A funnel-shaped percolator is useful for the percolation of drugs that swell a great deal during the maceration process, since the large upper surface permits the expansion of the drug column with little risk of a too tightly packed column or breakage of a glass percolator.

Tinctures

Tinctures are alcoholic or hydroalcoholic solutions prepared from vegetable materials or from chemical substances. They vary widely in their method of preparation, the strength of their active ingredient, their alcoholic content, and their intended use in medicine or pharmacy. When they are prepared from chemical substances (e.g., iodine, thimerosal, etc.) tinctures are prepared by simple solution of the chemical agent in the solvent.

Depending upon the preparation, tinctures contain alcohol in amounts ranging from approximately 15 to 80%. The alcoholic content protects against microbial growth and keeps the alcohol-soluble extractives in solution. In addition to alcohol, other solvents, as glycerin, may be employed. The solvent mix of each tincture is important in maintaining the integrity of the product. Tinctures cannot generally be mixed successfully with liquids too diverse in solvent character without the likelihood of inducing the precipitation of the solute. For example, compound benzoin tincture, prepared with alcohol as the sole menstruum, contains alcohol-soluble principles that are immediately expelled from solution upon the addition of water.

Because of the alcoholic content, tinctures must be tightly stoppered and not exposed to excessive temperatures. Also, because many of the constituents found in tinctures undergo a photochemical change upon exposure to light, many tinctures must be stored in light-resistant containers and protected from sunlight.

Medicated tinctures taken orally are a thing of the past. For one thing, they are bad-tasting. A person requiring oral medication nowadays would prefer to take a tablet or capsule or a pleasant-tasting elixir or syrup. Secondly, physicians prefer to prescibe single drugs and not preparations of plant extractives which contain many plant constituents, both active and inactive. Thirdly, since tinctures generally have a rather high alcoholic content, some physicians and patients alike prefer other forms of medication.

Fluidextracts

Fluidextracts are liquid preparations of vegetable drugs, prepared by percolation. They contain alcohol as a solvent or as a preservative, or both, and are made so that each mL contains the therapeutic constituents of 1 g of the standard drug that it represents. Because of their concentrated nature, many fluidextracts are considered too potent to be taken safely in self-administration by the patient and their use *per se* is almost nonexistent in medical practice. Also, many fluidextracts are simply too bitter tasting or otherwise unpalatable to be accepted by the patient. Therefore, most fluidextracts today are either modified by the addition of flavoring or sweetening agents before use, or are used pharmaceutically as the drug source component of other liquid dosage forms, such as syrups.

Extracts

Extracts are concentrated preparations of vegetable or animal drugs obtained by removal of the active constituents of the respective drugs with suitable menstrua, evaporation of all or nearly all of the solvent, and adjustment of the residual masses or powders to the prescribed standards.

Extracts are potent preparations, usually between two and six times as potent on a weight basis as the crude drug used as the starting material. They contain primarily the active constituents of the crude drug, with a great portion of the inactive constituents and structural components of the crude drug having been removed. Their function is to provide in small amounts and in convenient, stable physical form the medicinal activity and character of the more bulky plants that they represent. As such, they have use in product formulation.

In the manufacture of most extracts, percolation is employed to remove the active constituents from the drug, with the percolates generally being reduced in volume by evaporation of the solvent by distillation under reduced pressure, the latter being used to reduce the degree of heat and to protect the drug substances against thermal decomposition. The extent of the removal of the solvent determines the final physical character of the extract. Extracts are made in three forms: (a) *semiliquid extracts* or those of a syrupy consistency prepared without the intent of removing all or even most of the menstruum, (b) *pilular* or *solid extracts* of a plastic consistency prepared with nearly all of the menstruum removed, and (c) *powdered extracts* prepared to be dry by the removal of all of the menstruum insofar as is feasible or practical. Pilular and powdered extracts differ only by the slight amount of remaining solvent in the former preparation, but each has its pharmaceutical advantage because of its physical form. For instance, the pilular extract is preferred in compounding a plastic dosage form such as an ointment or paste or one in which a pliable material facilitates compounding, whereas the powdered form is preferable in the compounding of such dosage forms as powders, capsules, and tablets.

Aromatic Waters

Aromatic waters are clear, aqueous solutions generally saturated with volatile oils or other aromatic or volatile substances. Aromatic waters are no longer in widespread use. In years past, aromatic waters were prepared from a number of volatile substances including the following: orange flower oil, peppermint oil, rose oil, anise oil, spearmint oil, wintergreen oil, camphor and chloroform. Naturally, the odors and tastes of aromatic waters are of the volatile substances from which they are prepared.

Most of the aromatic substances in the preparation of aromatic waters have very low solubilities in water, and even though a water may be saturated, its concentration of aromatic material is still rather small. Aromatic waters may be used for perfuming and/or flavoring.

Diluted Acids

Diluted acids are aqueous solutions prepared by diluting the corresponding concentrated acids with purified water. The strength of a diluted acid is generally expressed on a per cent weight-to-volume (% w/v) basis, that is, the weight in grams of solute per 100 mL of solution, whereas the strength of a concentrated acid is generally expressed in terms of per cent weight-to-weight (% w/w), which indicates the number of grams of solute per 100 g of solution. In order to prepare a diluted acid from a concentrated one, it is first necessary to calculate the amount of solute required in the diluted product. Then, the amount of concentrated acid required to supply the needed amount of solute can be determined.

To illustrate, concentrated hydrochloric acid contains not less than 35 g and not more than 38 g of solute (absolute HCl) per 100 g of acid and therefore is considered to be, on the average, 36.5% w/w in strength. Diluted hydrochloric acid contains between 9.5 and 10.5 g of solute per 100 mL of solution and is therefore considered to be approximately 10% w/v in strength. If, for example, one wished to prepare 100 mL of the diluted acid from the concentrated acid, he would require 10 g of solute. The amount of concentrated hydrochloric acid required to supply this amount of solute may be calculated by the following proportion:

$$\frac{36.5\text{ g (solute)}}{100\text{ g (conc. acid)}} = \frac{10\text{ g (solute)}}{\times\text{(g conc. acid)}}$$

solving for x:

$$36.5x = 1000\text{ g}$$

$$x = 27.39\text{ g (conc. acid)}$$

Thus, 27.39 g of concentrated acid are required to supply 10 g of solute needed for the preparation of 100 mL of the diluted acid. Although the required amount of concentrated acid may be accurately weighed, it is a cumbersome task, and as a rule pharmacists prefer to measure liquids volumetrically. Therefore, in the preparation of diluted acids, the calculations are generally carried one step further to determine the *volume* of concentrated acid that corresponds with the calculated weight. Because this additional step requires the use of the concentrated acid's specific gravity, a brief review of specific gravity seems appropriate.

By definition, specific gravity is a ratio, expressed decimally, of the weight of a substance to the weight of an equal volume of a standard, both substances having the same temperature or the temperature of each being known. Water is used as the standard for liquids and solids; hydrogen or air, for gases. In pharmacy, specific gravity calculations mainly involve liquids and solids, and water is an excellent choice for a standard, because it is readily available and easily purified.

At 4°C, the density of water is 1 g per cubic centimeter (cc). Because the USP states that 1 mL may be considered the equivalent of 1 cc, in pharmacy, water is assumed to weigh 1 g per mL. By the following equation, used to calculate specific gravity, a substance having a density the same as water would have a specific gravity of 1.0:

$$\text{sp gr} = \frac{\text{weight of a substance}}{\text{weight of an equal volume of water}}$$

In solving this equation, the same units of weight must be used in each part of the ratio. These units cancel out, and the ratio is expressed decimally.

Specific gravity indicates the relative weight of a substance compared to an equal volume of water. For example, if 10 mL of a liquid weigh 20 g, an equal volume of water would weigh 10 g, and the ratio in the equation would be 20 g/10 g yielding a specific gravity of 2.0. This would indicate that the liquid is twice as heavy as water in equal volume. By the same token, a liquid having a specific gravity of 0.5 would be half as heavy as water; a liquid with a specific gravity of 0.8 would be eight-tenths as heavy as water, etc.

If both the volume of a liquid and its specific gravity are known, its weight may be calculated. For instance, if concentrated hydrochloric acid has a specific gravity of 1.17, it is that number times as heavy as water, and 100 mL of the acid would weigh 1.17 times as much as 100 mL of water. Since 100 mL of water weigh 100 g, 100 mL of the acid would weigh 1.17 times that or 117 g.

If one knows the weight of a liquid and its specific gravity, the volume of the liquid may be determined. For example, a liquid that is twice as heavy as water would have a specific gravity of 2.0 and would occupy half the volume that an equal weight of water would occupy. If one had 100 g of this liquid and substituted in the above equation as indicated below, the volume of the liquid could be arrived at:

$$2.0 = \frac{100\text{ g}}{\text{weight of an equal volume of water}}$$

$$\text{weight of an equal volume of water} = \frac{100\text{ g}}{2.0}$$

$$= 50\text{ g}$$

Since 50 g is the weight of an equal volume of water, it follows that the water must measure 50 mL. Since the volume of the water is an "equal volume" to the other liquid, that liquid must also measure 50 mL.

The volume represented by 27.39 g of the concentrated hydrochloric acid may be similarly determined by dividing the specific gravity of the concentrated acid into its weight and equating the answer of weight of an equal volume of water to the volume of the acid:

$$\frac{27.39\ \text{g}}{1.17} = 23.41\ \text{g, weight of equal volume of water.}$$

Thus, because 23.41 g of water measures 23.41 mL and because it is equal in volume to the concentrated acid, the latter also measures 23.41 mL and would be required to prepare 100 mL of the 10% w/v diluted acid.

Once the aforementioned is thoroughly understood, the following simplified formula can be used to calculate the amount of a concentrated acid required in the preparation of a specific volume of the corresponding diluted acid:

$$\frac{\text{Percentage strength (w/v) of diluted acid} \times \text{Volume of diluted acid to be prepared}}{\text{Percentage strength (w/w) of concentrated acid} \times \text{Specific gravity of concentrated acid}} = \text{Volume of concentrated acid to use}$$

Recalculating the preparation of 100 mL of diluted hydrochloric acid from the concentrated acid gives the following:

$$\frac{10 \times 100\ \text{mL}}{36.5 \times 1.17} = 23.41\ \text{mL of concentrated acid to use.}$$

Most diluted acids have a strength of 10% w/v, with the exception of diluted acetic acid which is 6% w/v. The strengths of these acids are commensurate with the concentrations generally used for medicinal or pharmaceutical purposes. The concentrations of the corresponding concentrated acids vary widely from one acid to another, depending upon various properties of the solute such as solubility, stability, and ease of preparation. For instance, concentrated sulfuric acid is generally between 95 and 98% w/w, nitric acid between 69 and 71% w/w, and concentrated phosphoric acid between 85 and 88% w/w. As a result, the amounts of each concentrated acid required to prepare the corresponding diluted acid vary widely and must be calculated on an individual basis.

There is very little use of diluted acids in medicine today. However, because of its antibacterial effects, acetic acid finds application as 1% solutions in surgical dressings, as an irrigating solution to the bladder in 0.25% concentration, and also as a spermatocidal in some proprietary contraceptive preparations.

Spirits

Spirits are alcoholic or hydroalcoholic solutions of volatile substances. Generally, the alcoholic concentration of spirits is rather high, usually over 60%. Because of the greater solubility of aromatic or volatile substances in alcohol than in water, spirits can contain a greater concentration of these materials than the corresponding aromatic waters. When mixed with water or with an aqueous preparation, the volatile substances present in spirits generally separate from solution and form a milky preparation.

Spirits may be employed pharmaceutically as flavoring agents and medicinally for the therapeutic value of the aromatic solute. As flavoring agents they are used to impart the flavor of their solute to other pharmaceutical preparations. For medicinal purposes, spirits may be taken orally, applied externally, or used by inhalation, depending upon the particular preparation. When taken orally, they are generally mixed with a portion of water to reduce the pungency of the spirit. Depending upon the materials utilized, spirits may be prepared by simple solution, solution by maceration, or distillation. The spirits most recently official in the USP/NF were aromatic ammonia spirit, camphor spirit, compound orange spirit, and peppermint spirit.

Effervescent Salts

Effervescent salts, as previously defined in Chapter 5, are prepared by two general methods: (1) the *wet method,* and (2) the *dry* or *fusion method.* Irrespective of the method used, the initial step is the determination of the proper formula for the preparation that will result in effective effervescence, efficient utilization of the acids and base present, a stable granulation, and a pleasant tasting and efficacious product.

Effervescent salts are usually prepared from a combination of citric and tartaric acids rather than from a single acid because the use of either acid alone presents difficulties. When tartaric acid is the sole acid, the resulting granules lose their firmness readily and crumble. Citric acid alone results in a sticky mixture difficult to granulate. Granulation is due to the presence of one molecule of water of crystallization in each molecule of citric acid, a feature that is taken advantage of and utilized in the preparation of granules by the fusion method using the combination of acids and sodium bicarbonate. Although the proportion of acids may be varied, so long as the total acidity is maintained and the bicarbonate completely neutralized, a general guideline of usual proportions of these materials can be shown from the formula of effervescent sodium phosphate:

Dried Dibasic Sodium Phosphate, dried and powdered	200 g
Sodium Bicardbonate, in dry powder	477 g
Tartaric Acid, in dry powder	252 g
Citric Acid, monohydrate	162 g
To make about	1000 g

From this formula it can be observed that of the effervescence-producing agents, about 53% of the mixture is sodium bicarbonate, 28% is tartaric acid, and about 19% is citric acid. The reactions between citric and sodium bicarbonate (1) and tartaric acid and sodium bicarbonate (2) may be shown as follows:

$$(1)\quad \underset{\text{citric acid}}{H_3C_6H_5O_7{\cdot}H_2O} + \underset{\text{sodium bicarbonate}}{3NaHCO_3} \rightarrow \underset{\text{sodium citrate}}{Na_3C_6H_5O_7} + \underset{\text{water}}{4H_2O} + \underset{\text{carbon dioxide}}{3CO_2}$$

$$(2)\quad \underset{\text{tartaric acid}}{H_2C_4H_4O_6} + \underset{\text{sodium bicarbonate}}{2NaHCO_3} \rightarrow \underset{\text{sodium tartrate}}{Na_2C_4H_4O_6} + \underset{\text{water}}{2H_2O} + \underset{\text{carbon dioxide}}{2CO_2}$$

It should be noted that it requires 3 molecules of sodium bicarbonate to neutralize 1 molecule of citric acid (1) and 2 molecules of sodium bicarbonate to neutralize 1 molecule of tartaric acid (2). In preparing a pharmaceutical formula of an effervescent salt from these components, one can determine the precise amounts of reactants to employ. For instance, using the official formula for effervescent sodium phosphate, one can calculate from information of the above reactions and the molecular weights of the three reactants the amount of sodium bicarbonate required to neutralize 252 g of tartaric acid and 162 g of uneffloresced citric acid:

(1) For the amount of sodium bicarbonate required to neutralize 162 g of citric acid:

$$\frac{162\text{ g citric acid}}{210.13\text{ g m.w. citric acid}} = \frac{\times\text{ g sodium bicarbonate}}{\begin{array}{l}(252.03\text{ g m.w. sodium bicarbonate}\\(84.01)\text{ times 3 (molecules)}\end{array}}$$

$$\times = \textit{194.3 g of sodium bicarbonate}$$

(2) For the amount of sodium bicarbonate required to neutralize 252 g of tartaric acid:

$$\frac{252\text{ g tartaric acid}}{150.09\text{ g m.w. tartaric acid}} = \frac{\times\text{ g sodium bicarbonate}}{\begin{array}{l}168.02\text{ g m.w. sodium bicarbonate}\\(84.01)\text{ times 2 (molecules)}\end{array}}$$

$$\times = \textit{282.1 g of sodium bicarbonate}$$

Total: 194.3 + 282.1

$$= \textit{476.4 g of sodium bicarbonate}$$

The amount of medicinal agent in effervescent preparations is determined by the intended dose of the medication. Generally the dose of the drug is contained in a teaspoonful or two of the dry effervescent salt. After the formula has been determined, the powders are uniformly mixed, being certain that the powders are dry to avoid premature chemical reaction. Then the granules are prepared.

FUSION METHOD. In the fusion method, the one molecule of water present in each molecule of citric acid acts as the binding agent for the powder mixture. Just before mixing the powders, the citric acid crystals are powdered and then mixed with the other powders (previously passed through a number 60 sieve) to ensure uniformity of the mixture. The sieves and the mixing equipment should be made of stainless steel or other material resistant to the effect of the acids. The mixing of the powders is performed as rapidly as is practical, preferably in an environment of low humidity to avoid the absorption of moisture from the air by the chemicals and a premature chemical reaction. After mixing, the powder is placed on a plate or glass or a suitable dish in an oven (or other suitable source of heat) previously heated to between 93°F and 104°F. During the heating process, an acid-resistant spatula is used to turn the powder. The heat causes the release of the water of crystallization from the citric acid, which in turn dissolves a portion of the powder mixture, setting of the chemical reaction and the consequent release of some carbon dioxide. This causes the softened mass of powder to become somewhat spongy, and when of the proper consistency (as bread dough), it is removed from the oven and rubbed through an acid-resistant sieve to produce granules of the desired size. A No. 4 sieve may be used to produce large granules, a No. 8 sieve to produce medium size granules, and a No. 10 sieve to prepare small granules. When all of the mass has passed through the sieve, the granules are immediately dried at a temperature not exceeding 54° and immediately transferred to containers which are then promptly and tightly sealed.

The fusion method is used in the preparation of most commercial effervescent powders and in the preparation of the effervescent sodium phosphate.

WET METHOD. The wet method differs from the fusion method in that the source of binding agent is not necessarily the water of crystallization from the citric acid but may be water added to the nonsolvent (such as alcohol), which is employed as the moistening agent, to form the pliable mass of material for granulation. In this method all of the powders may be anhydrous so long as water is added to the moistening liquid. Just enough liquid is added (in portions) to prepare a mass of proper consistency; then the granules are prepared and dried in the same manner as described above.

Divided Powders

Divided powders, as previously defined in Chapter 5, are prepared as follows.

Depending upon the potency of the drug substance, the pharmacist decides whether to weigh each portion of powder separately before enfolding in a paper or to approximate each portion by using the so-called *block-and-divide method*. By this method, used only for nonpotent drugs, the pharmacist places the entire amount of prepared powder on a flat surface such as a porcelain or glass plate or pill tile or a large sheet of paper on the prescription counter and with a large spatula forms a rectangular or square-shaped block of powder having a uniform depth. Then, using the spatula, he partially cuts into the powder vertically and horizontally to delineate the appropriate number of smaller, uniform blocks, each representing a dose or unit of medication. Each of the smaller blocks is then separated from the main block with the spatula and transferred to a powder paper and wrapped.

The powder papers may be of any convenient size to hold the amount of powder issued, but the most popular sizes are commercially available and include $2\frac{3}{4} \times 3\frac{3}{4}$ inches, $3 \times 4\frac{1}{2}$ inches, $3\frac{3}{4} \times 5$ inches, and $4\frac{1}{2} \times 6$ inches. The papers may be (1) simple bond paper, white or colored; (2) vegetable parchment, a thin, semiopaque paper having limited moisture-resistant qualities; (3) glassine, a glazed, transparent paper, also having limited moisture-resistant qualities; and (4) waxed paper, a transparent, waterproof paper. The selection of the type of paper is based primarily on the nature of the powder. If the powder contains hygroscopic or deliquescent materials, a waterproof or a waxed paper should be used. In practice, such powders are double-wrapped in waxed paper, and then for aesthetic appeal they are finally wrapped in bond paper. Glassine and vegetable parchment papers may be used when only a limited barrier against moisture is necessary. Powders containing volatile components should be wrapped in waxed or in glassine papers. Powders containing neither volatile components nor ingredients adversely affected by air or moisture are usually wrapped in white bond paper.

A certain degree of expertise is required in the folding of a powder paper, and the student should practice until he becomes proficient at preparing neat and uniform papers. Basically the steps in the folding of a powder paper are as follows:

1. Place the paper flat on a hard surface and fold toward you a uniform flap of about $\frac{1}{2}$ inch of the long side of the paper. To ensure uniformity of all of the papers, this step should be performed on all the required papers concurrently, using the first folded paper as the guide (Fig. 14–2A).
2. With the flap of each paper away from you and pointing upward, place the weighed or divided amount of powder in the center of each paper.
3. Being careful not to disturb the powder ex-

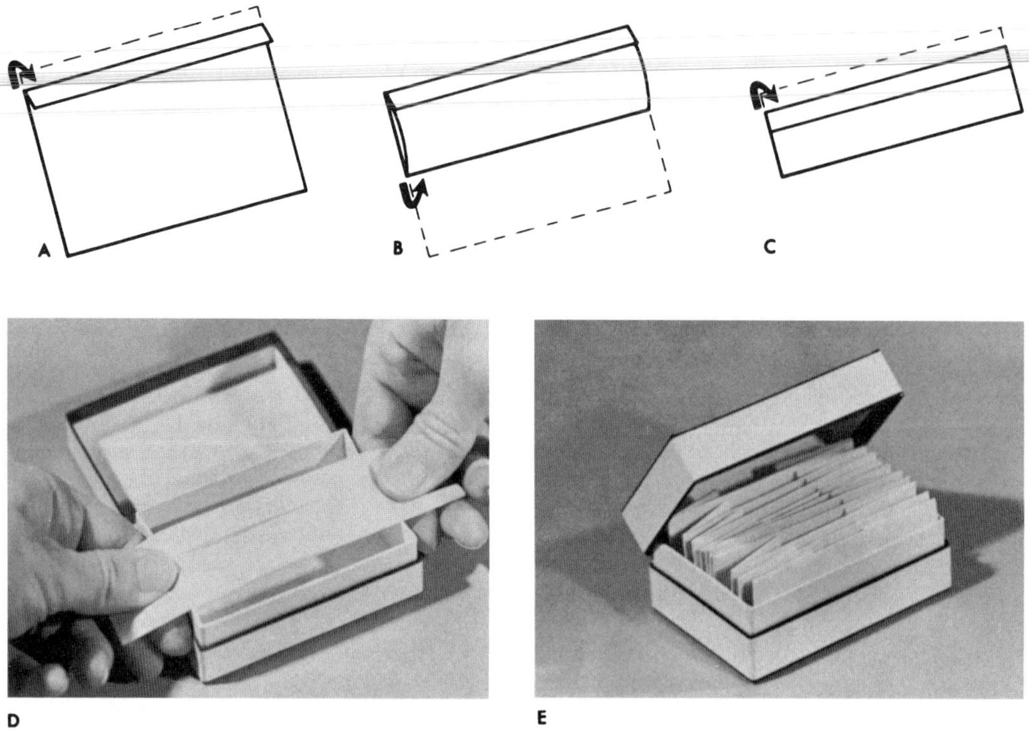

Fig. 14–2. *Steps in the folding of powder papers.*

cessively, bring the lower edge of the paper upward, and place it proximate to the crease of the flap (Fig. 14–2B).

4. Grasp the flap, press it down upon the tucked-in bottom edge of the paper and fold again toward you an amount of paper equal to the size of the original flap (½ inch) (Fig. 14–2C).
5. Pick the paper up with the flap upward and facing you, being careful not to disturb the position of the powder, and place the partially folded paper over the open powder box (to serve as the container) so that the ends of the paper extend equally beyond the sides (lengthwise) of the open container. Then, press the sides of the box slightly inward and the ends of the paper gently downward along the sides of the box to form a crease on each end of the paper. Lift the paper from the box and fold the ends of the paper along each crease sharply so that the powder cannot escape (Fig. 14–2D).
6. The folded papers are then each placed in the box so that the double-folded flaps are at the top, facing the operator, and the ends are folded away from the operator (Fig. 14–2E).

Papers folded properly should fit snugly in the box, have uniform folds, and should be of uniform length and height. There should be no powder in the folds, and none should be capable of escape with moderate agitation. Powder boxes, which are generally pasteboard and of the hinged type, should close easily without coming in contact with the tops of the papers. The label for the powders may be placed on the container, but some pharmacists affix a label of directions to each individual paper.

For convenience and uniformity of appearance, some pharmacists use commercially available cellophone or plastic envelopes to enclose individual doses or units of powders rather than folding individual papers. These envelopes are usually moisture resistant, and their use results in handsome and efficacious products.

References

1. Kowalsky, R.J. and Perry, J.R.: *Radiopharmaceuticals in Nuclear Medicine Practice,* Appleton and Lange, Los Altos, CA, 1987.
2. Mintun, M.A. *et al:* Breast Cancer: PET imaging of Estrogen Receptors. *Radiology, 169:*45–48, 1988.
3. Positron Emission Tomography—A New Approach to Brain Chemistry. The Report of the Positron Emission Tomography Panel, Jacobson, H.G., Section Editor, *JAMA, 260:*2704–2710, 1988.

Appendix I

Definitions of Selected Drug Categories*

Abradent—an agent that removes an external layer, such as dental plaque. (Pumice)

Absorbent—a drug that takes up other chemicals into its substance, used to reduce the free availability of toxic chemicals. (Polycarbophil, gastrointestinal absorbent)

ACE Inhibitor—see Angiotensin Converting Enzyme Inhibitor.

Acidifier, Systemic—a drug that lowers internal body pH, useful in restoring normal pH in patients with systemic alkalosis. (Ammonium Chloride)

Acidifier, Urinary—a drug that lowers the pH of the renal filtrate and urine. (Sodium Dihydrogen Phosphate)

Adrenergic—a drug that activates organs innervated by the sympathetic nervous system; a sympathomimetic drug. (Epinephrine)

Adrenocorticosteroid, Anti-inflammatory—an adrenal cortex hormone that regulates organic metabolism and inhibits inflammatory response; a glucocorticoid. (Prednisolone)

Adrenocorticosteroid, Salt-regulating—an adrenal cortex hormone that regulates sodium/potassium balance in the body; a mineralocorticoid. (Desoxycorticosterone Acetate)

Adrenocorticotropic Hormone—a hormone that stimulates the adrenal cortex to produce glucocorticoids. (Corticotropin)

Adsorbent—a drug that binds other chemicals onto its surface, used to reduce the free availability of toxic chemicals. (Kaolin, gastrointestinal adsorbent)

Agonist—a drug that reacts with and activates physiologic receptors, and induces the associated biological response. (Morphine, opiate receptor agonist; Isoproterenol, beta adrenergic receptor agonist)

Alcohol-Abuse Deterrent—a drug that alters physiology so that unpleasant symptoms follow ingestion of ethanol-containing products. (Disulfiram)

Alkalinizer, Systemic—a drug that raises internal body pH, useful in restoring normal pH in patients with systemic acidosis. (Sodium Bicarbonate)

Alkylating Agent—an antineoplastic drug that attacks malignant cells by reacting covalently with their DNA. (Chlorambucil)

* Prepared by H. Douglas Johnson, Ph.D., Professor Emeritus of Pharmacology/Toxicology, College of Pharmacy, University of Georgia.

Alpha Receptor Agonist—a drug that activates sympathetic nervous system alpha receptors, e.g., to induce vasoconstriction. (Norepinephrine)

Alpha Receptor Antagonist—a drug that reacts asymptomatically with sympathetic nervous system alpha receptors and prevents their endogenous activation, e.g., to induce vasodilation. (Phentolamine)

Anabolic Steroid—an androgen analogue with relatively greater anabolic activity, used to treat catabolic disorders. (Methandrostenolone)

Analeptic—a central nervous system stimulant, sometimes used to stimulate respiration during severe CNS depression. (Doxapram)

Analgesic—a drug that suppresses pain perception (nociception) without inducing unconsciousness. (Morphine Sulfate, narcotic analgesic; Aspirin, nonnarcotic analgesic)

Androgen—a hormone that stimulates and maintains male reproductive function and sex characteristics. (Testosterone)

Anesthetic, General—a drug that eliminates pain perception by inducing unconsciousness. (Ether, inhalation anesthetic; Thiopental Sodium, intravenous anesthetic)

Anesthetic, Local—a drug that eliminates pain perception in a limited body area by local action on sensory nerves. (Procaine)

Anesthetic, Topical—a local anesthetic that is effective upon application to mucous membranes. (Tetracaine)

Angiotensin Converting Enzyme Inhibitor—a drug that inhibits biotransformation of Angiotensin I into vasoconstricting Angiotensin II, used to treat hypertension. (Captopril)

Anorexic—a drug that suppresses appetite usually by elevating mood. (Phenmetrazine)

Antacid—a drug that neutralizes excess gastric acid. (Aluminum Hydroxide Gel)

Antagonist—a drug that reacts asymptomatically with physiologic receptors and prevents their endogenous activation. (Naloxone, opioid receptor antagonist; Propranolol, beta adrenergic receptor antagonist)

Anthelmintic—a drug that eradicates intestinal worm infestations. (Thiabendazole)

Antiacne Agent—a drug that combats the lesions of acne vulgaris. (Tretinoin)

Antiadrenergic—a drug that inhibits response to sympathetic nerve impulses and adrenergic drugs; a sympatholytic drug. (Phentolamine, alpha adrenergic antagonist; Propranolol, beta adrenergic antagonist)

Antiamebic—a drug that kills or inhibits protozoan parasites such as *Entamoeba histolytica*, causative agent of amebiasis. (Metronidazole, intestinal antiamebic; Chloroquine, extraintestinal antiamebic)

Antiandrogen—a drug that inhibits response to androgenic hormones. (Cyproterone)

Antianginal—a coronary vasodilator useful in preventing or treating attacks of angina pectoris. (Nitroglycerin)

Antiarrhythmic—a cardiac depressant useful in suppressing rhythm irregularities of the heart. (Procainamide)

Antiarthritic—a drug that reduces the joint inflammation of arthritis. (Prednisolone, glucocorticoid; Indomethacin, NSAID)

Antibacterial—a drug that kills or inhibits pathogenic bacteria. (Penicillin G, systemic antibacterial; Nitrofurantoin, urinary antibacterial; Bacitracin, topical antibacterial)

Anticholesterol Agent—a drug that lowers plasma cholesterol level. (Colestipol)

Anticholinergic—a drug that inhibits response to parasympathetic nerve impulses and cholinergic drugs; a parasympatholytic drug. (Atropine)

Anticholinesterase Antidote—a drug that reactivates cholinesterase enzyme after its inactivation by organophosphate poisons. (Pralidoxime)

Anticoagulant Antagonist—a drug that opposes overdosage of anticoagulant drugs. (Phytonadione, supplies vitamin K to oppose vitamin K-antagonist anticoagulants)

Anticoagulant, Systemic—a drug administered to slow clotting of circulating blood. (Warfarin)

Anticoagulant, for Storage of Whole Blood—a nontoxic agent added to collected blood to prevent clotting. (Anticoagulant Citrate Dextrose Solution)

Anticonvulsant—an antiepileptic drug administered prophylactically to prevent seizures, or a drug that arrests convulsions by inducing general CNS depression. (Phenytoin, antiepileptic prophylactic; Diazepam, CNS depressant anticonvulsant)

Antidepressant—a centrally acting drug that induces mood elevation, useful in treating mental depression. (Amitriptyline)

Antidiabetic—a drug that supplies insulin, or stimulates secretion of insulin, useful in treating diabetes mellitus. (Insulin Injection, supplies insulin; Tolbutamide, stimulates insulin secretion)

Antidiarrheal—a drug that inhibits intestinal peristalsis, used to treat diarrhea. (Diphenoxylate)

Antidiuretic—a drug that promotes renal water reabsorption, thus reducing urine volume, used to treat neurogenic diabetes insipidus. (Desmopressin)

Antianemic—a drug used to treat anemia; see Hematopoietic, Hematinic.

Antibiotic—a drug, originally of microbial origin, used to kill or inhibit bacterial and other infections. (Penicillin, Tetracycline)

Antidote, General Purpose—a drug that reduces the effects of ingested poisons (or drug overdoses) by adsorpting toxic material. (Activated Charcoal)

Antidote, Specific—a drug that reduces the effects of a systemic poison (or drug overdose) by a mechanism that relates to the particular poison. (Dimercaprol, specific antidote for arsenic, mercury and gold poisoning)

Antieczematic—a topical drug that aids in control of chronic exudative skin lesions. (Coal Tar)

Antiemetic—a drug that suppresses nausea and vomiting. (Prochlorperazine)

Antienuretic—a drug that aids in control of bedwetting (enuresis). (Imipramine)

Antiepileptic—a drug that prevents epileptic seizures upon prophylactic administration. (Ethosuximide)

Antiestrogen—a drug that inhibits action of estrogenic hormones. (Tamoxifen)

Antifibrinolytic—a drug that promotes hemostasis by inhibiting clot dissolution (fibrinolysis). (Aminocaproic Acid)

Antifilarial—a drug that kills or inhibits pathogenic filarial worms. (Diethylcarbamazine)

Antiflatuent—a drug that reduces gastrointestinal gas. (Simethicone)

Antifungal, Systemic—a drug that kills or inhibits pathogenic fungi. (Griseofulvin)

Antifungal, Topical—a drug applied externally to kill or inhibit pathogenic fungi. (Tolnaftate)

Antiglaucoma Agent—a drug that lowers intraocular fluid pressure, used to treat glaucoma. (Methazolamide reduces fluid formation; Isofluorophate promotes fluid drainage)

Antigonadotropin—a drug that inhibits anterior pituitary secretion of gonadotropins, used to suppress ovarian malfunction. (Danazol)

Antigout Agent—a drug that reduces tissue deposits of uric acid in chronic gout, or suppresses the intense inflammatory reaction of acute gout. (Allopurinol for chronic gout; Indomethacin for acute gout)

Antihemophilic—a drug that replaces blood clotting factors absent in the hereditary disease hemophilia. (Antihemophilic Factor)

Antiherpes Agent—a drug that inhibits replication of *Herpes simplex* virus, used to treat genital herpes. (Acyclovir)

Antihistaminic—a drug that antagonizes histamine action at H-1 histamine receptors, useful in suppressing the histamine-induced symptoms of allergy. (Chlorpheniramine)

Antihyperlipidemic—a drug that lowers plasma cholesterol and lipid levels. (Clofibrate)

Antihypertensive—a drug that lowers arterial blood pressure, especially the elevated diastolic pressure of hypertension. (Guanethidine)

Antihypocalcemic—a drug that elevates plasma calcium level, useful in treating hypocalcemia. (Parathyroid Injection)

Antihypoglycemic—a drug that elevates plasma glucose level, useful in treating hypoglycemia. (Glucagon)

Anti-infective, Topical (or Local)—a drug that kills or inhibits pathogenic microorganisms and is suitable for sterilizing skin and wounds. (Hexachlorophene Liquid Soap)

Anti-inflammatory—a drug that inhibits physiologic response to cell damage (inflammation). (Prednisolone, adrenocorticosteroid; Ibuprophen, nonsteroid)

Antileishmanial—a drug that kills or inhibits pathogenic protozoa of the genus *Leishmania.* (Hydroxystilbamidine Isethionate)

Antileprotic—a drug that kills or inhibits *Mycobacterium leprae,* causative agent of leprosy. (Dapsone)

Antimalarial—a drug that kills or inhibits protozoa of the genus *Plasmodium,* causative agents of malaria. (Chloroquine)

Antimanic—a drug that suppresses the excitement phase (mania) or manic-depressive psychosis. (Lithium Carbonate)

Antimetabolite—a drug that attacks malignant cells or pathogenic cells by serving as a nonfunctional substitute for an essential metabolite. (Fluorouracil, antineoplastic antimetabolite)

Antimigraine Agent—a drug that reduces incidence of severity of migraine vascular headaches. (Methylsergide)

Antimotion Sickness Agent—a drug that suppresses motion-induced nausea, vomiting, and vertigo. (Dimenhydrinate)

Antimuscarinic—an anticholinergic drug that inhibits symptoms mediated by acetylcholine receptors of visceral organs (muscarinic receptors). (Atropine)

Antinauseant—a drug that suppresses nausea and vomiting; an antiemetic. (Triethylperazine)

Antineoplastic—a drug that attacks malignant (neoplastic) cells in the body. (Chlorambucil, alkylating agent)

Antiparasitic—a drug that eradicates parasitic arthropods, helminths, protozoa, etc. (Lindane for scabies; Thiabendazole for intestinal worms; Metronidazole for amebic dysentary)

Antiparkinsonian (antidyskinetic)—a drug that suppresses the neurologic disturbances and symptoms of Parkinsonism. (Levodopa)

Antiperistaltic—a drug that inhibits intestinal motility; an antidiarrheal drug. (Diphenoxylate)

Antiplatelet Agent—a drug that inhibits aggregation of blood platelets, used prophylactically to prevent heart attack. (Aspirin)

Antiprotozoal—a drug that kills or inhibits pathogenic protozoa. (Metronidazole)

Antipruritic—a drug that reduces itching (pruritus). (Trimeprazine, systemic antipruritic; Menthol, topical antipruritic)

Antipsoriatic—a drug that suppresses the lesions and symptoms of psoriasis. (Methotrexate, systemic antipsoriatic; Anthralin, topical antipsoriatic)

Antipsychotic—a drug that suppresses symptoms of psychoses of various diagnostic types. (Haloperidol)

Antipyretic—a drug that restores normal body temperature in the presence of fever. (Acetaminophen)

Antirachitic—a drug with vitamin D activity, useful in treating vitamin D deficiency and rickets. (Cholecalciferol)

Antirheumatic—an anti-inflammatory drug used to treat arthritis and rheumatoid disorders. (Indomethacin)

Antirickettsial—a drug that kills or inhibits pathogenic microorganisms of the genus *Rickettsia.* (Chloramphenicol)

Antischistosomal—a drug that kills or inhibits pathogenic flukes of the genus *Schistosoma.* (Oxaminiquine)

Antiscorbutic—a drug with vitamin C activity, useful in treating vitamin C deficiency and scurvy. (Ascorbic Acid)

Antiseborrheic—a drug that aids in the control of seborrheic dermatitis (dandruff). (Selenium Sulfide)

Antispasmodic—a drug that inhibits motility of visceral smooth muscles. (Atropine)

Antithyroid Agent—a drug that reduces thyroid hormone action, usually by inhibiting hormone synthesis. (Methimazole)

Antitreponemal—a drug that kills or inhibits *Treponema pallidum,* causative agent of syphilis. (Penicillin)

Antitrichomonal—a drug that kills or inhibits pathogenic protozoa of the genus *Trichomonas.* (Metronidazole)

Antitubercular—a drug that kills or inhibits *Mycobacterium tuberculosis,* causative agent of tuberculosis. (Isoniazid)

Antitussive—a drug that suppresses coughing. (Dextromethorphan)

Antiviral—a drug that kills or inhibits viral infections. (Idoxuridine, Ophthalmic Antiviral)

Antiviral, Prophylactic—a drug useful in preventing (rather than treating) viral infections. (Amantadine, prophylactic for influenza)

Antixerophthalmic—a drug with vitamin A activity, useful in treating vitamin A deficiency and xerophthalmia. (Vitamin A)

Anxiolytic—a drug that suppresses symptoms of anxiety. (Diazepam)

Astringent—a drug used topically to toughen and shrink tissues. (Aluminum Acetate Solution)

Astringent, Ophthalmic—a mild astringent suitable for use in the eye. (Zinc Sulfate)

Barbiturate—a sedative-hypnotic drug that contains the barbituric acid moiety in its chemical structure. (Pentobarbital)

Belladonna Alkaloid—a plant principle derived from *Atropa belladonna* and related species, with anticholinergic action. (Atropine)

Benzodiazepine—a sedative-anxiolytic-muscle relaxant drug that contains the benzodiazepine moiety in its chemical structure. (Diazepam)

Beta Receptor Agonist—a drug that activates sympathetic nervous system beta receptors, e.g., to induce bronchodilation. (Isoproterenol)

Beta Receptor Antagonist—a drug that reacts asymptomatically with sympathetic nervous system beta receptors and prevents their endogenous activation, e.g., to oppose sympathetic stimulation of the heart. (Propranolol)

Bone Metabolism Regulator—a drug that slows calcium turnover in bone, used to treat Paget's disease. (Edidronate)

Bronchodilator—a drug that expands bronchiolar airways, useful in treating asthma. (Isoproterenol, adrenergic bronchodilator; Oxytriphylline, smooth muscle relaxant bronchodilator)

Calcium Channel Blocker—an antianginal drug that acts by impairing function of transmembrane calcium channels of vascular smooth muscle cells. (Verapamil)

Carbonic Anhydrase Inhibitor—a drug that inhibits the enzyme carbonic anhydrase, the therapeutic effects of which are diuresis and reduced formation of intraocular fluid. (Acetazolamide)

Cardiac Depressant, Antiarrhythmic—a drug that depresses myocardial function, useful in treating cardiac arrhythmias. (Procainamide)

Cardiac Glycoside—a plant principle derived from *Digitalis purpurea* and related species, with cardiotonic action. (Digoxin)

Cardiotonic—a drug that increases myocardial contractile force, useful in treating congestive heart failure. (Digoxin)

Catecholamine Synthesis Inhibitor—a drug that inhibits biosynthesis of catecholamine neurotransmitters such as norepinephrine. (Metyrosine)

Cathartic—a drug that promotes defecation, usually considered stronger in action than a laxative. (Danthron)

Caustic—a topical drug that destroys tissue on contact, useful in removing skin lesions. (Toughened Silver Nitrate)

Centrally Acting Drug—a drug that produces its therapeutic effect by action on the central nervous system, usually designated by type of therapeutic action (sedative, hypnotic, anticonvulsant, etc.)

Cephalosporin—an antimicrobial drug that contains the cephalosporin moiety in its chemical structure. (Cefotaxime)

Chelating Agent—a complexing agent that binds metal ions into stable ring structures (chelates), useful in treating poisoning. (Edetate Calcium Disodium, chelating agent for lead)

Cholelitholytic—a drug that promotes dissolution of gallstones. (Ursodoxycholic acid)

Choleretic—a drug that increases bile secretion by the liver (Dehydrocholic Acid)

Cholinergic—a drug that activates organs innervated by the parasympathetic nervous system; a parasympathomimetic drug. (Neostigmine, systemic cholinergic; Pilocarpine, ophthalmic cholinergic)

Chrysotherapeutic—a drug containing gold, used to treat rheumatoid arthritis. (Auranofin)

Coagulant—see Hemostatic, Systemic.

Contraceptive, Oral—an orally administered drug that prevents conception. Currently available oral contraceptives are for use by females. (Norethindrone Acetate and Ethinyl Estradiol Tablets)

Contraceptive, Topical—a spermicidal agent used topically in the vagina to prevent conception. (Nonoxynol-9)

Cycloplegic—an anticholinergic drug used topically in the eye to induce paralysis of accommodation (cycloplegia) and dilation of the pupil. (Cyclopentolate)

Decongestant, Nasal—an adrenergic drug used orally or topically to induce vasoconstriction in nasal passages. (Phenylpropanolamine)

Demulcent— a bland viscous liquid, usually water-based, used to coat and soothe damaged or inflamed skin or mucous membranes. (Methylcellulose)

Dental Caries Prophylactic—a drug applied to the teeth to reduce the incidence of cavities. (Stannous Fluoride)

Dentin Desensitizer—a drug applied to the teeth to reduce the sensitivity of exposed subenamel dentin. (Zinc Chloride)

Depigmenting Agent—a drug that inhibits melanin production in the skin, used to induce general depigmentation in certain splotchy depigmented conditions (e.g., vitiligo). (Hydroquinone)

Detergent—an emulsifying agent used as a cleanser. (Hexachlorophene Liquid Soap, anti-infective detergent)

Diagnostic Aid—a drug used to determine the functional state of a body organ, or to determine the presence of disease. (Peptavlon, gastric secretion indicator; Fluorescein Sodium, corneal trauma indicator)

Digestive Aid—a drug that promotes digestion, usually by supplementing a gastrointestinal enzyme. (Pancreatin)

Disinfectant—an agent that destroys microorganisms on contact and suitable for sterilizing inanimate objects. (Formaldehyde Solution)

Diuretic—a drug that promotes renal excretion of electrolytes and water, useful in treating generalized edema. (Furosemide, loop diuretic; Hydrochlorothiazide, thiazide diuretic; Triamterene, potassium-sparing diuretic)

Dopamine Receptor Agonist—a drug that activates dopamine receptors, e.g., to inhibit anterior pituitary secretion of prolactin. (Bromocryptine)

Emetic—a drug that induces vomiting, useful in expelling ingested but unabsorbed poisons. (Ipecac Syrup)

Emollient—a topical drug, especially an oil or fat, used to soften the skin and make it more pliable. (Cold Cream)

Ergot Alkaloid—a plant principle derived from the fungus *Claviceps purpura* grown on rye or other grains. (Ergonovine, uterine contractant; Ergotamine, migraine therapy)

Estrogen—a hormone that stimulates and maintains female reproductive organs and sex characteristics, and functions in the uterine cycle. (Ethinyl Estradiol)

Expectorant—a drug that increases respiratory tract secretions, lowers their viscosity and promotes removal. (Potassium Iodide)

Fecal Softener—a drug that promotes defecation by softening the feces. (Docusate)

Fertility Agent—a drug that promotes ovulation in women of low fertility, or spermatogenesis in men of low fertility. (Clomiphene)

Fibrinolytic-proteolytic—an enzyme drug used topically to hydrolyze exudates of infected and inflammatory lesions. (Fibrinolysin and Desoxyribuonuclease, Bovine)

Galactokinetic—a drug used to initiate lactation after childbirth. (Oxytocin Nasal Spray)

Glucocorticoid—an adrenocortical hormone that regulates organic metabolism and inhibits inflammatory response. (Betamethasone)

Gonadotropin—a drug that supplies the gonad-stimulating actions of follicle-stimulating hormone (FSH) and/or luteinizing hormone (LH), used to promote fertility. (Menotropins contains FSH and LH; Human Chorionic Gonadotropin has LH-like activity)

Growth Hormone, Human—a drug that duplicates endogenous growth hormone, used in children to treat growth failure due to growth hormone lack. (Somatrem)

Heavy Metal Antagonist—a drug used to antidote poisoning with toxic metals such as arsenic, mercury, etc. (Dimercaprol)

Hematopoietic—a vitamin that stimulates formation of blood cells, useful in treating vitamin-deficiency anemia. (Cyanocobalamin)

Hematinic—a drug that promotes hemoglobin formation by supplying iron. (Ferrous Sulfate)

Hemorheologic Agent—a drug that improves the flow properties of blood by reducing viscosity. (Pentoxyfylline)

Hemostatic, Local—a drug applied to a bleeding surface to promote clotting or to serve as a clot matrix. (Thrombin, clot promoter; Oxidized Cellulose, clot matrix)

Hemostatic, Systemic—a drug that stops bleeding by inhibiting systemic fibrinolysis. (Aminocaproic Acid)

Histamine H-1 Receptor Antagonist—a drug used to combat the histamine-induced symptoms of allergy; an antihistaminic (Chlorpheniramine)

Histamine H-2 Receptor Antagonist—a drug that inhibits histamine-mediated gastric acid secretion, used to treat peptic and duodenal ulcers. (Cimetidine)

Hormone—a drug that duplicates action of a physiologic cell regulator (hormone). (Insulin, Estradiol, Thyroxine)

Hydantoin—an antiepileptic drug that contains the hydantoin moiety in its chemical structure. (Phenytoin)

Hydrolytic, Injectible—an enzyme drug that promotes the diffusion of other injected drugs through connective tissues. (Hyaluronidase)

Hyperglycemic—a drug that elevates blood glucose level. (Glucagon)

Hypnotic—a central nervous system depressant used to induce sleep. (Flurazepam)

Hypotensive—see Antihypertensive.

Immune Globulin—Antibody proteins derived from blood serum, used to confer passive immunity to infectious diseases. (See Immunizing Agent, Passive)

Immunizing Agent, Active—an antigen that induces antibody production against a pathogenic microorganism, used to provide permanent but delayed protection against infection. (Tetanus Toxoid)

Immunizing Agent, Passive—a drug containing antibodies against a pathogenic microorganism, used to provide immediate but temporary protection against infection. (Tetanus Immune Globulin, Rabies Immune Globulin)

Immunosuppresant—a drug that inhibits immune response to foreign materials, used to suppress rejection of tissue grafts. (Azathioprine)

Inotropic Agent—a drug that increases the contractile strength of heart muscle; a cardiotonic. (Digitoxin, Dopamine)

Ion Exchange Resin—a drug that in the gastrointestinal tract takes up ions present in a toxic amount with equivalent release of nontoxic ions. (Sodium Polystyrene Sulfonate, takes up potassium ions with release of sodium ions)

Irritant, Local—a drug that reacts weakly and nonspecifically with biological tissue, used topically to induce a mild inflammatory response. (Camphor)

Keratolytic—a topical drug that softens the superficial keratin-containing layer of the skin and promotes desquamation. (Salicylic Acid)

Keratoplastic—a topical drug that toughens and protects skin. (Compound Benzoin Tincture)

Laxative—a drug that promotes defecation, usually considered milder in action than a cathartic. (Methylcellulose, bulk laxative; Mineral Oil, lubricant laxative; Sodium Phosphates Oral Solution, saline laxative)

Leprostatic—see Antileprotic

Loop Diuretic—a diuretic with renal site of action in the thick ascending loop of Henle. (Furosemide)

MAO Inhibitor—see Monoamine Oxidase Inhibitor.

Metal Complexing Agent—a drug that binds metal ions, useful in treating metal poisoning. (Dimercaprol, complexing agent for arsenic, mercury, and gold)

Mineralocorticoid—an adrenocortical hormone that regulates sodium/potassium balance in the body. (Desoxycorticosterone Acetate)

Miotic—a cholinergic drug used topically in the eye to induce constriction of the pupil (miosis). (Pilocarpine)

Monoamine Oxidase Inhibitor—an antidepressant drug that inhibits the enzyme monoamine oxidase, thereby increasing catecholamine levels of neurons. (Isocarboxazid)

Monoclonal Antibody—a highly specific immunoglobulin produced by cell culture cloning. (Muromonab-CD3, inactivates T-lymphocytes that reject tissue grafts)

Mucolytic—a drug that hydrolyzes mucoproteins, useful in reducing the viscosity of pulmonary mucus. (Acetylcysteine)

Muscle Relaxant, Skeletal—a drug that inhibits contraction of voluntary muscles. (Dantrolene, Succinylcholine)

Muscle Relaxant, Smooth—a drug that inhibits contraction of visceral smooth muscles. (Aminophylline)

Mydriatic—an adrenergic drug used topically in the eye to induce dilation of the pupil (mydriasis). (Phenylephrine)

Narcotic—a drug that induces action by reacting with opioid receptors of the central nervous system, or a drug legally classified as a narcotic with regard to prescribing regulations.

Narcotic Antagonist—a drug that reacts with opiate receptors asymptomatically, used to terminate the action of narcotic drugs. (Naloxone)

Neuromuscular Blocking Agent—a drug that paralyzes skeletal muscles by preventing transmission of neural impulses to them. (Succinylcholine)

Nonsteroidal Anti-inflammatory Drug—an analgesic, anti-inflammatory drug that inhibits prostaglandin synthesis. (Indomethacin)

NSAID—see Nonsteroidal Anti-inflammatory Drug.

Opiate—see Narcotic.

Opiate Antagonist—see Narcotic Antagonist.

Oxytoxic—a drug that stimulates uterine motility, used in obstetrics to initiate labor or to control postpartum hemorrhage. (Oxytocin)

Parasympatholytic—a drug that inhibits response to parasympathetic nerve impulses and to parasympathomimetic drugs; an anticholinergic drug. (Atropine)

Parasympathomimetic—a drug that activates organs innervated by the parasympathetic nervous system; a cholinergic drug. (Neostigmine)

Pediculicide—an insecticide suitable for eradicating louse infestations (pediculosis). (Lindane)

Penicillin Adjuvant—a drug that extends systemic duration of penicillin by inhibiting its renal excretion. (Probenecid)

Phenothiazine—an antipsychotic drug or an antidepressant drug that contains the phenothiazine nucleus in its chemical structure. (Chloropromazine, antipsychotic; Imipramine, antidepressant)

Photosensitizer—a drug that increases cutaneous response to ultraviolet light, used with ultraviolet light to treat certain skin diseases (e.g., psoriasis). (Methoxsalen)

Pigmenting Agent—a drug that promotes melanin synthesis in the skin. (Trioxsalen, oral pigmenting agent; Methoxsalen, topical pigmenting agent)

Posterior Pituitary Hormone, Antidiuretic—a hormone that promotes renal reabsorption of water, useful in treating diabetes insipidus. (Vasopressin injection)

Potassium-sparing Diuretic—a diuretic that does not induce systemic potassium depletion as a side effect. (Triamterene)

Potentiator—an adjunctive drug that enhances the action of a primary drug, the total response being greater than the sum of the individual actions. (Hexafluorenium, potentiator for Succinylcholine)

Progestin—a progesterone-like hormone that stimulates the secretory phase of the uterine cycle. (Norethindrone)

Prostaglandin—a drug from the classes of cell-regulating hormones cyclized from arachidonic acid. (Alprostadil, maintains ductus arteriosus patency in newborn infants pending corrective surgery for congenital heart defects)

Prostaglandin Synthetase Inhibitor—a drug that inhibits prostaglandin synthesis and prostaglandin-induced symptoms such as inflammation; a nonsteroidal anti-inflammatory drug. (Ibuprofen)

Protectant—a topical drug that provides a physical barrier to the environment. (Zinc Gelatin, skin protectant; Methylcellulose, ophthalmic protectant)

Proteolytic, Injectable—an enzyme drug for injection into herniated lumbar intervertebral discs to reduce interdiscal pressure. (Chymopapain)

Prothrombogenic—a drug with vitamin K activity, useful in treating the hypoprothrombinemia of vitamin K deficiency or overdosage with a vitamin K antagonist. (Phytonadione)

Psychedelic—a drug (especially a street drug) that induces vivid sensory phenomena and hallucinations. (Mescaline)

Psychotherapeutic—A drug used to treat abnormal mental or emotional processes. (Chlorpromazine, Haloperidol)

Rauwolfia Alkaloid—a plant principle derived from *Rauwolfia serpentina* and related species, with antihypertensive and antipsychotic actions. (Reserpine)

Radiographic Agent—see X-ray Contrast Medium.

Radiopharmaceutical—a drug containing a radioactive isotope, used for diagnostic or therapeutic purposes. (Iodinated Albumen, with I-125 or I-131)

Resin, Electrolyte Removing—see Ion Exchange Resin.

Rubefacient—a topical drug that induces mild skin irritation with erythema, and used as a toughening agent. (Rubbing Alcohol)

Salt Substitute—a sodium-free alternative to NaCl used for flavoring foods. (Potassium Chloride)

Scabicide—an insecticide suitable for eradication of the itch mite *Sarcoptes scabiei* (scabies). (Lindane)

Sclerosing Agent—an irritant drug suitable for injection into varicose veins to induce their fibrosis and obliteration. (Morrhuate Sodium Injection)

Sedative—a central nervous system depressant used to induce mild relaxation. (Phenobarbital)

Specific—a drug specially adapted to its indicated use, usually because of a functional relationship between drug mechanism and disease pathophysiology.

Stimulant, Central—a drug that increases the functional state of the central nervous system, sometimes used in convulsive therapy of mental disorders. (Flurothyl)

Stimulant, Respiratory—a drug that selectively stimulates respiration, either by peripheral initiation of respiratory reflexes, or by selective central nervous system stimulation. (Carbon Dioxide, reflex respiratory stimulant; Ethamivan, central respiratory stimulant)

Sun Screening Agent—a skin protectant that absorbs light energy at wave-lengths that cause sunburn. (Aminobenzoic Acid)

Sulfonylurea—an oral antidiabetic drug that contains the sulfonylurea moiety in its chemical structure. (Tolazamide)

Suppressant—a drug that inhibits the progress of a disease but does not cure it.

Sympatholytic—a drug that inhibits response to sympathetic nerve impulses and to sympathomimetic drugs; an antiadrenergic drug. (Phentolamine, alpha sympatholytic; Propranolol, beta sympatholytic)

Sympathomimetic—a drug that activates organs innervated by the sympathetic nervous system; an adrenergic drug. (Epinephrine)

Systemically Acting Drug—a drug administered so as to reach systemic circulation, from which the drug diffuses into all tissues, including the site of therapeutic action.

Thiazide Diuretic—a diuretic that contains the benzothiadiazide (thiazide) moeity in its chemical structure. (Hydrochlorothiazide)

Thrombolytic—an enzyme drug administered parenterally to solubilize blood clots. (Urokinase)

Thyroid Hormone—a hormone that maintains metabolic function and normal metabolic rate of tissues. (Levothyroxine)

Topically Acting Drug—a drug applied to the body surface for local therapeutic action.

Toxoid—a modified antigen from an infectious organism used as a vaccine. (Tetanus Toxoid)

Tranquilizer, Minor—an old term for an anxiolytic drug.

Tranquilizer, a drug (such as antipsychotic) used to suppress an acutely disturbed emotional state. (Trifluoperazine, antipsychotic)

Tricyclic Antidepressant—an antidepressant that contains the tricyclic phenothiazine nucleus in its chemical structure. (Imipramine)

Tuberculostatic—see Antitubercular.

Uricosuric—a drug that promotes renal excretion of uric acid, useful in treating chronic gout. (Probenecid)

Uterine Contractant—an obstetric drug used after placenta delivery to induce sustained uterine contraction to reduce bleeding. (Methylergonovine)

Uterine Contraction Inhibitor—a drug that inhibits uterine muscle contraction, used in preterm labor to prolong gestation. (Ritodrine)

Vaccine—an antigen-containing drug used to induce active immunity against an infectious disease. (Hepatitis B Vaccine, Rabies Vaccine)

Vasoconstrictor—a drug that narrows arterioles, usually to elevate blood pressure. See Vasopressor.

Vasodilator, Coronary—a drug that expands blood vessels in the heart and improves coronary blood flow, useful in treating angina pectoris; an antianginal drug. (Nitroglycerin)

Vasodilator, Peripheral—a drug that expands peripheral blood vessels and improves blood flow to the extremities of the body. (Minoxidil)

Vasopressor—an adrenergic drug administered to constrict arterioles and elevate arterial blood pressure. (Norepinephrine)

Vinca Alkaloid—a plant principle derived from *Vinca rosea* and related species, with antineoplastic action. (Vincristine)

Vitamin—an organic chemical essential in small amounts for normal metabolism, used therapeutically to supplement the vitamin content of foods.

Xanthine Alkaloid—a plant principle chemically related to xanthine, with central nervous system stimulant, smooth muscle relaxant, and diuretic actions. (Caffeine)

X-Ray Contrast Medium—a drug opaque to x rays that assists visualization of an internal organ during radiographic examination. (Barium Sulfate, Iopanoic Acid)

Appendix II

Systems and Techniques of Pharmaceutical Measurement

THE PHARMACIST'S knowledge and application of accurate pharmaceutical measurement are essential to his practice of pharmacy. Whether practicing in the community or institutional pharmacy or in the large industrial pharmaceutical manufacturing firm, accuracy of measurement is a prime requisite in the preparation of medications.

Pharmaceuticals prepared industrially pass numerous inspections and assays during the course of their manufacture to ensure conformance to standards of quality. However, prescriptions and medication orders filled extemporaneously in the community and institutional pharmacy usually lack the advantage of such control by assay, and the pharmacist must be absolutely certain that his calculations and measurements are accurate. He should double check his work, and when possible he should have a colleague check it as well. An error in the placement of a decimal point, for instance, represents an error of a *minimum* factor of ten.

The student must have a working knowledge of the systems of pharmaceutical measurement as presented in this appendix, including factors of conversion between the systems used, and the methods of applying these systems in pharmaceutical measurement.

Systems of Pharmaceutical Measurement

Although pharmacy has moved toward the exclusive use of the metric system, two other systems may be encountered on occasion. They are the *apothecary system*, and the *avoirdupois system*. The metric and apothecary systems include units of weight and volume measure with the metric system additionally having units of linear measure. The pharmacist utilizes these systems in his pharmaceutical measurements. The avoirdupois system is the common commercial system of weight used in the United States that is slowly being replaced by the metric system. The avoirdupois system may be used by the pharmacist in his purchase of bulk chemicals and commercial packages from manufacturers.

The Metric System

The metric system is the most widely used system in pharmacy. It is the system used by the official compendia and in the labeling of most of the commercial pharmaceutical products. Most of the prescriptions and medication orders written today are in the metric system.

In the metric system, the *gram* is the main unit of weight, the *liter* the main unit of volume, and

Table A–1. Metric System Unit Prefixes*

Multiplication Factor	*Prefix*	*Symbol*	*Term (USA)*
1 000 000 000 000 000 000 = 10^{18}	exa	E	one quintillion
1 000 000 000 000 000 = 10^{15}	peta	P	one quadrillion
1 000 000 000 000 = 10^{12}	tera	T	one trillion
1 000 000 000 = 10^{9}	giga	G	one billion
1 000 000 = 10^{6}	mega	M	one million
1 000 = 10^{3}	kilo	k	one thousand
100 = 10^{2}	hecto	h	one hundred
10 = 10	deka	da	ten
0.1 = 10^{-1}	deci	d	one tenth
0.01 = 10^{-2}	centi	c	one hundreth
0.001 = 10^{-3}	milli	m	one thousandth
0.000 001 = 10^{-6}	micro	μ	one millionth
0.000 000 001 = 10^{-9}	nano	n	one billionth
0.000 000 000 001 = 10^{-12}	pico	p	one trillonth
0.000 000 000 000 001 = 10^{-15}	femto	f	one quadrillionth
0.000 000 000 000 000 001 = 10^{-18}	atto	a	one quintillionth

* Adapted from *Metric Editorial Guide,* 4th Ed., American National Metric Council, Washington, D.C., 20005. The table is based on The International System of Units ("SI," from the French "Le Systeme International System of Unites"), as modified for use in the United States by the Secretary of Commerce.

the *meter* the main unit of length. Subunits and multiples of these basic units are indicated by the following prefix notations and symbols shown in Table A–1.

The following are most commonly used in pharmaceutical measurement:

units of weight, expressed in terms of the kilogram (kg), gram (g), milligram (mg), or microgram (μg).

units of liquid measure, expressed in terms of the liter (L) or milliliter (mL).

units of linear measure, expressed in terms of the meter (m), centimeter (cm), or millimeter (mm).

units of area measure, expressed in terms of the square meter (m^2) or square centimeter (cm^2).

The "metric weight scale" in Figure A–1 is

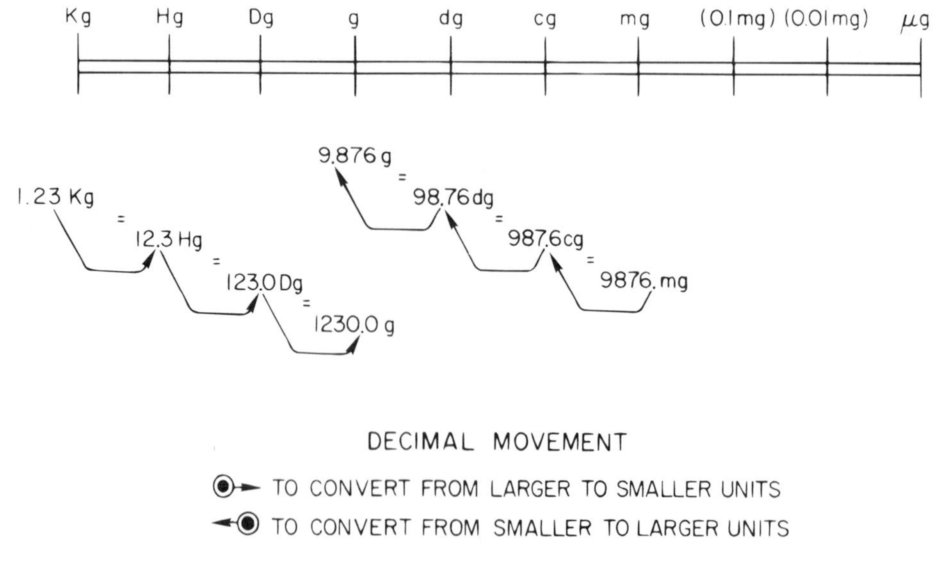

Fig. A–1. *Metric Weight Scale*

intended to depict the relationship between the units of weight in the metric system and to provide an example of an easy method of converting from one unit to another. In the example, 1.23 kilograms (kg) are to be converted to grams (g). On the scale, the gram position is three decimal positons from the kilogram position. Thus, the decimal point is moved three places toward the right. In the other example, the conversion from milligrams (mg) to grams also requires the movement of the decimal point three places, but this time to the left. The same method may be used to convert metric units of volume or length.

Table of Metric Weight:

1 kilogram (Kg or kg)	=	1000.000 grams
1 hektogram (Hg or hg)	=	100.000 grams
1 dekagram (Dg or dg)	=	10.000 grams
1 gram (Gm, gm or g)	=	1.000 gram
1 decigram (dg)	=	0.100 gram
1 centigram (cg)	=	0.010 gram
1 milligram (mg)	=	0.001 gram
1 microgram (μg or mcg)	=	0.000,001 gram
1 nanogram (ng)	=	0.000,000,001 gram
1 picogram (pg)	=	0.000.000.000.001 gram

or

1 gram = 0.001 kilogram
= 0.010 hektogram
= 0.100 dekagram
= 10 decigrams
= 100 centigrams
= 1000 milligrams
= 1,000,000 micrograms
= 1,000,000,000 nanograms
= 1,000,000,000,000 picograms

Table of Metric Volume:

1 kiloliter (Kl or kl)	=	1000.000 liters
1 hektoliter (Hl or hl)	=	100.000 liters
1 dekaliter (Dl)	=	10.000 liters
1 liter (L or l)	=	1.000 liter
1 deciliter (dl)	=	0.100 liter
1 centiliter (cl)	=	0.010 liter
1 milliliter (mL)	=	0.001 liter
1 microliter (μL)	=	0.000,001 liter

or

1 liter = 0.001 kiloliter
= 0.010 hektoliter
= 0.100 dekaliter
= 10 deciliters
= 100 centiliters
= 1000 milliliters
= 1,000,000 microliters

Table of Metric Length:

1 kilometer (Km or km)	=	1000.000 meters
1 hektometer (Hm)	=	100.000 meters
1 dekameter (Dm)	=	10.000 meters
1 meter (M or m)	=	1.000 meter
1 decimeter (dm)	=	0.100 meter
1 centimeter (cm)	=	0.010 meter
1 millimeter (mm)	=	0.001 meter
1 micrometer (μm)	=	0.000,001 meter
1 nanometer (nm)	=	0.000,000,001 meter

or

1 meter = 0.001 kilometer
= 0.010 hektometer
= 0.100 dekameter
= 10 decimeters
= 100 centimeters
= 1000 millimeters
= 1,000,000 micrometers
= 1,000,000,000 nanometers

The Apothecary System

The apothecary system provides for the measurement of both weight and volume. The tables of the system are presented below.

TABLES OF APOTHECARY SYSTEM

Tables of Apothecaries' Fluid Measure:

60 minims (♏)	= 1 fluidrachm (fZ or Z)*
8 fluidrachms (480 minims)	= 1 fluidounce (f℥ or ℥)*
16 fluidounces	= 1 pint (pt or 0)
2 pints (32 fluidounces)	= 1 quart (qt)
4 quarts (8 pints)	= 1 gallon (gal or C)

Table of Apothecaries' Measure of Weight:

20 grains (gr)	= 1 scruple (℈)
3 scruples (60 grains)	= 1 drachm (Z)
8 dram (480 grains)	= 1 ounce (℥)
12 ounces (5760 grains)	= 1 pound ℔

The Avoirdupois System

The avoirdupois system is used in commerce generally in the supplying of drugs, chemicals, and other materials by weight. The pharmacist who purchases bulk or prepackaged amounts of chemicals, as sodium bicarbonate powder or epsom salts, purchases them in the avoirdupois system. When he resells them "over the counter" in their original packages, he likewise sells them in the avoirdupois system. The "grain" in each of the apothecary and avoirdupois systems is equivalent. The other units (ounce and pound) are of different weights. It should also be noted that the symbols for the ounce and pound are different in the two systems.

Table of Avoirdupois Measure of Weight

437.5 grains (gr)	= 1 ounce (oz)
16 ounces (7000 grains)	= 1 pound (lb)

Intersystem Conversion

It is possible for the pharmacist to convert the weight, volume, or dimensions of length from one system to another. Depending upon the circumstances and requirements of accuracy, conversion equivalents of different exactness may be used. The following is a table of those equivalents commonly used in prescription practice. They are not the exact equivalents, but are over 99% accurate and suffice nicely for most pharmaceutical measurements. Exact equivalents may be found in the USP.

Conversion Equivalents of Weight

1 g	= 15.432 gr
1 Kg	= 2.2 Avoirdupois lb
1 gr	= 0.0648 g or 64.8 or 65 mg
1 Z	= 31.1 g
1 oz (Avoir)	= 28.35 g
1 ℔ (Apoth)	= 373.2 g
1 lb (Avoir)	= 453.6 or 454 g

Conversion Equivalents of Volume

1 mL	= 16.23 minims
1 minim	= 0.06 mL
1 fZ	= 3.69 mL
1 fZ	= 29.57 mL
1 pt	= 473 mL
1 gal (U.S.)	= 3785 mL
1 gal (British Imperial)	= 4546 mL

Conversion Equivalents of Length

1 inch	= 2.54 cm
1 meter	= 39.37 inches

Today there are very few occasions in which intersystem conversion is needed, owing to the almost exclusive use of the metric system in both product formulation and prescription compounding. However, when conversion is necessary or desired, it is a simple matter of selecting and applying the appropriate intersystem conversion factor.

For example, if one wishes to determine the number of milliliters present in 8 fluid ounces of a liquid, the conversion factor that most directly relates milliliters and fluid ounces is selected. That factor is one fluidounce = 29.57 mL; thus 8 fluidounces contain 8 × 29.57 mL, or 236.56 mL.

Another example: how many 30 mL containers may be filled from 10 gallons of a formulation? One gallon is equivalent to 3785 mL. Thus 10 gallons have 10 × 3785 mL, or 37,850 mL. By dividing this total number of milliliters by 30 mL, the number of containers that may be filled is found to be 1,261.

Another example: how many ½ grain tablets may be prepared from 1 kilogram of a drug substance? Since one grain is equivalent to 64.8 mg,

---

* When there is no doubt that the material referred to is a liquid, the *f* is usually omitted from this symbol. *Drachm* is also spelled *dram*.

½ grain is equal to 32.4 mg. One kilogram is equal to 1000 g, or 1,000,000 mg. Since 32.4 mg are required for one tablet, dividing 1,000,000 mg by 32.4 mg shows that 30,864 tablets may be prepared.

A final example: if a transdermal patch measures 30 mm square, what is this dimension in inches? The conversion factor, 1 inch equals 2.54 cm, may be expressed as 1 inch equals 25.4 mm. Thus, by dividing 30 mm by 25.4 mm/inch, one finds the patch is 1.18 inches square.

Quantitative Product Strength

The quantitative composition of certain pharmaceuticals, particularly liquids and semisolid dosage forms, often is expressed in terms of the *percentage strength* of the active, and sometimes inactive, ingredients. For some dilute solutions, the strength may be expressed in terms of its *ratio strength.* For most injections, many oral liquids, and some semisolid dosage forms, the quantity of active ingredient commonly is expressed on a weight (of drug) per unit volume basis, as "milligrams of drug per milliliter" (of injection or oral liquid), or on a weight (of drug) per unit weight of preparation, as "milligrams of drug per gram" (of ointment). The strength of solid dosage forms is given as the drug content (e.g., 5 mg) per dosage unit (e.g., tablets and capsules).

Percent, by definition, means parts per hundred. In pharmacy, percentage concentrations have specific meanings based on the physical character of the particular product or formulation. That is:

Percent weight-in-volume. Expressed "% w/v," this defines the number of grams of a constituent in 100 mL of a preparation (generally a liquid);

Percent volume-in-volume. Expressed "% v/v," this defines the number of milliliters of a constituent in 100 mL of a preparation (generally a liquid); and,

Percent weight-in-weight. Expressed "% w/w," this defines the number of grams of a constituent in 100 g of a preparation (generally a solid or semisolid, but also for liquid preparations prepared by weight).

Thus, a 5% w/v solution or suspension of a drug contains 5 g of the substance in each 100 mL of product; a 5% v/v preparation contains 5 mL of the substance in each 100 mL of product; and, a 5% w/w preparation contains 5 g of the substance in each 100 g of product.

In the manufacture or compounding of pharmaceutical preparations, the pharmacist may (1) calculate the strength of an individual component in a product, or (2) calculate the amount of a component needed to achieve a desired percentage strength.

For example, what is the percentage strength, w/v, of a solution containing 15 g of drug in 500 mL? Since, by definition, percentage strength is parts per hundred, we simply need to determine how many grams of drug are present in each 100 mL of solution. Solving by proportion: 15 g/500 mL = (x) g/100 mL, the answer is 3 g, and thus the solution is 3 % w/v in strength.

Other examples: 3 mL of a liquid in a liter of solution represents 0.3% v/v; 4 g of drug in 250 mL represents 1.6% w/v; and 8 g of drug in 40 g of product represents 20% w/w.

How many grams of drug are needed to prepare 400 mL of a 5% w/v preparation? In w/v problems, the specific gravity *of the preparation* is assumed to be the same as water (sp. gr. 1.0) and thus 1 mL is assumed to weigh 1 g. Therefore, in the problem example, the 400 mL is assumed to weigh 400 g; and, 5% of 400 g = 20 g, the amount of drug needed.

A v/v problem example: How many mL of a liquid are needed to make one pint of a 0.1% v/v solution? One pint contains 473 mL and 0.1% of that is 0.473 mL, the answer.

A w/w problem example: How many grams of zinc oxide powder should be used in preparing 120 g of a 20% w/w ointment? Twenty percent of 120 g is 24 g, the answer.

Ratio strength is sometimes used to express the strength of, or to calculate the amount of, a component needed to make a relatively dilute preparation. Compared to percentage strength designations, for example, a 0.1% w/v preparation (0.1 g per 100 mL) is equivalent to 1 g per 1000 mL, and may be expressed as a ratio strength of 1:1000 w/v. Ratio strength expressions utilize the w/v, v/v, and w/w designations in the same manner as percentage strength expressions, for example:

A 1:1000 w/v preparation of a solid constituent in a liquid preparation = 1 g of the solid constituent in 1000 mL of preparation;

A 1:1000 v/v preparation of a liquid constituent in a liquid preparation = 1 mL of constituent in 1000 mL of preparation; and

A 1:1000 w/w preparation of a solid constituent

in a solid or semisolid preparation = 1 g of constituent in 1000 g of preparation.

A ratio strength calculation example: what is the ratio strength of 6000 mL of solution containing 3 g of drug? Whenever possible, it is preferable for ratio strengths to be expressed as 1:____. In this example, if 3 g of drug are in 6000 mL of solution, 1 g of drug would be contained in 2000 mL, and thus the ratio strength of 1:2000 w/v. Sometimes the answers do not come out as evenly; for example, what is the ratio strength of 0.3 mL of a liquid in a liter of solution? In this instance, there would be 0.3 mL in 1000 mL, equivalent to 3 mL in 10,000 mL, or a ratio strength of 3:10,000 v/v, or 1:3,333.3 v/v.

Another ratio strength calculation example: How many grams of drug are needed to make 5 L of a 1:400 w/v solution? By definition (of 1:400 w/v), there would be 1 g of drug needed for each 400 mL of solution. Since 5 liters, or 5000 mL, of solution are to be prepared, the amount of drug required is found by solving 1 g/400 mL = (x) g/ 5000 mL, or 12.5 g, the answer.

Rather than being expressed in terms of percentage strength or ratio strength, the strength of some pharmaceutical preparations, particularly injections and sometimes oral liquids, is based on drug content per unit of volume, as "mg per mL." Thus flexibility in dosing can be achieved by administering the volume of preparation that contains the desired dose.

Reducing and Enlarging Formulas

In the course of pharmaceutical manufacturing, and in professional practice activities, it is often necessary to reduce or enlarge a pharmaceutical formulation in order to prepare the desired amount of product. A standard manufacturing formulation, or *master formula,* contains the quantitative amounts of each ingredient needed to prepare a specified quantity of product. When preparing other quantities, larger or smaller, the *quantitative relationship* of each component to the other in the formula must be maintained. For example, if there are 2 g of ingredient A and 10 mL of ingredient B (among other ingredients) in a formula for 1000 mL, then there needs to be 0.2 gram of ingredient A and 1 mL of ingredient B used when only 100 mL, or $\frac{1}{10}$ of the formula, is prepared. If, on the other hand, a formula is to be enlarged—for example, from a liter (1000 mL) of product to a gallon (3785 mL)—the amount of each ingredient required would be 3.785 times that needed to prepare the liter of product.

In these examples the quantity of product prepared is reduced or enlarged, but the quantitative relationship between each ingredient and the product strength remains unchanged.

Dosage Units

Drug dosage is selected by the prescriber based upon clinical considerations and the characteristics of the pharmacologic agent. Dosage forms (tablets, injections, transdermal patches) are used to administer the drug to the patient. Solid dosage forms, such as tablets and capsules, are generally prepared in various strengths to allow flexibility in dosing. The desired dose for a drug prepared in a liquid dosage form may be provided by the volume administered. For example, if a liquid dosage form contains 5 mg of drug per milliliter, and if a dose of 25 mg of drug is desired, 5 mL of the liquid may be administered. Commercially manufactured products are formulated to provide the drug in dosage forms and amounts convenient for administration. In instances where the desired dosage or dosage form is commercially unavailable, the community pharmacist may be called upon the compound the desired preparation.

Common Household Measure

Liquid and powdered medications which are not packaged in unit dose systems are usually measured at home by the patient with common household measuring devices as the teaspoon, tablespoon, and various cooking measure utensils. Although the household teaspoon may vary in volume capacity from approximately 3 to 8 mL, the American Standard Teaspoon has been established as having a volume of 4.93 ± 0.24 mL by the American National Standards Institute. For practical purposes, most pharmacy practitioners and pharmacy references utilize 5 mL as the capacity of the teaspoon. This is approximately equivalent to $1\frac{1}{3}$ fluid drams although physicians commonly utilize the dram symbol (ʒ) to indicate a teaspoonful in their prescription directions to be transcribed by the pharmacist to the patient. The tablespoon is considered to have a capacity of 15 mL, equivalent to three teaspoonfuls or approximately one-half fluid ounce.

Occasionally the pharmacist will dispense a special medicinal spoon which the patient may use in measuring this medication. These spoons

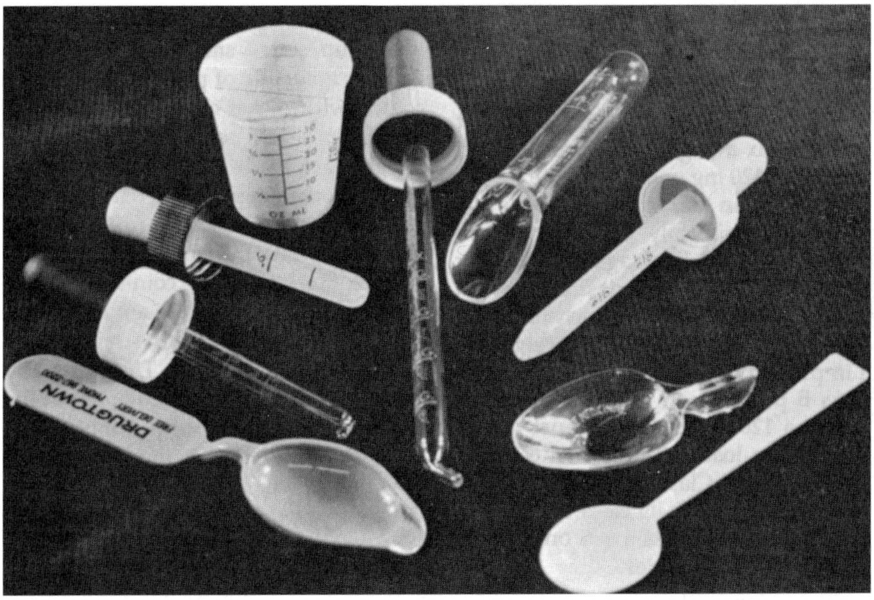

Fig. A–2. *Examples of medicinal spoons of various shapes and capacities, calibrated medicine droppers, an oral medication tube, and a disposable medication cup.*

are available in half-teaspoon, teaspoon, and tablespoon capacities. Some manufacturers provide specially designed devices to be used by the patient in measuring his medication. These include specially calibrated droppers, oral syringes, measuring wells or tubes, and calibrated bottle caps. In health care institutions, disposable measuring cups and unit-dose containers are commonly employed in administering liquid medication. Examples of measuring devices are shown in Fig. A–2.

Techniques of Pharmaceutical Measurement

Weighing and the Prescription Balance

In weighing materials, the selection of the instrument to use is based on the amount of material involved and the accuracy desired. In the large scale manufacture of pharmaceuticals, large industrial *scales* of varying capacity and sensitivity are employed, and later, highly sensitive analytical balances are utilized in the quality control and analytical work.

In the hospital and community pharmacy, most weighings are made on the *prescription balance.* Two examples of these balances are shown in Figure A–3. Prescription balances are termed *Class III* (formerly Class A) balances, which meet the prescribed standards of the National Institute of Standards and Technology. Every prescription department is required by law to have a prescription balance. The sensitivity of a balance is usually represented by the term *sensitivity requirement* (SR) which is defined as the maximum change in load that will cause a specified change, one subdivision on the index plate, in the position of rest of the indicating element(s) of the balance.[1] A Class III balance has an SR of 6 mg with no load as well as with 10 g on each pan. This means that under the above conditions, the addition of 6 mg of weight to one pan of the balance will disturb the equilibrium and move the balance pointer one division marking on the scale.

The USP directs that to avoid errors in weighing of 5% or greater, which may be due to the limits of accuracy of the prescription balance, one must weigh a minimum of 120 mg of any material in each weighing (5% of 120 mg being the 6 mg SR or error inherent with the balance). If a smaller weight of material is desired, it is directed that the pharmacist mix a larger, calculated weight of the ingredient (120 mg or over), dilute it with a known weight of an inert dry diluent (as lactose), mix the two uniformly, and

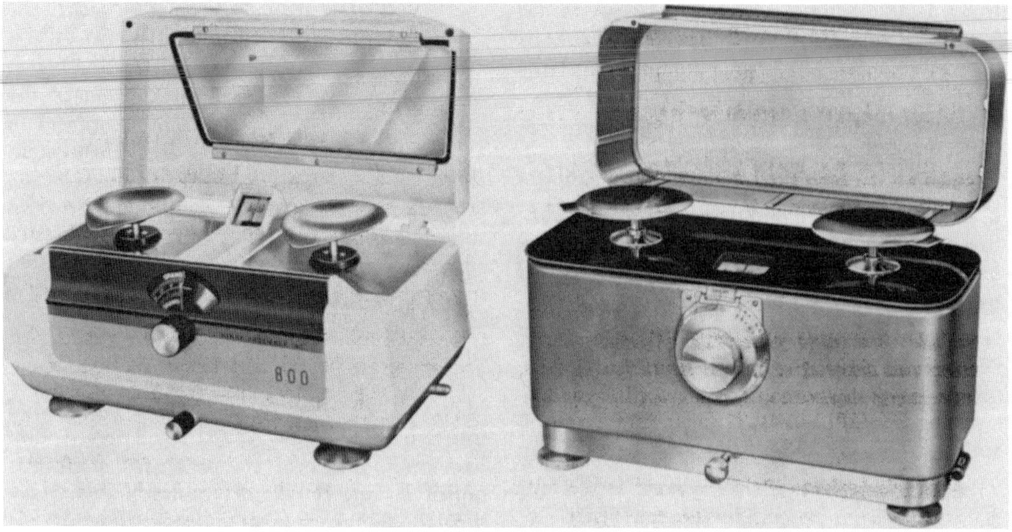

Fig. A–3. *Examples of commonly used Class III prescription balances. On left is the Troemner Model 800 Prescription Balance (Courtesy of Henry Troemner, Inc.); on right, the Model DRX2 Torsion balance (Courtesy of Torsion Balance Company.).*

weigh an aliquot portion of the mixture (again 120 mg or over) calculated to contain the desired amount of agent. The Class III balance which has a capacity of 120 g should be used for all weighings required in prescription compounding.

Weights

Today, pharmacies usually have a metric set of weights. Some commercial weight sets contain both the metric and apothecaries' systems of weights in a single container. Prescription weights meet the National Bureau of Standards' specifications for analytical weights. Metric weights of 1 g and greater, and apothecaries' weights of 1 scruple and greater, are generally conical in shape with a narrow neck and head which allows them to be easily grasped and picked up with a small forceps. Most of these weights are made of polished brass, with some coated with nickel or chromium or other materials to resist corrosion. Fractional gram weights are made of aluminum and are generally square-shaped and flat with one raised end or corner for picking up with the forceps (Fig. A–4). Apothecaries' weights of one-half scruple are frequently coin-shaped brass and those of 5 grains and less are usually bent aluminum wires, with each straight side representing 1 grain of weight. The half-grain weight is usually a smaller gauge wire bent in half.

To prevent the deposit of moisture and oils from the fingertips being deposited on the weights, all weights should be transferred with the forceps provided in each weight set.

Care and Use of a Prescription Balance

First and foremost, the prescription balance should be located in a well-lighted location, placed on a firm, level counter approximately waist-high to the operator. The area should be as free from dust as is possible and in an area that is draft-free. There should be no corrosive vapors present nor high humidity or vibration. When not in use, the balance should be clean and covered with the balance cover. Any agent spilled on the balance during use should be wiped off immediately with a soft brush or cloth. When not in use, the balance should be always

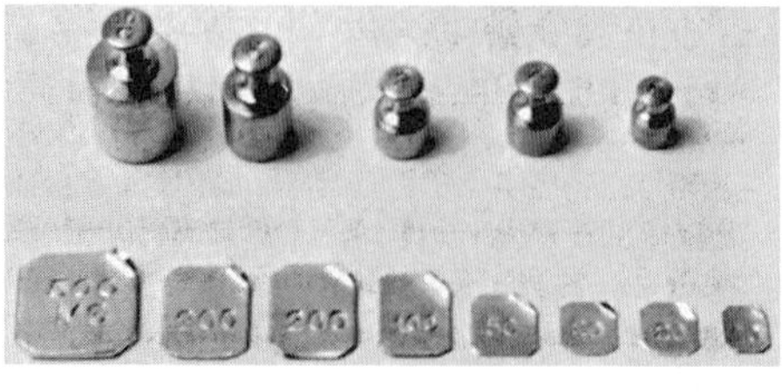

Fig. A–4. *Examples of some metric weights, showing their shape and markings.*

be maintained with the weights off and the beam in the fixed or locked (arrested) position.

Before weighing an article, the balance must be made level. This is acomplished with the leveling screws on the bottom of the balance, according to the instructional materials accompanying the balance. The balance should be level, front-to-back and side-to-side, as indicated by the leveling bubble of the balance.

In using a prescription balance, neither the weights nor the substance to be weighed should be placed on the balance while the beam is in the *un*arrested position and free to oscillate. Before weighing, powder papers of equal size should be placed on both pans of the balance and the equilibrium of the balance tested by releasing the arresting knob. If the balance is unbalanced due to differences in the weight of the powder papers, additional weight may be added to the "light pan" by adding small tearings of powder papers. When balanced, the balance is placed in the arrested position and the desired weight added to the right-hand pan. Then, an amount of substance, considered to be approximately the desired weight, is carefully placed on the left hand pan, with the assistance of a spatula. The beam should then be slowly released by means of the locking device in the front of the balance. If the substance is in excess, the beam is fixed again and a small portion of the substance removed with the spatula. The process is continued until the two pans balance, as indicated by central position of the balance pointer. If the amount of weight on the balance is initially too little, the reverse process is undertaken. The powder paper used on the left hand pan, intended to hold the substance to be weighed, is usually folded either diagonally or with the edges of the sides folded upwards to contain the material being weighed.

In transferring material by spatula, the material may be lightly tapped from the spatula when the correct amount to be measured is approached. Usually this is done by holding the spatula with a small amount of material on it in the right hand, and tapping the spatula with the forefinger. As material comes off the spatula, the left hand is working the balance arresting mechanism and the status of the weight observed alternately with the tappings of the spatula. Most balances have a "damping" mechanism which slows down the balance oscillations and permits more rapid determinations of the balance or imbalance positions of the pans.

Once the material has been weighed, the balance beam is again put in the fixed position and the paper holding the weighed substance carefully removed. If more than a single weighing is to be performed, the paper is usually marked with the name of the substance it holds. After the final weighing, all weights are removed with the forceps and the balance cleaned, closed, and the balance cover placed over the balance.

Most prescription balances contain built-in mechanisms whereby external weights are not required for weighings under 1 gram. Some balances utilize a rider, which may be shifted from the zero position toward the right side of the balance to add increments of weight marked on the scale in 10-mg units, up to 1 g. Another type of balance uses a centrally located dial, calibrated in 10-mg units, to add weight up to 1 gram. Both types of devices add the weight internally to the right-hand pan. In each case, the pharmacist may use a combination of the internal weights and external weights in his weighings. For instance, if 1.2 g are to be weighed, the pharmacist can place a 1-g weight on the right hand pan and place the rider or adjust the dial to add 0.2 g additionally. Care must always be exercised to bring the rider or dial to zero between weighings to avoid the inadvertent weighing of rider- or dial-amounts on subsequent weighings.

Most weighings on the prescription balance involve the weighing of powders or semisolid materials, as ointments. However, liquids may also be weighed through the use of tared (weighed) vessels of appropriate size, by placing the liquid inside of the vessel. The pharmacist must always be certain that he has accounted for the weight of the vessel in calculating the amount of liquid weighed.

Materials should never be "downweighed;" that is, substances should never be placed on the pan with the balance in the unarrested position forcing the pan to drop suddenly and forcefully as the excess maerial is placed on it. The sudden slamming down of the pan can do serious damage to the balance, affecting its sensitivity and the accuracy of subsequent weighings.

The two most popular types of prescription balances are the compound lever balance and the torsion balance. The former type operates through the use of a series of knife edges held in delicate contact and suspension. The torsion type operates on the tension of taut wires, which when twisted through the addition of weight, tend to twist back to the original balance position. The compound level principle is the basis for the Troemner balance and the torsion principle is applied in the Torsion Balance (Fig. A–3).

Measuring Volume

The common instruments for pharmaceutical measurement are presented in Figure A–5. Two types of graduates are used in pharmacy, those which are *conical* in shape and those which are *cylindrical.* Cylindrical graduates are generally calibrated in metric units, whereas conical graduates may be graduated in both the metric and apothecaries' units (dual scale) or with a single scale of either of the systems. Graduates of both shapes are available in a wide variety of capacities, ranging from 5 to 1000 mL or more. Most graduates in use are made of a good quality, heat-treated glass, although graduates of polypropylene are also available. In measuring small volumes of liquids, as less than 1.5 mL, the pharmacist should utilize a pipet as the one shown in Figure A–5. The bulk-like device shown with the pipet is a pipet filler, used for drawing acids or other toxic solutions into the pipet without the necessity of using the mouth. The device, without being removed from the pipet, also allows for the accurate delivery of the liquid.

In measuring volumes of liquids, the pharmacist should select the measuring device most appropriate to the volume of liquid to be measured and the degree of accuracy desired. It should be recognized that in measuring liquids, the more narrow the column of liquid, the more accurate is likely to be the measurement. Figure A–6 demonstrates this point. A reading error of the same dimension will produce a small volume-error when using a pipet, a greater volume-error when using a cylindrical graduate, and the greatest volume-error when using a conical graduate. The greater the flair in the design of the conical graduate, the greater is the volume-error due to an error in reading.

In reading the level of liquid in a graduate, it is important to recognize the error which could result due to the error of parallax. Figure A–7 depicts this point. A liquid in a graduate tends to be drawn to the inner surface of the graduate

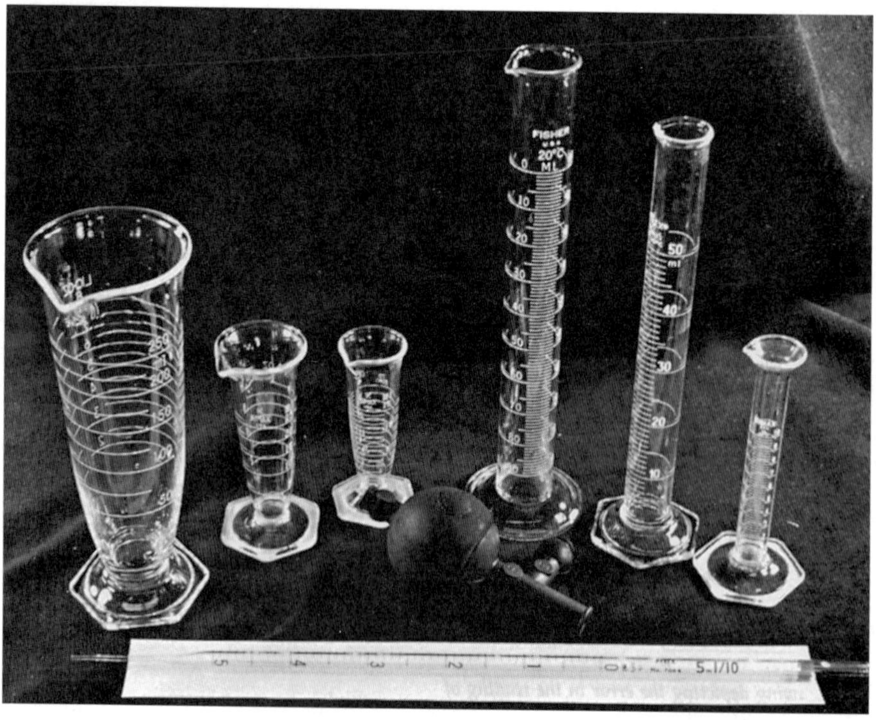

Fig. A–5. *Typical equipment for the pharmaceutical measurement of volume. On the left are conical graduates and on the right, cylindrical graduates. In the front is a pipet for the measurement of small volumes. Behind the pipet is a pipet filler, used instead of the mouth to draw acids and other dangerous liquids into the pipet.*

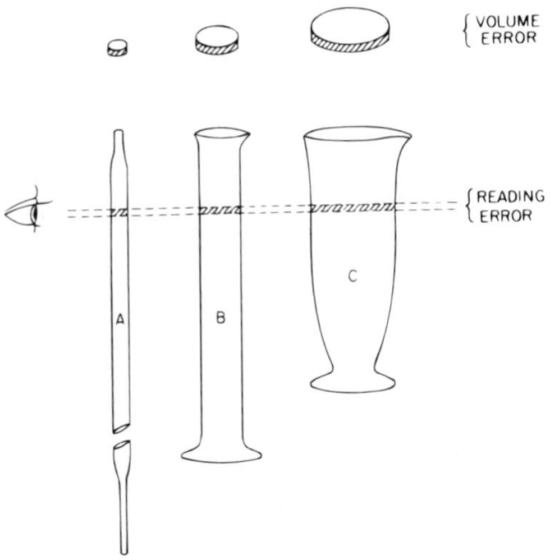

Fig. A–6. *Drawing showing the difference in the volume-error occurring with the same reading-error in measuring devices of different diameters.*

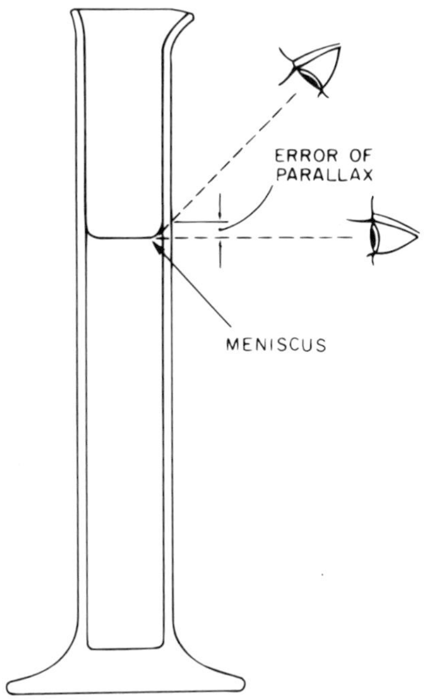

Fig. A–7. *Drawing depicting the error in the reading of the meniscus of a liquid in a graduate cylinder when the reading is made from above the level of the liquid rather than at the same level.*

and rises slightly against that surface and above its true meniscus. If one measured looking downward, it would appear as though the meniscus of the liquid is at this upper level, whereas it is slightly lower, at the actual level of the liquid within the center of the graduate. Thus, measurements of liquids in graduates should be taken with the eyesight level with the liquid in the graduate.

If a pharmacist was in error in his reading of a graduate, the *percentage of error* of his measurement would be affected by the volume of liquid that he was measuring. According to the USP, an acceptable 10-mL graduate cylinder with an internal diameter of 1.18 cm contains 0.109 mL of liquid in each 1 mm of column. A reading error of 1 mm in magnitude would cause a percentage error in the measurement of only 1.09% when 10 mL were being measured, 2.18% when 5 mL were being measured, 4.36% when 2.5 mL were being measured, and 7.26% when 1.5 mL were being measured. It is apparent that the greatest percentage error occurs when the smallest amount is being measured. Thus, the rule of thumb for measuring liquids in graduates is that a graduate should be used having a capacity *equal to or just exceeding* the volume to be measured.

According to Goldstein and Mattocks,[2] based on a deviation of 1 mm from the mark and an allowable error of 2.5%, the smallest amounts that should be measured in the following size cylindrical graduates having the stated internal diameters are as follows:

Graduate Cylinder Size	*Internal Diameter*	*Deviation in Actual Volume*	*Minimum Volume Measurable*
5 mL	0.98 cm	0.075 mL	3.00 mL
10 mL	1.18 cm	0.109 mL	4.36 mL
25 mL	1.95 cm	0.296 mL	11.84 mL
50 mL	2.24 cm	0.394 mL	15.76 mL
100 mL	2.58 cm	0.522 mL	20.88 mL

For a 5% error, the minimum volumes measurable would be one-half of those stated. It is apparent that for accuracy, one should not select a graduate for use when the measurement involves utilization of only the bottom portion of the scale.

In using graduates, the pharmacist pours the liquid into the graduate slowly, observing the level as he proceeds. In measuring viscous liquids, adequate time must be allowed for the liquid to settle in the graduate, as some may run slowly down the inner sides of the graduate. It is best to attempt to pour such liquids toward the center of the graduate, avoiding contact with the sides. In emptying the graduate of its measured contents, adequate drain time should be allowed.

When pouring liquids from bottles, it is considered good pharmaceutical technique to keep the label on the bottle facing upwards; this avoids the possibility of drops of liquid running down the label as the bottle is righted after use. Naturally, the bottle orifice should be wiped clean after each use.

Notes

1. The *sensitivity requirement* (SR) of a balance is determined in the following manner: (1) level the balance, (2) determine the rest point, (3) place a 6-mg weight on one of the empty pans, (4) the rest point is shifted *not less than* one division on the index plate. The entire operation is repeated with a 10-g weight placed in the center of each balance pan.
2. Goldstein, S.W., and Mattocks, A.M.: How to Measure Accurately, *J. Am. Pharm., 12*:421, 1951.

Index

Page numbers in *italics* indicate figures; numbers followed by "t" indicate tables; numbers followed by "c" indicate Physical Pharmacy Capsules.